*To our husbands and families
for your constant love, support, unflagging faith, and endless patience.
We thank you.*

and

*To our dear friend Gail, whose unfailing support and infinite wisdom
we will cherish forever. We love you and miss you.*

This textbook is a result of many years of hard work and dedication. In 1993, Melinda Manore and Gail Butterfield developed the idea for an advanced sport nutrition textbook that would be appropriate for students who already had courses in nutrition and exercise physiology. As an advanced level textbook did not exist, these two pioneers in sport nutrition set forth on an adventure to develop a book that would provide an instructive guide that includes the most recent references and research findings in sport nutrition. Joined by their colleague, Janice Thompson, and with unflagging support from Human Kinetics Publishers, development of this textbook progressed. Although Gail was not a primary author, she provided inspiration, advice, moral support, and invaluable editorial input throughout the writing period.

Sadly, Gail Butterfield passed away on December 27, 1999, of a brain tumor. Although she did not live to see this textbook in print, she was able to write the foreword to this book prior to her passing. Gail's contributions to this book and to the field of sport nutrition are immeasurable. Her indomitable spirit and undying passion for science have served as an inspiration to all who have been blessed to work with her. As authors of this textbook, we want to formally recognize Gail's significant contribution to this body of work.

SPORT NUTRITION for HEALTH and PERFORMANCE

Melinda Manore, PhD, RD
Arizona State University

Janice Thompson, PhD
University of New Mexico

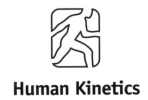

Human Kinetics

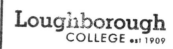

Library of Congress Cataloging-in-Publication Data

Manore, Melinda, 1951-
    Sport nutrition for health and performance / Melinda Manore & Janice Thompson.
      p. cm.
    Includes bibliographical references and index.
    ISBN 0-87322-939-8
      1. Athletes--Nutrition. 2. Physical fitness--Nutritional aspects.   I. Thompson, Janice,
1962- II. Title.
TX361.A8 M37 2000
613.2'024'794--dc21

                                  00-023158

ISBN: 0-87322-939-8

Permission notices for material reprinted in this book from other sources can be found on page(s) xix-xxii.

Acquisitions Editor: Michael S. Bahrke, PhD; **Developmental Editors:** Kristine Enderle, Amy N. Pickering; **Assistant Editors:** Derek Campbell, Amy Flaig; **Copyeditor:** Brian Mustain; **Proofreader:** Erin Cler; **Indexer:** Craig Brown; **Permission Manager:** Heather Munson; **Graphic Designer:** Robert Reuther; **Graphic Artist:** Denise Lowry; **Photo Manager:** Clark Brooks; **Cover Designer:** Robert Reuther; **Photographer (cover):** Tony Demin/International Stock; **Art Manager:** Craig Newsom; **Illustrator:** Kristin King, Denise Lowry; **Printer:** United Graphics; **Binder:** Dekker & Sons

Printed in the United States of America   10   9   8   7   6   5   4   3   2   1

Human Kinetics
Web site: http://www.humankinetics.com/

United States: Human Kinetics, P.O. Box 5076, Champaign, IL 61825-5076
800-747-4457
e-mail: humank@hkusa.com

Canada: Human Kinetics, 475 Devonshire Road Unit 100, Windsor, ON N8Y 2L5
800-465-7301 (in Canada only)
e-mail: humank@hkcanada.com

Europe: Human Kinetics, P.O. Box IW14, Leeds LS16 6TR, United Kingdom
+44 (0)113-278 1708
e-mail: humank@hkeurope.com

Australia: Human Kinetics, 57A Price Avenue, Lower Mitcham, South Australia 5062
(08) 82771555
e-mail: liahka@senet.com.au

New Zealand: Human Kinetics, P.O. Box 105-231, Auckland Central
09-309-1890
e-mail: humank@hknewz.com

Contents

Foreword

It is with great enthusiasm and admiration that I celebrate the accomplishment of *Sport Nutrition for Health and Performance!* Drs. Manore and Thompson are both experts in exercise science and nutrition. Dr. Manore is one of our foremost sport nutritionists, training student athletes and doing cutting edge research into the topic. Likewise, Dr. Thompson is highly qualified as a practicing exercise physiologist, noted for her teaching abilities and her research program.

Together they bring a text that is extremely well referenced and contains the most up-to-date information available. With their added highlights that shed light on important topics in the field dispersed throughout the text, this book is second to none.

The organization of the book is particularly exciting. Nutrients of a similar function are put into chapters (e.g., energy releasers, blood forming, bone forming, antioxidant, fluid, electrolytes) to provide students with a framework for remembering the details related to each nutrient.

I have taught nutrition using this paradigm for the last 10 years, and it seems to keep students from memorizing. Instead it helps them to understand so they can remember or "figure" things out for themselves. This approach adds to the uniqueness and usefulness of this book. It helps the students gain an understanding of the importance of integrating nutrition into the health and performance of the athlete.

In addition to the organization of the book, the assessment tools that are included are very useful and can be utilized by both students and practitioners. These tools take from the theoretical foundations of the book and create a practical application that will be useful to many.

I know the hours of time and the anguish that went into writing, editing, and rewriting this volume, and I know it will pay off for the readers. I am extremely pleased to help send this book forward!

Sincerely,

Gail Butterfield, PhD
Director of Sports Nutrition
Program in Sports Medicine
Stanford University Medical School

Preface

Now, more than ever, there is an increased demand for accurate sport nutrition information. From the elite athlete attempting to win an Olympic gold medal to the recreational athlete trying to improve a personal best, nutrition can play a vital role in helping active individuals achieve their fitness and performance goals. Nutrition can help them maximize performance, prevent injury, enhance recovery from exercise, achieve and maintain optimal body weight, improve daily training workouts, and maintain overall good health.

For the health, nutrition, or fitness professional working with active individuals, keeping up with sport nutrition information can be an overwhelming task. Currently, consumers get their sport nutrition information from a variety of sources, including magazines, television, advertisements, product labels, and the Internet. Unfortunately, some of this information has little or no scientific basis. Thus, our goal in writing this text is to provide you with a clear, concise, authoritative review of current exercise and nutrition research. We hope this book will help you sort the fact from the fiction and provide you with a scientific foundation from which to evaluate future claims and to make sound sport nutrition recommendations.

TOPICS COVERED

This text begins with an overview of sport nutrition and the role that good nutrition can play in sport and exercise. We think it is important that sport nutrition recommendations be consistent with general nutrition recommendations made to all individuals for good health. We then cover the macronutrient requirements of sport and the role carbohydrate, fat, and protein play in fueling the system at rest and during exercise (chapters 2-4). Special attention is given to showing the metabolic pathways used during exercise and how these pathways are altered with exercise intensity, duration, and training. Understanding these metabolic pathways, and how exercise changes them, will also help the health professional evaluate the myriad of performance enhancing and weight loss products marketed to active individuals. We have also covered the topics of energy balance, methods for achieving an optimal body weight, and body composition measurements in detail (chapters 5-7). It is rare to find an athlete or any active individual who is not concerned to some extent about body weight and composition. Because many sports "demand" a certain body shape or size, weight control issues frequently plague athletes in lean-build or aesthetic sports. The various components of energy balance are discussed in detail, and factors that may alter each of these are given. In addition, we give specific guidelines for helping an active individual either gain or lose weight and review the body composition issues associated with weight change. Since assessment of body composition is becoming more common, it is important that athletes understand how these data are derived and what they mean.

Poor fluid balance, especially dehydration, is a major nutritional concern of any active individual. We have provided the most recent information related to the physiology of fluid and electrolyte balance and make recommendations for maintaining good fluid balance before and during exercise and rehydrating after exercise is over (chapter 8). Chapters 9-13 detail the vitamin and mineral concerns most frequently associated with sport and exercise. The micronutrients are grouped according to their functions. For example, in chapter 12 the nutrients involved in blood formation are discussed. The other functional groups included in these chapters are vitamins important in energy metabolism, antioxidant nutrients and exercise, nutrients for bone health, and minerals and exercise. This functional grouping of the micronutrients provides an easy framework for understanding how these nutrients can influence exercise performance and good health. In addition, this framework should improve one's ability to remember the functions and interactions of these micronutrients. The final section of the book covers the practical side of working with a recreational or elite athlete or an athletic team. Topics covered in this section include nutrition and fitness assessment (chapter 14), nutrition and exercise issues specific to the active female (chapter 15), and evaluating ergogenic aids (chapter 16). The appendix provides a variety of useful resources and references frequently used by people working with active individuals. Some of these resources include the 1989 RDA and the new DRIs, various ethnic Food Guide Pyramids, equations for determining energy expenditure, prediction equations for resting metabolic rate, nutrition assessment tools, energy costs of various activities, commonly reported clinical blood biochemical values, and methods for assessing energy expenditure.

UNIQUE FEATURES

One way we have provided you with additional insights into the nutrition and exercise research is through our chapter "highlights." These highlights will give you in-depth information on a topic or critically evaluate issues surrounding a myth or controversy in sport nutrition. To facilitate understanding of the topics presented, each chapter begins with the key points to be covered and ends with a summary highlighting the key points presented. For those individuals who may want more in-depth information on a specific topic, additional key readings appear at the end of each chapter. Finally, this book bridges the gap between the scientific literature and the practical application of this information to the athlete or active individual. We have provided numerous charts, figures, and tables giving useful information that you can use to help athletes and active individuals make decisions regarding daily intakes of food and supplements. For example, we have provided information on the nutrient content of various sport foods, diet composition recommendations for athletes at various energy intakes, when to use nutritional supplements, and how to evaluate an ergogenic aid.

WHO THE BOOK IS FOR

This book is written for the health professional guiding the athlete or active individual through the sport nutrition maze. Thus, we assume the reader has a basic understanding of nutrition, exercise science, physiology, and metabolic pathways used in the metabolism of fuel substrates. The primary audiences for this text include:

- Undergraduate and graduate students in either nutrition, exercise physiology, health, or wellness programs with a strong science background and an interest in nutrition as it relates to sport, exercise, and fitness.
- Athletic trainers or physical therapists working with athletes, athletic teams, or teaching future athletic trainers or therapists.
- Nutritionists who have completed an undergraduate or graduate degree in nutrition and are interested in sport nutrition.
- Health fitness specialists, personal trainers, fitness practitioners, and physical therapists who are working in spas, gyms, or fitness and rehabilitation facilities. These individuals frequently provide nutrition information to clients.
- Sports medicine specialists who are working with athletes or athletic teams.

Melinda M. Manore
Janice L. Thompson

Acknowledgments

As first-time authors, we felt that writing a book was a great idea until we began the process. We had no idea how difficult it would be to write, review, and edit book chapters when our days were already too busy. Although it was a long and arduous process, we were able to complete this book due to the contributions and support of many people. First, we would like to thank the Human Kinetics publication team, especially Mike Bahrke and Amy Pickering, who constantly urged us on with encouraging words, unbelievable patience, and good humor. Second, we would like to thank Dr. Linda Houtkooper, who graciously agreed to write the Body Composition chapter (chapter 7). As an expert in this area, she has presented the most current body composition research along with practical recommendations. She certainly made our life a lot easier. Third, we would like to thank Carmen Febus, who spent countless hours getting permissions for the many tables and figures you find in each chapter and checking the references to make sure they were correct. Without her effort this book would never have been finished. Fourth, we would like to thank our many students, who sat through many reviews of the book material, read through our chapters, pointed out our mistakes, and made wonderful suggestions. Fifth, we would like to thank the many active individuals, including athletes and research subjects, who have taught us so much about the subject we love over the last 15 years. Finally, we would like to thank our families, friends, and colleagues, as they listened to us complain, gave us valuable advice, edited our work, encouraged us to finish, and continually asked, "When is your book going to be done?" We can finally say, "We are FINISHED!"

Credits

Table 1.1 Reprinted, by permission, from A.E. Harper, 1999, Defining the essentiality of nutrients. In *Modern Nutrition in Health and Disease*, 9th ed., M.E. Shils, J.A. Olson, M. Shike, and A.C. Ross, eds. (Baltimore, MD: Williams & Wilkins), 3-10.

Figure 1.1 Reprinted, by permission, from International Food Information Council, 2000, "Nutrient requirements get a makeover: The evolution of the recommended dietary allowances," *Food Insight* [Online], Sept./Oct. 1998. Available: **http://www.ificinfo.health.org/insight/septoct98/rdas.htm** [April 28, 2000].

Table 1.2 Reprinted, by permission, from E. Kennedy, L. Meyers, and W. Layden, 1996, "The 1995 dietary guidelines for Americans: an overview," *Journal of the American Dietetic Association* 96: 234-237.

Table 1.5 Reprinted, by permission, from Cheryl Achterberg, 1992, "A perspective: challenges of teaching the dietary guidelines graphic," *Food and Nutrition News* 64 (4): 23-30 © National Cattlemen's Beef Association.

Figure 1.4 Food Guide Pyramid for Athletes. Reproduced with permission from Houtkooper L. Winning Sports Nutrition Training Manual. Tucson, AZ: University of Arizona Cooperative Extension and University of Arizona Board of Regents, 1994, p. 1-2.

Table 2.1 Reprinted, by permission, from K. Foster-Powell and J. Brand Miller, 1995, *American Journal of Clinical Nutrition* 62: 871S-93S.

Figure 2.1 Reprinted, by permission, from G.A. Brooks and J. Mercier, 1994, "Balance of carbohydrate and lipid utilization during exercise: The "crossover" concept," *Journal of Applied Physiology* 76 (6): 2254.

Figure 2.2 Reprinted, by permission, from P.C. Champe and R.A. Harvey, 1994, *Lippincott's Illustrated Reviews: Biochemistry*, 2nd ed. (Philadelphia, PA: JB Lippincott Co.), 99.

Figure 2.3 Reprinted, by permission, from P.C. Champe and R.A. Harvey, 1994, *Lippincott's Illustrated Reviews: Biochemistry*, 2nd ed. (Philadelphia, PA: JB Lippincott Co.).

Figure 2.4 Reprinted, by permission, from P.C. Champe and R.A. Harvey, 1994, *Lippincott's Illustrated Reviews: Biochemistry*, 2nd ed. (Philadelphia, PA: JB Lippincott Co.), 87.

Figure 2.5 Reprinted, by permission, from P.C. Champe and R.A. Harvey, 1994, *Lippincott's Illustrated Reviews: Biochemistry*, 2nd ed. (Philadelphia, PA: JB Lippincott Co.).

Figure 2.6 Reprinted, by permission, from James Leklem, 1985, Physical activity and vitamin B- metabolism in men and women: interrelationship with fuel needs. In *Vitamin B-6: It's Role in Health and Disease* Copyright © 1985, Wiley-Liss, Inc. (New York: Wiley-Liss, Inc., a division of John Wiley & Sons, Inc.) 222.

Figure 2.7 Reprinted, by permission, from E.F. Coyle, 1995, "Substrate utilization during exercise in active people," *American Journal of Clinical Nutrition* 61(suppl.): 968-979. © Am. J Clin. Nutr. American Society for Clinical Nutrition.

Figure 2.8 Reprinted, by permission, from E.F. Coyle, A.R. Coggen, M.K. Hemmert, and J.L. Ivy, 1986, "Muscle glycogen utilization during prolonged strenuous exercise when fed carbohydrate," *Journal of Applied Physiology* 61 (1): 165-172.

Figure 2.9 Reprinted, by permission, from P. Felig, A. Cherif, A. Minagawa, and J. Wahren, 1982, "Hypoglycemia during prolonged exercise in normal men," *The New England Journal of Medicine* 306: 895-900. Copyright © 1982 Massachusetts Medical Society. All rights reserved.

Figure 2.10 Reprinted, by permission, from P. Felig, A. Cherif, A. Minagawa, and J. Wahren, 1982, "Hypoglycemia during prolonged exercise in normal men," *The New England Journal of Medicine* 306: 895-900. Copyright © 1982 Massachusetts Medical Society. All rights reserved.

Figure 2.11 Reprinted, by permission, from R. Murray, G.L. Paul, J.G. Seifert, D.E. Eddy, and G.A. Halaby, 1989, "The effects of glucose, fructose, and sucrose ingestion during exerise," *Medical Science Sport Exercise* 21 (3): 275-282.

Figure 2.12 Reprinted, by permission, from E. Adopo, F. Peronnet, D. Massicotte, G.R. Brisson, and C. Hillaire-Marcel, 1994, "Respective oxidation of exogenous glucose and fructose given in the same drink during exercise," *Journal of Applied Physiology* 76: 1016.

Figure 2.13 Reprinted, by permission, from J.C. Simonsen, W.M. Sherman, D.R. Lamb, A.R. Dernback, J.A. Doyle, and R. Strauss, 1991, "Dietary carbohydrate, muscle glycogen, and power output during rowing training," *Journal of Applied Physiology* 70: 1505.

Figure 2.14 Reprinted, by permission, from P.C.S. Blom, A.T. Hostmark, O. Baage, K.R. Kardel, S. Maehlum, 1987, "Effect of different post-exercise sugar diets on the rate of muscle glycogen synthesis," *Medical Science Sport Exercise* 19: 491-496.

Figure 2.15 Reprinted, by permission, from K.M. Zawadzki, B.B. Yaspelkis, and J.L. Ivy, 1992, "Carbohydrate-protein complex increases the rate of muscle glycogen storage after exercise," *Journal of Applied Physiology* 72 (5): 1854-1859.

Table 2.9 Adapted from S.K. Baker, T. Rusynyk, and P.M. Tiidus, 1994, "Immediate post-training carbohydrate supplementation improves subsequent performance in trained cyclists," *Sports Medicine Training and Rehabilitation* 1: 133. Copyright OPA (Overseas Publishers Association) N.V., with permission from Gordon and Breach Publishers.

Figure 2.16 Reprinted, by permission, from W.M. Sherman and D.L. Costill, 1984, "The marathon: dietary manipulation to optimize performance," *American Journal of Sports Medicine* 12: 44-51.

Table 3.4 Reprinted, by permission, from USDA Center for Nutrition Policy and Promotion (CNPP), 1998, "Is total fat consumption really decreasing?," *Nutrition Insights* 5, April: 171-172.

Figure 3.2 Reprinted, by permission, from USDA Center for Nutrition Policy and Promotion (CNPP), 1998, "Is total fat consumption really decreasing?," *Nutrition Insights* 5, April: 171-172.

Figure 3.3 Reprinted, by permission, from USDA Center for Nutrition Policy and Promotion (CNPP), 1998, "Is total fat consumption really decreasing?," *Nutrition Insights* 5, April: 171-172.

Figure 3.4 Reprinted, by permission, from USDA Center for Nutrition Policy and Promotion (CNPP), 1998, "Is total fat consumption really decreasing?," *Nutrition Insights* 5, April: 171-172.

Figure 3.5 Reprinted, by permission, G. M. Fogelholm, R. Koskinen, J. Laakso, T. Rankinen, and I. Ruokonen, 1993, "Gradual and rapid weight loss: effects on nutrition and performance in male athletes," *Medical Science Sport Exercise* 25: 374.

Figure 3.7 Reprinted, by permission, from B.R. Wolfe, S. Klein, F. Carraro, and J.M. Weber, 1990, "Role of triglyceride-fatty acid cycle in controlling fat metabolism in humans during and after exercise," *American Journal of Physiology* 258: E385.

Figure 3.9 Reprinted, by permission, from J.A. Romijn, E.F. Coyle, L.S. Sidossis, A. Gastaldelli, J.F. Horowitz, and R.R. Wolfe, 1993, "Regulation of endogenous fat and carbohydrate metabolism in relation to exercise," *American Journal of Physiology* 265: E387.

Figure 3.11 Reprinted from *The Journal of Nutritional Biochemistry,* 2, "Pathways of Nutritional Biochemistry: Iron Pools," 374, Copyright © 1991, with permission from Elsevier Science.

Figure 3.13 Reprinted, by permission, from B. Saltin and P.-O. Astrand, 1993, "Free fatty acids and exercise," *American Journal of Clinical Nutrition* 57(suppl.): 752S-758S.

Figure 3.14 Reprinted, by permission, from B. Saltin and P.-O. Astrand, 1993, "Free fatty acids and exercise," *American Journal of Clinical Nutrition* 57(suppl.): 752S-758S.

Figure 3.15 Reprinted, by permission, from B. Kiens and J.W. Helge, 1998, "Effect of high-fat diets on exercise performance," *Proceedings of the Nutrition Society* 57: 73-75.

Figure 3.16 Reprinted, by permission, from T.E. Graham and L.L. Spriet, 1995, "Metabolic chatecholamine and exercise performance responses to various doses of caffeine," *Journal of Applied Physiology* 78: 867-874.

Table 4.1 Adapted, by permission, from D.E. Matthews, *Modern Nutrition in Health and Disease,* 9th ed., M.E. Shils, J.A. Olson, M. Shike, and A.C. Ross eds., 1999. (Baltimore, MD: Williams & Wilkins), 14.

Figure 4.1 Adapted, by permission, from D.E. Matthews, 1999, *Modern Nutrition in Health and Disease,* 9th ed., edited by M.E. Shils, J.A. Olson, M. Shike, and A.C. Ross. (Philadelphia: Williams & Wilkins), 30.

Figure 4.3 Reprinted, by permission, from P.W.R. Lemon, 1998, "Effects of exercise on dietary protein requirements," *International Journal of Sport Nutrition* 8: 428.

Figure 4.4 Adapted, by permission, from P.C. Champe and R.A. Harvey, 1994, *Lippincott's Illustrated Reviews: Biochemistry,* 3rd ed. (Philadelphia: J.B. Lippincott Co.), 244.

Figure 4.5 Reprinted, by permission, from P.W.R. Lemon, M.A. Tarnopolsky, J.D. MacDougall, and S.A. Atkinson, 1992, "Protein requirements and muscle mass/strength changes during intensive training in novice bodybuilders," *Journal of Applied Physiology* 73: 767-775.

Figure 4.6 Adapted, by permission, from Babij, Matthews, Rennie, 1983, "Changes in blood lactate and amino acids in relation to workload during bicycle...," *European Journal of Applied Physiology* 50: 405-411.

Figure 4.7 Adapted from *Nutrition Research* Vol. 11, No. 3, I. Gontzea, R. Sutzescu, and S. Dumitrache, "The influence of adaptation to physical effort on nitrogen balance in man," Page 163, Copyright 1985, with permission from Elsevier Science.

Figure 5.1, a-c Reprinted, by permission, from C.D. Thomas, J.C. Peters, G.W. Reed, N.N. Abumrad, M. Sun, and J.O Hill, 1992, "Nutrient balance and energy expenditure during ad libitum feeding of high-fat and high carbohydrate diets in humans," *American Journal of Clinical Nutrition* 55: 934-942.

Figure 5.3, a-c Adapted, by permission, from Y. Schutz, A. Tremblay, R.L. Weiner, and K.M Nelson, 1992, "Role of oxidation in the long-term stabilization of body weight in obese women," *American Journal of Clinical Nutrition* 55: 670-674.

Figure 5.3, d-f Adapted, by permission, from G.A. Butterfield and A. Tremblay, 1994, Physical activity and nutrition in the context of fitness and health. In *Physical Activity, Fitness and Health: International Proceedings and Consensus Statement,* C. Bouchard, R.J. Shepard, and S. Stephens, eds. (Champaign, IL: Human Kinetics), 257-260.

Figure 5.4 Adapted, by permission, from J. Thompson, M.M. Manore, and S.S. Skinner, 1993, "Resting metabolic rate and thermic effect of a meal in low- and adequate-energy intake male endurance athletes," *International Journal of Sport Nutrition* 3 (2): 194-206.

Figure 5.5 Reprinted, by permission, from E. Ravussin and B.A. Swinburn *Obesity: Theory and Therapy,* 2nd ed., 1993, A.J. Stunkard and T.A. Wadden, eds. (New York, NY: Raven Press Ltd.), 98.

Figure 5.6 Reprinted, by permission, from E. Ravussin and C. Bogardus, 1989, "Relationship of genetics, age, and physical fitness to daily energy expenditure and fuel utilization," *American Journal of Clinical Nutrition* 49: 968-975.

Figure 5.7 Reprinted, by permission, from E. Ravussin and C. Bogardus, 1989, "Relationship of genetics, age, and physical fitness to daily energy expenditure and fuel utilization," *American Journal of Clinical Nutrition* 49: 968-975.

Figure 5.8 Reprinted, by permission, from J.T. Bisbee, W.P.T. James, and M.A. Shaw, 1989, "Changes in energy expenditure during the menstrual cycle," *British Journal of Nutrition* 61: 187-199.

Figure 5.9 Adapted, by permission, from R.C. Bullough, C.A. Gillette, M.A. Harris, and C.L. Melby, 1995, "Interaction of acute changes in exercise energy expenditure and energy intake on resting metabolic rate," *American Journal of Clinical Nutrition* 61: 473-481.

Figure 5.11 Adapted, by permission, from D.A. Sedlock, J.A. Fissinger, and C.A. Melby, 1989, "Effect of exercise intensity and duration on post-exercise energy expenditure," *Medical Science Sport Exercise* 21: 662-666.

Figure 5.12 Reprinted, by permission, from G.A. Brooks, T.D. Fahey, T.P. White, and K.M. Baldwin, 1999, *Exercise physiology: Human bioenergetics and its applications*, 3d ed. (Mountain View, CA: Mayfield), 44.

Figure 5.14, a-b Adapted, by permission, from J. Thompson and M.M. Manore, 1996, "Predicted and measured resting metabolic rate of male and female endurance athletes," *Journal of the American Dietetic Association* 96: 30-4.

Figure 6.1 Reprinted, by permission, from Déprés, Ross, and Lemieux, 1996, Imaging techniques applied to the measurement of human body composition. In *Human Body Composition*, A.F. Roche, S.B. Heymsfield, and T.G. Lohman, eds. (Champaign, IL: Human Kinetics),

Figure 6.3 Reprinted, by permission, from T.B. Van Itallie, *Obesity*, B. Bjorntorp and B.N. Brodoff, eds., 1992 (Philadelphia, PA: Lippincott Co.), 363.

Figure 6.4 Reprinted, by permission, from George A. Bray, 1992, "Pathophysiology of obesity," *American Journal of Clinical Nutrition* 55 (suppl.): 488S-494S.

Table 6.2 Adapted, by permission, from T.B. Van Itallie, 1979, "Obesity: Adverse effects on health and longevity," *American Journal of Clinical Nutrition* 32: 2723.

Figure 6.5 Reprinted, by permission, from L. Lissner, D.A. Levitsky, B.J. Strupp, H.J. Kalkwarf, and D.A. Roe, 1987, "Dietary fat and the regulation of energy intake in human subjects," *American Journal of Clinical Nutrition* 46: 886-892.

Figure 6.6 Reprinted, by permission, from J.A. Romijn, E.F. Coyle, L.S. Sidossis, et al., 1993, "Regulation of engenous fat and carbohydrate metabolism in relation to exercise," *American Journal of Physiology* 265: E380-E391.

Figure 6.7 Reprinted, by permission, from K.N. Pavlou, S. Krey, and W.P. Steffee, 1989, "Exercise as an adjunct to weight loss and maintenance in moderately obese subjects," *American Journal of Clinical Nutrition* 49: 1115-1123.

Table 6.5 Reprinted, by permission, from M.M. Manore, 1993, "Diet and exercise strategies of a world-class bodybuilder," *International Journal of Sport Nutrition* 3 (1): 79.

Table 6.6 Reprinted, by permission, from M.M. Manore, 1993, "Diet and exercise strategies of a world-class bodybuilder," *International Journal of Sport Nutrition* 3 (1): 80.

Figure 7.2 Reprinted, by permission, from V.H. Heyward, 1998, *Advanced Fitness Assessment and Exercise Prescription*, 3rd edition. (Champaign, IL: Human Kinetics), 162.

Table 7.1 Reprinted, by permission, from T.G. Lohman, L. Houtkooper, and Going, 1997, "Body fat measurement goes high-tech," *ACSM Health & Fitness Journal* 7: 30-35.

Table 7.2 Reprinted, by permission, from T.G. Lohman, L. Houtkooper, and Going, 1997, "Body fat measurement goes high-tech," *ACSM Health & Fitness Journal* 7: 30-35.

Table 7.4 Reprinted, by permission, from T.G. Lohman, 1987, "Measuring body fat using skinfolds," videotape. (Champaign, IL: Human Kinetics)

Table 8.1 Reprinted, by permission, from L.I. Kleinman and J.M. Lorenz, 1996, *Clinical Chemistry*. (St. Louis, MO: Mosby, Co.), 367.

Table 8.2 Reprinted, by permission, from L.I. Kleinman and J.M. Lorenz, 1996, *Clinical Chemistry*. (St. Louis, MO: Mosby, Co.), 376.

Figure 8.1 Reprinted, by permission, from M.N. Sawka and K.B. Padolf, 1990, Effects of body water loss in physiological function and exercise performance. In *Perspectives in Exercise and Science and Sports Medicine: Fluid Homeostasis During Exercise,* edited by D.R Lamb and C.V. Gisolfi (Indianapolis: Benchmark Press), 1-38.

Figure 8.2 Reprinted, by permission, from C.V. Gisolfi and A.J. Ryan, *Exercise and Sport*, E.R. Buskirk and S.M. Puhl, eds., 1996, Copyright Lewis Publishers, an imprint of CRC Press. Boca Raton, Florida.

Table 8.3 Reprinted, by permission, from Robert Murray, 1995, "Fluid needs in hot and cold environments," *International Journal of Sports Medicine* 5: S62-S73.

Table 8.4 Adapted, by permission, from J.M. Pivarnik and R.A. Palmer, 1994, *Nutrition in Exercise and Sport,* 2nd ed., I. Wolinsky, ed. Copyright Lewis Publishers and imprint of CRC Press. Boca Raton, Florida.

Figure 8.5 Reprinted, by permission, from S. Shirreffs, A. Taylor, J. Leiper, and R. Maughan, 1996, "Post-exercise hydration in man: effects of volume consumed and drink sodium content," *Medical Science Sport Exercise* 28: 1260-1271.

Figure 9.2 Adapted, by permission, from K. Suboticanec, A. Stavljenic, W. Schalch, and R. Buzina, 1990, "Effects of pyridoxine and riboflavin supplementation on physical fitness in young adolescents," *International Journal for Vitamin and Nutrition Research* 60: 85.

Figure 10.1 Reprinted, by permission, from B. Alberts, D. Bray, J. Lewis, M. Raff, K. Roberts, and J.D. Watson, 1989, *Molecular biology of the cell*, 2nd ed. (New York: Garland Publishing), 363.

Figure 10.2 Adapted, by permission, from J. Karlsson, 1997, *Antioxidants and Exercise*. (Champaign, IL: Human Kinetics), 29.

Figure 10.3 Reprinted, by permission, from R.R. Jenkins, 1993, "Exercise, oxidative stress, and antioxidants: a review," *International Journal of Sport Nutrition* 3 (4): 360.

Table 10.4 Reprinted, by permission, from J. Karlsson, 1997, *Antioxidants and Exercise*. (Champaign, IL: Human Kinetics), 16.

Figure 11.1 Reprinted, by permission, from M.E. Shils, 1994, Magnesium. In *Modern Nutrition in Health and Disease*, 8th ed., edited by M.E. Shils, J.A. Olson, and M. Shike. (Philadelphia: Lea & Febiger), 172.

Figure 11.2 Reprinted, by permission, from Manore et al., 1993, *Journal of the American Dietetic Association* 93: 1165-1168.

Figure 12.1 Reprinted, by permission, from W.E. Schreiber, 1989, Iron, porphyrin and bilirubin metabolism. In *Clinical Chemistry*, 2nd ed., L.A. Kaplan and A.J. Pesce, eds. (St. Louis: Mosby), 496-509.

Figure 12.2 Reprinted, by permission, from C.M. Weaver and S. Rajaram, 1992, "Exercise and iron status," *Journal of Nutrition* 122: 782-787.

Figure 12.3 Reprinted from D.G. Savage and J. Lindenbaum, 1995, Folate-cobalamin interactions. In *Folate in health and disease*, edited by L.B. Bailey (New York: Marcel Dekker, Inc.), 240 by courtesy of Marcel Dekker, Inc.

Figure 12.4 Reprinted from *The Journal of Nutritional Biochemistry*, 2, "Pathways of Nutritional Biochemistry: Iron Pools," 247, Copyright © 1991, with permission from Elsevier Science.

Figure 13.1 Reprinted, by permission, from D.J. Baylink and J.C. Jennings, 1994, Calcium and bone homeostasis and changes with aging. In *Principles of Geriatric Medicine and Gerontology,* 3rd ed., W.R. Hazzard, E.L. Bierman, J.P. Blass, W.H. Ettinger, J.B. Halter, eds. (New York: McGraw-Hill), 888.

Table 13.1 Reprinted, by permission, from R.S. Gibson, 1990, *Principles of Nutritional Assessment* (New York: Oxford University Press), 487.

Table 13.4 Adapted, by permission, from A.A. Yates, S.A. Schlicker, and C.W. Suitor, 1998, "Dietary reference intake," *Journal of the American Dietetic Association* 98: 699-706.

Figure 13.2 Reprinted, by permission, from J.B. Anderson, 1991, "Nutritional biochemistry of calcium and phosphorus," *Journal of Nutritional Biochemistry* 2: 301.

Table 13.7 Reprinted, by permission, from C.H. Chestnut, 1994, Osteoporosis. In *Principles of Geriatric Medicine and Gerontology*, 3rd ed. (New York: McGraw-Hill), 899. Reproduced with permission of The McGraw-Hill Companies.

Figure 13.4 Reprinted, by permission, from D.J. Baylink and J.C. Jennings, 1994, Calcium and bone homeostasis and changes with aging. In *Principles of Geriatric Medicine and Gerontology,* 3rd ed., W.R. Hazzard, E.L. Bierman, J.P. Blass, W.H. Ettinger, J.B. Halter, eds. (New York: McGraw-Hill), 888.

Table 14.1 Adapted, by permission, from the American College of Sports Medicine, 1995, *ACSM's Guidelines for Exercise Testing and Prescription.* (Philadelphia: Williams & Wilkins), 18.

Table 14.5 From M.L. Wheeler and I.M. Buzzard, 1994, "How to report dietary assessment data." Copyright The American Dietetic Association. Adapted by permission from JOURNAL OF THE AMERICAN DIETETIC ASSOCIATION, Vol. 4: 1255.

Table 14.6 From M.L. Wheeler and I.M. Buzzard, 1994, "How to report dietary assessment data." Copyright The American Dietetic Association. Adapted by permission from JOURNAL OF THE AMERICAN DIETETIC ASSOCIATION, Vol. 4: 1255.

Figure 14.2 Reprinted, by permission, from J.P. Wallace, T.L. McKenzie, and P.R. Nader, 1985, "Observed versus recalled exercise behavior," *Res Q Exercise and Sport* 56: 161-165.

Table 14.9 Adapted, by permission, from the American College of Sports Medicine, 1995, *ACSM's Guidelines for Exercise Testing and Prescription.* (Philadelphia: Williams & Wilkins), 42.

Table 14.10 Adapted, by permission, from the American College of Sports Medicine, 1995, *ACSM's Guidelines for Exercise Testing and Prescription.* (Philadelphia: Williams & Wilkins), 17.

Table 14.11 Reprinted, by permission, from O. Inbar, O. Bar-Or, and J.S. Skinner, 1996, *The Wingate Aerobic Test.* (Champaign, IL: Human Kinetics), 5.

Table 14.12 Reprinted, by permission, from O. Inbar, O. Bar-Or, and J.S. Skinner, 1996, *The Wingate Aerobic Test.* (Champaign, IL: Human Kinetics), 6.

Table 15.1 Adapted, by permission, from M.M. Manore, 1997, "How do you know when you are eating enough," *USA Gymnastics Magazine* 26 (6): 8-9.

Figure 15.1 Adapted, by permission, from D. Teegarden, W.R. Proulx, B.R. Martin, et al., 1995, "Peak bone mass in young women," *Journal of Bone and Mineral Research* 10 (5): 711-715.

Figure 15.2 Adapted, by permission, from J.E. Donnelly, D.J. Jacobsen, J.M. Jakicic, and J.E. Whatley, 1994, "Very low calorie diet with delayed and sequential exercise," *International Journal of Obesity* 18: 469-475.

Table 15.3 Adapted, by permission, from M.M. Manore, 1996, "Chronic dieting in active women: What are the health consequences?" *Women's Health Issues* 6:332-41.

Table 15.4 Adapted, by permission, from C.L. Otis, 1998, "Amenorrheic, fracture-prone: the female athlete triad," *ACSM's Health and Fitness Journal* 2 (1): 21.

Figure 15.3 Reprinted, by permission, from C.A. Dueck, M.M. Manore, and K.S. Matt, 1996, "Role of energy balance in athletic menstrual dysfunction," *International Journal of Sport Nutrition* 6 (2): 176.

Figure 15.4 Adapted, by permission, from C.A. Dueck, M.M. Manore, and K.S. Matt, 1996, "Role of energy balance in athletic menstrual dysfunction," *International Journal of Sport Nutrition* 6 (2): 169.

Figure 15.5 Adapted, by permission, from P. Brukner and K. Bennell, 1997, "Stress fractures in female athletes," *Sports Medicine* 24 (6): 419-429.

Table 15.5 Adapted, by permission, from C.L. Otis, 1998, "Amenorrheic, fracture-prone: the female athlete triad," *ACSM's Health and Fitness Journal* 2 (1): 24.

Table 16.2 Reprinted, by permission, from D.M. Lightsey and J.R. Attaway, 1992, "Deceptive tactics used in marketing purported ergogenic aids," *National Strength and Conditioning Journal* 14 (2): 27.

Highlight, pages 443-444 Adapted, by permission, from D.M. Lightsey and J.R. Attaway, 1992, "Deceptive tactics used in marketing purported ergogenic aids," *NSCA Journal* 14 (2): 26-31.

Figure 16.1 Adapted, by permission, from O.J. Heinonen, 1996, "Carnitine and physical exercise," *Sports Medicine* 22 (2): 112.

Appendix A.3 Reprinted, by permission, from D. Gifford, 1998, "The Mediterranean diet as a food guide: the problem of culture and history," *Nutrition Today* 33 (6): 239.

Appendix A.4 Reprinted, by permission, from D. Gifford, 1998, "The Mediterranean diet as a food guide: the problem of culture and history," *Nutrition Today* 33 (6): 242.

Appendix A.5 Reprinted, by permission, from D. Gifford, 1998, "The Mediterranean diet as a food guide: the problem of culture and history," *Nutrition Today* 33 (6): 241.

Appendix A.6 Reprinted, by permission, from D. Gifford, 1998, "The Mediterranean diet as a food guide: the problem of culture and history," *Nutrition Today* 33 (6): 240.

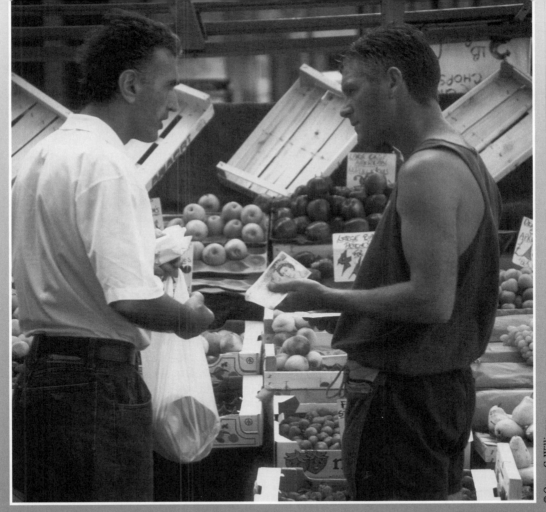

CHAPTER 1

Introduction to Nutrition for Exercise and Health

After reading this chapter you should be able to

- understand the role of nutrition in exercise and sport;
- identify the essential nutrients and the dietary recommendations for these nutrients;
- describe the various methods used in evaluating the diets of active individuals; and
- discuss the role of nutrition and exercise in the prevention of disease.

The goal of this book is to promote optimal health and sport performance by linking together information about nutrition and exercise. For competitive athletes this may mean determining fluid, nutrient, and energy needs required during times of intense training and competition. It may also mean determining the appropriate food and nutrient supplements required for various exercise situations or environmental conditions. For individuals who exercise for fitness or recreation, it may mean learning to eat to promote good health, maintain weight, and fuel exercise. No matter what one's fitness or exercise goals, good nutrition can help improve exercise performance, decrease recovery time from strenuous exercise, prevent exercise injuries due to fatigue, provide the fuel required during times of high-intensity training, and control weight. Combining good nutrition with exercise can also help reduce the risk of numerous chronic diseases such as diabetes, cardiovascular disease, hypertension, obesity, osteoporosis, and some cancers; moreover, physicians often recommend nutrition and exercise to treat individuals who already have these diseases. Learning how nutrition and exercise work together for optimal health is essential for health, nutrition, or fitness professionals who must teach the public how to maintain good health and reduce risks of chronic disease.

This chapter briefly outlines the various guidelines and tools nutritionists use to evaluate dietary intakes and to determine an individual's nutrient and energy needs. Knowing these general guidelines will help set the stage for the information covered later in this text. The more detailed guidelines for active individuals, discussed later in this book, are usually modifications—specific to the individual, sport, or situation—of these general nutrition recommendations.

Role of Nutrition in Exercise and Sport

Research on the role of nutrition in exercise and sport has increased dramatically over the last 15 years. Today there is no doubt that nutrition plays a vital role in exercise performance and training. Chapter 2 shows that carbohydrates are important for endurance exercise performance and during times of high-intensity training. Chapter 8 discusses the role fluid

intake plays in both short-term and endurance exercise. There is no question that competitive athletes can benefit from adequate energy, nutrient, and fluid intakes. Good nutrition can also help competitive or recreational athletes recover from strenuous physical activity: refueling and rehydrating the body, while providing nutrients to build and repair muscles, enable individuals to engage in the next bout of physical activity without adverse effects. This is especially important for athletes during sport tournaments, or for any individuals who engage in strenuous physical activity on a daily or more than daily basis. For example, a triathlete may do an hour swim in the morning and a 3-h cycle workout in the afternoon. Between these workouts, the athlete must replenish the body's glycogen stores and consume adequate fluid to ensure optimal exercise performance. Chapter 14 discusses methods for assessing both diet and fitness levels, so that individual recommendations can be made to improve energy and nutrient intakes based on activity levels.

Well-fueled and -hydrated athletes reduce their risk of injury during exercise—risk that increases as individuals become fatigued and lose their ability to concentrate, and as they deplete the substrates that fuel exercise. For example, chapter 15 discusses health problems that develop in female athletes who lack the energy and nutrients to fuel their activity. Proper nutrition can help speed the healing process for injured athletes; recovery from muscle or bone injuries or from surgery requires extra energy and nutrients, including protein, vitamins, and minerals. These points are discussed in detail in chapter 4 (protein), chapter 9 (B-complex vitamins), chapter 10 (antioxidants), chapter 11 (minerals), chapter 12 (blood nutrients), and chapter 13 (bone health). These chapters discuss the specific roles nutrients play in exercise, and whether exercise increases the need for the nutrients.

Nutrition also plays an important role in weight control and body composition. Few individuals today are happy with their weight, body fat levels, or body shape. Helping active individuals develop *realistic* approaches to weight maintenance (or weight loss/gain) can significantly improve health and reduce stress levels. For many active individuals, weight control is of primary concern. Chapter 3 (fat), chapter 5 (energy and macronutrient balance), chapter 6 (achieving optimal weight), and chapter 7 (body composition) address these issues. If concerns about weight and body image become overwhelming, an individual is at increased risk of disordered eating or even of developing a clinical eating disorder. Chapter 15 deals with these issues.

As interest in sport nutrition increases, the number of products promising improved exercise performance, gains in muscle strength, quick weight loss, and changes in body composition increases exponentially—which makes it difficult to sort fact from fiction. You cannot pick up a popular fitness, nutrition, or health magazine without being bombarded with advertisements for various nutrient supplements, ergogenic aids, and sport foods. If you combine these advertisements with the myriad of advertisements for weight loss or weight gain, it is not surprising that the public is confused and distrustful. Since nutrition and exercise research is still in its infancy, there are many unanswered questions. Chapter 16 presents ways to critically evaluate sport nutrition supplements and ergogenic aids.

Essential Nutrients and Dietary Recommendations

Over the last 70 years, nutrition research has identified a number of specific nutrients in foods that are essential to good health. Various organizations and governments have used this information to make dietary recommendations to ensure the health of their citizens. These dietary recommendations can also be used as general guidelines in designing diets for active individuals.

Essential and Nonessential Nutrients

The concept of essential nutrients evolved from observations that certain diseases occurred in populations that consumed poor diets, and that including certain foods in the diet could correct or prevent the diseases (Harper 1999). Food constituents that prevent diseases or health problems were classified as indispensable or **essential nutrients**. Nutrients that could be deleted from the diet with no adverse health effects were classified as dispensable or **nonessential nutrients**. These concepts are sometimes confusing because a nutrient can be *physiologically* essential for the body, but classified as nonessential for the diet since the body can synthesize it. Many nutritionists therefore prefer the terms **indispensable** (essential) or

dispensable (nonessential). Although all nutrients are important for growth and good health, they need not all come from the diet.

Classification of a nutrient as essential or indispensable clearly requires careful and extensive scientific examination. By the 1950s, 35 nutrients were identified as essential (indispensable) (see table 1.1). All of the nutrients listed in the Recommended Dietary Allowances (RDAs) and the Dietary Reference Intakes (DRIs) are currently accepted as essential for humans (see following section). However, as the science of human nutrition has developed, classifying nutrients as either essential or nonessential has not always worked.

Nutritionists have developed a list of criteria to determine whether a nutrient is considered essential (Harper 1999):

1. The substance is required in the diet for growth, health, and survival.
2. Inadequate intake of the substance leads

Table 1.1 Nutrients Essential for Humans

Water	Energy sources
Amino acids	Fatty acids
Histidine	Linoleic
Isoleucine	α-Linolenic
Leucine	Minerals
Lysine	Calcium
Methionine	Phosphorus
Phenylalanine	Magnesium
Threonine	Iron
Tryptophan	Trace minerals
Valine	Zinc
Vitamins	Copper
Ascorbic acid	Manganese
Vitamins A, D, E, K	Iodine
Thiamine	Selenium
Riboflavin	Molybdenum
Niacin	Chromium
Vitamin B_6 (pyridoxine)	Electrolytes
Pantothenic acid	Sodium
Folic acid/folate	Potassium
Biotin	Chloride
Vitamin B_{12} (cobalamin)	Ultratrace elements

Reprinted from Harper 1999.

to a characteristic deficiency disease, which can ultimately lead to death.

3. Growth failure and deficiency symptoms are prevented only by consuming the nutrient or specific precursors of it—*not* other substances.

4. If dietary intake of the nutrient drops below a critical level, growth responses and severity of deficiency symptoms are proportional to the amount consumed.

5. The substance is not synthesized in the body and is required for some critical function throughout life.

Conditionally Essential Nutrients

New research showed that the body could synthesize some "essential" nutrients from precursors, that interactions between nutrients could alter requirements, and that some disease states or genetic defects altered essential nutrient needs. A third category, **conditional essentiality,** has therefore been suggested. For example, a premature infant may require certain nutrients not required in a full-term infant. In order for the premature infant to grow and thrive, these nutrients must be added to the diet, even if they are not classified as essential nutrients for full-term infants. Rudman and Feller (1986) proposed three criteria, all of which must be present to establish the conditional essentiality of a nutrient:

1. The plasma concentration of the nutrient declines into the subnormal range, although the body should be able to synthesize the nutrient.

2. Chemical, structural, or functional abnormalities appear that are associated with low blood concentrations of the nutrient.

3. Dietary supplementation of the nutrient returns plasma concentrations to normal and corrects the chemical, structural, or functional abnormalities seen when blood concentrations were low.

Desirable and Beneficial Nutrients

In the last 20 years, the science of nutrition has taken a new direction. Nutritionists no longer focus only on preventing deficiency diseases—they now recognize many nutrients which, although not classified as essential nutrients, are important for good health and disease prevention. This has prompted research-

ers to suggest a fourth nutrient category called **"desirable or beneficial for health"** (Harper 1999). Nutrients that might fit into this category are fiber, various phytochemicals, beta-carotene, and fluoride. While many of these nutrients are now recommended for good health, they are not classified as essential nutrients. As the science of nutrition progresses, we may see this fourth category of nutrients evolve with specific inclusion criteria, which would then stimulate the rigorous research required for their inclusion.

Recommended Dietary Allowances (RDAs) and Dietary Reference Intakes (DRIs)

The Food and Nutrition Board (FNB) of the National Research Council last published a complete set of **Recommended Dietary Allowances** for essential vitamins and minerals in 1989 (see appendix A.1). The RDAs are defined as "the levels of intake of essential nutrients that, on the basis of scientific knowledge, are judged by the Food and Nutrition Board to be adequate to meet the known nutrient needs of practically all healthy persons" (FNB 1989). In the past, the RDAs were regularly updated to reflect new scientific knowledge (see figure 1.1). However, there is now a transition period in which the RDAs are being replaced with a set of dietary intake recommendations grouped by nutrient function and classification (e.g., B-complex vitamins, antioxidants and related nutrients, bone-building nutrients, trace elements, electrolytes, energy sources and macronutrients, other food components). These new recommendations are termed **Dietary Reference Intakes** or DRIs and are being developed jointly by Canadian and United States scientists. This change reflects the growing body of scientific evidence that *chronic diseases may alter nutrient requirements*. The DRI committee for each group of nutrients will establish reference intake values depending on the current scientific information available. At the present time, there are new guidelines only for the bone-building nutrients (calcium, vitamin D, phosphorus, magnesium, and fluoride) (FNB 1998a), and for the B-complex vitamins (thiamine, riboflavin, niacin, vitamin B_6, folate, vitamin B_{12}, pantothenic acid, biotin, and choline) (FNB 1998b) (see appendix A.2). The new guidelines account for physical activity as a factor affecting nutrient requirements. The reference intake values for the antioxidants and related nutrients will soon be published. A separate com-

Recommended Dietary Allowance (RDA)/Dietary Reference Intakes (DRI) time line

1941   First edition of the RDAs published

1941-1989 RDAs were periodically updated and revised based on cumulative scientific data. The 10th edition was published in 1989.

1993   The Food and Nutrition Board (FNB) held a symposium, "Should the RDAs be Revised?" Based on comments and suggestions from this meeting, FNB proposed changes to the development process of RDAs.

1995   The DRI Committee announced that seven expert nutrient group panels would review major nutrients, vitamins, antioxidants, electrolytes, and other food components.

1997   First DRI report issued on calcium, phosphorus, magnesium, vitamin D, and fluoride.

1998   Second DRI report issued on thiamine, riboflavin, niacin, vitamin B-6, folate, vitamin B-12, panthothenic acid, biotin, and choline.

2000   Third DRI report issued on vitamins C and E, betacarotene, and other selected antioxidants.

2000-2003 Estimated release dates for reports on trace elements (e.g. selenium, zinc), vitamins A and K; electrolytes and fluids; energy and macronutrients; and other food components (e.g., phytoestrogens, fiber, and phytochemicals found in foods such as garlic and tea). (Source: IFIC, 1998)

Figure 1.1   RDA/DRI time line.
Reprinted from International Food Information Council 2000.

mittee will help health professionals and the public to interpret and use the DRI values and to determine how these values can be used in various settings of clinical and public health.

These were the goals of the Food and Nutrition Board (FNB) in setting up the DRIs:

- Develop a comprehensive set of reference values for dietary nutrient intakes for the healthy population in the United States and Canada. These values will replace the RDAs for the United States and the Recommended Nutrient Intakes (RNIs) for Canada.
- Clearly document the derivation of the reference values, with emphasis on nutrient function.
- Consider the evidence concerning prevention of disease and developmental disorders in addition to prevention of nutrient deficiency.
- Examine data on nutrients that had not been previously considered essential nutrients.
- Make recommendations for future research to fill in the identified knowledge gaps.

As reference values, DRIs are quantitative estimates of nutrient intakes to be used for planning and assessing diets for healthy people (FNB 1998a, 1998b). Think of the DRI as an umbrella term that includes the specific definitions given below.

• ***Recommended Dietary Allowance (RDA):*** The intake that meets the nutrient requirement of almost all (97-98%) of the healthy individuals in a specific age and gender group. RDAs can help individuals achieve adequate nutrient intake in order to decrease risks of chronic disease. Values for RDAs are estimates of average requirements plus increases to account for variations within a particular group. Available scientific evidence allowed DRI committees to calculate RDAs for phosphorus, magnesium, thiamine, riboflavin, vitamin B_6, folate, and vitamin B_{12}.

• ***Adequate Intake (AI):*** Empirical intake levels of healthy people, used when sufficient scientific evidence is not available to estimate RDAs. AI values derive from experimental or observed intake levels that appear to sustain a desired indicator of health, such as calcium retention in bone for most members of a population group. For example, the average observed nutrient intake of populations of breast-fed infants defined AIs for infants through one year of age. Individuals should use AIs as goals for intake where no RDAs exist. To date, DRI committees have set AIs for calcium, vitamin D, fluoride, pantothenic acid, biotin, and choline.

• ***Estimated Average Requirement (EAR):*** The nutrient intake value that is estimated to meet the requirement of half the individuals in a specific group. This figure is used

5

as a basis for developing the RDA. Makers of nutrition policy used EARs to evaluate the adequacy of nutrient intakes of a group and to plan how much the group should consume. For example, the RDA for a particular nutrient is calculated as follows: $RDA = EAR + 2 SD_{EAR}$ where SD_{EAR} is the standard deviation of the EAR. If data about the variability in requirements are insufficient to calculate a standard deviation, a coefficient of variation (CV) for the EAR of 10% is ordinarily assumed.

• ***Tolerable Upper Intake Level (UL):*** The maximum intake by an individual that is unlikely to pose risks of adverse health effects to almost all healthy individuals in the general population. As intake increases above the UL, the risk of adverse effects increases. This figure is not intended to be a recommended level of intake. There is no established benefit for individuals to consume nutrients at levels above the RDA or AI. For most nutrients, the UL refers to total nutrient intake from food, fortified food, and nutrient supplements. The term "tolerable intake" was chosen to avoid implying a possible beneficial effect from this level of the nutrient.

Figure 1.2 graphically describes the relationships among the preceding terms and where they fall on an intake continuum.

Eating a Balanced Diet

What does it mean to eat a balanced diet? Do active individuals need a "different" balanced diet from that of sedentary individuals? What does a "balanced diet" mean if you are a vegetarian? Although the term "balanced diet" is

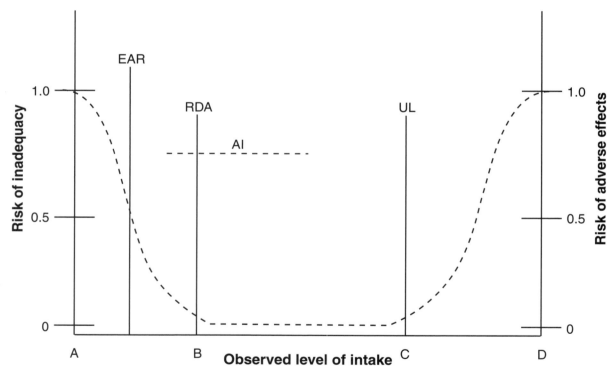

Figure 1.2 Dietary reference intakes. This figure shows that the Estimated Average Requirement (EAR) is the intake at which the risk of inadequacy is 0.5 (50%). The Recommended Dietary Allowance (RDA) is the intake at which the risk of inadequacy is very small—only 0.02 to 0.03 (2 to 3%). The Adequate Intake (AI) does not bear a consistent relationship to the EAR or the RDA because it is set without being able to estimate the requirement. At intakes between the RDA and the Tolerable Upper Intake Level (UL), the risks of inadequacy and of adverse effects are both close to 0. The UL is the highest level of daily nutrient intake that is likely to pose no risks of adverse health effects to almost all individuals in the general population. At intakes above the UL, the risk of adverse effects increases. A dashed line is used because the actual shape of the curve has not been determined experimentally. The distances between points A and B, B and C, and C and D may differ much more than is depicted in this figure. Reproduced from FNB 1998a.

frequently used by nutritionists, most consumers have no clue as to its meaning or how to change their diet so it is more "balanced." To help provide consumers with dietary guidelines and a simple way of evaluating their diets, the United States Department of Agriculture (USDA) and the Department of Health and Human Services (DHHS) developed the Dietary Guidelines for Americans and the Food Guide Pyramid. Similarly, the Canadian government has developed Canada's Guidelines for Healthy Eating (Health and Welfare Canada 1989) and Canada's Food Guide to Healthy Eating (1992).

Dietary Guidelines for Americans

The Dietary Guidelines for Americans has evolved over the last 15-20 years in an attempt to answer the question, "What should Americans eat to stay healthy?" (Kennedy 1998) (see table 1.2). The **Dietary Guidelines**—targeting healthy Americans age 2 years and older—provide advice about food choices that promote health, decrease the risk of chronic disease, meet nutrient requirements, and support active lives (Kennedy et al. 1996). The guidelines were developed by a panel of experts based on current science as well as on input from the public and from government agencies (Bialostosky and St. Jeor 1996). Yet while the Dietary Guidelines in table 1.2 provide general goals for all Americans (including active individuals), they do not provide the specific methods for achieving the goals. The **Food Guide Pyramid** translates the message of the Dietary Guidelines into specific daily dietary recommendations (see the next section).

Since the Dietary Guidelines were designed to convey dietary recommendations and not medical advice, it is the job of health professionals to help clients interpret and implement these guidelines into their own lifestyles. The following list briefly describes the recommendations for each of the 1995 Dietary Guidelines for Americans.

1. ***Eat a variety of foods.*** This guideline provides a link to all the others. Foods contain varying combinations of nutrients and other healthful substances, and no single food can supply all the nutrients in the amounts needed. This recommendation focuses on the *total* diet and counsels that *foods are the preferred form of nutrients,* since many healthful substances are present in foods (e.g., phytochemicals, isoflavones) but not in dietary supplements. In discussing the specific nutrient needs of special populations (e.g., growing children, teenage girls, women, elderly, vegetarians), this guideline suggests that in specific situations supplements or fortified foods may be necessary to meet the nutrient needs of these populations.

Table 1.2   Dietary Guidelines for 1980-1995

1980	1985	1990	1995
Eat a variety of foods.	Eat a variety of foods.	Eat a variety of foods.	Eat a variety of foods.
Maintain ideal weight.	Maintain desirable weight.	Maintain healthy weight.	Balance the food you eat with physical activity—maintain or improve your weight.
Avoid too much fat, saturated fat, and cholesterol.	Avoid too much fat, saturated fat, and cholesterol.	Choose a diet low in fat, saturated fat, and cholesterol.	Choose a diet with plenty of grain products, vegetables, and fruits.
Eat foods with adequate starch and fiber.	Eat foods with adequate starch and fiber.	Choose a diet with plenty of vegetables, fruits, and grain products.	Choose a diet low in fat, saturated fat, and cholesterol.
Avoid too much sugar.	Avoid too much sugar.	Use sugars only in moderation.	Choose a diet moderate in sugars.
Avoid too much sodium.	Avoid too much sodium.	Use salt and sodium only in moderation.	Choose a diet moderate in salt and sodium.
If you drink alcohol, do so in moderation.	If you drink alcoholic beverages, do so in moderation.	If you drink alcoholic beverages, do so in moderation.	If you drink alcoholic beverages, do so in moderation.

Reprinted from Kennedy, Meyers, and Layden 1996.

2. ***Balance the food you eat with physical activity—maintain or improve your weight.*** For the first time, the Dietary Guidelines emphasize that *both diet and physical activity are important for weight control.* Although the weight guidelines stress both weight maintenance and weight loss, they emphasize the importance of weight maintenance over weight loss as a more realistic goal that people are more likely to attempt and achieve (Kennedy et al. 1996). This guideline specifically states, "Many Americans gain weight in adulthood, increasing their risk of high blood pressure (hypertension), heart disease, stroke, diabetes, certain types of cancers, arthritis, breathing problems, and other illnesses. Therefore, most adults should NOT gain weight. If you are overweight and have one of these problems, you should try to lose weight, or at the very least not gain weight." Specific recommendations are given for increasing energy expenditure and reducing energy intake to help maintain or lose weight.

3. ***Choose a diet with plenty of grain products, vegetables, and fruits.*** This guideline was moved up to third place in the bulletin to emphasize its increasing importance in health and disease prevention (Kennedy et al. 1996). Grains are mentioned first, to ensure consistency with the ordering of the food groups in the Food Guide Pyramid. The Dietary Guidelines state that "grain products, vegetables, and fruits are key parts of a varied diet. They are emphasized in this guideline because they provide vitamins, minerals, complex carbohydrates (starch and dietary fiber), and other substances that are important for good health. They are also generally low in fat, depending on how they are prepared and what is added to them at the table. Most Americans of all ages eat fewer than the recommended number of servings of grain products, vegetables, and fruits, even though consumption of these foods is associated with a substantially lower risk of many chronic diseases, including certain types of cancers."

4. ***Choose a diet low in fat, saturated fat, and cholesterol.*** The 1995 Dietary Guidelines continue to recommend reducing dietary fat to no more than 30% of total energy intake, and saturated fat to no more than 10%. Dietary cholesterol intake should be no more than 300 mg/d. Although Americans have lowered the percentage of energy from fat over the last 10 years, absolute fat intake has not changed and Americans continue to gain weight (see chapter 3). For the first time, the Dietary Guidelines indicate

that children between the ages of 2 and 5 years should gradually decrease their fat intake to 30% of total energy intake by the time they enter school. This recommendation was included to help guard against overzealous dietary fat restrictions in preschool-age children. As children begin to eat less fat, they will gain energy by eating more grain products, fruits, vegetables, low-fat dairy products, beans, and lean meats.

5. ***Choose a diet moderate in sugars.*** This recommendation represents a change of wording from the 1990 Dietary Guidelines to clarify the role of sugars in health and weight maintenance. The guidelines state that, "There is no scientific evidence indicating that diets high in sugars cause hyperactivity or diabetes. The most common type of diabetes occurs in overweight adults. Avoiding sugars alone will not correct overweight. To lose weight reduce the total amount of calories from the food you eat and increase your level of physical activity." Just reducing sugar intake, without reducing total energy intake, will not lead to weight loss. The guidelines also discuss sugar substitutes and the role of sugar in dental caries.

6. ***Choose a diet moderate in salt and sodium.*** While describing the important role that sodium plays in the body, this guideline emphasizes that *most Americans eat more sodium than is needed, which may contribute to hypertension.* It is recommended that Americans reduce their sodium intake to less than 2400 mg/d. (One level teaspoon of table salt provides ~2300 mg of sodium.) This recommendation may not apply to very physically active individuals exercising in hot climates, since they can lose large amounts of sodium through perspiration (see chapter 8). The guideline states that, "In the body, sodium plays an essential role in regulation of fluids and blood pressure. Many studies in diverse populations have shown that a high sodium intake is associated with higher blood pressure. Most evidence suggests that many people at risk for high blood pressure reduce their chances of developing this condition by consuming less salt or sodium." The guideline also discusses other factors that affect blood pressure—such as weight, physical activity, potassium, calcium, and alcohol intake.

7. ***If you drink alcoholic beverages, do so in moderation.*** Although the wording of this guideline is the same as in the 1990 edition, there are slight changes in the text ac-

companying it (Kennedy et al. 1996). The guideline acknowledges that current research associates moderate drinking with lower risks of heart disease, and that many societies use alcoholic beverages to enhance the enjoyment of meals. However, there is still a strong emphasis on the negative effects of high levels of alcohol intake, which can increase risks of high blood pressure, stroke, heart disease, certain cancers, accidents, violence, suicides, birth defects, cirrhosis of the liver, inflammation of the pancreas, and overall mortality (deaths). High alcohol intake also increases the risk of malnutrition, because the energy in alcohol may replace other more nutritious foods. Finally, the guidelines give a list of individuals who should not drink.

The Food Guide Pyramid

The USDA first released the Food Guide Pyramid in 1992, intending to translate the Dietary Guidelines recommendations on nutrient intake into practical recommendations for food intake (Cronin 1998; Welsh et al. 1992; Nestle 1998). The Pyramid provides the conceptual framework for selecting specific kinds and amounts of food to eat on a daily basis. It is not a rigid prescription of what people must eat, but rather a general guide for healthful eating that allows people to fit a variety of dietary patterns into the Pyramid framework (Kennedy 1998). Figure 1.3 shows the Food Guide Pyramid, with the specific servings recommended for each food group. Canada's Food Guide to Healthy Eating was also released in 1992, to help translate the

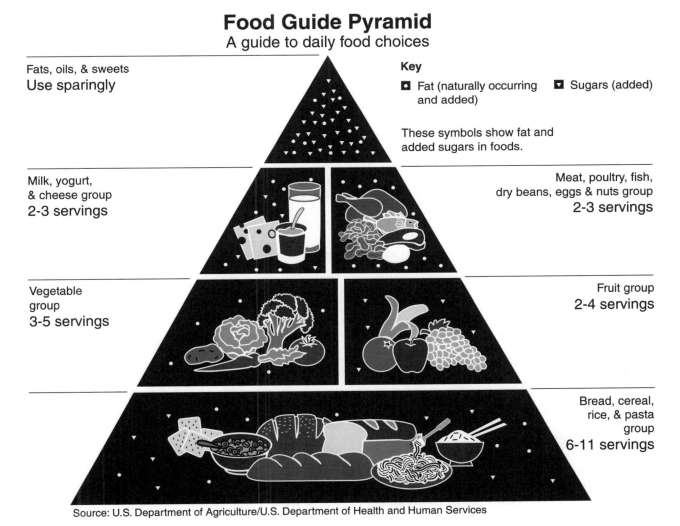

Figure 1.3 USDA Food Guide Pyramid.
Reproduced from USDA 1992.

Canadian Guidelines for Healthy Eating (Health and Welfare Canada 1989) into practical eating guidelines for the consumer.

Using the Food Guide Pyramid

A key to using the Food Guide Pyramid is understanding what constitutes a serving size for each of the food groups and how many servings from each group should be consumed. Tables 1.3 and 1.4 provide this information.

Table 1.5 outlines some of the specific food and nutrition messages carried in the Food Guide Pyramid diagram—the primary messages being the importance of dietary variety; of moderation in fat, oil, and sugar intake; and

of balance (serving size and number of servings within each food group). As a health professional, you can decide which of these specific messages you want to emphasize with your client. The Pyramid provides an excellent way to quickly review an individual's dietary intake, and to recommend dietary changes that combine their food preferences with their specific energy and nutrient needs (see "Building Your Own Food Guide Pyramid," page 14).

Variations of the Food Guide Pyramid

For active individuals, Dr. Linda Houtkooper at the University of Arizona has modified the Food Guide Pyramid to include fluids as a new

Table 1.3 Serving Sizes for the Food Guide Pyramid: What Counts As a Serving?

Bread, cereal, rice, and pasta

1 slice of bread, 6 in. diameter tortilla, 1/2 bun or bagel, 1/2 medium doughnut	1 oz of ready-to-eat cereal	1/2 cup of cooked cereal, rice, or pasta; 3-4 small plain crackers; 2 cookies

Vegetable

1 cup of raw leafy vegetables	1/2 cup of other vegetables, cooked or chopped raw	3/4 cup of vegetable juice

Fruit

1 medium apple, banana, or orange; 1/4 cup of dried fruit	1/2 cup of chopped, cooked, or canned fruit	3/4 cup of fruit juice

Milk, yogurt, and cheese

1 cup of milk or yogurt	1 1/2 oz of natural cheese	2 oz of processed cheese

Meat, poultry, fish, dry beans, eggs, and nuts

2-3 oz of cooked lean meat, poultry, or fish. A 3-oz piece of meat is about the size of an average hamburger, or the amount of meat on a medium chicken breast half.	1/2 cup of cooked dry beans, 1 egg, or 2 tbsp of peanut butter count as 1 oz of lean meat (about 1/3 serving)

Fats, oils, and sweets

Limit calories from this food group, especially if you need to lose weight or maintain a low body weight. Foods in this category include full-fat salad dressing, cream cheese, sour cream, butter, margarine, shortening, lard, sugars, soft drinks, fruit drinks, candies, sweet snack foods, or desserts. These foods provide calories but few vitamins and minerals. Note that some fat and sugar symbols are shown in the other food groups. This means that some of the foods in these groups can also be high in fat and sugars, such as cheese or ice cream in the milk group or fried foods from any group.

Source: The Food Guide Pyramid, USDA, Human Nutrition Information Service, Washington, DC, Home and Garden Bulletin Number 252, 1992.

Table 1.4 Food Guide Pyramid:
Sample Diets for a Day at Four Different Energy Intake Levels

Directions: Eat at least the lowest recommended number of servings for each food group in the Pyramid. Very active athletes will need to eat more than the highest recommended number of servings for each group. Choosing an energy intake: 1600 kcal/d is about right for very sedentary women and some older adults. 2200 kcal/d is about right for most children, teenage girls, moderately active women, and many sedentary men. Women who are pregnant or breastfeeding may need somewhat more. 2800 kcal/d is about right for teenage boys, many active men, and some very active women. 3500 kcal/d is about right for active teenage boys, active men, and some unusually active women. Very active men will need more than 3500 kcal/d.

	Energy intake			
	Low ~1600 kcal/d[1]	Moderate ~2200 kcal/d[1]	High ~2800 kcal/d[1]	Very High ~3500 kcal/d[1]
Bread group servings	6	9	11	21
Vegetable group servings	3	4	5	6
Fruit group servings	2	3	4	10
Milk group servings	2-3[2]	2-3[2]	2-3[2]	5
Meat group[3] servings (oz)	5	6	7	7
Total fat[4] (g)	**53**	**73**	**93**	**~105**
Total added sugar[5] (tsp)	**6**	**12**	**18**	**~28**

[1]These are the calorie levels if you choose low-fat, lean foods from the five major food groups and use foods from fat, oils, and sweet group sparingly.

[2]Women who are pregnant or breastfeeding, teenagers, and young adults to age 24 need 3 servings per day.

[3]Meat group amounts are in total ounces.

[4]These are estimates based on the common fat content of foods (1 pat of butter or margarine = 4 g of fat).

[5]These are estimates based on the common added sugar content of foods (1 tsp = 4 g of sugar).

Adapted from The Food Guide Pyramid, USDA, Human Nutrition Information Service, Washington, DC, Home and Garden Bulletin Number 252, 1992.

food category (see figure 1.4, page 15). This adaptation of the Pyramid helps active individuals see the importance of daily fluid replacement and understand the sources of fluids in their diets.

Nutritionists have developed food guide pyramids for vegetarians, Asians, Latin Americans, and individuals who want to follow the "Mediterranean diet" (see appendixes A.3-A.6, pages 457-460). These adaptations are somewhat similar in that all are based on the same building blocks—grains, vegetables, and fruit (Kennedy 1998; Nestle 1998)—and they all include daily physical activity as part of the pyramid. Before recommending these modifications of the Food Guide Pyramid to your clients, however, be sure you understand how your clients are interpreting the messages in these pyramids (Crotty 1998a, 1998b; Gifford 1998; Nestle 1998; Wilson 1998). As with any general nutri-

tion guideline, you can adapt information from any of the Pyramids for use with a specific individual. In general, the Pyramids provide a visual educational tool that can help consumers make wise daily food choices.

Role of Nutrition and Exercise in Disease Prevention

The role that nutrition and exercise play in reducing chronic disease risk factors is well established—yet most Americans are sedentary, overweight, and eat too much fat and sugar and too few fruits, vegetables, whole grains, and low-fat protein. In order to communicate positive nutrition and exercise messages to all Americans, various public and private organizations have jointly developed diet and

Table 1.5 Some Content Messages Carried by the Food Guide Pyramid Graphic

Message	Anticipated level of appropriateness
Foods can be divided into distinct groups.	Relatively easy and appropriate for even young children.
There are five "major" food groups.	Appropriate for elementary school-aged children.
Some food from each of the major food groups should be eaten every day.	Appropriate for elementary school-aged children.
No one food group is more or less important than another.	A more abstract concept to teach, probably not interpretable until upper elementary grades.
There is another category labeled fats, oils, and sweets.	Young children will probably only understand portions of this message.
Different food groups have different numbers of servings recommended.	This message assumes an understanding of serving size, which can be taught in upper elementary grades.
All the recommendations are made as daily recommendations.	Can be easily understood by all, if emphasized.
Some foods or food groups should be eaten more often than other food groups.	Can be understood at the elementary level.
Each food group has a range of servings recommended for it.	This may be difficult for even adult audiences to interpret correctly.
The icons represent an unstated range of products in each food group.	Young children may not generalize beyond the literal exemplars.
Fat may be naturally occurring or added.	Most children and many adults are unaware of this concept, especially those inexperienced in food preparation.
Naturally occurring and added fat should be used sparingly.	This is an abstract concept as presented. More concrete examples will be needed to make it comprehensible.
Sugars can be added or naturally occurring (an inference).	This statement assumes an understanding of "sugars" that most children and many adults do not understand.
Added sugars should be used sparingly.	This will be easier to teach for sugar than for fat. Suitable at an elementary level.
Naturally occurring sugars are (apparently) not a problem.	Can be understood, but needs to be taught specifically (i.e., not left to an assumption).
Fats can be found in the milk group, meat group, vegetable group, and the bread group.	Upper elementary grades and above.
Sugars can be found in the milk, yogurt, and cheese group; the fruit group; and the bread, cereal, rice, and pasta group.	Upper elementary grades and above.
Sugars are not found in the vegetable group.	Upper elementary grades and above.

Reprinted from Achterberg 1992.

physical activity goals, as described in the following two sections.

Healthy People 2000

Healthy People 2000 is a national initiative to increase years of healthy life, reduce health disparities among different populations, and achieve access to preventive services for all Americans (Crane et al. 1998). Healthy People 2000 consists of 319 specific health promotion and disease prevention objectives, organized into 22 priority areas, all targeted for achievement by the year 2000. The broad nature of the goals, however, makes them desirable and relevant for decades into the future. Because both nutrition and physical activity have primary roles in promoting health and reducing premature death and disability from chronic disease, they are included in the first three priority areas. There are 27 nutritional and 13 physical activity and fitness objectives in Healthy People 2000, as outlined in table 1.6.

Table 1.6 Healthy People 2000 Nutrition and Physical Activity and Fitness Objectives

Year 2000 objectives: Nutrition	Year 2000 objectives: Physical activity and fitness
1. Reduce coronary heart disease deaths.	1. Reduce coronary heart disease deaths.
2. Reverse the rise in cancer deaths.	2. Reduce overweight prevalence.
3. Reduce overweight prevalence.	3. Preserve independent functioning in older adults.
4. Reduce growth retardation.	4. Increase moderate physical activity.
5. Reduce dietary fat intake.	5. Increase vigorous physical activity.
6. Increase complex carbohydrate and fiber-containing foods.	6. Reduce sedentary lifestyle.
7. Increase sound weight-loss practices.	7. Increase activities that enhance muscular strength, endurance, and flexibility.
8. Increase calcium intake.	8. Increase sound weight-loss practices.
9. Decrease salt and sodium intake.	9. Increase participation in school physical education.
10. Reduce iron deficiency.	10. Increase activity level in school physical education.
11. Increase breastfeeding.	11. Increase work site fitness programs.
12. Decrease baby bottle tooth decay.	12. Increase availability and accessibility of community fitness facilities.
13. Increase use of food labels.	13. Increase physical activity counseling by primary care providers.
14. Achieve useful nutrition labeling.	
15. Increase availability of low-fat foods.	
16. Increase low-fat, low-calorie food choices.	
17. Increase school and child care menus consistent with the Dietary Guidelines.	
18. Increase home-delivered meals.	
19. Increase nutrition education in schools.	
20. Increase nutrition education and weight-management programs at work sites.	
21. Increase nutrition assessment, counseling, and referrals.	
22. Reduce stroke deaths.	
23. Reduce colorectal cancer deaths.	
24. Reduce diabetes incidence/prevalence.	
25. Reduce prevalence of high blood cholesterol.	
26. Increase blood pressure screening.	
27. Reduce adult mean serum cholesterol.	

Source: U.S. Department of Health and Human Services. Healthy People 2000: national health promotion and disease prevention objectives. DHHS Publication No. (PHS)91-50212. Washington, DC: Public Health Service, 1991.

As the Healthy People 2000 goals are evaluated and the Healthy People 2010 objectives determined, check the following web sites for the latest information.

Web site: **http://web.health.gov/healthypeople/2010**

Web site: **http://odphp.osophs.dhhs.gov/pubs/hp2000**

For general information on Healthy People 2000 and Healthy People 2010:
Office of Disease Prevention and Health Promotion
U.S. Public Health Service
330 C Street, SW, Room 2132
Washington, DC 20201; 202-205-8583

For Healthy People 2000 and 2010 publications, please write to:
ODPHP National Health Information Center
P.O. Box 1133
Washington, DC 20013-1133

Building Your Own Food Guide Pyramid

Help your clients build their own Food Guide Pyramid for good health and weight maintenance (see figure 1.4). Eating smart and exercising are not just for today; they are lifetime commitments. Below are some guidelines for helping your clients make gradual changes in diet and exercise that will translate into a lifetime of positive health behaviors. Get them to start building their pyramid now!

1. **Modify food choices gradually.** This is easier than overhauling your whole diet at once. For example, begin selecting 1% or 2% milk instead of whole milk. When the time is right, you can make the big jump to skim milk or stay with 1% milk. This substitution will help reduce both fat and energy intake. Another easy change is to substitute whole wheat bread for white bread or add beans to a meal. These changes will help improve micronutrient and fiber intakes.

2. **Choose foods from the five major foods groups on a daily basis.** If you are vegetarian, choose beans, legumes, tofu, or other high-protein foods instead of meat. Learn to build your pyramid from the bottom up—with plenty of whole grains, fruits, and vegetables! Use the Food Guide Pyramid to help make meal selections. If it is dinnertime and you have not eaten any vegetables yet, this would be a great time to have a big salad or a bowl of stir-fried vegetables instead of a hamburger.

3. **Use moderation as your goal.** Do not set out to eliminate all your favorite foods. This will not work and may cause you to binge on these foods after days of deprivation. Try to eat foods lower in fat and sugar more often than foods high in these items. Work to keep your meals and snacks in balance. Learn to pack healthy snacks with you to help reduce the urge to eat from the vending machine. Pick juice and water over soda pop.

4. **Spice up your life.** Try new foods. Besides the nutritional benefits, a variety of foods adds interest to meals and snacks. For example, add new vegetables to your shopping list, try new menu items in restaurants, or add the seasonal fruits to your diet. If you are real adventurous, try adding a new recipe each week to your standard menu. It can make eating more interesting for everyone sitting around your dinner table. If you do not cook, start. You may find you love the adventure.

5. **Drink lots of fluids.** Water is an important nutrient we often forget about. Learn to drink water throughout the day and at meal times. In addition, eating fruits, vegetables, soups, coffee, tea, and fruit juices adds fluid to the body. Remember that thirst is not a good indicator of fluid needs. Drink even when you are not thirsty, especially on hot days. Sport beverages are a great way to keep hydrated when you exercise.

6. **Evaluate your lifestyle.** Are you active? Is your weight stable? Do you want to gain or lose weight? Consider the number of calories or the amount of food you need to maintain your current lifestyle. Then from each food group, eat enough servings—at least the minimum—to reach or keep your healthy weight.

7. **Get active.** If you are not already, begin adding physical activity into your day. For example, take the stairs instead of the elevator, walk briskly on your next errand instead of driving the car, work in the yard, briskly walk the dog, take a walk on your lunch hour, or try exercising in front of the TV. If you are already physically active, try increasing the intensity at which you exercise, adding a new sport or activity to your exercise routine, or start strength training. Exercise helps keep your muscles toned, burns calories, and makes you feel great! Remember, weight is maintained when you burn all the calories consumed each day.

Food Guide Pyramid for Athletes
A plan for daily training food choices

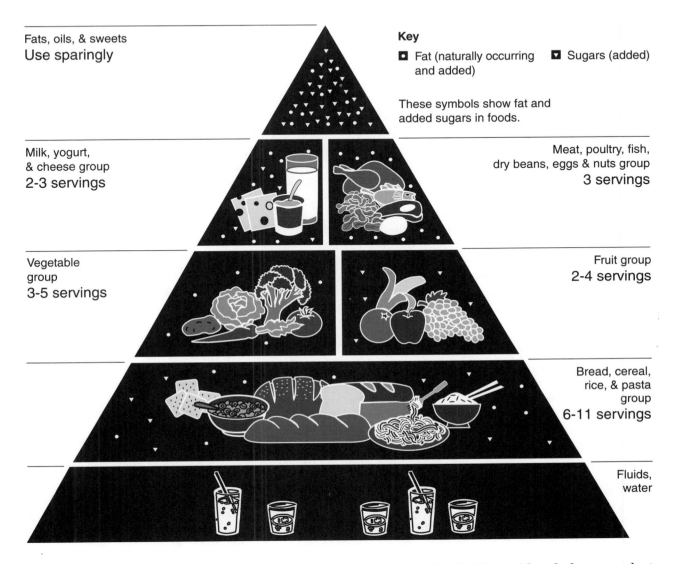

Fats, oils, & sweets
Use sparingly

Key
◨ Fat (naturally occurring and added)   ◩ Sugars (added)

These symbols show fat and added sugars in foods.

Milk, yogurt, & cheese group
2-3 servings

Meat, poultry, fish, dry beans, eggs & nuts group
3 servings

Vegetable group
3-5 servings

Fruit group
2-4 servings

Bread, cereal, rice, & pasta group
6-11 servings

Fluids, water

Figure 1.4 Food Guide Pyramid for athletes. Use the Food Guide Pyramid to help you select foods you need for top performance. Start with plenty of whole grain bread, cereals, rice, and pasta; vegetables; and fruits. Add two to three servings from the Milk group and two to three servings from the Meat group. Each of these food groups provides some, but not all, of the nutrients you need. No one food group is more important than another for top performance. You need tham all! Go easy on fats, oils, and sweets, the foods in the small tip of the Pyramid.

Reprinted from Houtkooper 1994.

Many of the objectives for nutrition and exercise overlap, emphasizing the role that both play in promoting health and preventing chronic disease. For example, reducing the risk of coronary heart disease deaths is listed as the number-one objective for both nutrition and physical activity, while reducing overweight prevalence is listed as the number-three objective for nutrition and the number-two objective for physical activity. The Healthy People

2000 documents (see appendix A.7) describe each of the nutrition and fitness objectives, with suggested ways to implement them. Appendix A also provides a complete list of public and private organizations involved in developing and implementing the objectives—agencies that, by the year 2000, expected to publish even newer objectives for Healthy People 2010.

Physical Activity and Public Health

The greatest emphasis in the Healthy People 2000 objectives is on getting the American population more physically active. The Centers for Disease Control and Prevention (CDC) and the American College of Sports Medicine (ACSM) assembled an international group of experts to review the pertinent scientific evidence and develop a clear "public health message" regarding physical activity (Pate et al. 1995). This public health message for physical activity is analogous to the Dietary Guidelines

and Food Guide Pyramid developed by the Departments of Agriculture and Health and Human Services. The CDC/ACSM workshops recommended the following for Americans:

- Every adult should accumulate 30 min or more of moderate-intensity physical activity on most, preferably all, days of the week. Table 1.7 provides examples of moderate-intensity activities.
- The recommended 30 min of activity can be accumulated in short bouts of activity throughout the day, such as walking up stairs instead of taking the elevator, walking instead of driving, or doing calisthenics.

The above recommendations deviate from earlier recommendations that suggested that 20-60 min of continuous moderate- to high-intensity activity (60-90% of maximum heart rate) is needed to reduce the risk of cardiovascular disease. Although exercising at a greater intensity

Table 1.7 Examples of Common Physical Activities for Healthy U.S. Adults

Light (<3.0 METs or <4 kcal/min)	Moderate (3.0-6.0 METs or 4-7 kcal/min)	Hard/Vigorous (>6.0 METs or >7 kcal/min)
Walking, slowly (strolling) (1-2 mph)	Walking, briskly (3-4 mph)	Walking, briskly uphill or with a load
Cycling, stationary (<50 W)	Cycling for pleasure or transportation (≤10 mph)	Cycling, fast or racing (>10 mph)
Swimming, slow treading	Swimming, moderate effort	Swimming, fast treading or crawl
Conditioning exercise, light stretching	Conditioning exercise, general calisthenics	Conditioning exercise, stair ergometer, ski machine
- - -	Racket sports, table tennis	Racket sports, singles tennis, racketball
Golf, power cart	Golf, pulling cart or carrying clubs	- - -
Bowling	- - -	- - -
Fishing, sitting	Fishing, standing/casting	Fishing in stream
Boating, power	Canoeing, leisurely (2.0-3.9 mph)	Canoeing, rapidly (≥4 mph)
Home care, carpet sweeping	Home care, general cleaning	Home care, moving furniture
Mowing lawn, riding mower	Mowing lawn, power mower	Mowing lawn, hand mower
Home repair, carpentry	Home repair, painting	- - -

Activities are classified according to kilocalories (kcal) per minute. The METs (work metabolic rate/resting metabolic rate) are multiples of the resting rate of oxygen consumption during physical activity. One MET represents the approximate rate of oxygen consumption of a seated adult at rest, or about 3.5 ml/min/kg. The equivalent energy cost of 1 MET in kcal/min is about 1.2 for a 70-kg person, or approximately 1 kcal/kg/h.

Reproduced from Pate et al. 1995.

and for a longer duration will certainly improve physical fitness and provide definite health benefits, *most of the health benefits can be gained by performing* moderate *physical activity.* Moreover, most people are more likely to work toward accumulating 30 min of total activity each day than to achieve 30 min of activity in one session. The current low participation in physical activity may occur in part because individuals assume they will reap health benefits only if they engage in vigorous continuous activity for 30-60 min. We now know this is not true. Health benefits gained from increased physical activity depend on one's initial activity level. Figure 1.5 shows that sedentary individuals realize the most benefit from increasing their activity to recommended levels. Exercises that improve strength and flexibility are important not only for cardiovascular fitness, but for overall health, and should become part of everyone's total fitness program (see chapter 14). However, clients always have excuses as to why they cannot start a fitness program. "Ten Great Reasons to Get More Active" (next page) tells why your clients should start exercising. Give this list to your clients to help motivate them to be more active.

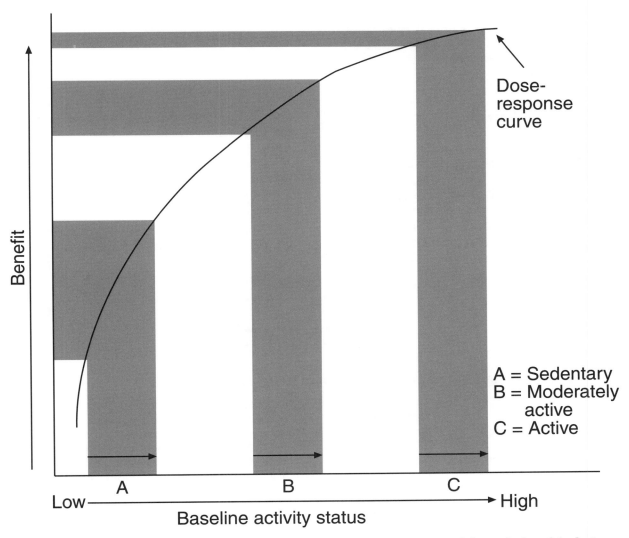

Figure 1.5 The dose-response curve represents the best estimate of the relationship between physical activity (dose) and health benefit (response). The lower the baseline of physical activity, the greater will be the health benefit from a given increase in physical activity (arrows A, B, and C).

Reproduced from Pate et al. 1995.

■ HIGHLIGHT ■

Ten Great Reasons to Get More Active

1. Helps you lose weight, especially fat weight.
2. Helps increase your level of muscle strength and lean tissue.
3. Improves posture and decreases risk of lower back pain.
4. Reduces your level of anxiety and stress.
5. Reduces your risk of cardiovascular disease, stroke, diabetes, hypertension, and some cancers.
6. Helps you maintain a healthy body weight and become a better fat burner.
7. Improves appearance and self-esteem.
8. Helps you sleep better.
9. Improves your immune function and reduces the number of sick days.
10. Improves overall quality of life.

Chapter in Review

Diet and exercise play an important role in health, sport performance, and the reduction of chronic disease risk factors. Numerous government and professional agencies have identified essential dietary nutrients, recommended appropriate nutrient intakes, and defined goals for nutrition and exercise for all North Americans. They have also developed educational tools to help implement these recommendations into people's daily lives. The goal now is to learn how to motivate individuals to make positive diet and exercise changes. While this is a tremendous challenge, this book will give you the knowledge, understanding, and tools necessary to help you teach your clients how to make healthy lifestyle changes.

KEY CONCEPTS

1. Understand the role of nutrition in exercise and sport.

Good nutrition can improve exercise performance, decrease recovery time from strenuous exercise, prevent exercise injuries due to fatigue, provide the fluid and fuel required during times of high-intensity training, and help maintain an appropriate body weight and composition for one's sport. Optimal energy, fluid, and nutrient intakes also help keep athletes healthy, which in turn helps them perform their best in training and competition. Finally, combining good nutrition with exercise can help reduce the risk of chronic diseases such as diabetes, cardiovascular disease, hypertension, obesity, osteoporosis, and some cancers.

2. Identify the essential nutrients and the dietary recommendations for these nutrients.

Food constituents that prevent disease or health problems are classified as essential nutrients, while nonessential nutrients are those that can be deleted from the diet without adverse effects on growth or health. The RDAs and the DRIs are dietary guidelines that help determine the amount of an essential nutrient required for good health.

3. Describe the various methods used in evaluating the diets of active individuals.

Both the United States and Canada have developed dietary guidelines for healthy eating. These guidelines provide advice about food choices that promote health, decrease the risk of chronic disease, meet nutrient requirements, and support active lives. The U.S. Food Guide Pyramid and Canada's Good Guide for Healthy Living were developed to help translate these guidelines into everyday eating behaviors. These tools allow individuals to monitor their food selections to improve overall nutrient intakes.

4. Discuss the role of nutrition and exercise in the prevention of disease.

The roles of nutrients and exercise in disease prevention are well documented in scientific literature. Appropriate levels of exercise combined with a healthy diet can help reduce the risk of coronary heart disease, stroke, hypertension, diabetes, osteoporosis, and cancer, and help maintain a healthy body weight and composition throughout life. Diet and exercise affect these diseases by lowering blood pressure, improving blood lipid profiles, improving blood glucose and insulin levels, improving cardiac function, improving bone mineral density, and helping to maintain a healthy body weight. Physical activity also helps maintain muscular strength, endurance, and flexibility—which in turn help preserve independence in older adults.

KEY TERMS

Adequate Intake
conditional essentiality
desirable or beneficial for health
Dietary Guidelines
Dietary Reference Intake (DRI)
essential/indispensable nutrient

Estimated Average Requirement (EAR)
Food Guide Pyramid
Healthy People 2000
nonessential/dispensable nutrient
Recommended Dietary Allowance (RDA)
Tolerable Upper Intake Level (UL)

References

Achterberg C. A perspective: challenges of teaching the dietary guidelines graphic. Food & Nutrition News 1992;64:23-6.

Bialostosky K, St. Jeor ST. The 1995 Dietary Guidelines for Americans. Nutr Today 1996;31:6-11.

Canada's Food Guide to Healthy Eating. Ottawa: Minister of Supply and Services Canada, 1992.

Crane NT, Hubbard VS, Lewis CJ. National nutrition objectives and the Dietary Guidelines for Americans. Nutr Today 1998;33:49-58.

Cronin FJ. Reflections on food guides and guidance systems. Nutr Today 1998;33:186-8.

Crotty P. The Mediterranean diet as a food guide. Nutr Today 1998a;33:227-32.

Crotty P. Point/counterpoint: Response to K. Dun Gifford. Nutr Today 1998b;33:224-45.

Food and Nutrition Board, Institute of Medicine. Recommended Dietary Allowances, 10th ed. Washington, DC: National Academy Press, 1989.

Food and Nutrition Board, Institute of Medicine. Dietary Reference Intakes: Calcium, phosphorus, magnesium, vitamin D, and fluoride. Washington, DC: National Academy Press, 1998a.

Food and Nutrition Board, Institute of Medicine. Dietary Reference Intakes: Thiamin, riboflavin, niacin, vitamin B-6, folate, vitamin B-12, pantothenic acid, biotin, and choline. Washington, DC: National Academy Press, 1998b.

Gifford D. The Mediterranean diet as a food guide: the problem of culture and history. Nutr Today 1998;33:233-43.

Harper AE. Defining the essentiality of nutrients. In: Shils ME, Olson JA, Shike M, Ross AC, eds. Modern Nutrition in Health and

Disease. Baltimore, MD: Williams & Wilkins, 1999:3-10.

Health and Welfare Canada. Nutrition Recommendations....A Call for Action: Summary Report of the Scientific Review Committee and the Communications/Implementation Committee. Ottawa: Minister of Supply and Services Canada, 1989.

Houtkooper L. Winning sports nutrition training manual. Tucson: University of Arizona Cooperative Extension, 1994.

International Food Information Council (IFIC) Foundation. Nutrient Requirements Get a Makeover: The Evolution of the Recommended Dietary Allowances. Food Insight, 1998.

Kennedy E. Building on the pyramid—where do we go from here? Nutr Today 1998;33:183-5.

Kennedy E, Meyers L, Layden W. The 1995 Dietary Guidelines for Americans: an overview. J Am Diet Assoc 1996;96:234-7.

Nestle M. In defence of the USDA Food Guide Pyramid. Nutr Today 1998;33:189-97.

Pate RR, Pratt M, Blair SN, et al. Physical Activity and Public Health. A Recommendation from the Centers for Disease Control and Prevention and the American College of Sports Medicine. JAMA 1995;273:402-7.

Rudman D, Feller A. Evidence for deficiencies of conditionally essential nutrients during total parenteral nutrition. J Am Coll Nutr 1986;5:101-6.

United States Department of Agriculture (USDA). The Food Guide Pyramid. Washington, DC: Human Nutrition Information Service, Home and Garden Bulletin Number 252, 1992.

Welsh S, Davis C, Shaw A. Development of the Food Guide Pyramid. Nutr Today 1992;Nov/Dec:12-23.

Wilson CS. Mediterranean diets: once and future? Nutr Today 1998;33:246-9.

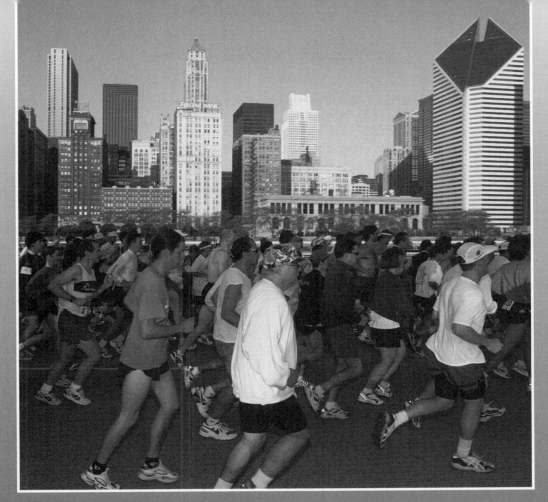

CHAPTER 2

Carbohydrate As a Fuel for Exercise

After reading this chapter you will be able to

- describe the function, classification, and dietary sources of carbohydrate;
- discuss carbohydrate metabolism during exercise;
- discuss carbohydrate reserves and dietary intake;
- describe recommendations for carbohydrate feeding before exercise;
- describe recommendations for carbohydrate feeding during exercise;
- describe carbohydrate feeding recommendations for post-exercise and during training periods; and
- explain the concept of muscle glycogen supercompensation.

It is common knowledge that carbohydrate is important for athletic performance. High levels of stored glycogen before endurance exercise can decrease the risk of fatigue during the exercise. Carbohydrate intake during exercise can increase performance and further prolong the time to fatigue. After exercise, diets high in carbohydrate help replenish muscle glycogen levels. For active people, it appears prudent to consume a diet high in carbohydrates. Unfortunately, many athletes and active people consume inadequate levels of carbohydrate. Optimum dietary carbohydrate levels depend on total energy intake; body size; health status; and the duration, intensity, and type of exercise in which an individual participates.

Function, Classification, and Dietary Sources of Carbohydrate

Carbohydrates are a primary source of energy, and they provide the substrate (glucose) necessary for glycogen replacement. Consumed during exercise, they help maintain blood glucose levels and prevent premature fatigue. Athletes in training are encouraged to eat high-carbohydrate diets (60-65% of energy from carbohydrate) and use carbohydrate-containing sport drinks during periods of heavy exercise training.

We can classify dietary carbohydrates in a number of ways—according to the type of carbohydrate in the food, the level of commercial processing it has undergone, or the blood glucose or glycemic responses to the carbohydrate within the body. Carbohydrate-containing foods comprising long complex chains of sugars linked together are frequently termed **complex carbohydrates.** Nutritionists often use the term "complex carbohydrate" for carbohydrate-containing foods such as fruits, vegetables, whole grains (breads, cereals, pasta), and legumes (beans, peas, lentils) because they are a good source of vitamins, minerals, and fiber. The dominant digestible carbohydrate in these foods is starch, except for fruits that contain primarily simple sugars. Carbohydrates from processed foods (sweetened cereals, breakfast bars) or foods high in sugar (candy, sodas, desserts) are frequently termed **simple carbohydrates**. These foods contain primarily glucose, sucrose, fructose, and high-fructose corn syrup,

and are generally low in vitamins, minerals, and fiber, unless they are fortified.

In general, complex carbohydrates have a more complex chemical structure, are less processed, and contain more nutrients and fiber than simple carbohydrates. Although this classification of carbohydrates (complex versus simple) was previously used to describe the body's glycemic response to these carbohydrates, this categorization is no longer appropriate. Research now shows that the glycemic responses to both simple and complex carbohydrate foods can vary greatly, and that some complex carbohydrates (i.e., foods high in starch) can be hydrolyzed and absorbed as quickly as simple sugars (Cummings and Englyst 1995; Foster-Powell and Miller 1995).

As table 2.1 indicates, we can now classify foods as producing a high, moderate, or low glycemic response. Foods that produce a high glycemic response—a large and rapid rise in blood glucose and insulin—increase muscle glycogen more than foods that produce a low glycemic response. See "Calculating the Glycemic Index of a Food," page 24, for more information.

Table 2.2 outlines the primary carbohydrates found in our diet. Foods generally classified as simple carbohydrates are made up of mono-, di-, and oligosaccharides, while foods generally classified as complex carbohydrates are made up of starch and fiber (e.g., grains, cereals, and legumes). Most of these carbohydrates occur naturally in foods, while others, such as high-fructose corn syrup, are produced commercially and used as sweeteners in processed foods.

The various types of dietary carbohydrate listed in table 2.2 should not be confused with low-calorie sweeteners, which do not add significant amounts of energy or carbohydrate to the diet, and are used solely to enhance flavor. Artificial sweeteners are found in a number of foods marketed as reduced-calorie or reduced-fat. Appendix B.1 describes the most common low-calorie sweeteners used in the United States. Some of these sweeteners, such as sorbitol and xylitol, can cause gastrointestinal distress if used in large quantities. Some people may need to avoid these sweeteners.

Carbohydrate Metabolism During Exercise

Muscles require carbohydrate as a fuel source during exercise. The amount of carbohydrate

Table 2.1   The Glycemic Index (GI) of Some Common Foods*

High glycemic index foods (GI > 85)

Angel food cake	Croissant	Muffins	Melba toast
Cake doughnut	Soft drinks	Waffles	Cheese pizza
Bagel, white	Barley flour bread	White bread	Rye flour bread
Whole wheat bread	Cheerios	Corn bran cereal	Corn Chex cereal
Cornflakes	Cream of wheat	Crispix cereal	Grape-nuts
Raisins	Mueslix	Rice Krispies	Shredded Wheat
Cornmeal	Millet	Ice cream	Brown rice
Rice cakes	Soda crackers	Oatmeal	Total cereal
Couscous	Watermelon	Potatoes	Hard candy
Sucrose	Carrots	Glucose	Maltose
Corn chips	Honey/syrups	Sport drinks	Molasses

Moderate glycemic index foods (GI = 60-85)

Sponge cake	Pastry	Popcorn	Oat bran bread
Rye kernel bread	Pita bread, white	Bulgur bread	Mixed grain bread
All-Bran cereal	Bran Chex cereal	Oat bran cereal	Special K cereal
Cracked barley	Buckwheat	Bulgur	Sweet corn
White rice (long-grain)	Basmati rice	Parboiled rice	Wild rice
Sweet potato/yams	Wheat, cooked	Ice cream, low-fat	Banana
Fruit cocktail	Grapefruit juice	Grapes	Kiwi fruit
Mango/papaya	Orange (whole/juice)	Durum spaghetti	Linguine

Low glycemic index foods (GI < 60)

Barley kernel bread	Barley	Rice bran	Wheat kernels
Milk (whole/skim)	Yogurt (all types)	Apples	Apricots (dried)
Cherries	Grapefruit	Peaches (fresh)	Pears (fresh)
Plums	Beans (all types)	Lentils	Dried peas
Spaghetti	Peanuts	Tomato soup	Fructose

*White bread (50 g) was used as the reference food and has a GI = 100.

Reprinted from Foster-Powell and Brand Miller 1995.

Table 2.2   Primary Carbohydrates and Sugars in the Diet

Monosaccharides (glucose, fructose, galactose) are the simplest forms of sugar.

- Glucose—The main carbohydrate in the blood; the substrate used to make the glycogen stored in the liver, muscles, and other organs; the main carbohydrate energy source in the cell.
- Fructose—The simple sugar found primarily in fruit and honey. Sweeter than common table sugar (sucrose).
- Galactose—The simple sugar found in milk.

Disaccharides (sucrose, lactose, and maltose) are sugars made up of two simple sugars.

- Sucrose—Common table sugar, made up of one glucose and one fructose unit. Extracted from sugar cane and beet sugar. The most common disaccharide in our diet.
- Lactose—Sugar found in milk products, made up of one glucose and one galactose unit. Many adults, especially Asians, Native Americans, Hispanics, and Blacks, cannot digest this sugar and are termed lactose intolerant.
- Maltose—Sugar made up of two glucose units. Made from the breakdown of starch.

(continued)

Table 2.2   (continued)

Oligosaccharides are short chains of 3-10 monosaccharides linked together.

- Maltodextrins—A glucose polymer manufactured by breaking long starch units into smaller groups. Found frequently in sport drinks and many processed foods.
- Corn syrup—A sweet syrup made up of glucose and short-chain glucose polymers, produced by enzymatic hydrolysis of corn starch.
- High-fructose corn syrup (HFCS)—An especially sweet corn syrup in which 45-55% of the corn syrup's carbohydrate is enzymatically hydrolyzed to the simple sugars, glucose and fructose. HFCS is less viscous than traditional corn syrup, yet has nearly twice the concentration of mono- and disaccharides than regular corn syrup. Currently the predominant sweetener found in commercially sweetened foods.

Polysaccharides are foods that contain starch and fiber. These foods are often called complex carbohydrates.

- Starch—Found in plants, seeds, and roots. Made up of straight chains of glucose polymers called amylose and some branching chain polymers called amylopectin. When complex carbohydrates (composed primarily of starch and fiber) are digested, they yield glucose and fiber. The extent of starch digestion in the small intestine is variable; some starch escapes digestion in the small intestine and enters the colon.
- Dietary fiber—A part of the plant that cannot be digested by human gut enzymes. Dietary fiber passes through the small intestine to the colon, where it is expelled as fecal material or fermented and used as a food source for gut bacteria. Thus, some fibers are broken down in the colon. Diets high in fiber generally increase the amounts of fecal material and of flatulence.

■ HIGHLIGHT ■

Calculating the Glycemic Index of a Food

The term **glycemic response** refers to the body's increase in blood glucose and insulin after consuming a given food or combination of foods. The glycemic response is determined by measuring the area under the glucose curve using sophisticated computer software. The greater the blood glucose response to a particular carbohydrate food, the greater the area under the glucose response curve. For example, what would be the glucose response to feeding an individual two very different carbohydrates such as white bread or lentils? Because blood sugar rises higher and stays elevated longer with white bread compared to lentils, white bread is said to produce a greater glycemic response. To standardize the glycemic response between individuals, researchers have categorized foods using the glycemic index. The **glycemic index** is determined for any particular food or combination of foods by feeding 50 g of the food and determining the blood glucose response over a 2-h period. The glycemic index is then calculated using the following formula (Burke et al. 1999):

Glycemic index (GI) =
[(blood glucose area of test food)/(blood glucose area of reference food)] × 100

In the example here, GI = (blood glucose area, lentils)/(blood glucose area, white bread) × 100.

The reference food is typically white bread and has a glycemic index of 100, although sometimes glucose is used as the reference food (glycemic index = 100). Table 2.1 gives common foods and their glycemic index values. The glycemic index of a meal or of a total diet can be calculated from the weighted means of the glycemic index values for the component foods of the meal or diet (Wolever et al. 1991). The weighting is based on the proportion of the total carbohydrate provided by each food within the meal. Thus, if a food represents 60% of the carbohydrate consumed in the meal, the contribution of this food to the total glycemic index of the meal is the food glycemic index multiplied by 60%. After this calculation is done for each carbohydrate-containing food in the meal, the values are added to give a total meal glycemic index.

required depends on the frequency, intensity, and duration of the exercise and on the individual's fitness level. Figure 2.1 illustrates how carbohydrate use changes with exercise intensity. The carbohydrate used during exercise can come from any of the following sources:

- Endogenous production of glucose by the liver (gluconeogenesis)
- Blood glucose
- Muscle and liver glycogen stores
- Carbohydrate consumed during exercise

The amount of gluconeogenesis that occurs during exercise depends on the available carbohydrate reserves before exercise begins, the amount of carbohydrate provided during exercise, and the duration and intensity of the exercise bout. Thus the total amount of carbohydrate used during exercise (as well as the source of this carbohydrate) depends on a number of factors, some of which can be manipulated with exogenous carbohydrate intake either before or during exercise.

Endogenous Glucose Production During Exercise

The substrates for **gluconeogenesis** during exercise are lactate, alanine, glycerol, and pyruvate. In general, these substrates come primarily from the muscle, with small amounts of glycerol coming from adipose cells. These substrates are transported to the liver for glucose production. Figure 2.2 reviews the gluconeogenic pathway.

The primary source of lactate during exercise is from the metabolism of glucose to lactate, through glycolysis, in both the working and nonworking muscle. (See figures 2.3 and 2.4 for a quick review of intermediate metabolism and **glycolysis**.) The lactate is transported to the liver for glucose production through the **Cori cycle** (figure 2.5, page 29), or it may be used directly by adjoining cells as an energy source. As glycogen depletes in the working muscle, the nonworking muscles can give up some of their stored carbohydrate by releasing lactate. This phenomenon was first demonstrated in humans by Ahlborg and Felig (1982). They showed that

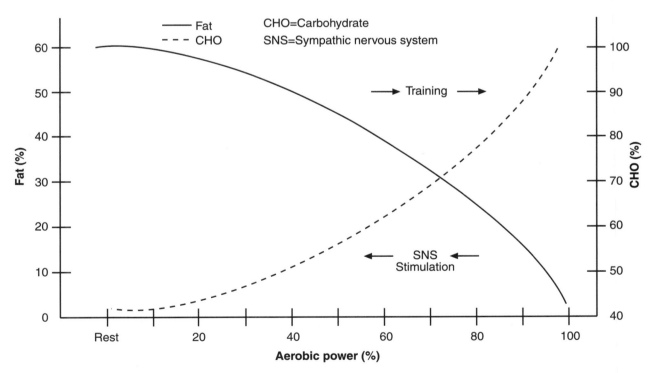

Figure 2.1 The crossover concept of fuel use during exercise. At low- to moderate-intensity exercise, CHO and lipids both play major roles as energy substrates. However, when relative aerobic power output reaches 60-65%, then CHO becomes increasingly important and lipids become less important. Because of the crossover phenomenon, in most athletic activities glycogen stores provide the greatest fuel for exercise. Lipids become important energy sources during recovery.

Reprinted from Brooks and Mercier 1994.

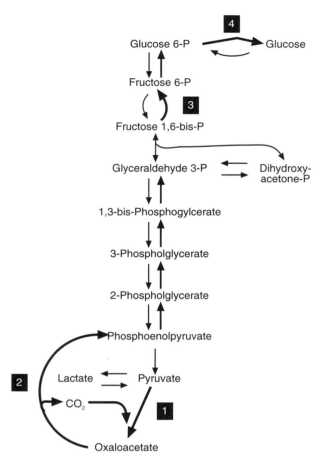

Figure 2.2 Gluconeogenesis pathway shown as part of the essential pathways of energy metabolism. Numbered reactions are unique to gluconeogenesis.

Reprinted from Champe and Harvey 1994.

lactate release from the arms increased both during and after 3.0-3.5 h of leg exercise (cycling), providing substrate for gluconeogenesis.

A second major gluconeogenic precursor is alanine. Alanine is the primary amino acid released by working muscle during exercise. The rate of alanine appearance can increase 60-96% after 40 min of strenuous exercise (Felig and Wahren 1971). It is synthesized by combining nitrogen (released from the breakdown of amino acids in the muscles) with pyruvate (see chapter 4). Alanine is transported to the liver where it is broken back down into pyruvate and nitrogen. This pathway is called the **glucose-alanine cycle** (figure 2.6, page 29). The pyruvate can be used as a gluconeogenic substrate, while the nitrogen is converted into urea and eliminated through the kidneys.

The third gluconeogenic precursor the liver uses is glycerol, the three-carbon backbone of triglyceride (also called triacylglycerols). When adipose tissue or muscle triglycerides are broken down, they yield three fatty acids and glycerol (see chapter 3). The fatty acids from the adipose tissue can be transported to the muscles for energy production, but glycerol is transported to the liver for gluconeogenesis. Finally, some pyruvate leaks from the working cells into the blood and is transported to the liver. Like glycerol, this three-carbon compound can be used by the liver to make glucose.

During prolonged exercise, gluconeogenesis is a major source of glucose for the working muscles. Ahlborg and Felig (1982) estimated that after 3 h of endurance exercise (58% $\dot{V}O_2$ max), the uptake of lactate, pyruvate, and glycerol by the liver accounts for 60% of the glucose output.

The amount of lactate coming from working muscle during prolonged exercise decreases as muscle glycogen is depleted. The body then must rely on lactate from nonworking muscles and from amino acid metabolism to make glucose (Ahlborg 1985; Ahlborg and Felig 1982). Thus, *an increase in gluconeogenesis late in exercise requires that the body use amino acids from the breakdown of protein as an energy substrate.* The amount of protein used for energy during exercise depends on a number of factors, including the amount of carbohydrate stores available at the beginning of exercise, whether exogenous carbohydrate is provided during exercise, and the intensity and duration of the exercise bout (see chapter 4).

Another source of blood glucose during exercise is the breakdown of liver glycogen (liver glycogenolysis). **Glycogenolysis** is the chemical process by which glucose is freed from glycogen. Unlike with muscle glycogen, glucose from liver glycogen can be released directly into the blood stream, thus helping to maintain blood glucose levels during exercise. As with muscle glycogen, however, liver glycogen can become depleted if exercise is strenuous and of long duration. As both liver and muscle glycogen become depleted, blood glucose levels fall, and the body must rely on gluconeogenesis to maintain blood glucose levels.

Hormonal Control of Carbohydrate Metabolism During Exercise

During exercise a number of hormonal changes occur that signal the body to break down stored energy for fuel, which can then be used by the working muscles for energy. Table 2.3 (page 30)

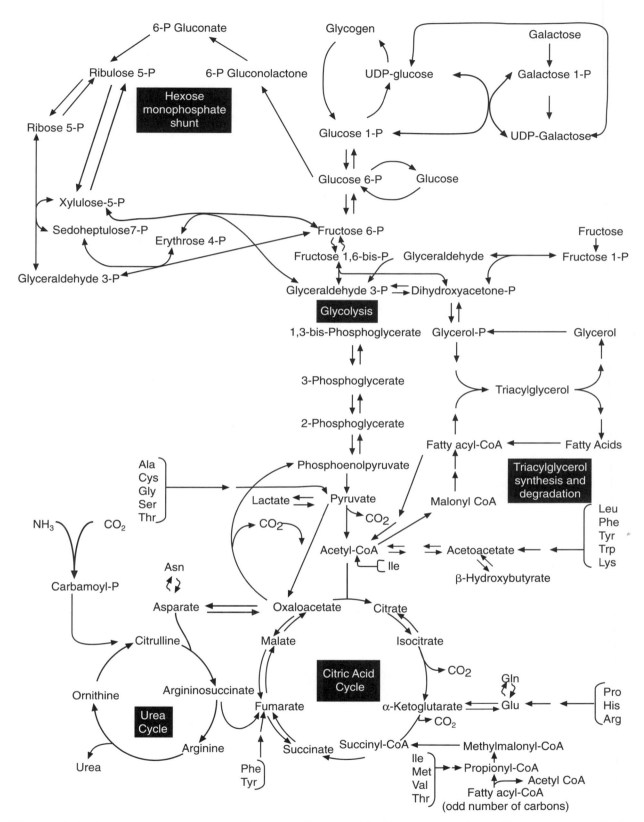

Figure 2.3 Important reactions of intermediary metabolism. Curved reaction arrows indicate forward and reverse reactions, which are catalyzed by different enzymes.

Reproduced from Champe and Harvey 1994.

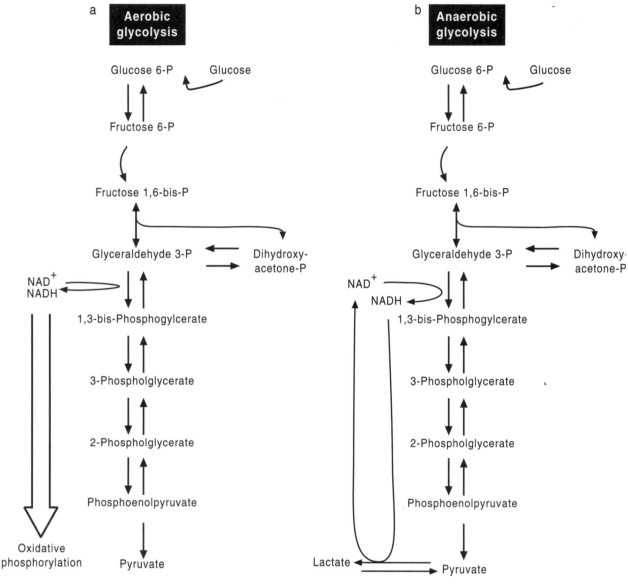

Figure 2.4 *(a)* Reactions of aerobic glycolysis. *(b)* Reactions of anaerobic glycolysis. Reproduced from Champe and Harvey 1994.

outlines these hormonal responses, which depend on a variety of factors including the intensity and duration of the exercise and the individual's level of physical fitness. Thus, trained individuals may have different responses than untrained individuals.

Blood levels of norepinephrine and epinephrine rise dramatically within seconds of the initiation of exercise (table 2.4). These hormones stimulate the breakdown of stored fat (in both adipose and muscle tissue) and carbohydrate (both liver and muscle glycogen), making these fuels available to the working muscles. Insulin levels decrease or are main-

tained at a low concentration during exercise, while glucagon levels increase. Glucagon, released from the pancreas in response to the low blood glucose levels that may occur with exercise, is a potent stimulator of glycogenolysis and gluconeogenesis. Both of these metabolic processes help maintain blood glucose levels by increasing the release of glucose into the blood. Exercise also increases the sensitivity of the skeletal muscle to the action of insulin. Finally, exercise has an "insulin-like" effect on the muscle, increasing the uptake of glucose without the need for insulin (Brooks et al. 1995). Thus, adequate glucose can be delivered to the

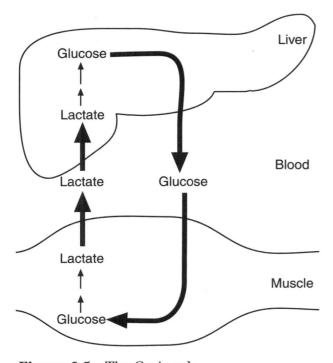

Figure 2.5 The Cori cycle.
Reprinted from Champe and Harvey 1994.

muscle in spite of the lower blood insulin levels usually observed during exercise.

All of these hormonal changes create an optimal environment for the breakdown and oxidation of both fat and carbohydrate for energy during exercise. In many ways, the acute hormonal response to exercise is similar to that seen in fasting. In both exercise and fasting, the body must provide energy to working muscles from the body's energy reserves: body energy reserves must be broken down and provided to cells and tissues that require energy.

Carbohydrate Reserves and Dietary Intake

During exercise the primary sources of energy are carbohydrate (glucose) and fat (fatty acids). The relative amounts of each of these substrates used depend on exercise intensity and

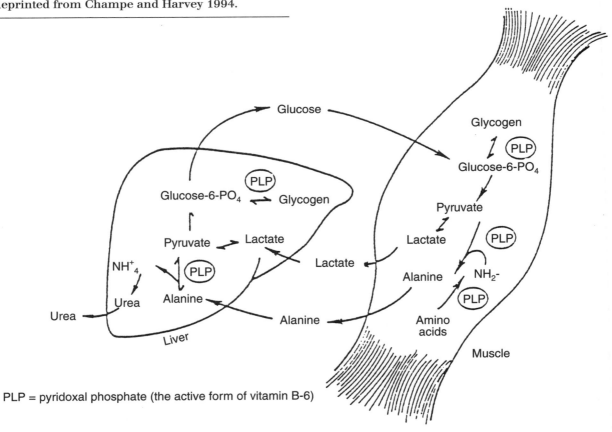

PLP = pyridoxal phosphate (the active form of vitamin B-6)

Figure 2.6 The glucose-alanine cycle and the involvement of vitamin B_6 (PLP) in glucose and alanine metabolism.
Reprinted from Leklem 1985.

Table 2.3 **Effect of Various Hormones on Fuel Production During Exercise**

Cortisol—Produced in the adrenal cortex. Stimulates gluconeogenesis and helps to mobilize free fatty acids and amino acids.

Epinephrine—Produced mainly by the adrenal medulla. Affects target tissues by increasing cyclic AMP concentrations in the cells. Promotes glycogenolysis in the muscle and liver, activates lipolysis in adipose tissue, and raises blood glucose concentrations and fatty acid levels.

Norepinephrine—Produced in sympathetic nerves and released in response to nerve stimulation, acting as a neurotransmitter. Also found in the adrenal medulla. Stimulates the breakdown of stored fat and glucose for energy; produces metabolic effects on peripheral tissues similar to those evoked by epinephrine.

Glucagon—Secreted by α-cells of the pancreas. Responds to low levels of blood glucose by activating cyclic AMP in the liver, stimulating both gluconeogenesis and glycogenolysis.

Insulin—Secreted by β-cells of the islets of Langerhans in the pancreas. Enhances uptake of glucose by peripheral tissues and helps maintain blood glucose within normal limits (80-120 mg/dL). Also increases the synthesis of glycogen from glucose, decreases gluconeogenesis, and promotes lipogenesis in fat cells. Thus, insulin acts as an anabolic hormone. During exercise, insulin levels are low because the body needs fuel to be released, not stored.

Table 2.4 **Hormonal Changes That Stimulate the Breakdown of Stored Energy During Exercise**

Increased with exercise	Decreased with exercise
cortisol	insulin
epinephrine	
norepinephrine	
glucagon	

duration (see figure 2.1, page 25). *Compared to protein and fat stores, the body's carbohydrate reserves are severely limited—the total amount of energy stored as glycogen ranges from 800-2000 kcal,* depending not only on diet and on the size and the fitness level of the individual, but also on the time of day. Dietary recommendations for active people usually focus on making sure the diet is adequate in carbohydrate to replace these limited and easily depleted reserves. Carbohydrate may also be consumed during exercise to supplement these reserves.

Muscle and Liver Glycogen

The body's carbohydrate reserves are primarily in liver and muscle glycogen. **Glycogen** concentrations are highest in the liver—the amount in the typical liver (about 1.5 kg) after an overnight fast is ~4% of the liver's total weight, or 60 g. After a meal, the amount of glycogen can double to ~8% of the liver's weight, or 120 g (Flatt 1995). Thus, the amount of carbohydrate stored in the liver ranges from 60-120 g (250-500 kcal), depending on the time of day and the amount of carbohydrate in the last meal consumed. Liver glycogen plays a major role in maintaining blood glucose levels throughout the night. A morning meal helps replenish glycogen stores.

The amount of carbohydrate stored in muscle is lower than that in the liver and requires deliberate carbohydrate loading to increase the amount to more than 2% of muscle weight. Since muscle typically accounts for 20-30% of total body weight, the absolute amount of glycogen stored in the muscle can range from roughly 200-500 g (800-2000 kcal) in a person weighing 154 lb (70 kg). Muscle glycogen levels can be dramatically increased under certain conditions, however, such as by eating a high-carbohydrate meal after exercise has depleted the stores of muscle glycogen (see "Muscle Glycogen Supercompensation," page 53).

The body's total glycogen reserve (that found in liver, muscle, and other organs) is not much greater than the amount of carbohydrate usually consumed each day (Flatt 1995). For people consuming 2000 kcal/d with 50% of the energy coming from carbohydrate, this represents approximately 250 g of carbohydrate. Maintenance of glycogen stores within a desirable range requires that the body balance carbohydrate oxidation to carbohydrate intake (Flatt 1995). After a typical meal, about one-fourth to one-third of the carbohydrate consumed is converted to liver glycogen; about one-third to one-half is converted to muscle glycogen; and the remainder is oxidized for energy in the hours after eating (Flatt 1995).

Use of muscle glycogen during exercise depends primarily on the intensity of an exercise bout, with more glycogen used at higher intensities (see figure 2.1, page 25). For example, the rate of glycogen breakdown is 0.7, 1.4, and 3.4 mmol/kg/min at 50%, 75%, and 100% of $\dot{V}O_2$max, respectively (Sherman 1995). Higher-intensity exercises use muscle glycogen more quickly, since the availability of fat for fuel is limited. In exercise events lasting greater than 90 min at intensities of 65-85% $\dot{V}O_2$max, fatigue usually occurs concurrently with the depletion of glycogen stores. *The time to fatigue is directly related to initial glycogen levels.* Thus, a person with higher glycogen stores at the beginning of an endurance event will fatigue later than someone who begins the event with poor glycogen stores, assuming that other factors affecting carbohydrate use are equal. The pattern of muscle glycogen use during exercise appears to be curvilinear—the highest rate of glycogenolysis occurs during the first 20-30 min of an exercise bout lasting 60 min at an intensity of 75% $\dot{V}O_2$max (Sherman 1995). Remember, however, that muscle glycogen depletion is not the only factor involved with the onset of fatigue during exercise. Other physiological, psychological, and environmental factors also have significant effects.

Dietary Carbohydrate Intakes of Active Individuals

Active men and women usually report carbohydrate intakes similar to those of weight-matched, inactive individuals: 45-55% of total energy generally comes from carbohydrate (~5 g/kg body weight/d) (Hawley et al. 1995). For recreational or fitness athletes, these intakes may be adequate to meet the carbohydrate demands of moderate exercise for less than 1 h per day. These carbohydrate intake levels may be too low, however, for endurance athletes engaging in daily intense training, where glycogen stores need to be replenished rapidly.

If intake of energy is reduced for any reason, carbohydrate intake may be dramatically reduced (e.g., when energy intake is restricted for weight loss). For active women, energy intakes less than 1800-1900 kcal/d provide carbohydrates below recommended levels (Manore 1996); these low carbohydrate intakes are not adequate to replenish the glycogen used during endurance exercise. Active females require at least 5 g of carbohydrate/kg body weight to maintain glycogen stores (O'Keeffe et al. 1989). During intense (≥90 min/d) daily training, the carbohydrate needs may be 8-10 g of carbohydrate/kg body weight for men and 6-8 g/kg for women. Of course, if activity increases, energy intake usually increases also, allowing more carbohydrate to be consumed.

Carbohydrate Feeding Before Exercise

Most trainers and sport nutritionists recommend that athletes consume a high-carbohydrate diet during periods of intense training, including the days before an exercise competition. While these recommendations differ little from those for the general population (58-60% of energy from carbohydrate), many athletes want dietary and carbohydrate recommendations specific for the day of competition and for the hours immediately before competition.

Pre-Exercise and Between-Competition Meals

The goals of a pre-exercise meal, or of any food consumed just before competition, are to promote additional glycogen synthesis, to supply the body with glucose for use during exercise, and to minimize fatigue during exercise. Many active individuals and athletes frequently compete or train after an overnight fast. This fast lowers liver glycogen levels since the liver provides glucose to the body during the sleeping hours. The pre-exercise meal helps replenish liver glycogen and provides the body with additional carbohydrate to help prevent or delay the onset of fatigue during exercise. Consumption of carbohydrate before exercise can indeed improve performance, especially for individuals who have eaten poorly the 24 h before competition.

Athletes usually consume their pre-exercise meal 2 to 6 h before the exercise event; yet in many cases it can be safely eaten as late as 1 h before exercise. The meal should be small, easy to digest, and familiar to the individual; it should contain foods that do not cause gastrointestinal distress; and it should provide carbohydrate to improve glycogen reserves and blood glucose. For these reasons the pre-exercise meal is usually high in carbohydrate (~200-300 g), moderate in protein, low in fat and fiber, and moderate in size. Although it takes approximately 4-6 h to digest a meal consumed on an empty stomach and for blood hormone levels to return to baseline, current research reveals no reason for individuals to fast this long before an exercise event. There is no evidence that blood glucose and hormone levels need to return to baseline levels before exercise begins. Individuals differ in the volume of food they want in their stomachs during competition. Athletes engaging in early morning competitions may want to schedule a very early morning (2:30-4:30 A.M.) snack or carbohydrate beverage instead of eating immediately before competition. The timing and amount of food consumed depend on individual preferences and on the type, intensity, and duration of the sport.

Nervousness before an exercise event can cause gastrointestinal distress and loss of appetite. If athletes are too nervous to consume a meal before competition, they can use fruit juices, sport drinks, or glycogen replacement products to provide the energy and carbohydrate needed.

Athletes sometimes must perform more than one exercise event within a 24 h period. The type of food or drink provided in these situations depends on the athlete's preferences, the type of event, and the amount of time between events. If the time is short, water, fruit juices, or sport drinks are most appropriate—they provide the fluid and carbohydrate required to prepare the body for the next exercise bout, while being rapidly absorbed from the gut without having to be digested. People with longer times (1-4 h) between events can consume small meals similar to the pre-event meal (see "Key Points to Remember When Feeding Athletes Before Competition" [below] and "Practical Dietary Guidelines for Pre-Exercise or Between-Competition Meals" [page 34]).

Effects of Pre-Exercise Feedings on Performance and Fatigue

Research examining the effects of feeding carbohydrate before exercise usually focuses on the following questions: Can the pre-exercise meal enhance exercise performance? Can active individuals eat within 30-60 min before exercise without impairing athletic performance?

There is increasing evidence that a high-carbohydrate pre-exercise meal 3-4 h before exercise can improve performance. If this meal is then combined with carbohydrate intake during exercise, the performance improvements are even greater. Wright et al. (1991) fed either no carbohydrate (controls), a pre-exercise carbohydrate meal (3 h before exercise), carbohydrate during exercise, or a combination of carbohydrate feedings before and during exercise to well-trained male cyclists who exercised at 70% $\dot{V}O_2$max to exhaustion. Subjects also completed performance and work production tests. The pre-exercise meal averaged 333 g of carbohydrate (5 g carbohydrate/kg body weight), and

■ HIGHLIGHT ■

Key Points to Remember When Feeding Athletes Before Competition

- The meal usually should be consumed 2-6 h before competition, depending on the athlete and the time of day the competition occurs.
- The meal should be high in carbohydrate, moderate in protein, and low in fat and fiber. The carbohydrate promotes additional glycogen synthesis before the competition, while lower fat and fiber content help prevent gastrointestinal (GI) distress.
- The meal should be easy to digest, familiar to the athlete, and should not contain foods that cause GI distress.
- If an athlete is too nervous to eat before competition, experiment with high-carbohydrate products that are easy to digest—such as juice, sport drinks, meal replacement products, or glycogen replacement beverages.

an 8% carbohydrate solution was provided during exercise, providing a total of 175 g of carbohydrate. Total work performance during exercise was 19-46% higher when carbohydrate was fed. As compared with the controls, average time to exhaustion was 44% greater when carbohydrate was consumed both before and during exercise, 32% greater when fed during exercise, and 18% higher when fed 3 h before exercise. Neufer et al. (1987) reported a 22% improvement in cycling power when carbohydrate was consumed 4 h before exercise (200 g) plus immediately before exercise (43 g). Sherman et al. (1989) reported a 15% improvement in exercise performance time (8.3 min improvement on cycling performance test) when subjects consumed 312 g of carbohydrate 4 h before exercise. *Thus, feeding active individuals a pre-exercise meal high in carbohydrate extends endurance time to exhaustion and improves work output.* In addition, the pre-exercise meal may be especially helpful for individuals who pay little attention to their diet or who have had a poor diet during the 24 h period before an exercise event.

Carbohydrate Consumption Immediately Before Exercise

Controversy exists over whether carbohydrates eaten immediately before exercise can cause hypoglycemia during exercise. It has been hypothesized that the high blood insulin levels that result from carbohydrate consumption immediately before exercise (~30 min) may cause a decline in blood glucose (**hypoglycemia**) at the onset of exercise, resulting in premature fatigue. Blood glucose decreases because elevated blood insulin levels—due to carbohydrate feeding—stimulate the uptake of glucose by tissues at the same time that exercise causes an uptake of glucose, and the liver output of glucose may be low. Although research indicates that blood glucose declines if carbohydrate is eaten 30 min before exercise, there appears to be no adverse effect of this change on exercise performance—in fact, most people do not perceive a change in their blood glucose levels. Controversy also exists on the effect that changes in blood glucose can have on muscle glycogen levels. A number of studies have now addressed these issues and have found that carbohydrate feeding immediately (30-45 min) before exercise has no adverse effect on performance or perceived exertion. Horowitz and Coyle (1993) fed foods with both moderate

(rice, potatoes + margarine, rice + margarine) and high (potatoes, sucrose, candy bars) glycemic indexes to nine fit males 30 min before a 75-85 min exercise bout. Although blood glucose levels significantly declined with all foods after 20 min of moderate-intensity exercise (60% $\dot{V}O_2max$), the subjects completed each trial without adverse effects, and ratings of perceived exertion were similar among the trials. Other researchers (Alberici et al. 1993; Devlin et al. 1986; Neufer et al. 1987) also have found either no difference or improved performance in treatment groups fed carbohydrate immediately before exercise compared with the control groups. Feeding carbohydrate immediately before exercise appears to have little adverse effect on performance and may even enhance performance in some cases. Carbohydrate fed before exercise is most likely oxidized by the muscle during exercise. This exogenous carbohydrate may be especially beneficial for the people who have low glycogen stores at the beginning of the exercise.

Carbohydrate Feeding During Exercise

It has long been recognized that individuals fatigue when they engage in moderate exercise (60-80% $\dot{V}O_2max$) of long duration (>90 min)—a result, in part, of a decrease in blood glucose and a depletion of muscle and liver glycogen stores. Depletion of these stores requires increased reliance on liver gluconeogenesis to provide the glucose necessary to sustain exercise. Ingestion of exogenous carbohydrate can delay fatigue but cannot prevent it. Researchers hypothesized that exogenous carbohydrates during exercise would spare muscle glycogen, which in turn would increase time to fatigue. Studies examining the effect of exogenous carbohydrate ingestion on muscle glycogen use during exercise have produced mixed results. Some have shown that carbohydrate use during exercise spares muscle glycogen (Erickson et al. 1987; Leatt and Jacobs 1989), while others have not (Bosch et al. 1994; Coyle et al. 1986; Coyle et al. 1991; Fielding et al. 1985; Flynn et al. 1987). However, most studies show an improvement in exercise performance or time to fatigue with carbohydrate ingestion during exercise, regardless of the change in muscle glycogen stores. Studies reporting no muscle

■ HIGHLIGHT ■

Practical Dietary Guidelines for Pre-Exercise or Between-Competition Meals

Feeding competitive or recreational athletes before or during competition requires planning and (sometimes) experimentation. The following guidelines will be helpful:

- Provide foods that are familiar to the athletes and that are high in carbohydrate (~200-300 g), moderate in protein, and relatively moderate in fat and fiber. Avoid foods that may cause gastrointestinal distress (e.g., milk products for lactose-intolerant athletes, acidic fruit juices, highly fortified meal replacement beverages or energy bars).

- Meals should be moderate in size. The exact size of the meal will depend on the size of the athlete, the nature of the sport, and the length of time until exercise. For example, the pre-exercise meal for a football player may provide 1000-2000 kcal, while that for a gymnast may be 400-600 kcal. Most athletes do not like to exercise on a full stomach.

- Many athletes like to use drinks containing caffeine (coffee, tea, cola) before competition. This generally is not a problem as long as the athletes are accustomed to the practice, and the quantity is within the limits allowable under drug testing procedures. The International Olympic Committee allows a maximum caffeine concentration of 12 µg/ml in the urine. To reach this level, one would have to consume ~897-1965 mg of caffeine—equivalent to ~8 cups of coffee (Nehlig and Debry 1994) or 20-45 12-oz cola drinks.

- The type of meal or snack fed between competitions depends primarily on the amount of time available. If the time is short, replace fluids as well as carbohydrates by using a sport drink, glycogen replacement product, or fruit juice. Small, moderate-protein, high-carbohydrate, low-fat meals (sandwiches, bagels, cereal) or snacks (fruit, candy bars, energy or sport bars) are appropriate when more time is available. Smaller adults or children may need to eat small frequent meals between competitions. Athletes should experiment with between-competition meals to find out what works best for them.

- Because many athletes have strong preferences about the types of foods they eat before or during competition, it may be more convenient to pack a cooler with those preferred foods. If packing a cooler is not possible, check with the sponsoring organization to find out what types of foods will be available to the athletes at the competition.

glycogen-sparing effect with exogenous glucose suggest that the observed improvement in exercise performance may be due to a sparing of liver glycogen and the reduced need for gluconeogenesis during exercise. Bosch et al. (1991, 1994) observed a 59% reduction in liver glucose production during prolonged exercise (3 h, 70% $\dot{V}O_2$max) when a 10% carbohydrate drink was ingested. Exogenous carbohydrate intake also helps to maintain blood glucose levels throughout exercise (Coggan and Coyle 1989; Coyle et al. 1986). Exercising muscles rely heavily on blood glucose for energy late in exercise—thus, carbohydrate ingestion during exercise may complement the body's muscle glycogen rather

than replacing it (Tsintzas et al. 1996). The consumption of carbohydrate during exercise should help maintain blood glucose levels and ensure that the muscles have adequate glucose when muscle glycogen sources are low or depleted.

Figure 2.7 illustrates changes in energy substrate use by working muscles during moderate exercise (65-75% $\dot{V}O_2$max) lasting 4 h. The subjects in this study were endurance-trained males who had fasted overnight before the exercise performance test. This figure shows that, as muscle glycogen levels decline, the muscles increasingly rely on blood glucose for carbohydrate—by the end of 4 h of exercise, about half of the energy required to sustain exercise is

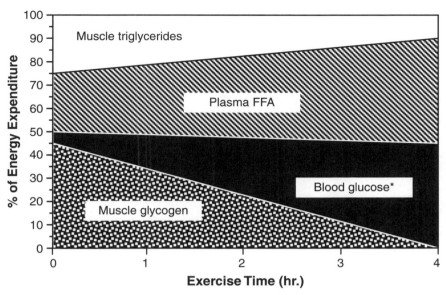

Figure 2.7 Percentage of energy derived from the four major substrates during prolonged exercise at 65-75% of maximal oxygen uptake. Initially, approximately one-half of the energy is derived each from carbohydrate and fat. As muscle glycogen concentration declines, blood glucose becomes an increasingly important source of carbohydrate energy for muscle. *After 2 h exercise, carbohydrate ingestion is needed to maintain blood glucose concentrations and carbohydrate oxidation. FFA = free fatty acids.

Reprinted from Coyle 1995.

coming from blood glucose. This glucose must be provided by the liver, via gluconeogenesis, or from an exogenous carbohydrate source.

Carbohydrate Feeding During Exercise Prevents Hypoglycemia

For some individuals, exhaustive exercise (60-75% $\dot{V}O_2$max for 2.5-3.5 h) without exogenous carbohydrate intake can result in hypoglycemia, a condition where blood glucose levels decrease to less than 45 mg/dL (<2.5 mmol/L). Some people may experience light-headedness, dizziness, inability to concentrate, nausea, irritability, and fatigue. Coyle et al. (1986) found that hypoglycemia leads to a decline in total body glucose oxidation and eventually to exhaustion (see figure 2.8). In this study, as plasma glucose concentrations decreased, so did total carbohydrate oxidation. Once mean plasma glucose values were between 45-54 mg/dL (2.5-3.0 mmol/L), exhaustion occurred and subjects could no longer exercise.

Hypoglycemia occurs during strenuous exercise when glucose output from the liver can no longer keep up with glucose uptake by the working muscles. Felig et al. (1982) had 19 healthy, active males exercise on a cycle ergometer until exhaustion (~2.5 h, 60-65% $\dot{V}O_2$max) while consuming water, a 5% glucose drink, or a 10% glucose drink. During the water trial, the mean blood glucose decreased from 80 to 60 mg/dL (4.5 to 3.3 mmol/L), with seven subjects developing hypoglycemia (blood glucose levels <45 mg/dL). Figure 2.9 shows the changes in mean blood glucose levels during exercise for each of the three treatments; figure 2.10 shows individual data for each of the subjects who became hypoglycemic. Ingestion of glucose (either a 5% or 10% solution) prevented the fall in blood glucose observed during the water-only period. Exogenous carbohydrate clearly prevented the drop in blood glucose frequently seen with exhaustive exercise. It also decreased the body's reliance on gluconeogenesis for glucose production, thereby possibly sparing body protein.

Carbohydrate Feeding During Exercise Improves Performance and Reduces Fatigue

During prolonged exercise in which no exogenous carbohydrate is provided, the body has difficulty maintaining blood glucose levels within the normal range (80-120 mg/dL). Feeding carbohydrate during prolonged exercise

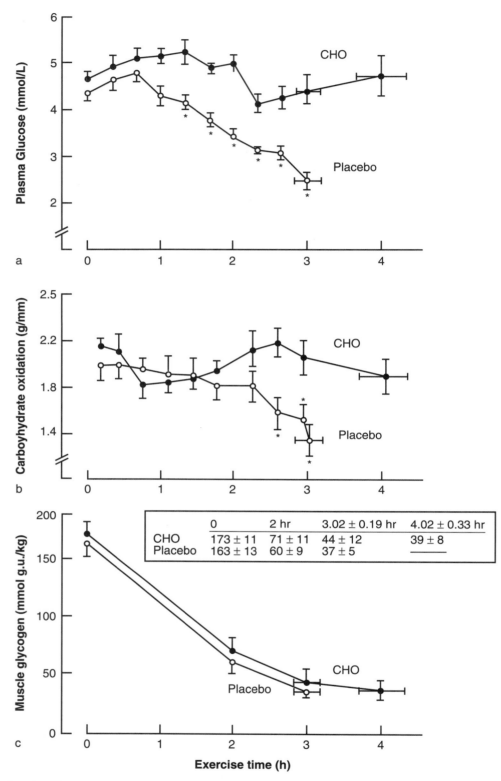

Figure 2.8 *(a)* Plasma glucose, *(b)* carbohydrate oxidation, and *(c)* muscle glycogen responses when cycling at 74% of maximal oxygen uptake when ingesting a placebo (flavored water) or carbohydrate (CHO) every 20 min. Values are mean ± SE. *Significantly different from carbohydrate; $p < 0.05$; g.u. = glucose used.

Reprinted from Coyle et al. 1986.

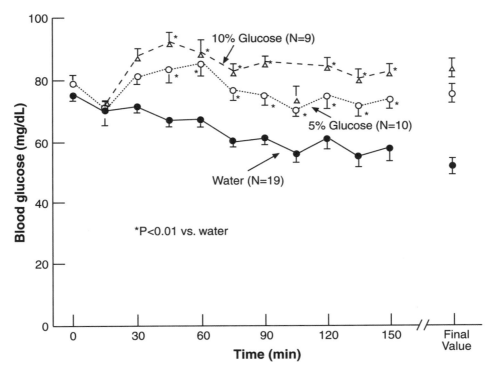

Figure 2.9 Blood glucose response to prolonged exercise with ingestion of either water or glucose (40 or 80 g/h as either a 5% or 10% solution, respectively). "Final value" refers to the specimens obtained at exhaustion. Bars indicate SEM. Figures in parentheses indicate the number of subjects in each group. To convert blood glucose values to millimoles per liter, multiply by 0.05551. Reprinted from Felig et al. 1982.

improves performance and lengthens the time an athlete can exercise before becoming fatigued. Coyle et al. (1986) measured the plasma glucose and muscle glycogen levels in seven trained cyclists exercising at 70-75% $\dot{V}O_2$ max to fatigue during two sessions, one with and one without exogenous carbohydrate. Fatigue was defined as the point when subjects were unable to maintain the designated workload. Muscle biopsies were taken before exercise began, after 2 h of exercise, and 5 min after cessation of exercise. When the subjects consumed only flavored water during exercise (the placebo group), both blood glucose (mmol/L) and carbohydrate oxidation (g/min) declined significantly—and the subjects fatigued 1 h sooner than when they consumed carbohydrate (at 3 vs. 4 h). When a carbohydrate drink was provided during exercise (~400 g carbohydrate over the 4-h period), blood glucose and carbohydrate oxidation remained high and subjects were able to exercise 1 h longer. Thus the consumption of carbohydrate improved exercise time to fatigue by 33% and maintained blood glucose values within normal ranges. Muscle glycogen use was

similar between the treatments throughout the study, with minimal muscle glycogen being used during the last hour of the carbohydrate trial— suggesting that blood glucose is a primary fuel substrate during the late stages of exercise when muscle glycogen is depleted. It appears, then, that carbohydrate feeding during exercise may benefit individuals participating in endurance events lasting more than 90 min.

Although most studies documenting the benefit of carbohydrate intake during exercise have been done in the laboratory, there is ample evidence that it works in "real-life" situations. Tsintzas et al. (1993) measured performance time in two 18.6-mi (30-km) races with and without exogenous carbohydrate (5% maltodextrin or a placebo of flavored water). The seven subjects were experienced runners, four men and three women, who competed against each other during the races. Diets were controlled before the races, and treatments were randomly assigned so that the runners did not know which drink they were consuming. Performance time for the carbohydrate trial was significantly faster (128.3 min) compared with the placebo

37

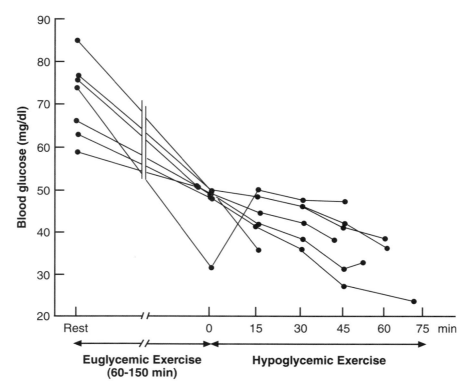

Figure 2.10 Individual blood glucose values in the seven subjects whose blood glucose concentrations fell below 45 mg/dL (2.5 mmol/L) during the water-ingestion phase of the study. "Euglycemic exercise" refers to the period of exercise during which blood glucose levels remained above 50 mg/dL (2.8 mmol/L). "Hypoglycemic exercise" refers to the duration of exercise after the blood glucose concentration fell below 50 mg/dL (2.8 mmol/L). To convert blood glucose values to millimoles per liter, multiply by 0.05551.

Reprinted from Felig et al. 1982.

trial (131.2 min); and the runners maintained their speed throughout the race in the carbohydrate trial, whereas those receiving the placebo decreased their speed after 15.5 mi (25 km). Below and Coyle (1995) had male cyclists consume a carbohydrate drink (providing 78 g of carbohydrate) while exercising for 1 h at high intensity (80-90% $\dot{V}O_2$max). The drink increased mean exercise performance time by 6.3% compared to water only. This is one of the first studies to show that carbohydrate feeding during high-intensity exercise that lasts only 1 h can be beneficial. It also showed that performance can be even further enhanced if the carbohydrate is consumed with a large volume of fluid (>1000 ml). However, this study was done on athletes who had undergone an overnight fast, which reduces liver glycogen stores. The results might have been different if the athletes had been tested in the afternoon, after eating breakfast and lunch.

Currently, there is little evidence to indicate that carbohydrate ingestion during low to mod-

erate activity lasting less than 1 h is beneficial for people who are well fed before beginning exercise. Remember, however, that the amount of carbohydrate used during an exercise bout depends on a variety of factors: the intensity, duration, and type of exercise; the environmental temperature; the fitness level of the individual; and the pre-exercise glycogen stores in the body. The decision to use exogenous carbohydrate during exercise, regardless of duration and intensity, may need to be individually determined, but research evidence suggests it can be beneficial.

Timing and Rate of Carbohydrate Feeding During Exercise

Carbohydrate ingestion generally should begin early in an exercise event, to ensure that adequate carbohydrate is available during the later stages of exercise. If athletes wait until the onset of fatigue before consuming carbohydrate, they may be unable to absorb it rapidly enough to prevent fatigue. Coggan and Coyle (1987) demonstrated that the latest an individual can consume carbohydrate and still prevent fatigue is 30 min before the onset of fatigue. Tsintzas et al. (1996) found that ingestion of carbohydrate (48 g) during the first hour of an exhaustive exercise bout increased time to exhaustion by 14% (~13 min more) compared to a water placebo.

The goal of carbohydrate feeding during exercise is to provide working muscle with an additional 1 g of exogenous glucose per minute late in exercise (Coyle 1995; Wagenmakers et al. 1993)—or approximately 40-65 g of carbohydrate per hour (Coggan and Coyle 1991; Coyle 1995; Sherman 1995). Any sport drink containing at least 6-8% carbohydrate would provide 60-80 g of carbohydrate per liter. Thus, consuming 18-34 oz (500-1000 ml) per hour of these drinks should provide adequate carbohydrate and fluid. It is generally recommended that fluid intake be approximately 4-6 oz (120-180 ml) for each 15-20 min period, depending on body size and environmental conditions. If this rate of carbohydrate (using a 6% solution) and fluid ingestion is followed, one would consume approximately 500-1000 ml and 30-60 g of carbohydrate per hour, meeting the carbohydrate requirements of most individuals doing moderate activity. If the activity level is very high and the duration is long (e.g., a marathon, ironman race, ultraendurance event), or if the temperature is extreme (e.g., either hot [>90°F] or cold [< 33°F]), additional carbohydrate and fluid may be needed to maintain body temperature and prevent disturbances in fluid homeostasis (Murray 1995; Yaspelkis and Ivy 1991).

Type of Carbohydrate

What type of carbohydrate should be consumed during exercise? Does one type of carbohydrate absorb more quickly than another? All simple sugars, such as glucose, sucrose, and maltodextrin (e.g., Polycose, glucose polymers), are absorbed rapidly from the gut. These carbohydrate sources are also equally effective in maintaining blood glucose levels during exercise (Flynn et al. 1987; Murray et al. 1989). Choosing one source over another depends more on personal preference and the availability of the carbohydrate. There appears to be no physiological advantage of one type of simple sugar over the other. Maltodextrins are frequently added to sport drinks because they are less sweet than sucrose or glucose—the lower sweetness level permits a higher concentration of carbohydrate without making the product unbearably sweet. Most sport drinks on the market today use a combination of sugars with glucose, sucrose, fructose, and maltodextrin. Drinks containing 6-8% carbohydrate plus sodium are generally well absorbed during exercise and provide adequate carbohydrate to maintain blood glucose if 17-34 oz (500-1000 ml) of fluid are consumed per hour.

Fructose (usually from high-fructose corn syrup) is absorbed more slowly from the gut than glucose because it is absorbed through facilitated diffusion instead of active absorption. Large doses of fructose can overload the absorption capabilities of the gut and cause gastrointestinal distress, such as cramping and diarrhea. When fructose is consumed in moderate amounts, however, absorption from the gut is rapid and without adverse effects.

Once fructose is absorbed, it is transported to the liver where it is converted to glucose. This process slows the release of glucose into the blood stream. The glucose response to a fructose load is lower than to an equal amount of glucose or sucrose, as demonstrated by a study in which subjects consumed different sugar solutions (6% sucrose, 6% glucose, or 6% fructose) during a 2-h period in which they cycled intermittently (65-80% $\dot{V}O_2$max). Blood glucose responses for glucose and sucrose were similar, while fructose produced very little change in blood glucose (figure 2.11). When a fructose drink (60-85 g) is fed 60 min before exercise, the change in blood glucose during exercise is similar to that seen with water only (Okano et al. 1988). Thus, fructose produces no major change in blood glucose levels. While this effect may benefit active people who are sensitive to blood glucose fluctuations before exercise or during the first 15-30 min of exercise, fructose alone is not as effective as other sugars in preventing the drop in blood glucose that can occur with exhaustive endurance exercise.

The oxidation rate of fructose fed during exercise is much lower than that of either glucose or glucose polymers (Adopo et al. 1994; Massicotte et al. 1989). However, if fructose is fed in combination with glucose (50 g fructose + 50 g glucose), the oxidation of the combined sugars is significantly higher (25-38% higher) than when a 100-g dose of either fructose or glucose is fed alone (figure 2.12) (Adopo et al.

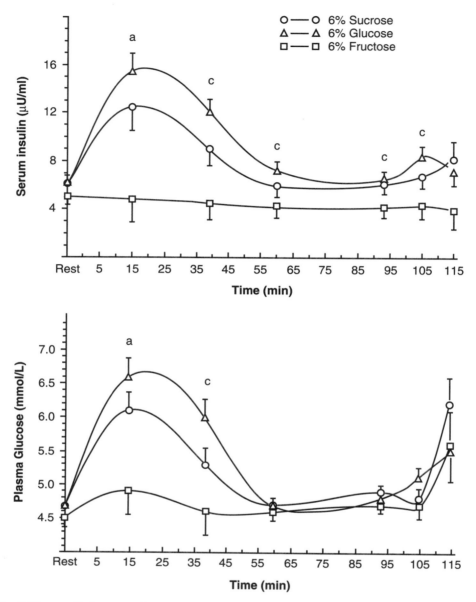

Figure 2.11 Effects of glucose, fructose, and sucrose ingestion during exercise. Data represent mean blood glucose and insulin values for all subjects. Bars represent standard error of the mean.
a = glucose and sucrose significantly different from fructose, $p < 0.05$
c = glucose significantly different from fructose, $p < 0.05$
Reprinted from Murray et al. 1989.

1994). Feeding *small amounts* of fructose in combination with other sugars may thus be beneficial both before and during exercise.

Fructose does not appear to replace muscle glycogen stores as well as other carbohydrates (e.g., glucose, sucrose, or maltodextrin), which elicit a greater glycemic response than fructose. This increase in blood insulin stimulates the enzymes involved in glycogen synthesis and enhances the uptake of glucose by muscle cells.

Drinks containing only high fructose, therefore, are not recommended during or immediately after exercise. However, fructose works well in combination with other sugars in effectively replacing liver glycogen after exercise.

Although athletes often consume carbohydrate as a liquid during exercise, some prefer solid foods. Researchers have compared the glucose response during exercise of solid (energy or sport bars, whole fruit) to liquid carbohydrate sources

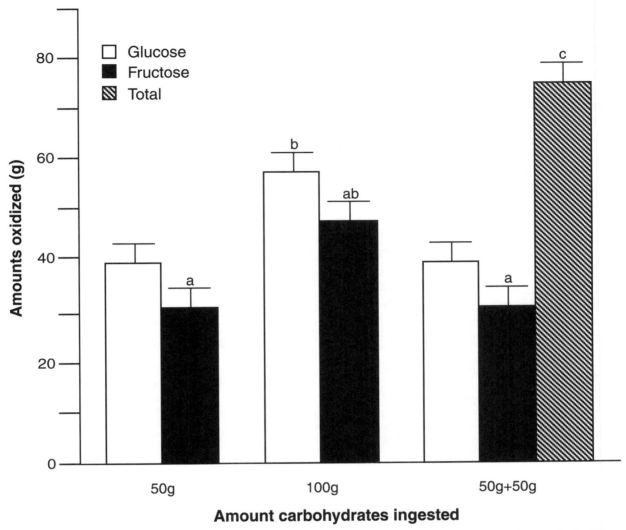

Figure 2.12 Amounts of exogenous glucose and fructose oxidized over exercise period (2 h on cycle ergometer at 61% $\dot{V}O_2$max) after ingestion of 50 or 100 g of glucose or fructose, or a mixture of 50 g each of glucose and fructose. Significantly different ($p < 0.05$) from: [a]glucose; [b]50 g; [c]100g. Reprinted from Adopo et al. 1994.

(sport drink or blended fruit) with similar amounts of carbohydrate (Mason et al. 1993; Murdoch et al. 1993). The studies found no significant difference in blood glucose levels during exercise with solid versus liquid carbohydrate—both produce similar blood glucose and insulin responses. Thus, the form of carbohydrate consumed during exercise is a matter of availability and personal preference. Since people consuming solid carbohydrate during exercise should drink appropriate amounts of fluid to ensure adequate hydration, use of solid carbohydrates is not always practical during some strenuous activities or sports. Table 2.6 lists various types of energy sources frequently used by athletes.

Practical Guidelines for Carbohydrate Intake During Exercise

The following guidelines may be helpful to active individuals who consume carbohydrate during exercise:

- People respond differently to various types of carbohydrate foods or drinks. To avoid unexpected gastrointestinal disturbances during competition, athletes should use the carbohydrate supplement during training that they will use during competition.

- Athletes should ingest carbohydrate early in an exercise session, to prevent the decrease

Table 2.6   **Energy and Nutrient Composition of Sport, Energy, and Breakfast Bars**

Product	Size (oz)	Energy (kcal)	CHO (g)	Fat (g)	Protein (g)	Fortified with vitamins and minerals
American Body Building Hi-Protein Steel Bar	3	380	68	5	16	Yes
Balance Food Bar	1.76	200	22	6	14	Yes
Clif Bar (chocolate chip)	2.4	250	45	4	10	Yes
EAS Myoplex Plus Deluxe	3.2	340	43	7	24	Yes
Kellogg's Nutri-Grain Cereal Bar (raspberry)	1.3	140	27	3	2	Yes
Meta-Rx Source One Food Bar (devil's food cake)	2.2	190	30	3	15	Yes
Meta-Rx (fudge brownie)	3.53	320	48	2.5	27	Yes
Nature Valley Granola Bar	1.5	180	29	6	5	No
PowerBar Essential Energy Bar (chocolate)	1.87	180	28	4	10	Yes
PowerBar (chocolate)	2.25	225	42	2	10	Yes
PowerBar Harvest (chocolate)	2.3	240	45	4	7	Yes
PowerBar Protein Plus (chocolate)	3	290	15	8	32	Yes
PR Bar Ironman	2	230	24	7	17	Yes
Tiger Sport Bar (chocolate)	2.3	230	43	2	10	Yes
Tiger's Milk Bar	1.2	130	24	2.5	4	Yes

CHO = carbohydrate; Information taken from packages of products sold.

in blood glucose often seen during endurance events. This practice is especially helpful for those who come into an exercise event with poor glycogen stores (e.g., individuals involved in very heavy training or who have followed a low-kilocalorie or a high-fat diet).

• Sport drinks or other carbohydrate-containing drinks should have a concentration of 6-8% carbohydrate (60-80 g per 1000 ml). Drinks with higher concentrations are less well absorbed and do not replace lost fluids during exercise as efficiently. An additional advantage to sport drinks is that they contain sodium, which helps in the absorption of carbohydrate across the gut mucosa.

• Athletes should drink 4-8 oz (120-240 ml) of fluid every 15-20 min—a volume that provides about 500-1000 ml of fluid and 30-60 g of carbohydrate per hour if a 6% carbohydrate drink is used. Exercise events of long duration or during extreme temperatures may require higher fluid and carbohydrate intakes.

• When using body weight to determine carbohydrate intake during exercise, prescribe a minimum of 0.05-0.1 g of carbohydrate per lb body weight (0.1-0.2 g/kg) every 20 min. For a 154-lb (70-kg) male, this provides 7-14 g of carbohydrate every 20 min or 21-42 g/h. Plasma glucose may be oxidized late in exercise at rates in excess of 1 g/min.

Carbohydrate Feeding Post-Exercise and During Training Periods

After an exercise session, one must replenish muscle glycogen and refuel the body for the next exercise event. Athletes with 24 h or more before the next activity can replenish glycogen stores more easily than if they will exercise sooner. Yet, since 24 h rarely pass between exercise sessions, post-exercise feeding is critical. The types and amounts of food used and the timing of the meals after exercise depend in part on when the next exercise bout will occur. In addition to refueling the body, post-exercise feeding

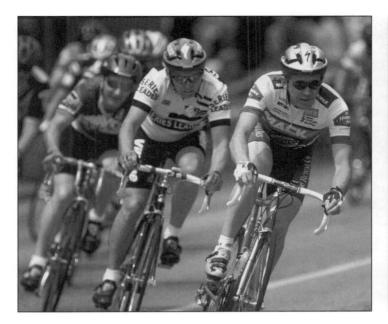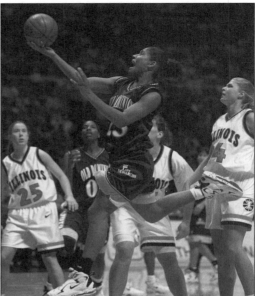

Both high-intensity and endurance exercise can deplete glycogen stores.

should also provide the energy and nutrients to repair and strengthen muscle tissue that may have been damaged during the previous exercise session and fluids to rehydrate the body.

Glycogen Synthesis Post-Exercise

Glycogen depletion can occur after 2-3 h of continuous exercise performed at 60-80% $\dot{V}O_2$max, or after high-intensity exercise (90-130% $\dot{V}O_2$ max) that occurs intermittently over a shorter time (15-60 min); thus, both endurance exercise (e.g., cycling or running) and intermittent exercise (e.g., tennis, basketball, soccer, swimming) can deplete glycogen stores. Glucose is the only substrate the body can use for glycogen synthesis. Muscle glycogen replacement occurs at approximately 5-6 mmol/kg of muscle per hour (Blom et al. 1987; Coyle 1995). Normal glycogen levels of trained male athletes on a mixed diet (consuming 6-10 g carbohydrate per kg body weight) are ~130-160 mmol/kg of muscle, while those of untrained individuals range from ~80 to 110 mmol/kg of muscle. Male athletes who attempt to supercompensate glycogen can increase stored glycogen to ~200 mmol/kg of muscle. Since the amount of glycogen that can be resynthesized within a given period is limited, one goal of post-exercise feeding is to provide adequate carbohydrate for liver and muscle glycogen replacement before the next exercise bout.

A number of factors determine the rate of glycogen synthesis—including the degree of muscle glycogen depletion, the degree of insulin activation of **glycogen synthase**, and the carbohydrate content of the post-exercise diet. Without adequate dietary carbohydrate, muscle glycogen cannot be replaced to normal levels (Bogardus et al. 1981). Nearly 90% of the dietary carbohydrate (digested primarily to glucose) consumed post-exercise is deposited in muscle glycogen, which predominates over liver glycogen synthesis. Greater muscle glycogen depletion enhances glycogen resynthesis, as do high insulin levels. Bonen et al. (1985) found that, during the first 4 h after exercise, glycogen synthesis increased 43% after exhaustive exercise (producing an 80% decrease in leg muscle glycogen) compared with only a 13% increase after nonexhaustive exercise (producing a 35% decrease in leg muscle glycogen).

High-Carbohydrate Diets During Training Improve Performance and Power Output

We have established that high-carbohydrate diets fed post-exercise increase the level of stored glycogen in the body, while high-carbohydrate intake during periods of high-intensity training will keep glycogen levels high. The question remains: do these higher levels of glycogen lead to improved performance?

To examine this question, Simonsen et al. (1991) fed male (n = 12) and female (n = 10) rowers two different carbohydrate levels over a 4-week period of intense training that included rowing twice a day. The subjects were randomly assigned to either a high-carbohydrate diet (10 g/kg body weight, 70% of energy) or a moderate-carbohydrate diet (5 g/kg body weight, 42% of energy) (figure 2.13). Dietary protein intake was 2 g/kg body weight (13% of energy) for both groups, and fat intake was adjusted to maintain body weight throughout the period. The subjects exercised daily for 65 min at 70% peak VO_2 and 38 min at ≥90% peak VO_2. Although muscle glycogen levels increased by 65% in the high-carbohydrate group as compared to the moderate-carbohydrate group, the moderate-carbohydrate group maintained their baseline glycogen levels

(119 mmol/kg) throughout the training period. Carbohydrate at 5 g/kg body weight apparently was sufficient to maintain, but not increase, glycogen levels during this period of intense training. However, the mean power output in the time trials increased by 10.7% in the high-carbohydrate group, but by only 1.6% in the moderate-carbohydrate group after 4 weeks of intense training. Thus, the high-carbohydrate diet increased glycogen levels and power output, when compared to the moderate-carbohydrate diet. These data are supported by Jenkins et al. (1993), who found a 5.6% increase in total work done during high-intensity interval cycling when a

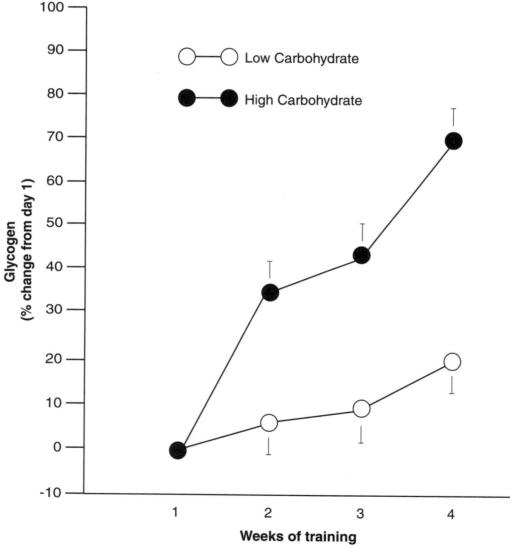

Figure 2.13 Percent change in muscle glycogen from day 1 of a moderate-carbohydrate diet (5 g carbohydrate/kg body mass/d) and from day 1 for a high-carbohydrate diet (10 g carbohydrate/kg body mass/d) during 4 weeks of intense twice-daily rowing exercise.

Reprinted from Simonsen et al. 1991.

high-carbohydrate diet was fed for 10 d (83% energy from carbohydrate) versus a moderate-carbohydrate diet (58% from carbohydrate).

Type and Amount of Carbohydrate

Glucose, sucrose, and maltodextrins appear to replace muscle glycogen equally well. To exam-ine both quantity and type of carbohydrate re-quired to restore muscle glycogen after exhaus-tive exercise, Blom and colleagues (1987) fed carbohydrate immediately after exercise and then at 2, 4, and 6 h post-exercise. In one ex-periment (figure 2.14a), they tested three levels of glucose (high, medium, and low concentra-tions); in another (figure 2.14b), they tested three

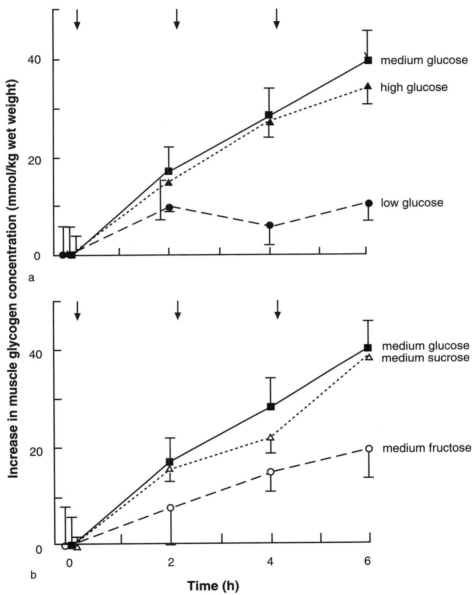

Figure 2.14 Changes in muscle glycogen during post-exercise recovery when different sugar loads were given. *(a)* Different amounts of glucose. *(b)* Different kinds of sugars. Arrows indicate sugar loads. Mean values are shown; one SEM is indicated by the length of the vertical bar. ● = low glucose (LG) (0.35 g/kg body weight); ■ = medium glucose (MG) (0.70 g/kg body weight); ▲ = high glucose (HG) (1.40 g/kg body weight); △ = medium sucrose (MS) (0.70 g/kg body weight); and □ = medium fructose (MF) (0.70 g/kg body weight). Medium glucose appears on both panels. Mean values are shown. One SEM is indicated by the length of the vertical bar.

Reprinted with permission from Blom et al. 1987.

types of sugars (glucose, sucrose, and fructose) at equal concentrations (0.7 g/kg body weight). They took muscle biopsies at rest; 5 min after exercise; and 2, 4, and 6 h after exercise. The high and medium glucose solutions replaced glycogen equally (~5.7 mmol/kg), as did glucose and sucrose fed at the same concentrations (0.7 g/kg body weight). Fructose, however, did not replace muscle glycogen nearly as well as the other sugars. As mentioned earlier, research suggests that fructose is better for the resynthesis of liver glycogen than of muscle glycogen.

Recently Burke et al. (1996) examined the effect of meal size on glycogen replacement in the 24-h period following exhaustive exercise. They fed eight well-trained triathletes either 4 large meals ("gorging") or 16 frequent, small meals ("nibbling") post-exercise. Subjects received the same types of carbohydrate foods, providing 10 g of carbohydrate per kg body weight, during each trial. The researchers hypothesized that "gorging" would elicit a greater glucose and insulin response than "nibbling," and thus be better at replacing muscle glycogen. There was no statistically significant difference between the groups in muscle glycogen storage over the 24-h period (gorging: 74 ± 8 mmol glycogen/kg wet muscle weight; nibbling: 95 ± 15 mmol glycogen/kg wet muscle weight). The size of the high-carbohydrate meal apparently had no influence on muscle glycogen levels. This research has practical implications. For many athletes, appetite is frequently suppressed following strenuous exercise, making a large post-exercise meal unappealing—yet this is the time when the glycogen storage potential is highest. This research provides a practical solution to this dilemma: small, frequent post-exercise high-carbohydrate snacks can be just as effective at replacing muscle glycogen as large post-exercise meals.

To determine the ability of protein or carbohydrate/protein combinations to replace muscle glycogen, Zawadzki et al. (1992) fed nine male cyclists either 112 g of carbohydrate (456 kcal), 41 g of protein (164 kcal), or 112 g of carbohydrate plus 41 g of protein (620 kcal), immediately after and 2 h after exhaustive exercise. Muscle biopsies were taken immediately after exercise and 4 h post-exercise to determine how much glycogen was replaced with each of the treatments. Glycogen replacement was 28% higher with the carbohydrate/protein combination than with the carbohydrate-only treatment. As expected, the protein-only treatment did a poor job of replacing muscle glycogen. Figure

2.15 shows the amount of muscle glycogen replacement for each treatment. The greater amount of glycogen stored with the combination of both protein and carbohydrate may have been due to the higher energy content of the combined treatment (more kilocalories were provided in this treatment) versus the carbohydrate or protein-only treatments. Thus, the amount of glycogen stored after exercise will be a function of total energy intake and the carbohydrate content of the diet as illustrated by Burke et al. (1995) in the next paragraph.

Burke et al. (1995) randomly assigned three different dietary regimens to eight well-trained triathletes after exhaustive exercise (2 h at 75% peak VO_2, followed by four 30-s sprints). The diets were fed one week apart. For 24 h after each exercise bout, the athletes were fed one of the following diets:

- High-carbohydrate diet (7 g/kg body weight/d)
- High-carbohydrate diet with added fat and

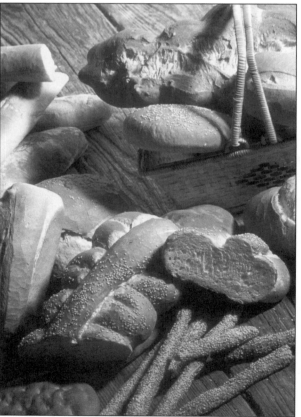

Whole-grain breads are excellent sources of carbohydrate, vitamins, and minerals.

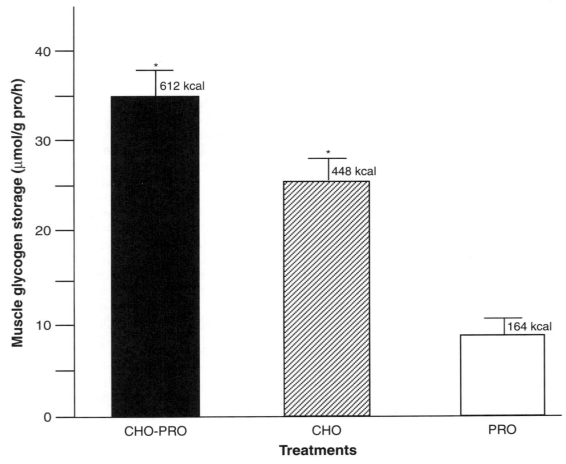

Figure 2.15 Rates of muscle glycogen storage during 4-h recovery period for trained male cyclists (mean $\dot{V}O_2$max = 73 ml/kg/min) receiving 112 g carbohydrate (CHO) plus 41 g of protein (PRO); CHO only (112 g); or PRO only (41 g). Supplements were provided immediately and 2 h after exhaustive exercise (cycling) designed to deplete muscle glycogen.

Reprinted from Zawadzki et al. 1992.

protein (protein: 1.6 g/kg body weight/d; fat: 1.2 g/kg body weight/d)

- Matched energy diet (carbohydrate diet + 4.8 g/kg body weight/d additional carbohydrate).

There were no significant differences between the trials in muscle glycogen storage over a 24-h period. It appears that, as long as carbohydrate and energy intake are adequate, addition of protein or fat does not enhance glycogen storage. Yet it is still important to feed both protein and carbohydrate during the 24-h period following strenuous exercise—the protein provides the necessary amino acids for building and repairing muscle tissue and to maintain positive nitrogen balance, while the carbohydrate provides the substrate for glycogen storage.

Researchers have also examined whether solid or liquid forms of carbohydrate are better at replacing muscle glycogen. When Reed et al. (1989) fed solid and liquid carbohydrate (1.5 g/kg body weight) immediately after exercise and at 2-h intervals after exercise, they found similar rates of muscle glycogen synthesis. It appears that solid and liquid forms of carbohydrate replace muscle glycogen equally well.

Glycogen Replacement Using High Glycemic Index Foods

Most research examining the effects of different types of carbohydrates on muscle glycogen replacement categorizes foods as either simple or complex carbohydrates. This approach assumes that simple carbohydrates (higher in sugar) elicit a large, rapid rise in blood glucose, while complex carbohydrates (high in starch) produce a slower, flatter blood glucose response curve. This simplistic approach to classifying carbohydrate foods is incorrect. Carbohydrate foods with quite similar chemical structures (e.g., spaghetti and white bread are both high in starch), can produce different blood glucose responses (see table 2.1, page 23).

If the previous assumptions were true, feeding high glycemic index foods post-exercise would produce a greater increase in muscle glycogen storage compared to low glycemic foods. To test this hypothesis, Burke et al. (1993) had five well-trained cyclists perform 2 h of exhaustive exercise on two different occasions, 1 week apart. For 24 h after each trial, the cyclists rested and consumed a high-carbohydrate diet. They consumed a low glycemic index diet in the first trial, and a high glycemic index diet for the second. Both diets provided 10 g of carbohydrate/kg body weight (730 g carbohydrate; 74% of energy) over the 24-h period, and both were similar in energy content (~3900 kcal/d). Muscle biopsies were taken immediately after exercise and 24 h after consuming the experimental diets. The degree of muscle glycogen depletion was similar in the two trials (26-34 mmol/kg wet weight). Muscle glyco-

gen content 24 h after recovery was significantly greater with a high glycemic diet (106 ± 12 mmol/kg wet muscle weight) than with the low glycemic diet (72 ± 7 mmol/kg wet muscle weight). The authors attributed the higher glycogen content to the significantly higher glucose and insulin response on the high compared to the low glycemic diet. It appears that high glycemic index foods are indeed preferable for replacing muscle glycogen immediately after exercise.

Although high glycemic index foods are excellent for replacing muscle glycogen, planning all the meals of an athlete around such foods in the 24 h after exercise may be difficult or impossible—the athlete may be traveling and need to purchase food from restaurants or grocery stores. It may be more practical to provide 100 g of high glycemic index carbohydrate (either food or commercially available product) immediately after exercise and simply to encourage the athlete to eat high-carbohydrate foods for the remainder of the day. Table 2.1 (page 23) lists glycemic indexes of a number of foods that can be used immediately after exercise. A more convenient way to consume a high glycemic index food post-exercise is to use glycogen replacement products available on the market. Table 2.7 lists some of these products and the

Table 2.7 **Examples of Carbohydrate-Loading Products**

The following information is based on a 12-oz serving except where indicated differently. All products are made from maltodextrin, glucose polymers, fructose, high-fructose corn syrup, and/or glucose.

Product	Carbohydrate (g/serving)	Carbohydrate (% concentration)	Carbohydrate (% of energy)	Energy (kcal)
CarboPower[a]	64	15	100	255
CarboFuel	80	35	89	360
CarboSurge	36	16	100	144
Gatorlode	71	20	100	280
Exceeds High CHO	88	26	100	350
PowerFuel	50	22	100	200
Reload[b]	20	54	100	80
UltraGel[b]	24	65	72	130
UltraFuel[c]	75	22	100	300

CHO = carbohydrate; Information taken from packages of products sold and SCAN's Pulse 1997;16(3):13.

[a]Sold in 16-oz serving that contains 85 g carbohydrate.

[b]Reload—a gel form of carbohydrate sold in 0.75 fl oz servings—contains concentrated carbohydrate in the form of maltodextrin and dextrose. It is recommended that it be consumed with 8-10 oz of fluid. UltraGel, a gel form of carbohydrate, is sold in 1.3-oz servings and contains concentrated carbohydrate like Reload; however, UltraGel also contains 4 g of fat and 1 g of protein.

[c]Sold in 16-oz serving that contains 100 g carbohydrate.

amount of carbohydrate they provide per serving. These products are especially convenient for active people who prefer not to eat immediately following strenuous exercise or for occasions when food is not readily available postexercise. For athletes wanting inexpensive ways to provide small meals containing a known amount of carbohydrate, table 2.8 gives individual foods and combinations of foods that provide either 50 or 100 g of carbohydrate. Finally, many active individuals like the convenience of the energy and sport bars currently on the market. These products usually provide some protein, fat, and micronutrients, along with carbohydrate. They are not designed exclusively for glycogen replacement but as a snack to

Table 2.8 **Foods and Combinations of Foods Containing Either 50 or 100 g of Carbohydrate**

Food or combination foods	Amount	Carbohydrate (g)	Energy from carbohydrate (%)	Protein (g)	Fat (g)	Total energy (kcal)
Sweetened applesauce	1 cup	50	97	0.5	0.5	207
Whole wheat bread	1 oz slice					
Jelly	4 tsp					
Skim milk	12 fl oz	50	71	16	2	282
Brown rice (cooked)	1 cup					
Tomato sauce	1/4 cup	50	83	6	2	242
Spaghetti noodles (cooked)	1 cup					
Tomato sauce	1/4 cup	50	75	8	4	268
Large apple	1					
Saltine crackers	8	50	82	3	4	248
Grape-nuts cereal	1/2 cup					
Raisins	3/8 cup					
Skim milk	8 fl oz	100	84	16	1	473
Large bagel	1 (3.5 oz)					
Jelly	8 tsp					
Skim milk	8 fl oz	100	81	19	2	494
Brown rice (cooked)	1 cup					
Mixed vegetables	1/2 cup					
Apple juice	12 fl oz	100	88	8	2	450
Large apple	1					
Raisins	1/3 cup					
Saltine crackers	14	100	84	6	6	460
Sandwich/Salad:						
Whole wheat bread	2 slices					
Skinless chicken	2 oz					
Medium whole tomato	1					
Loose-leaf lettuce	1 cup					
Low-cal salad dressing	1 tbsp					
Pinapple juice	16 oz	104	73	26	4	565

supplement meals. Table 2.6 (page 42) lists the amount of carbohydrate and energy provided in commonly available sport, energy, and breakfast bars.

Timing and Rate of Post-Exercise Carbohydrate Feedings

The timing and rate of carbohydrate consumption after exercise can influence the amount of glycogen stored. Glycogen synthesis rates are highest immediately after exercise when the muscle is depleted and glycogen synthase activation is high. One goal of post-exercise feeding is therefore to get carbohydrate into the system quickly, especially in the first 2 h after exercise. Baker et al. (1994) monitored the diets of seven highly trained, competitive cyclists for 3 d before and 24 h after exhaustive exercise. Subjects were then given either a flavored high-carbohydrate drink (12% maltodextrin) or a flavored placebo. They completed another exhaustive exercise bout the following day. This protocol was repeated 2 weeks later until all athletes had completed both the carbohydrate and placebo trials (table 2.9). Athletes receiving the additional carbohydrate after the first exercise session improved their time to exhaustion on the following day by an average of 11%. The athletes' typical diet contained only 4 g of carbohydrate per kg body weight, with carbohydrate representing 50% of their total energy intake. The athletes who received the additional

high-carbohydrate drink immediately after exercise significantly increased their total carbohydrate intake for the day to 68% of total energy intake (7 g/kg body weight). The additional carbohydrate increased their total energy intake ~500 kcal/d. Thus, the simple addition of a high-carbohydrate replacement drink to the athletes' diet immediately after exercise significantly improved their overall carbohydrate and energy intake, even when the athletes self-selected their diets. High-carbohydrate replacement products like those used in this study (see table 2.7) are convenient and make it easy to ensure that adequate carbohydrate is provided post-exercise. However, they need to be used in combination with nutritious foods and should not replace the post-exercise meal.

Since the rate of muscle glycogen synthesis is linear during the first 6 h after glycogen-depleting exercise, most researchers have used this time period to determine the effects of timing on glycogen replacement. Ivy, Katz et al. (1988) found that a 2-h delay in feeding carbohydrate after exercise reduced the rate of glycogen synthesis by 47% compared with feeding carbohydrate immediately after exercise. In a follow-up study, eight male cyclists were fed carbohydrate (either 1.5 or 3.0 g/kg body weight) immediately and 2 h after exhaustive exercise. Muscle biopsies were taken immediately, 2 h, and 4 h after exercise to determine muscle glycogen levels. They found that providing >1.5 g of carbohydrate per kg body

Table 2.9 **Energy and Carbohydrate Intake, and Cycling Performance Times, of Cyclists With and Without Carbohydrate (CHO) Supplementation 24 h Post-Exercise**

	Energy intake on 3-d typical diet (kcal/kg BW)	Energy intake 24-h post-typical diet (kcal/kg BW)	CHO intake 24-h post-exercise (g/kg BW)	CHO intake 24-h post-exercise (% of energy intake)	Ride time (min)
CHO supp	34.3 ± 6.3	41.8 ± 9.7	$6.8 \pm 0.9*$	$68 \pm 6*$	$72 \pm 8**$
Placebo	29.3 ± 8.5	34.8 ± 19.2	4.7 ± 2.5	55 ± 5	64 ± 11

- CHO supplement = 3.0 g carbohydrate/kg body weight; placebo = a noncaloric drink; BW = body weight.
- Subjects performed two exercise tests: (1) after recording their diet for 3 d, they exercised at 70% $\dot{V}O_2$max to exhaustion; (2) subjects then received either a placebo or a carbohydrate supplement during the next 24 h; (3) the next day, subjects exercised for 1 h of cycling at 70% $\dot{V}O_2$max, then to exhaustion at 85% $\dot{V}O_2$max.

*Diets 24 h post-exercise were significantly higher in CHO than self-selected diets before exercise ($p < 0.05$).

** Ride time with the carbohydrate supplement was significantly longer than placebo condition ($p < 0.05$). Exercise was 1 h or cycling at 70% $\dot{V}O_2$max, then to exhaustion at 85% $\dot{V}O_2$max.

Adapted from Baker et al. 1994.

weight added no additional increase in muscle glycogen levels (Ivy, Lee et al. 1988). In another study, Doyle et al. (1993) reported that the highest level of glycogen resynthesis (10 mmol/kg/h) occurred after feeding 0.4 g of maltodextrin per kg body weight every 15 min over a 4-h period immediately following exhaustive exercise. This higher glycogen storage may be due to the higher insulin response observed when carbohydrate is consumed more frequently (every 15 min) compared to less frequent feedings (every 1-2 h). Insulin stimulates the uptake of glucose by the cells for glycogen storage and stimulates glycogen synthase. If a 176-lb (80-kg) male consumed the amount of carbohydrate required to achieve the highest level of glycogen replacement (0.4 g of carbohydrate every 15 min for 4 h), he would need to ingest 128 g of carbohydrate per hour or 512 g of carbohydrate in 4 h. This level of carbohydrate intake after exhaustive exercise may be difficult for many athletes to achieve, but certainly could be achieved over a longer time period of 6-8 h.

The more frequent feeding (1-2 h) in the Doyle et al. (1993) study is comparable to the "nibblers" (fed every 1.5 h) discussed earlier in this chapter (Burke et al. 1996). However, Burke and colleagues saw no difference in glycogen storage between individuals fed high-carbohydrate diets every 1.5 h versus every 6 h over a 24-h period. The differences in these two studies may be due to the timing of the muscle biopsies done to assess glycogen levels. Burke's group determined glycogen levels 24 h after exhaustive exercise, while Doyle's group did their measurements 4 h after exhaustive exercise. Thus it appears that as long as adequate carbohydrate is fed within 24 h, glycogen replacement will occur.

Determining Overall Carbohydrate Intake for Individuals

Although it is frequently recommended that athletes consume diets containing 60-65% of the energy from carbohydrate, this may be an unrealistic goal for some individuals. Making carbohydrate recommendations based on grams of carbohydrate per kilogram body weight is probably an easier and more realistic approach (see table 2.10). The total amount of carbohydrate consumed in a diet containing 65% of its energy from carbohydrate varies dramatically with the total calories consumed. For example, a 176-lb (80-kg) male athlete consuming 5000 kcal per day with 65% of the energy coming from carbohydrate would consume 813 g (3252 kcal) of carbohydrate. This is equivalent to ~10 g of carbohydrate/kg body weight and more than exceeds the amount of carbohydrate needed to replace glycogen at a maximum rate. For this person, a diet providing 55% of its energy from carbohydrate would still provide 688 g of carbohydrate, or 8.5 g of carbohydrate/kg body weight (see the complete diet composition for these two diets in table 2.10). For many male athletes this level of carbohydrate intake would be a more realistic and achievable goal and would easily replace muscle glycogen during heavy training periods.

For many female athletes, who typically report consuming 2200-2500 kcal/d, it is almost impossible to consume the 500-600 g of carbohydrate per day frequently recommended for adequate glycogen replacement in men. For example, a 121-lb (55-kg) woman who consumed 6-7 g carbohydrate/kg body weight would need 330-385 g of carbohydrate/d (see table 2.10). This is equivalent to 1320-1540 kcal just from carbohydrate (or 66-77% of energy coming from carbohydrate based on a 2000 kcal/d diet). This total carbohydrate intake is below the 500-600 g/d recommendation for men, but the percentage of energy from carbohydrate is at or above the recommended level. Diets high in carbohydrate prevent the onset of fatigue in active females during exercise. For example, O'Keeffe et al. (1989) found that, compared to subjects' typical diets (<4.5 g of carbohydrate/kg body weight), a diet providing 6-7 g of carbohydrate/kg body weight significantly increased time to exhaustion in female cyclists. Athletes who are dieting may find it easy to consume a high-carbohydrate diet (60-70% of energy from carbohydrate), but the amount of carbohydrate per kg body weight will be low. For example, if a 121-lb (55-kg) woman decided to consume only 1500 kcal/d, a 65% carbohydrate diet would provide only 4.4 g of carbohydrate per kg body weight. This level of carbohydrate intake is too low to prevent premature fatigue during endurance exercise or to adequately replace muscle glycogen on a daily basis during periods of intense exercise training. Carbohydrate recommendations are more accurate when based on grams of carbohydrate per kilogram body weight than on percentage of total energy from carbohydrate. This concept is also easier for most athletes to understand and follow since they can readily eat from a

Table 2.10 **Examples of High- and Moderate-Carbohydrate Diets of Different Energy Levels for Male and Female Athletes**

	Male (176 lb or 80 kg) % of energy from carbohydrate						Female (121 lb or 55 kg) % of energy from carbohydrate					
Energy (kcal/d)	5000	5000	4000	4000	3000	3000	3000	3000	2500	2500	2000	2000
Carbohydrate (%)	65	55	65	55	65	55	65	55	65	55	65	55
g/d	813	688	650	550	488	413	488	413	438	344	325	275
g/kg body wt.	10.2	8.6	8.1	6.9	6.1	5.2	8.9	7.5	7.9	6.3	5.9	5.0
Protein (%)	12	15	12	15	12	15	12	15	12	15	12	15
g/d	150	188	120	150	90	113	90	113	75	94	60	75
g/kg body wt.	1.9	2.4	1.5	1.9	1.1	1.4	1.6	2.1	1.4	1.7	1.1	1.4
Fat (%)	23	30	23	30	23	30	23	30	23	30	23	30
g/day	128	167	102	133	78	100	78	100	64	83	51	67
g/kg body wt.	1.5	2.1	1.3	1.7	1.0	1.3	1.4	1.8	1.2	1.5	0.9	1.2

recommended list of foods to attain the required carbohydrate intake (see table 2.8).

To illustrate the above points, two studies were conducted at Ohio State University (Lamb et al. 1990; Sherman et al. 1993): male athletes consumed either high-carbohydrate diets (80-84% of energy from carbohydrate) or low-carbohydrate diets (42-43% of energy from carbohydrate) for 7-9 d, then either exercised to exhaustion (runners and cyclists) or swam various distances (ranging from 50-m interval sets to continuous 3000-m swims). For the swimmers, there were no differences in mean swim velocities for any interval distances, and mean velocities for all swims were identical on both diets. For the runners and cyclists, there were no differences in time to exhaustion on either diet, although the high-carbohydrate diet maintained a higher muscle glycogen level. The low-carbohydrate diet reduced muscle glycogen by 30-36% over the test period. Thus, consuming a lower-carbohydrate diet had no apparent deleterious effects on training capacity or high-intensity exercise performance over the 7-9 d this study was conducted. However, in terms of carbohydrate consumed per kg body weight, the low-carbohydrate diet provided 5.0-6.5 g of carbohydrate per kg body weight, while the high-carbohydrate diet provided 10-12 g. Thus even the lower-carbohydrate diet (42-43% of energy from carbohydrate, 370-470 g carbohydrate/d) appeared to provide adequate carbohydrate to maintain high-intensity work since the subjects were consuming 3600-4700 kcal/d. Because the study period was short (7 d), we

do not know what effect a "low"-carbohydrate diet such as this would have on muscle glycogen stores over a longer period of time. Would glycogen levels continue to decrease and eventually inhibit exercise performance?

The results of this study may have been very different if it had tested active females consuming only 2500 kcal/d. For women with energy needs of 2000-2500 kcal/d, a diet containing 43% of energy from carbohydrate would not provide adequate carbohydrate for muscle glycogen replacement. These diets would provide only 215-268 g of carbohydrate per day, or 3.9-4.8 g of carbohydrate per kg body weight for a 121-lb (55-kg) woman. This level of carbohydrate is too low for most active people during training.

Practical Guidelines for Feeding Carbohydrate Post-Exercise and During Training Periods

The research described above suggests the following recommendations for post-exercise carbohydrate feedings. These recommendations assume that the athlete is in training or competition and thus requires maximum glycogen replacement. Athletes frequently train twice a day for a total of 12-20 h per week of exercise. Less stringent carbohydrate recommendations are appropriate for recreational or fitness athletes who exercise only 4-10 h per week.

- Feed approximately 100-150 g of carbohydrate within the first hour after exercise, depending on body size. Combine this carbohydrate with some dietary protein if possible.

- Over a 24-h period, feed 6-8 g of carbohydrate per kg body weight for women and 8-10 g carbohydrate per kg body weight for men. Male athletes consuming more than 3500 kcal per day should be able to consume 500-600 g carbohydrate/d. Smaller individuals or those who need fewer calories may find it impossible to consume this much carbohydrate postexercise. A diet providing 6-8 g per kg body weight should be adequate for glycogen replacement for these people.

- If you need a more specific post-exercise recommendation based on body size, try the following: feed approximately 1.5 g of carbohydrate per kg body weight the first hour after exercise. For a 176-lb (80-kg) man this would be approximately 120 g of carbohydrate; for a 121-lb (55-kg) woman, it would be 83 g. Follow the above guidelines for the recommended 24-h carbohydrate intake.

- Within the first 6 h after exercise, high glycemic index foods or simple carbohydrates (glucose, sucrose, maltodextrin) provide the best glycogen replacement. These types of foods increase insulin levels in the blood, which stimulate both glucose transport into the cells and glycogen resynthesis.

- Provide a carbohydrate replacement beverage containing 70-90 g of carbohydrate (Gatorlode, Exceed High Carbohydrate Source) immediately after exercise if athletes are eating self-selected diets, are unable to eat within 2 h, or do not feel hungry after strenuous exercise. The beverage should provide enough additional carbohydrate to replace muscle glycogen when added to the carbohydrate consumed in the self-selected diet. This recommendation is very useful to coaches or trainers who have little control over athletes' diets, as it promotes adequate glycogen replacement even if athletes have poor diets.

- Consider individual athletes' dietary preferences. You can set carbohydrate recommendations and goals, but they will not be achieved if they do not fit well into an individual's daily diet. Your recommendations must be acceptable to the athletes' time and money constraints as well as their cooking abilities. Great diet plans are useless if they are not implemented.

Muscle Glycogen Supercompensation

Many endurance athletes know the benefits of maximizing muscle glycogen levels before an exercise event to help prevent fatigue. This practice is called **muscle glycogen supercompensation** or **glycogen loading.** Bergstrom et al. (1967) first introduced the concept of glycogen loading in 1967 with their "classical" routine, which began 1 week before an endurance exercise event (see figure 2.16). On the first 3 d, athletes ate a low-carbohydrate diet (<10% of energy from carbohydrate) and performed a glycogen depleting exercise. This was followed by 3 d of a high-carbohydrate diet (>90% of energy from carbohydrate) with little or no activity. This routine supercompensated the muscles with glycogen and water in preparation for the exercise event that occurred on the seventh day. Because of the adverse side effects associated with this routine (increased risk of injury, irritability, decreased ability to train, dizziness, fluid loss), Sherman and Costill (1984) modified it. In this routine the athletes consumed a modified carbohydrate diet (50% of energy from carbohydrate, 353 g carbohydrate/3000 kcal) for 3 d, performing a more tapered exercise protocol; then came 3 d of high-carbohydrate intake (70% of energy from carbohydrate, 542 g carbohydrate/3000 kcal) and little or no exercise. As with the classical routine, this routine supercompensated the muscles with glycogen and water for the exercise event on the seventh day. Figure 2.16 compares the modified with the classical glycogen-loading regime. Both provide similar amounts of muscle glycogen replacement. The modified routine is easier for athletes to follow, however, since eating either an extremely high- or low-carbohydrate diet can be difficult—especially if they are eating meals away from home. The modified routine can also reduce the risk of injury during the first 3 d of the regimen since it does not totally deplete the athlete of glycogen.

Athletes can maximize muscle glycogen loading by ingesting high-carbohydrate foods or liquid carbohydrate supplements made of maltodextrin (Lamb et al. 1991) during their training period or during the taper period before competition. One advantage of using a liquid carbohydrate supplement is that it may produce less gastrointestinal distress than extreme high-carbohydrate diets (80-90% of

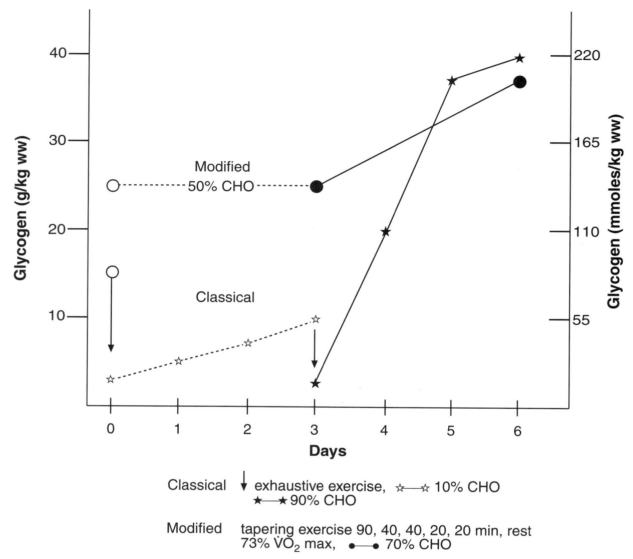

Figure 2.16 Schematic representation of the "classical" regimen of muscle glycogen supercompensation described by Scandinavian investigators; and the "modified" regimen of muscle glycogen supercompensation, which elevates muscle glycogen stores to comparably high levels with normal diets and a tapering sequence of exercise.

Reprinted from Sherman and Costill 1984.

___

energy from carbohydrate) derived solely from food.

Maximizing muscle glycogen levels before an endurance exercise event (>2 h) may improve performance (Karlsson and Saltin 1971), power, output, and speed (Rauch et al. 1995). High initial levels of muscle glycogen appear to increase endurance by postponing muscle glycogen depletion rather than by sparing liver glycogen (Bosch et al. 1993). An example of how maximizing muscle glycogen can improve work performance was demonstrated by

Rauch et al. (1995) in a study using eight well-trained male endurance cyclists (mean peak VO_2 = 66.3 ml/kg/min). Subjects were randomly assigned to one of two experimental treatments (carbohydrate loading or normal carbohydrate) for 3 d before exercise. They then performed a 2-h submaximal ride (~75% VO_2 peak) with five 60-s sprints (100% VO_2 peak) at 20-min intervals. This was then followed by a 60-min performance ride. Order of treatment was randomly assigned, and all subjects completed both treatments with a 4-

d rest period between each. The carbohydrate-loading trial provided a mean carbohydrate intake of 10.5 g per kg body weight per day, while the normal carbohydrate trial provided 6.2 g. The carbohydrate-loading trial also provided significantly more energy (4283 kcal/d) than the normal carbohydrate trial (3045 kcal/d). The carbohydrate-loading trial significantly increased mean power output (W) by 6% and speed (km/hr) by 3% compared with the normal carbohydrate trial. Simonsen et al. (1991) observed similar results: athletes with higher muscle glycogen levels exhibited significantly improved exercise performance compared to those with lower muscle glycogen levels (figure 2.13, page 44).

It should be noted that glycogen loading before exercise does not always improve performance. Some athletes experience extreme gastrointestinal distress, including diarrhea, when attempting this procedure. Because leg muscles become heavier with the addition of extra glycogen and water, many athletes complain that they feel heavy and sluggish, and may experience a slight weight gain. Athletes should experiment with glycogen loading during practice before trying it for competitions.

Chapter in Review

Carbohydrate is an important component in the diets of active individuals because it is required for glycogen synthesis and for the maintenance of blood glucose levels during exercise. During intense exercise training, the diet should provide the following level of carbohydrate:

- 8-10 g of carbohydrate per kg body weight for men
- 6-8 g of carbohydrate per kg body weight for women

This level of carbohydrate should be adequate to replace muscle glycogen and help to optimize exercise performance. In addition, carbohydrate feedings before and during exercise help improve performance and prevent fatigue, especially in endurance events lasting longer than 1 h. During exercise, carbohydrate-containing drinks providing a 6-8% concentration will provide optimal gastric emptying and absorption. Finally, carbohydrate or glycogen loading before an endurance event lasting longer than 2 h may help reduce fatigue and improve exercise performance and mood.

KEY CONCEPTS

1. Describe the function, classification, and dietary sources of carbohydrate.

Carbohydrate is a primary energy source during exercise, is required for glycogen replacement, and helps maintain blood glucose levels during exercise. Dietary carbohydrates can be classified based on the type of carbohydrate in the food (starch, sugar, or fiber content), how the carbohydrate has been processed, or the glycemic index of the carbohydrate. Complex carbohydrates are higher in starch than simple carbohydrates, which contain more sugar. Carbohydrate foods such as whole grains, breads, cereals, fruits, and vegetables contain more vitamins, minerals, and fiber than carbohydrate foods high in simple sugars (candy, desserts, soda). The glycemic index of a carbohydrate food is determined by measuring the body's glycemic response to the carbohydrate when it is eaten. Foods with a high glycemic index cause a greater rise in blood glucose than foods with a low glycemic index.

2. Discuss carbohydrate metabolism during exercise.

Muscles require carbohydrate as a fuel source during exercise. This carbohydrate will come from exogenous (diet) and/or endogenous (gluconeogenesis and glycogenolysis) sources. The amounts and sources of carbohydrate used during exercise depend on the intensity and duration of the exercise, the athlete's fitness level and overall health, how well fed the athlete is before exercise, and the environmental temperature and conditions. The amount of gluconeogenesis that occurs during exercise depends on the carbohydrate reserves, the amount of carbohydrate provided before and during exercise, and the intensity and duration of the exercise.

3. Discuss carbohydrate reserves and dietary intake.

The body's carbohydrate reserves are primarily in liver and muscle glycogen. The amount of glycogen in each of these pools is limited and will provide <2000 kcal, depending on the level of carbohydrate in the diet, the size of the individual, and total energy intake. Activities that are high in intensity and longer in duration use more glycogen than low-intensity exercise. Although high-carbohydrate diets (60% of energy) are generally recommended for athletes, especially endurance athletes, most athletes consume between 45-55% of their energy from carbohydrate. It is more practical to make carbohydrate recommendations based on body size than on percent of energy from carbohydrate. During high-intensity training, make carbohydrate recommendations of 2.7-3.6 g/lb (6-8 g/kg) for women and 3.6-4.5 g/lb (8-10 g/kg) for men.

4. Describe recommendations for carbohydrate feeding before exercise.

The goal of the pre-exercise meal is to promote additional glycogen synthesis, supply the body with glucose for use during exercise, and to help minimize fatigue during exercise. The pre-exercise meal is usually fed 2-6 h before exercise, provides ~200-300 g of carbohydrate, is moderate in protein, and is low in fat and fiber. The meal should be easy to digest, familiar to the athlete, and should not cause GI distress. If food cannot be consumed before exercise, carbohydrate-containing sport beverages are easy to digest and will provide the needed energy.

5. Describe recommendations for carbohydrate feeding during exercise.

Carbohydrate feeding during exercise complements the body's own carbohydrate reserves by providing additional carbohydrate to the working muscles and by helping maintain blood glucose levels—both of which may diminish fatigue. Carbohydrate feeding during exercise should begin early in the exercise event to ensure that adequate carbohydrate is available during the later stages of exercise. Athletes generally should consume ~30-60 g of carbohydrate per hour during exercise. This can be provided by a sport beverage containing 60-80 g of carbohydrate per liter, if athletes consume 4-6 oz of this fluid every 15-20 min. If you use body weight to determine carbohydrate intake, feed ~0.05-0.1 g/lb body weight (0.1-0.2 g/kg) every 20-30 min.

6. Describe carbohydrate feeding recommendations for post-exercise and during training periods.

The purpose of the post-exercise feeding period is to replenish muscle glycogen and refuel the body for the next exercise event. The type and amount of carbohydrate fed depends on how soon the next exercise event occurs. How quickly the body replaces muscle glycogen depends on the level of muscle glycogen depletion, the degree to which insulin activates glycogen synthase, and the carbohydrate content of the post-exercise diet. In general, athletes should consume 100-150 g of carbohydrate during the first hour after exercise; within the following 24 h women should consume 2.7-3.6 g of carbohydrate per lb (6-8 g/kg), and men 3.6-4.5 g/lb (8-10 g/kg).

7. Explain the concept of muscle glycogen supercompensation (glycogen-loading).

Athletes can maximize muscle glycogen levels before exercise by following dietary and exercise practices that promote muscle glycogen loading. The glycogen-loading routine is followed for 6 d before competition, with competition occurring on the seventh day. It is now recommended that athletes follow a modified glycogen-loading routine in which they eat a diet containing 55% of the energy from carbohydrate for 3 d while performing a tapered exercise protocol. For the next 3 d, they should consume a high-carbohydrate diet (70% of energy) and do little or no exercise. Exercise competition occurs on the seventh day.

KEY TERMS

complex carbohydrates	glycogen loading
Cori cycle	glycogenolysis
gluconeogenesis	glycogen synthase
glucose-alanine cycle	glycolysis
glycemic index	hypoglycemia
glycemic response	muscle glycogen supercompensation
glycogen	simple carbohydrates

References

Adopo E, Peronnet F, Massicotte D, Brisson GR, Hillaire-Marcel C. Respective oxidation of exogenous glucose and fructose given in the same drink during exercise. J Appl Physiol 1994;76:1014-9.

Ahlborg G. Mechanism for glycogenolysis in nonexercising human muscle during and after exercise. Am J Physiol 1985; 248(Endocrinol Metab 11):E540-5.

Ahlborg G, Felig P. Lactate and glucose exchange across the forearm, legs, and splanchnic bed during and after prolonged leg exercise. J Clin Invest 1982;69:45-54.

Alberici JC, Farrell PA, Kris-Etherton PM, Shively CA. Effects of preexercise candy bar ingestion on glycemic response, substrate utilization, and performance. Int J Sport Nutr 1993;3:323-33.

Baker SK, Rusynyk T, Tiidus PM. Immediate post-training carbohydrate supplementation improves subsequent performance in trained cyclists. Sports Med Training Rehab 1994;5:131-5.

Below PR, Coyle EF. Fluid and carbohydrate ingestion individually benefit intense exercise lasting one-hour. Med Sci Sports Exerc 1995;27:200-10.

Bergstrom J, Hermansen L, Hultman E, Saltin B. Diet, muscle glycogen and physical performance. Acta Physiol Scand 1967;71:140-50.

Blom PCS, Hostmark AT, Vaage O, Kardel KR, Maehlum S. Effect of different post-exercise sugar diets on the rate of muscle glycogen synthesis. Med Sci Sports Exerc 1987; 19:491-6.

Bogardus C, LaGrange BM, Horton ES, Sims EAH. Comparison of carohydrate-containing and carbodydrate-restricted hypocaloric diets in the treatment of obesity. J Clin Invest 1981;68:399-404.

Bonen A, Ness GW, Belcastro AN, Kirby RL. Mild exercise impedes glycogen repletion in muscle. J Appl Physiol 1985;58:1622-9.

Bosch AN, Dennis SC, Noakes TD. Influence of carbohydrate loading on fuel substrate turnover and oxidation during prolonged exercise. J Appl Physiol 1993;74:1921-7.

Bosch AN, Dennis SC, Noakes TD. Influence of carbohydrate ingestion on fuel substrate turnover and oxidation during prolonged exercise. J Appl Physiol 1994;76:2364-72.

Bosch AN, Noakes TD, Dennis S. Carbohydrate ingestion during prolonged exercise: a liver glycogen sparing effect in glycogen loaded subjects. Med Sci Sports Exerc 1991; 23:S152.

Brooks GA, Fahey TD, White TP. Exercise Physiology. 2nd ed. Mountain View, CA: Mayfield Publishing Company, 1995.

Burke LM, Collier GR, Beasley SK, et al. Effect of co-ingestion of fat and protein with carbohydrate feedings on muscle glycogen storage. J Appl Physiol 1995;78:2187-92.

Burke LM, Collier GR, Davis PG, Fricker PA, Sanigorski AJ, Hargreaves M. Muscle glycogen storage after prolonged exercise: effect of the frequency of carbohydrate feeding. Am J Clin Nutr 1996;64:115-9.

Burke LM, Collier GR, Hargreaves M. Muscle glycogen storage after prolonged exercise: effect of the glycemic index of carbohydrate feeding. J Appl Physiol 1993;75:1019-23.

Burke LM, Collier GR, Hargreaves M. Glycemic Index —a new tool in sport nutrition? Inter J Sport Nutr 1999;8:401-15.

Champe PC, Harvey RA. Lippincott's Illustrated Reviews: Biochemistry. Philadelphia, PA: JB Lippincott Company, 1994.

Coggan AR, Coyle EF. Reversal of fatigue during prolonged exercise by carbohydrate infusion or ingestion. J Appl Physiol 1987;63:2388-95.

Coggan AR, Coyle EF. Metabolism and performance following carbohydrate ingestion late in exercise. Med Sci Sports Exerc 1989; 21:59-65.

Coggan AR, Coyle EF. Carbohydrate ingestion during prolonged exercise: effects on metabolism and performance. Exerc Sport Sci Rev 1991;19:1-40.

Coyle EF. Substrate utilization during exercise in active people. Am J Clin Nutr 1995; 61(suppl):968S-79S.

Coyle EF, Coggan AR, Hemmert MK, Ivy JL. Muscle glycogen utilization during prolonged strenuous exercise when fed carbohydrate. J Appl Physiol 1986;61(1):165-72.

Coyle EF, Hamilton MT, Alonso JG, Montain SJ, Ivy JL. Carbohydrate metabolism during intense exercise when hyperglycemic. J Appl Physiol 1991;72:834-40.

Cummings JH, Englyst HN. Gastrointestinal effects of food carbohydrates. Am J Clin Nutr 1995;61(suppl):938S-45S.

Devlin JT, Calles-Escandon J, Horton ES. Effects of preexercise snack feeding on endurance cycle exercise. J Appl Physiol 1986; 60:980-5.

Doyle AJ, Sherman WM, Strauss RL. Effects of eccentric and concentric exercise on muscle glycogen replenishment. J Appl Physiol 1993;74(4):1848-55.

Energy Bars and Gels. SCAN's Pulse 1997; 16(3):13.

Erickson MA, Schwartzkopf RJ, McKenzie RD. Effects of caffeine, fructose, and glucose ingestion on muscle glycogen utilization during exercise. Med Sci Sports Exerc 1987; 19:579-83.

Felig P, Cherif A, Minagawa A, Wahren J. Hypoglycemia during prolonged exercise in normal men. N Engl J Med 1982;306:896-900.

Felig P, Wahren J. Amino acid metabolism in exercising man. J Clin Invest 1971;50:2703-14.

Fielding RA, Costill DL, Fink WJ, King DS, Hargreaves M, Kovaleski JE. Effect of carbohydrate feeding frequencies and dosage on muscle glycogen use during exercise. Med Sci Sports Exerc 1985;17:472-6.

Flatt JP. Use and storage of carbohydrate and fat. Am J Clin Nutr 1995;61(suppl):952S-9S.

Flynn MG, Costill DL, Hawley JA, et al. Influence of selected carbohydrate drinks on cycling performance and glycogen use. Med Sci Sports Exerc 1987;19:37-40.

Foster-Powell K, Miller JB. International tables of glycemic indices. Am J Clin Nutr 1995; 62:871S-93S.

Hawley JA, Dennis SC, Lindsay FH, Noakes TD. Nutritional practices of athletes: are they suboptimal? J Sport Sci 1995;13:S75-S87.

Horowitz JP, Coyle EF. Metabolic responses to preexercise meals containing various carbohydrates and fat. Am J Clin Nutr 1993; 58:235-41.

Ivy JL, Katz AL, Cutler CL, Sherman WM, Coyle EF. Muscle glycogen synthesis after exercise: effect of time on carbohydrate ingestion. J Appl Physiol 1988;64:1480-5.

Ivy JL, Lee MC, Brozinick JT, Reed MJ. Muscle glycogen storage after different amounts of carbohydrate ingestion. Am J Physiol 1988; 65:2018-23.

Jenkins DG, Palmer J, Spillman D. The influence of dietary carbohydrate on performance of supramaximal intermittent exercise. Eur J Appl Physiol 1993;67:309-14.

Karlsson J, Saltin B. Diet, muscle glycogen, and endurance performance. J Appl Physiol 1971;31:203-6.

Lamb DR, Rinehardt KF, Bartels RL, Sherman WS, Snook JT. Dietary carbohydrate and intensity of interval swim training. Am J Clin Nutr 1990;52:1058-63.

Lamb DR, Snyder AC, Baur TS. Muscle glycogen loading with a liquid carbohydrate supplement. Int J Sport Nutr 1991:1:52-60.

Leatt PB, Jacobs I. Effect of glucose polymer ingestion on glycogen depletion during a soccer match. Can J Sports Sci 1989;14:112-6.

Manore MM. Chronic dieting in active women: what are the health consequences? Women Health Iss 1996;6:1-10.

Mason WL, McConell G, Hargreaves M. Carbohydrate ingestion during exercise: liquid vs. solid feedings. Med Sci Sports Exerc 1993; 25:966-9.

Massicotte D, Peronnet F, Brisson G, Bakkouch K, Hilliare-Marcel C. Oxidation of glucose polymer during exercise: comparison of glucose and fructose. J Appl Physiol 1989; 66:179-83.

Murdoch SD, Bazzarre TL, Snider IP, Goldfarb AH. Differences in the effects of carbohydrate food form on endurance performance to exhaustion. Int J Sport Nutr 1993;3:41-54.

Murray R. Fluid needs in hot and cold environments. Int J Sport Nutr 1995;5:S62-S73.

Murray R, Paul GL, Seifert JG, Eddy DE, Halaby GA. The effects of glucose, fructose, and sucrose ingestion during exercise. Med Sci Sports Exerc 1989;21:275-82.

Nehlig A, Debry G. Caffeine and sports activity: a review. Int J Sports Med 1994;15:215-23.

Neufer PD, Costill DL, Flynn MG, Kriwan JP, Mitchell JB, Houmard J. Improvements in exercise performance: effects of carbohydrate feedings and diet. J Appl Physiol 1987; 62:983-8.

Okano G, Takeda H, Morita I, Katoh M, Mu Z, Miyake S. Effect of pre-exercise fructose ingestion on endurance performance in fed men. Med Sci Sports Exerc 1988;20:105-9.

O'Keeffe KA, Keith RE, Wilson GD, Blessing DL. Dietary carbohydrate intake and endurance exercise performance in trained female cyclists. Nutr Res 1989;9:819-30.

Rauch LHG, Rodger I, Wilson GR, et al. The effects of carbohydrate loading on muscle glycogen content and cycling performance. Int J Sport Nutr 1995;5:25-36.

Reed MJ, Brozinick JT, Lee MC, Ivy JL. Muscle glycogen storage post-exercise: effect of mode of carbohydrate administration. J Appl Physiol 1989;66:720-6.

Reynolds RD, Leklem JE ed. Vitamin B-6: Its Role in Health and Disease. New York, NY: Alan R. Liss, 1985.

Sherman WM. Metabolism of sugar and physical performance. Am J Clin Nutr 1995; 62(suppl):228S-41S.

Sherman WM, Brodowicz G, Wright DA, Allen WK, Simonsen J, Dernback A. Effect of 4 h preexercise carbohydrate feedings on cycling performance. Med Sci Sports Exerc 1989; 21:598-604.

Sherman WM, Costill DL. The marathon: dietary manipulation to optimize performance. Am J Sports Med 1984;12:44-51.

Sherman WM, Doyle JA, Lamb DR, Strauss RH. Dietary carbohydrate, muscle glycogen, and exercise performance during 7 d of training. Am J Clin Nutr 1993;57:27-31.

Simonsen JC, Sherman WM, Lamb DR, Dernbach AR, Doyle AJ, Strauss R. Dietary carbohydrate, muscle glycogen and power output during rowing training. J Appl Physiol 1991;70:1500-5.

Tsintzas K, Liu R, Williams C, Campbell I, Gaitanos G. The effect of carbohydrate ingestion on performance during a 30-km race. Int J Sport Nutr 1993;3:127-39.

Tsintzas OK, Williams C, Wilson W, Burrin J. Influence of carbohydrate supplementation early in exercise on endurance running capacity. Med Sci Sports Exerc 1996;28:1373-9.

Wagenmakers AJM, Browns F, Saris WHM, Halliday D. Oxidation rates of orally ingested carbohydrates during prolonged exercise in men. J Appl Physiol 1993;75:2774-80.

Wolever TMS, Jenkins DJA, Jenkins AL, Josse RG. The glycemic index: methodology and clinical implications. Am J Clin Nutr 1991; 54:846-54.

Wright DA, Sherman WM, Dernback AR. Carbohydrate feedings before, during or in combination improve cycling endurance performance. J Appl Physiol 1991;71:1082-8.

Yaspelkis BB, Ivy JL. Effect of carbohydrate supplements and water on exercise metabolism in the heat. J Appl Physiol 1991; 71:680-7.

Zawadzki KM, Yaspelkis BB, Ivy JL. Carbohydrate-protein complex increases the rate of muscle glycogen storage after exercise. J Appl Physiol 1992;72:1854-9.

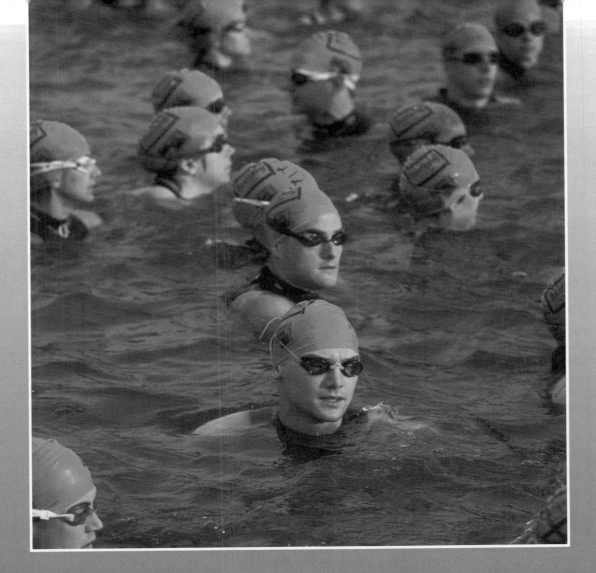

CHAPTER 3

Fat As a Fuel for Exercise

After reading this chapter you should be able to

- explain the functions, classifications, and dietary sources of fat;
- compare and contrast the current fat intake of active and inactive individuals;
- understand fat metabolism during exercise and the sources of this fat;
- identify factors that can enhance or inhibit fat oxidation during exercise; and
- discuss the current dietary fat recommendations for active individuals.

Although many people think of dietary fat as something to be avoided, fat is very important for athletic performance and good health. Fat and carbohydrate are the primary fuels used by the body during exercise. Both fuels are oxidized simultaneously, with the proportion of energy coming from each substrate dependent on the meal prior to exercise, the duration, intensity and type of exercise, and one's fitness level. Fat becomes the primary fuel source during endurance exercise events since the body's supply of carbohydrate in the form of glycogen and blood glucose is limited. Although diets high in carbohydrate are necessary to help replenish muscle glycogen levels after exercise, fat should not be eliminated from the diet. Research has helped us identify the best mix of dietary carbohydrate, fat, and protein for optimal exercise performance and good health. This mix may change slightly depending on individuals' personal food preferences and fitness levels, the sports they participate in, and their general health status—yet all macronutrients are important in the diet. For active people of all levels, it appears prudent to consume a diet high in carbohydrates, but also to include adequate amounts of protein and fat.

The 1995 U.S. Dietary Guidelines and the 1990 Nutrition Recommendations for Canadians encourages everyone to eat diets providing <30% of energy from fat. Because of the role carbohydrate plays in replenishing glycogen, athletes should consume less fat and more carbohydrate than sedentary individuals. Endurance athletes in training are often encouraged to eat moderate- to low-fat diets (20-25% of energy from fat), while athletes trying to lose weight (body fat) may be encouraged to obtain only ~20% of kcal from fat. But less is not always better. Low-fat foods are not always more nutritious. Ultralow-fat diets (≤15% of energy from fat) may not provide additional health or performance benefits over a moderate-fat diet and are usually very difficult to follow (Dreon et al. 1999; Lichtenstein and Van Horn 1998).

This chapter reviews the role of fat in the diet of athletes and active persons, and how fat is metabolized as an energy source during exercise. First, we discuss the function, classification, and dietary sources of fat, including the use of fat-modified foods. This is followed by discussion of the amount of fat typically consumed by all Americans and by active individuals. Next, we review fat metabolism during exercise and describe products and practices used to enhance fat oxidation during exercise. Finally, we provide dietary fat recommendations for active people.

Function, Classification, and Dietary Sources of Fat

Fat plays an important role in the diet of the physically active. It is a primary source of energy at rest and during exercise. It is twice as energy dense as carbohydrate or protein—providing 9 kcal/g, while carbohydrate and protein provide only 4 kcal/g. This means that 1 tbsp of butter or oil contains ~100 kcal, while it takes 4 cups of chopped broccoli or 1+ slices of whole wheat bread to provide 100 kcal from foods consisting primarily of carbohydrate. Fat also provides the essential fatty acids and fat-soluble vitamins (vitamins A, D, E, and K) our bodies need (see "Essential Fatty Acids," next page). The **essential fatty acids (linoleic and α-linolenic acid)** are the precursors for many regulatory compounds within the body, while fat-soluble vitamins are required for many essential metabolic processes (see chapters 10 and 13). Fats are part of the structural component of cell membranes, and part of brain and spinal cord tissue. They help keep the skin and other tissues soft and pliable. The body uses fat to store extra energy, which can be used to provide fuel to the working muscles. Fat stored as adipose tissue pads the body and protects the organs. Adipose tissue is also an efficient way to store extra energy in a small space. If all extra energy were stored as carbohydrate (stored glycogen), our bodies would be twice as large. Finally, we can't ignore the role fat plays in food preparation—fat tastes good! It makes our foods more palatable by adding texture and flavor. In summary, dietary fat is important for good health and for providing energy to the working muscles. It should not be eliminated from the diet, but used in moderation.

Fats or lipids are substances that are generally insoluble in water, but soluble in organic solvents (acetone or ether), and are very rich in methyl ($-CH_3$) or methylene ($-CH_2-$) groups (figure 3.1). That they do not mix well with water alters the way they are digested, absorbed, and transported in our bodies (as compared with protein and carbohydrate).

Dietary fats can be classified in a number of ways (see figure 3.1 and "Classification of Dietary Fats," page 66)—by their structure or chain length (number of carbons in each fatty

Essential Fatty Acids

As with essential vitamins and minerals, the body requires essential fatty acids for good health. Two essential fatty acids have been identified: **linoleic acid** (C18:2, n-6,9) and α-**linolenic acid** (C18:3, n-3,6,9). Linoleic is classified as an omega-6 or n-6 fatty acid, while α-linolenic acid is classified as an omega-3 or n-3 fatty acid. Linoleic acid occurs primarily in vegetable oils such as sunflower, safflower, corn, soy, and peanut oil; α-linolenic acid occurs mainly in leafy green vegetables, soy oil and other soy foods, seafood, and canola oil. Fish oils contain two n-3 fatty acids, **eicosapentaenoic acid (EPA)** and **docosahexaenoic acid (DHA),** that are metabolic derivatives of α-linolenic acid metabolism. Within the body, α-linolenic acid is metabolized to EPA and DHA. The essential fatty acids are required to make a family of hormone-like substances called eicosanoids, such as prostaglandins, thromboxanes, leukotrienes, and prostacyclins. These substances are important and potent mediators of many biochemical functions and play a critical role in coordinating a number of physiological functions—such as blood clotting, blood pressure, vascular dilation, heart rate, and immune response. Since essential fatty acids are necessary for the normal function of all tissue and cannot be synthesized in the body, deficiencies can develop. Some of the deficiency symptoms associated with poor essential fatty acid intakes are eczema, skin lesions, infertility, reduced growth, increased susceptibility to infection, and abnormal fetal growth and development (especially brain and retinal development) (Innis 1996; Linscheer and Vergroesen 1994). Dietary recommendations are for an upper limit of 2% of dietary energy from linoleic acid (n-6 fatty acid), and at least 1.3% of dietary energy (~3 g/d on a 2000-kcal diet) for α-linolenic, EPA, and DHA acids (n-3 fatty acids) (Simopoulos et al. 1999). Currently the consumption of n-3 fatty acids is very low (~0.15 g/d) in the United States (Harris 1997). Thus, one dietary goal should be to increase our intake of n-3 fatty acids, especially EPA and DHA, by incorporating more seafood into our diet. One problem with ultralow-fat diets is that, unless good food choices are made, they may not provide adequate amounts of the essential fatty acids, especially n-3 fatty acids. Table 3.1 lists various foods and the percentage of total fat kcal coming from omega-3 (n-3) and omega-6 (n-6) fatty acids. The following list provides you with the amount of n-3 fatty acids, primarily EPA and DHA, found in various foods, especially seafoods.

n-3 Fatty Acid Content Per Serving of Selected Foods

Food item	n-3 fatty acid (g/serving)
Tuna, light in water (3 oz, 85 g)	0.23 g
Canola oil (1 tbsp, 15 ml)	1.27 g
Salmon, smoked Chinook (3 oz, 85 g)	0.50 g
Salmon oil (fish oil) (1 tbsp, 15 ml)	4.39 g
Halibut, fillet baked (3 oz, 85 g)	0.58 g
Trout, rainbow fillet baked (3 oz, 85 g)	1.05 g
Shrimp, broiled (3 oz, 85 g)	1.11 g
Crab, Dungeness steamed (3 oz, 85 g)	0.34 g
Herring, Atlantic broiled (3 oz, 85 g)	1.52 g
Herring oil (1 tbsp, 15 ml)	1.52 g
Walnuts (1 tbsp, 15 ml)	0.51 g

1. Palmitic acid: satuated fatty acid (FA) with 16 carbons, no double bonds:

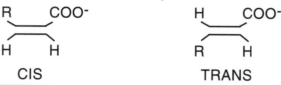

2. Oleic acid: Monounsaturated FA with 18 carbons; one double bond:

3. Sample structure of a triglyceride with a fatty acid (FA) attached at each carbon of the glycerol backbone.

C-FA (#1 position)

(#2 position)FA-C

C-FA (#3 position)

4. Example of a "cis" and a "trans" fatty acid:

CIS   TRANS

Figure 3.1 Structural differences between fatty acids (16-C saturated FA vs. 18-C monounsaturated FA). Example of a triglyceride (triacylglycerol–glycerol backbone with three FAs attached) and examples of the differences in shape between "cis" (H on same side) and "trans" (H on different sides) FAs. H = hydrogen; C = carbon; O = oxygen; FA = fatty acid; R = side chain of FA.

acid), by their level of saturation (number of hydrogen atoms attached to each carbon atom), by their shape, or by the commercial processing the fat has undergone (Grundy 1996). Chain length is important because it determines the method of digestion and absorption, the properties of the lipid, and its function within the body. Degree of fatty acid saturation also can determine function within the body, effect on health, and use within food products. The shape of a fatty acid can alter its characteristics and thus its function within the body: a fatty acid that has a *trans* configuration or shape will function differently from the same fatty acid with a *cis* configuration. For example, a *trans* fatty acid may have a negative effect on blood lipids, while the same fatty acid in the *cis* form does not. Finally, processing can change the saturation, chain length, and shape of fats. One of the most common fat processing methods is **hydrogenation** of oils, wherein the double bonds of fatty acids are broken and extra hydrogen is added, making the fat more saturated. This makes the fat more solid at room temperature and converts some *cis* fatty acids to *trans* fatty acids. Corn oil

margarine is an example of a partially hydrogenated fat—the double bonds found in the monounsaturated and polyunsaturated fatty acids in the corn oil are broken, and additional hydrogen is added. The more solid the form of margarine, the more hydrogenated the product. Thus, stick margarine has more highly saturated fat than tub or liquid margarine.

Dietary fat is found primarily in the form of **triacylglycerols** (frequently called triglycerides), where three **fatty acids** are attached to a **glycerol** backbone (figure 3.1). The fatty acids (FAs) can vary in chain length (the number of carbons) and in the degree of saturation. Food also contains other forms of lipids such as cholesterol, phospholipids, and sterols. In general, animal fats provide approximately 40-60% of their energy as saturated fats and 30-50% as monounsaturated and polyunsaturated fatty acids; fats from plants provide only 10-20% of their energy from saturated fatty acids with the rest monounsaturated and polyunsaturated. Table 3.1 lists examples of the primary fat-containing foods in our diet and the composition of the fat in these foods. For example, butter is considered a "saturated fat" because 65% of its fat is saturated; however, butter still contains some mono- and polyunsaturated fatty acids. Conversely, olive oil is considered "monounsaturated" because 74% of its fat is monounsaturated, yet it still contains some saturated and polyunsaturated FAs.

Fat-containing foods such as oils, butter, cream, margarine, or dressings (mayonnaise, salad dressings) are generally termed **visible fats** because almost 100% of the energy (kcal) in the food comes from fat (see table 3.1). These foods are frequently added as condiments to

prepared foods, such as butter on toast or mayonnaise on sandwiches, where consumers can clearly see that they are adding additional fat to their food. **Invisible fats** are those incorporated into prepared foods such as cookies, cakes, or casseroles, and are not easily discernible as fats. For example, croissants are much higher in fat (56% of kcal/serving from fat) than a slice of bread or a bagel (5-15% of kcal/serving from fat)—yet many consumers assume the fat content of these three "bread" foods are the same. The majority of the fat in most people's diets comes from invisible fat. Foods that can be high

Table 3.1 Composition of Common Fat-Containing Foods

Food	% Total kcal from fat	% Total fat kcal as omega-3 and -6	Distribution of fat by type		
			% Total fat kcal as SFAs	% Total fat kcal as MUFAs	% Total fat kcal as PUFAs
Butter	100	4	65	31	4
Milk, whole 3.3% fat	49	4	63	33	4
Milk, 2% fat	40	4	66	30	4
Milk, skim (nonfat)	4	>1	73	30	>1
Beef, ground 16% fat	54	4	45	51	4
Chicken, bonelesss	35	20	18	44	24
Turkey, boneless	26	28	32	25	35
Tuna, water packed	6	39	32	22	46
Tuna, oil packed	37	36	21	40	39
Salmon, Chinook	33	16	25	48	24
Egg, large	62	13	37	46	16
Canola oil	100	30	7	59	30
Safflower oil	100	74	9	12	74
Corn oil	100	60	13	25	60
Corn oil margarine	100	—	2	27	27
Sesame oil	100	42	15	42	44
Olive oil	100	10	14	74	10
Salmon oil (fish oil)	100	34	20	29	40
Cottonseed oil	100	50	26	20	52
Palm kernel oil	100	2	82	11	2
Coconut oil	100	2	87	6	2
Walnuts	86	63	10	23	64
Cashew nuts	72	17	20	59	17

SFAs = saturated fatty acids
MUFAs = monounsaturated fatty acids
PUFAs = polyunsaturated fatty acids

Data from Food Processor, Version 7.01, ESHA Research, Salem, OR.

■ HIGHLIGHT ■

Classification of Dietary Fats

Chain Length

Fatty acids come in various chain lengths. **Short-chain fatty acids (SCFAs)** are usually less than six carbons in length. **Medium-chain fatty acids (MCFAs)** are 6-12 carbons in length, while **long-chain fatty acids (LCFAs)** have 14 or more carbons. Chain length helps determine method of fat digestion, transport, and metabolism. SCFAs and MCFAs are digested and transported more quickly than LCFAs.

Saturation Level

A fatty acid is considered **saturated** (SFAs) if there are no double bonds in the fatty acids chain—all carbon atoms in the fatty acid chain have the maximum number of hydrogen atoms. **Monounsaturated** fatty acids (MUFAs) have one double bond, while **polyunsaturated** fatty acids (PUFAs) have more than one double bond (figure 3.1). Table 3.1 gives examples of various foods, and the distribution of fat kcal by SFAs, MUFAs, and PUFAs.

Shape

Fatty acids can be either *trans* or *cis*. These terms describe the positioning of the hydrogen atom around the double bond (figure 3.1). A *cis* fatty acid has both hydrogen atoms on the same side of the double bond. A *trans* fatty acid has the hydrogens attached to opposite sides of the double bond. *Cis* fatty acids are more common in nature, while *trans* fatty acids are rarely found in nature. Most of the *trans* fatty acids in the American diet are due to manipulation of fatty acids during food processing, such as the partial hydrogenation of vegetable oils. Thus, most margarine (excluding those that are not hydrogenated) has more *trans* fatty acids than butter. The health consequences of diets high in *trans* fatty acids have recently been questioned since research indicates that they can raise blood LDL-cholesterol levels (Grundy 1996) and increase the risk of coronary heart disease (FDA 1999).

Structure of Triacylglycerols

Fatty acids are attached to the glycerol backbone at one of three sites (figure 3.1). The type of fatty acids (either SFAs, MUFAs, PUFAs) attached at each of these sites determines how the fat is digested, absorbed, and transported.

---

in invisible fats are meat and meat products, dairy products, baked goods, and most convenience and fast foods.

Many similar foods are available with a wide range of fat contents. You can purchase full-fat, low-fat, or fat-free ice cream. The same is true for cookies. Table 3.2 lists a number of full-fat foods (the way the food was originally produced or found in nature) and their lower-fat alternatives. The latter products may significantly reduce the amount of fat in a person's diet, but do not always change total energy intake. For example, buying nonfat skim milk (86 kcal, 0.5 g of fat/8 oz serving) instead of whole milk (150 kcal, 8.2 g of fat/8 oz serving) will dramatically reduce both fat and energy intake; buying fat-free Fig Newton cookies (3 cookies = 204 kcal, 0 g fat) to replace regular Fig Newton cookies (3 cookies = 210 kcal, 4.5 g fat) reduces fat intake by 4.5 g per serving—but it does not significantly reduce energy intake.

Unfortunately many people think that, because a product is marked reduced-fat or fat-free, they can eat as much as they desire (the whole box instead of just two or three cookies). Since many active individuals choose to use reduced-fat products either for weight control or for health reasons, they should understand that, while total fat intake may decrease, energy intake may not (Callaway 1998). The Calo-

Table 3.2   Energy and Nutrient Composition of Full-Fat Products and Their Reduced- or Low-Fat Counterparts

Product	Serving size	Energy (kcal)	Protein (g)	Carbohydrate (g)	Fat (g)
Milk, whole (3.3% fat)	8 oz	150	8.0	11.4	8.2
Milk, 2% fat	8 oz	121	8.1	11.7	4.7
Milk, 1% fat	8 oz	102	8.0	11.7	2.6
Milk, skim (nonfat)	8 oz	86	8.4	11.9	0.5
Cheese, cheddar regular	1 oz	111	7.1	0.5	9.1
Cheese, cheddar low-fat	1 oz	81	9.1	0.0	5.1
Cheese, cheddar nonfat	1 oz	41	6.8	4.0	0.0
Mayonnaise, regular	1 tbsp	100	0.0	0.0	11.0
Mayonnaise, light	1 tbsp	50	0.0	1.0	5.0
Mayonnaise, fat-free	1 tbsp	10	0.0	2.0	0.0
Margarine, regular corn oil	1 tbsp	100	0.0	0.0	11.0
Margarine, reduced-fat	1 tbsp	60	0.0	0.0	7.0
Peanut butter, regular	1 tbsp	95	4.1	3.1	8.2
Peanut butter, reduced-fat	1 tbsp	81	4.4	5.2	5.4
Cream cheese, soft regular	1 tbsp	50	1.0	0.5	5.0
Cream cheese, soft light	1 tbsp	35	1.5	1.0	2.5
Cream cheese, soft nonfat	1 tbsp	15	2.5	1.0	0.0
Crackers, Wheat Thins regular	18 crackers	158	2.3	21.4	6.8
Crackers, Wheat Thins reduced-fat	18 crackers	120	2.0	21.0	4.0
Cookies, Oreo regular	3 cookies	160	2.0	23.0	7.0
Cookies, Oreo reduced-fat	3 cookies	130	2.0	25.0	3.5
Cookies, Fig Newton regular	3 cookies	210	3.0	30.0	4.5
Cookies, Fig Newton fat-free	3 cookies	204	2.4	26.8	0.0
Breakfast bars, regular	1 bar	140	2.0	27.0	2.8
Breakfast bars, fat-free	1 bar	110	2.0	26.0	0.0

The Food and Drug Administration and the U.S. Department of Agriculture have set specific regulations on allowable product descriptions for reduced-fat products. The following claims are defined for one serving: Fat-free—less than 0.5 g of fat; Low-fat—3 g or less of fat; Reduced- or less fat—at least 25% less fat as compared to a standard serving; Light—one-third fewer calories or 50% less fat as compared with standard serving size.
Data from Food Processor, Version 7.01, ESHA Research, Salem, OR.

rie Control Council (Atlanta, GA) has been studying U.S. dieting trends for 20 years. Their 1998 National Consumer Survey asked adults about their regular use (at least once every 2 weeks) of fat-modified foods. The results of the survey follow. The reduced-fat products are listed in descending order, with the most popular products listed first. The percentage of consumers who reported using the product at least once every 2 weeks appears in parentheses:

- Skim or low-fat milk (62%)
- Reduced-fat salad dressings, sauces, or mayonnaise (56%)
- Reduced-fat cheese/dairy products (50%)
- Reduced-fat margarine (44%)
- Reduced-fat chips/snack foods (40%)
- Reduced-fat meat products (39%)
- Reduced-fat ice cream/frozen desserts (36%)
- Reduced-fat cakes/baked goods (32%)
- Reduced-fat dinner entrees (30%)
- Reduced-fat candy (18%)

It is estimated that there are over 5000 different fat-modified foods on the market

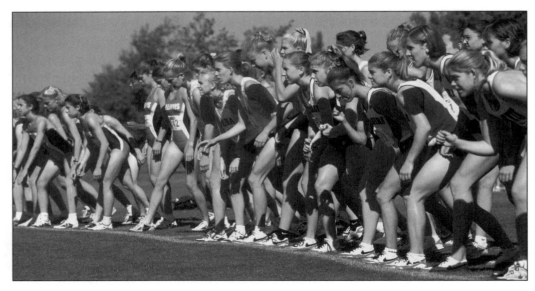

Endurance exercise uses stored fat in the muscles and the adipose tissue as an energy source.

(Callaway 1998; Sigman-Grant 1997); however, the degree to which these foods are used by consumers varies dramatically. Consumers appear more likely to use a reduced-fat version of a full-fat product (like milk) where only the fat has been removed, than to replace a full-fat snack (cookie or chips) with a lower-fat alternative in which a fat substitute or a fat replacer may have been used. Fat substitutes and fat replacers are now found in a number of foods, especially snack foods. Appendix B.2 describes the most common fat replacers used in the United States. Some of these products, such as olestra (brand name Olean), may cause gastrointestinal distress if used in large quantities. Since fat substitutes are new to the U.S. marketplace, the effect they will have on total fat intake and on the reduction of obesity and cardiovascular disease has yet to be seen.

Body Fat Reserves and Dietary Fat Intake

During exercise, the primary energy sources are carbohydrate (glucose) and fat (fatty acids). The relative amounts used of each depend on factors such as exercise intensity and duration, level of physical fitness, and composition of the meal prior to exercise. Compared to protein and carbohydrate stores, the body's fat reserves are almost unlimited. Table 3.3 gives an estimate of the amount of total fat and carbohydrate stored within a 176-lb (80-

kg) man. The total amount of energy stored as fat will varies with an individual's size and percentage of body fat. For example, a man weighing 176 lb (80 kg) with 15% body fat would have approximately 26 lb (~12 kg) of total body fat or ~100,000 kcal of energy stored as fat. Of course, not all of this fat would be available for energy since 3-4% of body fat is biologically essential and incorporated into cell membranes and tissues. Since women typically have higher amounts of body fat than men, their amount of stored energy is usually higher, even though body weight is less. A woman weighing 130 lb (59 kg) with 24% body fat would have approximately 31 lb (~14 kg) of body fat, representing ~110,000 kcal of stored energy. Thus, even though the female is on average 46 lb (21 kg) lighter than her male counterpart, she has more stored energy as fat. If we consider that a 130-lb (59-kg) woman may require ~100 kcal to run one mile at a moderate pace, this amount of stored fat would be enough for more than 1000 mi! In addition to adipose tissue fat (subcutaneous fat and deep visceral fat), the body also stores fat within the muscle as intramuscular triacylgly-cerol. The amount of fat stored here is difficult to estimate and varies with fitness level, daily training time, and dietary fat intake; but it appears that even lean people have plenty of stored energy in the form of adipose tissue. Therefore, dietary recommendations to active people usually focus on making sure the diet has adequate fat to replace muscle triacylgly-cerol stores and to meet energy and

Table 3.3 **Estimated Energy Stores of Fat and Carbohydrate in a 176-lb (80-kg) Man With 15% Body Fat**

Substrate		Weight (kg)	Energy (kcal)
Carbohydrates	Plasma glucose	0.02	78
	Liver glycogen	0.1	388
	Muscle glycogen	0.4	1550
	Total (approximately)	0.52	2000
Fat	Plasma fatty acid	0.0004	4
	Plasma triacylglycerols	0.004	39
	Adipose tissue	12.0	100,000
	Intramuscular triacylglycerols	0.3	2616
	Total (approximately)	12.3	106,500

Values given are estimates for a "normal" man of 176-lb (80-kg) and 15% body fat and not those of an athlete, who might be leaner and have more stored glycogen. The amount of protein in the body is not mentioned but this would be about 22 lb (10 kg, 40,000 kcal), mainly located in the muscles.

Adapted from Jeukendrup, Saris, and Wagenmakers 1998.

essential fatty acid requirements—but is not excessive. On rare occasions, fat may be consumed during exercise to supplement these reserves. We discuss the pros and cons of this practice later in this chapter.

Dietary Fat Intake in the United States

There appears to be a strong link between high dietary fat intake and risks of obesity, coronary heart disease, and some forms of cancer. Because of these links, the United States and Canadian governments formulated the 1995 Dietary Guidelines for Americans and the 1990 Nutrition Recommendations for Canadians. One recommendation in these documents is the reduction of total fat intake to <30% of total energy intake, and that saturated fat should be limited to <10% of total energy intake. Nutritionists have been recommending the reduction of dietary fat for a decade. Based on the most recent U.S. governmental data, it appears that *relative fat intake (% of energy from fat) has decreased from 45% in 1965 to 34% in 1995 for both men and women* (figure 3.2). However, total fat consumption (g/d) does not appear to be decreasing. As table 3.4 demonstrates, total fat consumption decreased in the 1960s and 70s but has been relatively constant since 1989. How can relative fat intake decrease while absolute fat intake remains the same? Figures

Table 3.4 **Average Total Fat Consumption in the United States: Individuals 19 to 50 Years of Age**

Years	Men	Women
	Grams per day	
1965	139	83
1977-78	113	73
1989	96	62
1990	89	64
1991	100	62
1994	101	62
1995	101	65

Reprinted from USDA Center for Nutrition Policy and Promotion (CNPP) 1998.

3.3 and 3.4 provide the answer: *total energy intake has increased in both men and women over the last 5-10 years.* For example, for men there was a 13% increase in fat intake from 1990 (89 g/d) to 1995 (101 g/d) (table 3.4), but a 21% increase in energy intake. Increasing energy intake (kcal/d) will reduce the percentage of kcal from fat even if absolute fat intake does not change (USDA 1998). "How Can One's

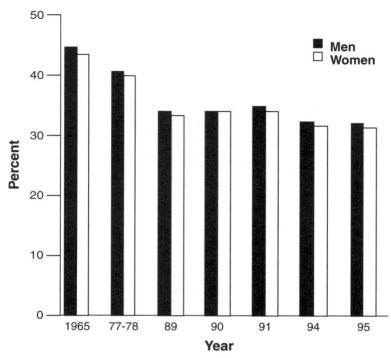

Figure 3.2 Percentage of calories (kcal) from total fat: individuals 19 to 50 years of age. Reprinted from USDA (CNPP) 1998.

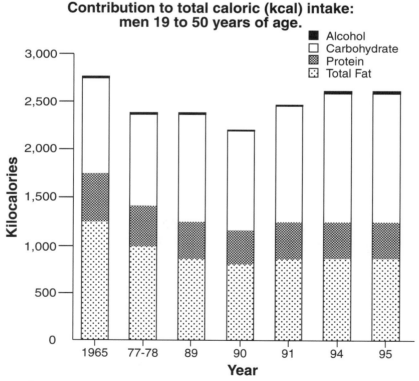

Figure 3.3 Contribution of total caloric (kcal) intake: men 19 to 50 years of age. Total caloric intake, as well as calories from fat, decreased between 1965 and 1990. Total caloric intake began to increase relatively more than the increase in calories from fat between 1991 and 1995.

Reprinted from USDA (CNPP) 1998.

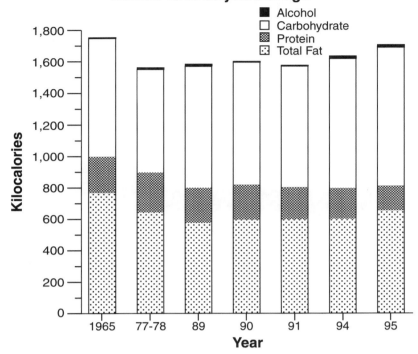

Contribution to total caloric (kcal) intake: women 19 to 50 years of age

Figure 3.4 Contribution of total caloric (kcal) intake: women 19 to 50 years of age. Total caloric intake, as well as calories from fat, decreased between 1965 and 1989. Total caloric intake increased between 1990 and 1995, whereas calories from fat consumption remained at a steady level.

Reprinted from USDA (CNPP) 1998.

Percentage of Energy From Fat Decrease While Absolute Fat Intake Increases?" (page 72) shows calculations that demonstrate the point made in figures 3.3 and 3.4. Many Americans have not reached the recommended fat goal of <30% of total energy intake from fat.

At the same time that percentage of energy from fat is declining, Americans appear to be getting fatter. A variety of factors contribute to obesity in any one person; high dietary fat intake is but one of many contributing factors, along with physical inactivity and overconsumption of energy (Prentice 1998). One cannot assume that only one factor is causing the rise of obesity in the United States. Obesity is a gradual problem that develops over years or decades. Once people become obese, there appear to be powerful metabolic forces that act to maintain the increased body weight. It is difficult to pinpoint a single factor as the major cause of our growing obesity. Obesity is a multifaceted problem that involves the interactive forces of genetics, physiology, metabolism, and the environment. (See chapter 5 on energy balance for more information about factors contributing to obesity.)

Dietary Fat Intake of Active Individuals

Although active individuals and athletes typically self-report carbohydrate intakes to be approximately 45-55% of energy intake, intakes of fat are much more variable depending on the sport and gender of the athlete. Athletes typically report consuming about 35% of their energy from fat (Hawley et al. 1995). However, athletes in endurance sports, such as runners, cyclists, or cross-country skiers, report lower fat intakes and higher carbohydrate intakes than sprinters and field event athletes (Fogelholm et al. 1992; Hawley et al. 1995; Saris et al. 1989). For example, Saris and colleagues monitored the energy and food intake of five male cyclists during the 22-d race of the Tour de France. Mean energy intake during the race was 5880 kcal/d, with 62% of the energy from carbohydrate, 15% from protein, and 23% from fat.

Athletes who are concerned about weight, or who participate in sports where they are required to "weigh in," have lower fat intakes—especially during periods of energy restriction. For example, Fogelholm and colleagues (1993) examined the diets of wrestlers and judo

How Can One's Percentage of Energy From Fat Decrease While Absolute Fat Intake Increases?

Here is a sample calculation to demonstrate how percentage of energy intake from fat can decrease while absolute total fat intake increases:

Example 1: A diet contains 2250 kcal/d, with 36% of energy coming from fat (90 g of fat/d); the rest of the energy is obtained from protein (15%, 84 g/d) and carbohydrate (49%, 276 g/d).

Example 2: Now increase the diet in example 1 by 300 kcal/d (9 g fat, 12 g protein, 49 g carbohydrate), for a total energy intake of 2550 kcal/d. This diet obtains 34% of its energy from fat (96 g of fat/d), with the rest obtained from protein (15%, 96 g/d) and carbohydrate (51%, 325 g/d).

Notice how the percentage of energy coming from fat has decreased (from 36% to 34%), but *the absolute amount of fat increased* (90 g/d to 96 g/d). This same scenario appears to be taking place in the United States. *Total energy intake is increasing, along with absolute intakes of fat,* but relative fat intake (% of energy from fat) is decreasing. Although at first glance it may appear that the American diet is improving, it is not. These dietary changes, combined with our abundance of good-tasting food and our inactivity, have contributed to increased obesity in the United States.

athletes at baseline and during gradual and rapid weight-loss regimens. The gradual weight-loss diet consisted of a 3-week period of diet restriction in which subjects reduced energy intake by 1000 kcal/d. The rapid weight-loss diet consisted of ~1400 kcal/d for 3 d. Figure 3.5 shows that both energy intake and the proportion of energy from fat decreased, while the proportion of energy from carbohydrate increased. Beals and Manore (1998) also reported that mean fat intake in female athletes with subclinical eating disorders (19% of energy intake, 43 g/d) was lower than that of control athletes (23% of energy intake, 61 g/d). Thus, if athletes are restricting energy intake, distribution of energy as carbohydrate, fat, and protein often compares favorably with recommended intakes; yet total energy intake is too low to maintain body weight and rigorous physical activity. Examination of an athlete's diet requires determining total energy intake and distributing energy from each of the macronutrients.

Fat Metabolism During Exercise

After reading chapter 2 on carbohydrates, one might feel there is little room for fat in the diet of an athlete or an active individual. Yet fat is a major energy source during exercise, and the ability to mobilize and use stored fat during exercise can improve exercise performance. Fat can be mobilized from any of the following sources: muscle fat, adipose tissue fat, blood lipoproteins, or fat consumed during exercise. A number of factors determine the amount and the source of the fat utilized during exercise:

- Fitness level
- Type of exercise
- Intensity and duration of exercise
- Available fat reserves in the muscles
- Ability to mobilize and transport fatty acids from adipose tissue to muscles
- Composition of the meal prior to exercise
- Availability of stored carbohydrate or amount of carbohydrate fed during exercise

In the following sections we outline the metabolic processes that stimulate the breakdown, mobilization, and transport of fat from storage to the working muscle for energy during exercise. We also discuss availability of intramuscular fat for energy during exercise. We then briefly review the oxidation of fat within muscle

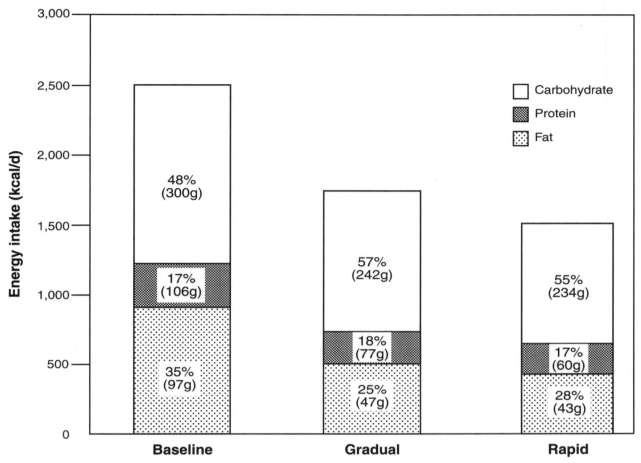

Figure 3.5 Daily energy intake and the proportion of dietary fat, protein, and carbohydrate for 10 male athletes (7 wrestlers, 3 judo athletes) during weight maintenance (baseline), and during both gradual and rapid weight reduction. Percentage of energy from protein, fat, and carbohydrate is indicated in each column.

Reprinted from Fogelholm et al. 1993.

and the numerous factors that can influence this process. Since we cannot discuss the biochemistry of fat metabolism in detail, we suggest these references as additional readings: Cortright et al. 1997; Jeukendrup, Saris, and Wagenmakers 1998a, b, c; Saltin and Åstrand 1993; Turcotte et al. 1995. Since the nomenclature used in discussing fat is frequently confusing, see "Fat and Fatty Acid Nomenclature" (page 74) for a review of terms.

Adipose Tissue Fat

Adipose tissue contains the largest reservoir of stored energy within the body. In order to use this fat as a fuel source during exercise, the body must mobilize and transport it to the working muscle. The use of fat during exercise involves numerous steps:

1. Breakdown of triacylglycerols to free fatty acids (FFAs) and glycerol
2. Mobilization and transport of FFAs within the fat cell
3. Transport of the FFAs out of the fat cell to the blood
4. Transport of the FFAs in the blood
5. Transport of the FFAs into the muscle cell
6. Transport of the FFAs to the muscle mitochondria
7. Oxidation to energy via the TCA cycle

Figure 3.6 illustrates lipolysis and mobilization within the fat cell, and the transport of fatty acids to the muscle cell for oxidation. The breakdown of fat in the adipose or muscle tissue to FFAs and glycerol occurs through a process call **lipolysis**. This metabolic process is

■ HIGHLIGHT ■

Fat and Fatty Acid Nomenclature

Fatty acids are stored in the body in the form of **triacylglycerol** or **triglycerides**, where three fatty acids are attached to a glycerol backbone. These fatty acids can vary in their level of saturation and length. If fatty acids are not esterified to form mono-, di-, or triacylglycerol, they are called nonesterified fatty acids or **free fatty acids (FFAs)**. However, the term FFA is sometimes ambiguous because the fatty acids found in the blood are frequently referred to as FFAs, when in actuality they are bound to albumin. There is a very small concentration of true (unbound) FFAs found in the plasma (< 0.01% of the plasma fatty acid pool) (Jeukendrup, Saris, and Wagenmakers 1998). Because FFAs are not soluble in water, they must be transported bound to some type of transport protein, both within the cell and across cell membranes. However, not all of these transport proteins or carriers have been identified for each step of the fat mobilization and oxidation process. Depending on the article you read, the exact method of FFA transport discussed may vary. Within this chapter, when FFAs are discussed it is assumed that they are not truly free, but bound to some type of transport protein or carrier. Review articles by Turcotte et al. (1995); Cortright et al. (1997); and Jeukendrup, Saris, and Wagenmakers (1998) discuss fatty acid transport proteins in more detail.

initiated when the sympathetic nervous system stimulates production of **hormone sensitive lipase (HSL)** and **epinephrine**. After exercise begins, blood concentrations of epinephrine rise—which in turn stimulate production of the phosphorylated (active) form of HSL in the adipose cell. HSL is activated when it is phosphorylated by a cyclic adenosine monophosphate (cAMP)-dependent protein kinase. This protein kinase is produced in the adipose cell when epinephrine binds to receptors on the cell membrane and activates adenyl cyclase (Champe and Harvey 1987). HSL splits off two of the fatty acids attached to the glycerol backbone of the triacylglycerol (fatty acids at positions 1 and 3), leaving a monoglyceride (glycerol with one fatty acid attached at position 2) (Turcotte et al. 1995). The final fatty acid is removed through the action of the enzyme **monoglyceride lipase (MGL).** Both enzymes, HSL and MGL, are needed for complete breakdown of the triacylglycerol. The end result of lipolysis is three FFA molecules and a glycerol molecule that must be transported across the adipose cell cytosol and the membrane into circulation. HSL is the rate-limiting step in this process; the activity of this enzyme depends on several inhibitory and stimulatory factors (Jeukendrup, Saris, and Wagenmakers 1998). These regulatory factors are discussed later.

The glycerol produced by lipolysis cannot be reused by the adipose tissue since the cell does not contain significant amounts of glycerol ki-

nase (Wolfe et al. 1990). Levels of glycerol in the blood are therefore an indirect measure of lipolysis, since one glycerol molecule is produced for each triacylglycerol broken down. Glycerol can then be transported to the liver where it is used as a gluconeogenic precursor.

The FFAs produced through lipolysis must either cross the adipose cell membrane passively or be transported out of the cell by a transport protein such as **fatty acid binding protein (FABP)** or **fatty acid translocase (FAT)** (Jeukendrup, Saris, and Wagenmakers 1998). FFAs released into the blood are bound to albumin and transported to the working muscles. These FFAs are eventually released from albumin and actively transported across the muscle membranes (Cortright et al. 1997; Turcotte et al. 1995). However, not all of the FFAs produced through lipolysis are used for energy. In the triacylglycerol-fatty acid cycle, FAs released during the process of lipolysis are re-esterified if they are not needed for energy. **Re-esterification** can occur within the adipose cell (intracellular recycling) or after the fatty acid is released from the adipose cell (extracellular recycling), in which case the fat is re-esterified elsewhere (e.g., the liver) (Wolfe et al. 1990). Thus, *if the fatty acids are not needed for energy, they can be re-esterified into triacylglycerols again, either in adipose tissue or in the liver.* At rest, re-esterification is high and blood concentrations of albumin-bound fatty acids are low. During exercise, re-esterifi-

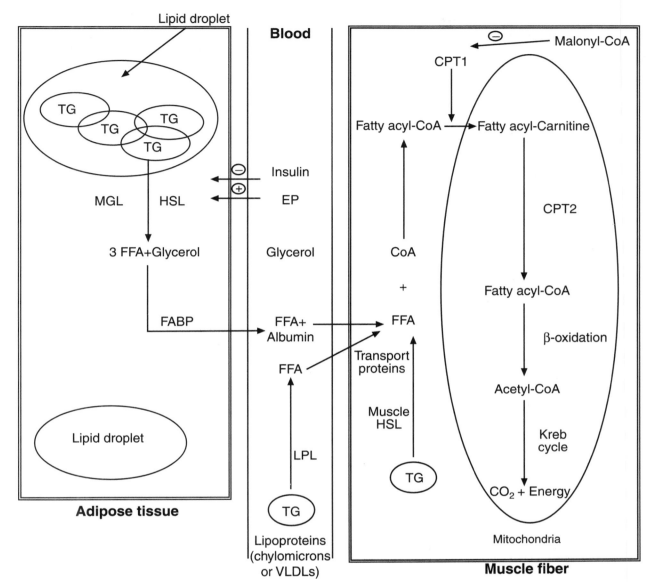

Figure 3.6 Mobilization and oxidation of fatty acids from adipose tissue, blood lipids, and intramuscular triglycerides. Adipose tissue: Hormone sensitive lipase (HSL) cleaves two fatty acids from the triglyceride (TG), while the final fatty acid is removed by the enzyme monoglyceride lipase (MGL). HSL is the rate-limiting step of lipolysis. Epinephrine (EP) stimulates production of active HSL, while insulin inhibits its production. The end product of this lipolysis is three free fatty acids (FFAs) and one glycerol molucule. The FFAs are transported from the adipose cell via fatty acid binding protein (FABP); a second protein-mediated transport system moves the FFA to the blood, where albumin transports the FFA to the muscle tissue. The FFA is then transported across the plasma membrane and into the muscle fiber via additional transport proteins. Glycerol can be transported to the liver for gluconeogenesis. Additional FFAs can be released from blood lipoproteins or from fat stored in the muscle fibers. The FFAs can now enter the mitochondria for β-oxidation. LPL = lipoprotein lipase; CPT1 = carnitine palmitoyl transferase 1; CPT2 = carnitine palmitoyl transferase 2; VLDL = very-low-density lipoprotein.

cation is suppressed at the same time that the rate of lipolysis is accelerated, and blood levels of FFAs bound to albumin increase dramatically (Jeukendrup and Saris 1998). Wolfe et al. (1990) measured re-esterification at rest and during 4 h of treadmill exercise at 40% $\dot{V}O_2$max. They found that 75% of the FAs were re-esterified at rest; but this value decreased to 25%

within the first 30 min of exercise and remained low throughout the exercise period.

Several factors affect the degree of re-esterification. Re-esterification increases if albumin is not available to transport the free fatty acids away from adipose cells. This may occur if blood levels of albumin are low (during periods of malnutrition or high blood loss), if blood flow through adipose tissue is decreased, or if available transport sites on albumin are full (Bulow and Madsen 1986). Each albumin molecule can bind only a finite number of FFAs; as albumin becomes saturated with FAs, there is less affinity for the acids (Bulow 1988). Thus, under any of the conditions described above, fewer FFAs are bound and transported away from the fat cell. High lactate levels also decrease FFA mobilization by increasing re-esterification without affecting lipolysis (Turcotte et al. 1995). During prolonged endurance exercise, however, lactate levels usually remain low and probably play a minimal role in regulating FFAs mobilization.

Effect of Exercise on Lipolysis

Exercise stimulates lipolysis sufficiently that the rate of lipolysis usually far exceeds the need for FAs for oxidation by the muscles. At rest, basal level of FFAs after a mixed diet will be ~0.2-0.4 mmol/L; while during exercise, arterial plasma FA concentrations can increase 10- to 20-fold over basal levels, depending on the exercise intensity and duration (Jeukendrup, Saris, and Wagenmakers 1998; Wolfe et al. 1990). Figure 3.7 shows the rate of appearance of FFAs and glycerol during 4 h of treadmill exercise at 40% of $\dot{V}O_2$max. The rate of FFA appearance rose dramatically (~sixfold) with even low-intensity exercise. The dramatic rise in glycerol appearance indicates an increase in lipolysis within fat cells during exercise. Respiratory exchange ratio also dropped over the 4-h period from 0.92 to 0.83, indicating an increase in fat oxidation (tenfold increase). Immediately after exercise stopped, almost 90% of the FAs released from lipolysis were re-esterified (Wolfe et al. 1990). This study clearly indicates that *the best way to mobilize and use stored fat for energy is to exercise.* Exercise is the greatest stimulator of fat lipolysis and oxidation currently available to the consumer; however, this stimulant cannot be purchased in a bottle.

Hormonal Control of Lipolysis

During exercise, a number of hormonal changes signal the body to break down stored energy to fuel the working muscles. These hormonal responses depend on a variety of factors including the intensity and duration of the exercise, level of physical fitness, and how recently food has been consumed.

The sympathetic nervous system and catecholamines are the strongest stimulators of lipolysis. Catecholamines stimulate the breakdown of both stored fat (both in adipose and muscle tissue) and carbohydrate (both liver and muscle glycogen), making these fuels available to the working muscles. Blood levels of the catecholamines norepinephrine and epinephrine rise dramatically within seconds of the initiation of exercise and activate cAMP—which then stimulates production of the active phosphorylated form of HSL. Other hormones, such as growth hormone, cortisol, and thyroid stimulating hormone, also stimulate lipolysis (Saltin and Åstrand 1993; Turcotte et al. 1995; Jeukendrup, Saris, and Wagenmakers 1998).

Insulin is the strongest inhibitor of lipolysis. It decreases the amount of active HSL produced by blocking cAMP from phosphorylating HSL. During exercise or times of starvation, when the need for fat as an energy source is high, insulin is typically low and lipolysis is high. The decrease in insulin concentrations during exercise occurs primarily because epinephrine and norepinephrine inhibit pancreatic insulin release (Jeukendrup, Saris, and Wagenmakers 1998). Insulin is high during times of feeding, when the need for mobilization of energy is low and the stimulation for fat storage is high. Thus, any increase in blood insulin either before or during exercise may inhibit fat lipolysis and oxidation. Horowitz et al. (1997) found that feeding either glucose or fructose (0.8 g/kg) 1 h before exercise (1 h of cycling at 44% $\dot{V}O_2$max) and after an overnight fast significantly increased plasma insulin concentrations compared to fasting. This increase in insulin also significantly decreased whole-body lipolysis and fat oxidation during exercise.

Independent of insulin, any increase in blood glucose concentrations (such as feeding carbohydrate during exercise) suppresses lipolysis and decreases FA turnover within adipose cells. This in turn changes the mix of fuels used for energy during exercise. Carlson et al. (1991) demonstrated that a hyperglycemic state in which insulin was held constant decreased FA turnover (i.e., the difference between lipolysis and FFA re-esterification) by 30%. Thus, blood

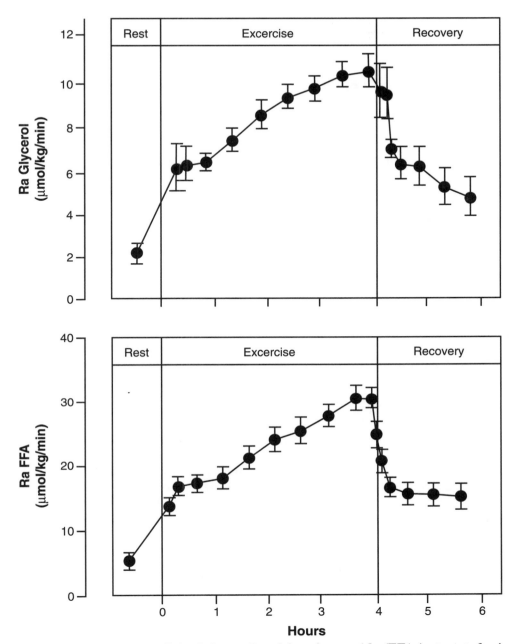

Figure 3.7 Rate of appearance (R_a) of glycerol and free fatty acids (FFAs) at rest, during exercise (40% $\dot{V}O_2$max for 4 h on the treadmill), and during recovery in five men. Exercise induced a sixfold increase in FFAs available for oxidation.

Reprinted from Wolfe et al. 1990.

glucose also appears to be a strong regulator of lipolysis and of the availability of FAs for energy during exercise.

Intramuscular Fat

Fat stored within skeletal muscle also appears to be an important source of energy during ex-ercise—although the significance of its contri-bution to total fat oxidation is still being de-bated. The initial hypothesis behind the use of muscle triacylglycerols as a fuel source during exercise came from the observation that the uptake and oxidation of plasma FFAs (albumin-bound fatty acids) cannot account for all the fat oxidized during exercise (Saltin and Åstrand

1993). One advantage to having triacylglycerols stored within muscle fiber is that the substrate (fat) is close to mitochondria, the site of lipid oxidation and energy production, and does not have to be transported through the blood. However, the exact amount of intramuscular fat stored appears to depend on muscle fiber type, nutritional status, and type of physical activity engaged in (Dyck et al. 1997; Jeukendrup, Saris, and Wagenmakers 1998). The amount of intramuscular fat oxidized during exercise has not been well determined. Depending on the research cited, it is estimated that endurance exercise decreases intramuscular fat concentrations from 25-50% (Oscai et al. 1990; Turcotte et al. 1995). Yet the purported contribution of intramuscular fat triacylglycerol breakdown to total fat oxidation during exercise may be 5-35%, depending on the study examined (Hurley et al. 1986; Romijn et al. 1993; Saltin and Åstrand 1993). Differences in estimates of how much intramuscular triacylgly-cerol is used during exercise most likely stem from differences in subject fitness levels, exercise protocols, and methods used to determine triacylglycerol content. Different types of exercise may recruit different muscle fibers with different fat oxidation rates. Methods for measuring changes in muscle triacylglycerol content are also difficult since fat is not distributed equally within the muscle fibers, and the two major types of muscle fibers oxidize fat differently (Saltin and Åstrand 1993; Turcotte et al. 1995). Exercise intensity and duration may also alter the amount of muscle triacylglycerol used, with higher intensities using more intramuscular fat. Finally, the fitness level of the subjects may alter the amount of intramuscular fat used during exercise since more fit individuals are better fat oxidizers.

The final two points discussed above are illustrated by two studies that measured changes in muscle triacylglycerol concentrations before and after exercise. In the first, Hurley et al. (1986) examined the effect of endurance exercise adaptation on muscle triacylglycerol depletion. They exercised nine untrained men for 2 h at 65% $\dot{V}O_2$max and measured changes in muscle triacylglycerol and glycogen concentrations. They found a 20% average decrease in muscle triacylglycerol concentration, and a 71% decrease in glycogen concentration, after the initial test. The subjects were retested after they had trained for 12 weeks. After exercise training, intramuscular triacylglycerol use in-

creased to 41%, twice that in the untrained state; and the amount of glycogen used decreased by nearly 60% (figure 3.8). Thus, *exercise training caused a shift in substrate use to more intramuscular fat and less carbohydrate.*

Exercise intensity can also change the amount of intramuscular triacylglycerol used on even a short-term basis. Romijn et al. (1993) measured substrate utilization at three different exercise intensities in trained male cyclists. The contribution of intramuscular fat was 7%, 26%, and 8% during exercise intensities of 25%, 65%, and 85% $\dot{V}O_2$max, respectively (figure 3.9). Both exercise training and intensity appear to alter the amount of intramuscular fat used during exercise.

However, not all research has demonstrated significant decreases in intramuscular triacylglycerol levels with endurance exercise or exercise training (Turcotte et al. 1995). Kiens et al. (1993) found no changes in intramuscular utilization with training. In this study they measured changes in muscle triacylglycerol and glycogen before and after training, using knee extensor exercises with one leg only (the other leg was not trained). Figure 3.10 shows no statistically significant change in muscle triacylglycerol concentrations (8% use before training, 12% after training) but significant changes in glycogen after training. The change in muscle glycogen was similar to that reported by Hurley et al. (1986). The differences between these two studies and others examining changes in muscle triacylglycerol use during exercise suggest that a number of factors control intramuscular triacylglycerol use. Additional research is needed to identify these regulatory factors and to determine under what exercise conditions muscle triacylglycerol use is high. Finally, differences in the methods used to measure intramuscular fat changes during exercise may also be contributing to the equivocal results. As researchers adopt new standardized methods of measuring intramuscular fat changes, we will have a better idea of the effects training and exercise intensity have on this fat storage system.

Blood Lipids

Blood lipids, transported in **lipoproteins**, can also contribute to the fat used during exercise (figure 3.6). The two lipoproteins highest in triacylglycerols are chylomicrons and very-low-density lipoproteins. If a person is exercising

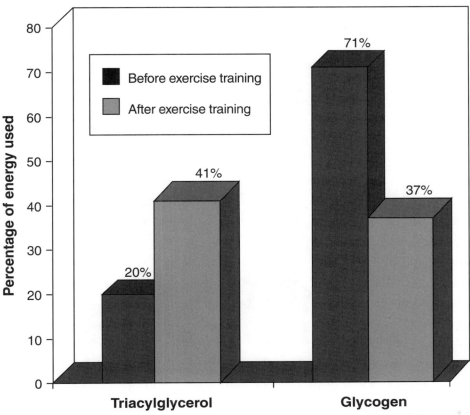

Figure 3.8 Percentage of intramuscular triacylglycerol and glycogen used for energy before and after a 12-week aerobic exercise training program. Subjects were nine men exercising for 2 h at 60% $\dot{V}O_2$max.

Reproduced from Hurley et al. 1986.

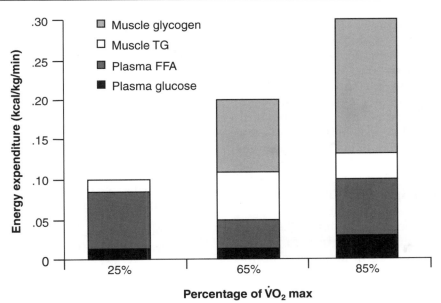

Figure 3.9 Substrate utilization at three different exercise intensities (25%, 65%, and 85% $\dot{V}O_2$max) in trained male cyclists exercising for 30 min at 85% $\dot{V}O_2$max or 120 min at 25% and 65% $\dot{V}O_2$max. FFA = free fatty acids; TG = triacylglycerol.

Reprinted from Romijn et al. 1993.

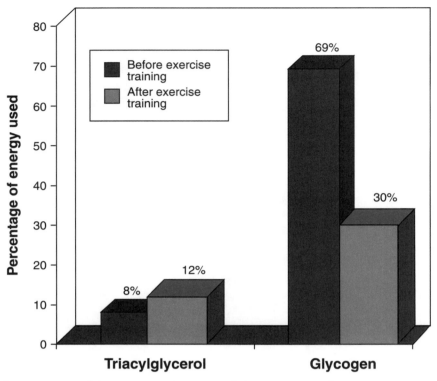

Figure 3.10 Percentage of intramuscular triacylglycerol and glycogen used for energy before and after a 12-week exercise training program using trained and untrained limbs (knee extensions with only one leg).

Adapted from Kiens et al. 1993.

after a meal, chylomicron levels in the blood can be high. **Chylomicrons** are responsible for transporting dietary fat to the tissues of the body for either energy production or storage as fat. Other blood lipoproteins, especially **very-low-density lipoproteins (VLDLs)**, can also carry triacylglycerols. See table 3.5 (page 81) for a brief description of the definitions, functions, and composition of the various blood lipoproteins. As with lipolysis in the adipose and muscle tissue, the fatty acids in lipoproteins must also be released from the triacylglycerols before they can enter the muscle cell. The enzyme **lipoprotein lipase (LPL)** is responsible for cleaving the fatty acids from the triacylglycerol molecules in blood lipoproteins. The FFAs are then available for transport into the muscle cells for energy production or for storage, or into adipose tissue for storage. From a practical standpoint, since most people do not exercise strenuously after eating a large meal (especially a high-fat meal), the amount of energy obtained from blood lipoproteins is generally small (Turcotte et al. 1995). If one exercises after an overnight fast, the contribution of li-

poprotein triacylglycerols is still minimal since in healthy individuals no chylomicrons would be present and VLDLs would be low.

Oxidation of Fatty Acids

Fatty acids released from adipose cells must go through a series of steps before they can be oxidized for energy within the muscle mitochondria. The steps are outlined below and illustrated in figure 3.6 (page 75). A more detailed description of this metabolic process can be found in Jeukendrup and Saris (1998); Jeukendrup, Saris, and Wagenmakers (1998); and Winder (1998).

1. Fatty acids are attached to albumin for transport in the plasma to the muscle. **Fatty acid binding proteins** within muscle cell membranes transport FAs across the membranes and into the cytoplasm of muscle cells.

2. Once fatty acids are in the cytoplasm of a muscle cell, they can either be re-esterified and stored into intracellular triacylglycerol

Table 3.5 Blood Lipoproteins: Synthesis, Functions, and Composition

Lipoprotein	Synthesis	Primary function	Composition
Chylomicrons	Formed in the gut mucosal cell after a meal and released into the intracellular space, where they enter the lymph system and are eventually dumped into the blood at the thoracic duct. Chylomicrons are the largest lipoproteins, with the lowest density. While circulating in the blood, chylomicrons can exchange apoproteins with other lipoproteins, especially HDLs. After the triglycerides are removed from this lipoprotein, a chylomicron remnant remains and is taken up by the liver.	Transport dietary fat (exogenous fat) into the blood and to the tissues of the body. Blood chylomicrons are high after a meal, but clear within 4-6 h depending on the fat content of the meal.	Triglycerides = 85% Phospholipids = 8% Cholesterol/CE = 5% Protein = 2%
Very-low-density lipoproteins (VLDLs)	Formed in the liver (80% of production) and the intestine (20%). As triglycerides are removed, the concentration of cholesterol increases until an intermediate-density lipoprotein (IDL) is formed.	Transport endogenous lipids, especially triglycerides, to tissues of the body.	Triglycerides = 50-60% Phospholipids = 15-18% Cholesterol/CE = 15-20% Protein = 10%
Low-density lipoproteins (LDLs)	Formed in the blood from VLDLs (VLDL → IDL → LDL). As the triglycerides are removed, the VLDLs become more dense with cholesterol and transition to IDLs. When cholesterol content becomes greater than the triglyceride content, IDLs transition to LDLs.	Transport cholesterol to the cells of the body. LDLs are recognized by an LDL receptor on the cell surface and taken up by the cells via endocytosis.	Triglycerides = 8% Phospholipids = 20% Cholesterol/CE = 50% Protein = 22%
High-density lipoproteins (HDLs)	Synthesized in the liver and release into the blood. They can move through the system picking up apoproteins and free cholesterol. HDLs transport their cholesterol back to the liver.	Transport cholesterol from tissues back to the liver.	Triglycerides = 3% Phospholipids = 30% Cholesterol/CE = 17% Protein = 50%

CE = cholesterol esters.

or be activated for transport into the mitochondria. Fatty acids are transported through the cytoplasm bound to a **cytoplasmic fatty acid binding protein.**

3. If a fatty acid is to be used for β-oxidation, it must first be activated by the enzyme **acyl-CoA synthetase.** This activation occurs outside the mitochondria.

4. The activated fatty acid must then be transported across the mitochondrial inner membrane by **carnitine palmitoyl transferase I (CPT 1)** and **carnitine palmitoyl transferase II (CPT 2),** which work in unison to accomplish this task. First, the CPT 1 located on the outer surface of the mitochondrial membrane converts the fatty acyl-CoA to **acylcarnitine** for transport. Then, on the inner mitochondrial membrane side, CPT 2 reconverts the acylcarnitine back to fatty

acyl-CoA for β-oxidation (Winder 1998). Figure 3.11 describes the process in detail. *As the rate-limiting enzyme in this process, CPT 1 activity regulates the amount of fatty acid entering the mitochondria for oxidation.* Malonyl-CoA, which is a potent inhibitor of CPT 1, is elevated when glucose availability is high (Winder 1998). Carnitine is synthesized in the body from two amino acids, lysine and methionine; the synthesis requires the essential nutrients vitamin C, niacin, iron, and vitamin B_6. In addition, we may obtain small amounts of carnitine from animal and dairy foods. In healthy individuals, supplemental carnitine does not improve fat oxidation since the body makes adequate carnitine (see "Does Carnitine Supplementation Enhance Performance and Reduce Body Fat?" on page 448).

The carnitine and fatty acid transport system

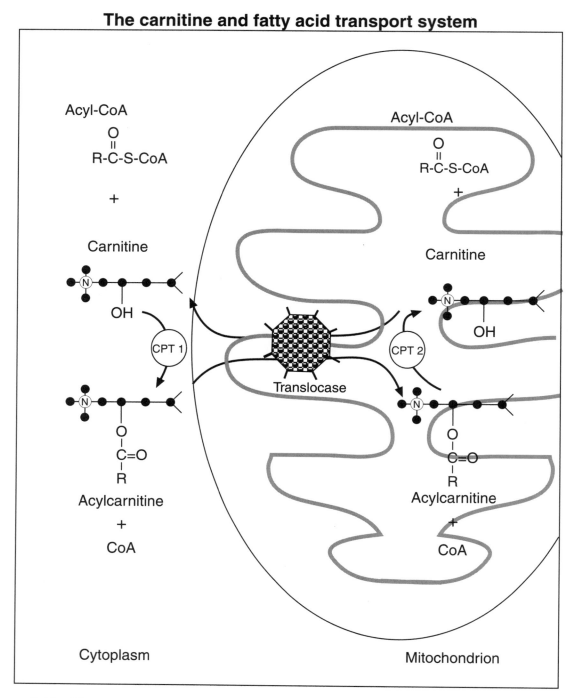

Figure 3.11 The carnitine and fatty acid transport system. R = carbon backbone of fatty acid. CPT 1 = carnitine palmitoyl transferase 1. CPT 2 = carnitine palmitoyl transferase 2.
Reprinted from *The Journal of Nutritional Biochemistry* 1991;2.

5. Fatty acyl-CoA undergoes β-oxidation in the mitochondria via a cyclic degradative pathway, with two-carbon units cleaved from the carboxyl end of the fatty acid in the form of **acetyl-CoA.** Each time the fatty acid goes through the cycle it loses a two-carbon unit, until there are only four carbons remaining. At this point, the four-carbon unit is degraded to produce two acetyl-CoA units. Each rotation of the

cycle produces one unit each of acetyl-CoA, FADH$_2$, and NADH. The acetyl-CoA units can then enter the TCA cycle for the production of energy (adenosine triphosphate [ATP]). If the acetyl-CoA is completely reduced to oxygen and water in the TCA cycle, 12 ATPs are produced for each unit of acetyl-CoA. The FADH$_2$ and NADH enter the electron transport cycle for further ATP production—each FADH$_2$ unit produces 2 ATPs, while each NADH yields 3 ATPs. The total production of ATP from the complete oxidation of one 16-C fatty acid yields 129 ATPs (2 ATPs are used up in this pathway) (Champe and Harvey 1987). Oxidation of fat produces three times the energy of an equal amount of glucose. Figure 3.12 shows the β-oxidation process in detail.

Regulation of Fat Oxidation

Since muscle and liver glycogen stores are limited, and depletion of these stores contributes to fatigue during exercise, maximization of fat oxidation during exercise might help prevent fatigue and improve exercise performance. Reducing body fat stores may also be appealing for health, fitness, or aesthetic reasons. Even though most people have relatively large fat stores, the ability to oxidize these stores during exercise is limited. While the exact reasons for this limited ability to burn fat has not been identified, Jeukendrup, Saris, and Wagenmakers (1998) have outlined a number of factors that might contribute to our limited ability to burn fat during exercise. There may be limitations in the ability to efficiently execute the steps of fat lipolysis or transport at any number of levels, including the following:

- Mobilization of fatty acids from the adipose tissue
- Transport of fatty acids to the muscles
- Uptake of fatty acids by the muscles, either from plasma or from the triacylglycerol in lipoproteins
- Mobilization of fatty acids from the intramuscular triacylglycerol pools

If any of the above steps is inhibited or limited, the ability to deliver fat to muscle cells for oxidation may be reduced. In addition, a number of factors regulate fatty acid transport and oxidation within the cell (Jeukendrup, Saris, and

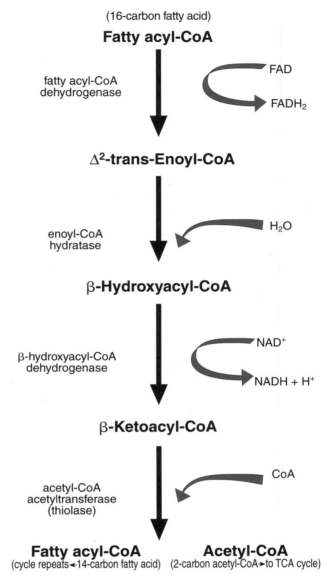

Figure 3.12 Initial steps in β-oxidation using palmitic acid, a 16-C fatty acid, as an example. Each turn of the cycle yields one acetyl-CoA unit and shortens the fatty acid by two carbons. The newly formed acetyl-CoA can then go to the TCA cycle for further metabolism, while the shorter fatty acid repeats through the cycle. When the fatty acid has been shortened to four carbons, the final turn of the cycle produces two acetyl-CoA units.

Adapted from Champe and Harvey 1987.

Wagenmakers 1998). Glucose availability appears to be a strong regulator of fat oxidation within the cell, with high glucose availability decreasing oxidation of long-chain fatty acids by inhibiting their transport into the mitochondria (Wolfe 1998). Glucose availability and oxidation

' closely coupled (i.e., if glucose is
; oxidized). The same is not true of
, acid availability is generally much
..... than required for oxidation. Plasma FFA concentrations during exercise greatly exceed the level needed to meet the fat oxidation capacity of the muscle. Research suggests that fatty acid oxidation rates within the muscle cell during exercise, controlled primarily at the site of oxidation, are determined by the availability of glucose, not by the availability of fatty acids via lipolysis or other transport mechanism (Carlson et al. 1991; Coyle et al. 1997; Wolfe 1998).

Enhancement of Fat Oxidation

What can a person do to increase burning of fat? Can a supplement like carnitine or a drug like caffeine really increase the burning of fat? A multitude of products are marketed with claims that they increase fat metabolism. Since such products are a multimillion dollar business in the United States, it is important to understand the science behind fat metabolism. Are these products legitimate or a waste of money? This section addresses training strategies, dietary changes, and ergogenic products thought to improve or enhance the ability to burn fat. Because of wide interest in this topic, a number of reviews have addressed in greater detail the issues we discuss in the next few paragraphs (Brouns and van der Vusse 1998; Hawley et al. 1998; Kiens and Helge 1998; Lambert et al. 1997; Sherman and Leenders 1995).

Exercise Training

Exercise training enables a person to work harder (higher oxygen uptake), while deriving more energy from fat (both plasma FFAs and intramuscular triacylglycerol) and less from carbohydrate (blood glucose and glycogen) (figure 3.13). A number of researchers have reported the specific physiological and metabolic adaptations that occur with training (Brouns and van der Vusse, 1998; Jeukendrup and Saris 1998; Saltin and Åstrand 1993), which are as follows:

1. Increased numbers of mitochondria and increased activity of enzymes within the mitochondria—including increased concentration of enzymes for the TCA cycle, fatty acid oxidation, and the electron transport system.

2. Increased fatty acyl-CoA synthesis and reduction in muscle; plus increased levels of LPL, lipase, carnitine, and carnitine transferase—all of which favor improved availability and transport of fatty acids to the mitochondria for β-oxidation.

3. Increased triacylglycerol storage and oxidation within muscle—more fat is stored closer to the site of oxidation, improving the availability of fat for oxidation during exercise.

4. Increased FFA uptake by the muscle. Exercise increases capillary density of muscle, which in turn improves blood flow and the exchange of FFAs and oxygen; exercise also increases transport of fatty acids through the sarcolemma. Figure 3.14 illustrates this improvement in FFA uptake, showing that the trained person has a higher FFA uptake compared to the untrained.

5. Alterations in the mobilization of FFAs from the adipose tissue. Exercise may increase the delivery of FFAs from the fat cell to the blood, due to increased blood flow in the adipose tissue.

6. Improved cardiovascular respiratory system that enhances oxygen delivery to the muscle for fat oxidation.

Taken collectively, the adaptations listed above enhance the body's ability to oxidize fat as a fuel, improve intramuscular fat storage, and increase fat flux (Brouns and van der Vusse 1998; Saltin and Åstrand 1993). At the same time, exercise training spares endogenous carbohydrate stores that may be needed for prolonged, high-intensity events (see chapter 2).

Exercise training is the best intervention one can recommend to improve a person's ability to burn fat. Unfortunately, many people do not want to put the time and energy into becoming more fit. They are looking for a pill or a potion to improve their fat burning ability. They want the quick fix! Unfortunately, there are no legitimate quick fixes available in the marketplace (but lots of illegitimate ones). This will become evident as you read the rest of this chapter.

High-Fat Diets and Fat Infusions

Both fat and carbohydrate are important energy substrates during exercise. *During moderate exercise (60-75% $\dot{V}O_2$max) of long duration (>90 min), however, fat becomes the primary*

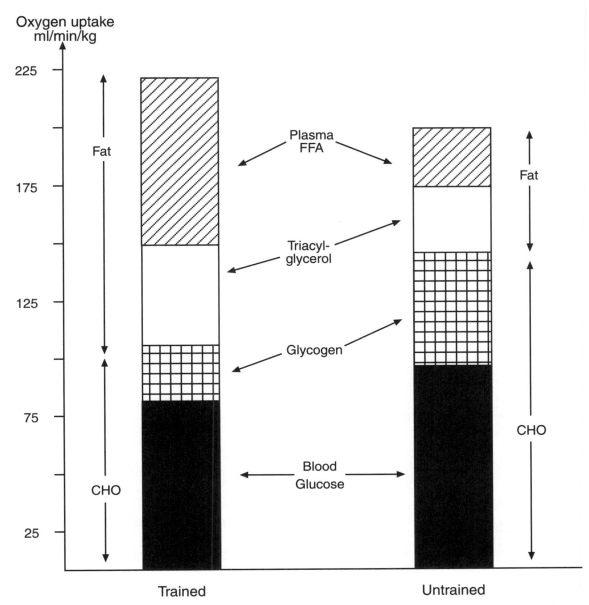

Figure 3.13 The estimated contribution of various substrates to energy metabolism during exercise when the limb is trained or untrained. There is greater dependence on plasma free fatty acids (FFAs) and triacylglycerol in the trained limb, and less reliance on carbohydrate (CHO). Reprinted from Saltin and Åstrand 1993.

energy substrate as carbohydrate stores are depleted. This depletion of the body's carbohydrate stores is usually manifested by a decrease in blood glucose over time and a depletion of muscle and liver glycogen stores. Depletion of these stores increases reliance on liver gluconeogenesis to provide the glucose necessary to sustain exercise. (See figure 2.2, page 26, to review the gluconeogenesis pathway.) Ingestion of exogenous carbohydrate can delay fatigue but

cannot prevent it (Coyle et al. 1986). But when carbohydrate is consumed during exercise, a shift in substrate utilization occurs—glucose feeding suppresses fat lipolysis, mobilization, and oxidation during exercise, thereby reducing the proportion of energy coming from fat. Consuming a short-term high-fat diet increases FFA levels in the plasma while resting; subsequently, during exercise, more fatty acids are taken up by the muscles than if a person had

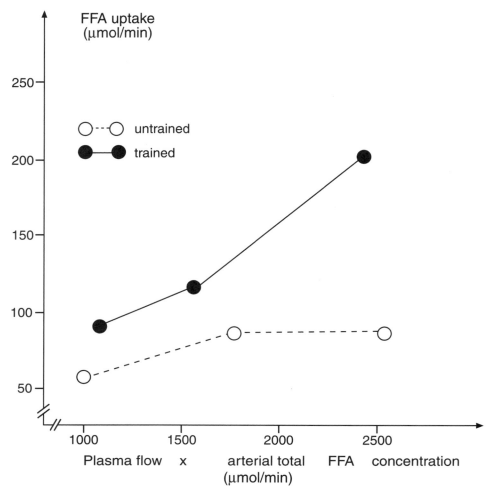

Figure 3.14   Uptake of free fatty acids (FFAs) by the contracting muscle in relation to the amount of FFAs offered to the limb. At a higher inflow of FFAs, the trained individual can utilize a larger fraction of the FFAs available.

Reprinted from Saltin and Åstrand 1993.

been following a high-carbohydrate diet (Jeukendrup and Saris 1998). Moreover, long-term fat consumption may induce skeletal muscle adaptations that increase the body's ability to oxidize fat as a fuel (Kiens and Helge 1998). Finally, some studies examining the effect of fat infusions (Intralipid) during exercise report decreases in muscle glycogen utilization compared to control trials (Odland et al. 1998; Vukovich et al. 1993).

Because of the factors mentioned above, a number of researchers hypothesized that high-fat diets would increase the availability of fat for oxidation and the ability to oxidize fat during exercise. This in turn would cause the body to become less reliant on carbohydrate for energy, thus sparing muscle glycogen. The body

appears to adapt to the lower carbohydrate availability by becoming a better fat oxidizer (Hawley et al. 1998; Jeukendrup and Saris 1998; Sherman and Leenders 1995). If these hypotheses are true, high-fat diets would improve exercise performance by sparing carbohydrates and improving fat oxidation. Research examining these issues has produced mixed results due to a number of factors, including differences in experimental designs, training status of the subjects, methods of measuring exercise performance, the percentage of energy derived from fat, and the length of time the high-fat diet was fed (Helge et al. 1998). The diets used by researchers examining effects of high-fat meals/diets on glycogen utilization and fat oxidation during exercise can be grouped roughly as follows:

- A single high-fat meal before exercise
- Short-term high-fat diets (3-5 d) before exercise
- Moderate-term high-fat diets (1-4 weeks) before exercise
- Long-term high-fat diets (>7 weeks) before exercise

Recent studies on the effect of high-fat meals (~60-75% of energy) 4 h before endurance exercise (90-120 min) show no differences in exercise performance or work production compared to high-carbohydrate meals (58-87% of energy). However, the effect of a high-fat meal on substrate utilization during exercise appears more variable. Whitley et al. (1998) reported no differences in substrate oxidation between their high-fat, high-carbohydrate, and control (fasting) trials, while Okano et al. (1998) observed a significantly lower respiratory exchange ratio during exercise when a high-fat meal was fed versus a high-carbohydrate meal. This lower respiratory exchange ratio suggests that a high-fat meal prior to exercise increases fat oxidation during exercise.

It appears that 2-4 weeks of high-fat meals does not negatively impact exercise performance compared to high-carbohydrate diets. Lambert et al. (1994) fed five endurance cyclists either a high-fat (76% of energy) or a high-carbohydrate diet (74% of energy) for 2 weeks in random order separated by 2 weeks of a normal diet. After each treatment period the athletes performed three exercise tests in the following order:

1. Wingate test—to test muscle power.
2. High-intensity exercise exhaustion test— cycle to exhaustion at 85% of peak power (90% $\dot{V}O_2$max).
3. Moderate-intensity exercise exhaustion test—cycling to exhaustion at 60% of $\dot{V}O_2$max.

The results showed that diet had no effect on muscle power output or on the high-intensity exercise exhaustion test. Muscle glycogen utilization during exercise was similar for both diets during the high-intensity exercise test, even though glycogen levels were significantly lower after the high-fat diet (68 mmol/kg/wet mass) compared to the high-carbohydrate diet (121 mmol/kg/wet mass). However, exercise time to exhaustion after moderate-intensity exercise was significantly longer after the high-fat diet

(80 min) compared to the high-carbohydrate diet (43 min). This longer endurance time was attributed to a lower respiratory exchange ratio (0.87) while athletes were on the high-fat diet compared to the high-carbohydrate diet (0.92). Two recent studies examining the effect of 4 weeks of a high-fat diet on endurance time report mixed results. Venkatraman and Pendergast (1998) reported improved time to exhaustion in runners fed a moderate-fat diet (32% of energy) compared to a low-fat diet (17% of energy), but no difference between the moderate-fat and the high-fat diet (41% of energy). Unfortunately, the diets were not randomly assigned, and there was no washout period between the diets. Thus, it is difficult to know if there was a carryover effect from one diet to the next. In addition, the level of fat fed in this study was significantly lower than the 60-70% fat diets typically fed in other studies. This makes it difficult to compare these results to those of other high-fat feeding research. Helge et al. (1998) reported no difference in endurance performance in untrained males going through a 4-week training period and consuming either a 4-week high-fat (62% of energy) or high-carbohydrate (65% of energy) diet. Time to exhaustion was similar between the groups (figure 3.15); however, the high-fat group did have a lower respiratory exchange ratio during exercise compared both to their own baseline values and to the high-carbohydrate group.

What about the effects of long-term fat feeding (7 weeks)? Helge et al. (1996) fed untrained men either a high-carbohydrate (n = 10, 65% of energy) or high-fat (n = 10, 62% of energy) diet for 7 weeks. All subjects went through endurance training three to four times per week for the duration of the study. At the end of the study, those receiving the high-carbohydrate diet significantly improved exercise endurance time from ~35 min at baseline to 102 min (191% improvement), while the high-fat group improved to only 65 min (85% improvement). Figure 3.15 compares the effect of moderate- and long-term fat feeding on exercise time to exhaustion. Long-term fat feeding appears not to benefit exercise performance.

To summarize current research (which admittedly is limited): high-fat meals before exercise have no effect on performance, while short-term high-fat diets (3-5 d) decrease exercise performance compared to high-carbohydrate diets. When high-fat diets are fed for 2-4

87

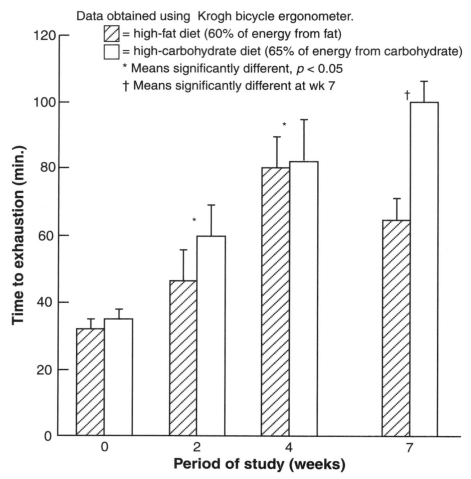

Figure 3.15 Endurance performance to exhaustion measured at baseline (time 0) before exercise training and after 2, 4, and 7 weeks of a high-fat diet compared to a high-carbohydrate diet. Mean values were significantly different from those at week 0 for both diets ($^*p < 0.05$). Mean value for the high-carbohydrate diet was significantly different from the high-fat diet at week 7 ($^\dagger p < 0.05$).

Reprinted from Kiens and Helge 1998.

weeks, allowing individuals to adapt metabolically to the high-fat diet, the effect on performance is similar to that seen when a high-carbohydrate diet is fed. In other words, both high-fat and high-carbohydrate diets produced the same results. However, when high-fat diets are fed for longer periods (7 weeks) and compared to high-carbohydrate diets, endurance performance is better on the high-carbohydrate diets (Helge et al. 1996; Kiens and Helge 1998). *At the present time there appears to be no advantage to feeding high-fat diets to athletes—* especially the levels of fat fed in experimental studies (~60-70% of energy from fat)! These levels of fat are generally not acceptable to most active individuals, can cause gastrointestinal distress, and are not practical. In addition, diets this high in fat are not recommended for

good long-term health. Fat infusions during exercise decrease glycogen use but are of no practical use to the active individual; and they are illegal in athletic competition (Sherman and Leenders 1995). In summary, based on the limited data available, extremely high-fat diets seem impractical and are not recommended for athletes or active individuals.

Long-Chain Triacylglycerols

During some endurance events (e.g., ultramarathons or triathlons) athletes eat food while competing. In general, the ingestion of **long-chain triacylglycerols (LCTs),** or tri-glycerides, during exercise events lasting less than 4 h is not recommended. LCTs comprise three long-chain fatty acids (LCFAs) and a glycerol backbone. Because LCTs slow gastric emptying, they stay in the gastrointestinal tract longer and enter the blood more slowly than other sources of energy typically used during exercise. Note also that, since they are insoluble in water, LCFAs must enter the general circulation via chylomicrons—a much slower process than carbohydrate digestion. Carbohydrate is much more readily digested and available for energy during exercise than LCTs. Chylomicrons are not major contributors of energy to the body during exercise but are thought to contribute to the replenishment of muscle intramuscular fat after exercise is over (Jeukendrup and Saris 1998).

In summary, LCT consumption is generally not recommended during intense exercise lasting less than 4 h. If the activity is long-lasting (e.g., an ultramarathon, a multiday exercise event, or even an all-day hike), foods with LCT are appropriate and even recommended. Even during these types of events, however, the level of fat consumed should usually be low, with the majority of energy coming from carbohydrate.

Medium-Chain Triacylglycerols

Since fat digestion is generally slower than that of carbohydrate, fat stays in the gastrointestinal tract longer before it enters circulation—thus decreasing the immediate availability of exogenous fat as an energy source during exercise. **Medium-chain triacylglycerols (MCTs)** are an exception to this rule since they are digested differently from typical dietary fats. MCTs comprise three **medium-chain fatty acids (MCFAs)** and a glycerol backbone; however, because MCFAs are only 6-12 carbons long, their smaller size alters the way they are digested, transported, and utilized for energy within the body (Linscheer and Vergroesen 1994). MCTs rapidly exit the stomach into the small intestine. They are digested into MCFAs, which are absorbed across the mucosal membrane almost as rapidly as glucose. Compared with LCFAs, MCFAs are more soluble in water, require less pancreatic lipase and bile salts for digestion, and diffuse rapidly through the unstirred water layer of the gut. Once inside the gut mucosal cells, they do not require resynthesis into triacylglycerols and incorporation into chylomicrons for transport into the blood, as LCFAs do. MCFAs enter the portal vein bound to albumin and are transported to the liver as rapidly as glucose. They enter systemic circulation and are available for metabolism 250 times more quickly than LCFAs (Linscheer and Vergroesen 1994). MCFAs are not stored in adipose tissue but are oxidized rapidly for energy by the cells, especially in the liver. Within muscle cells MCFAs are not dependent on carnitine for transport into the mitochondria. Finally, MCFAs are metabolized within the muscle about as rapidly as glucose, and preferentially over LCFAs. These unique characteristics of MCTs and MCFAs have lead researchers to suggest that MCTs could be a valuable source of energy during exercise, especially during extreme endurance events (Ivy et al. 1980). It has also been suggested that MCTs might be able to spare muscle glycogen since they are rapidly metabolized to energy.

A number of researchers have examined the effect of MCTs on exercise performance, glycogen sparing, and substrate utilization during exercise. One of the first was by Ivy et al. (1980), who studied 10 well-trained male volunteers during 1 h of exercise at 70% $\dot{V}O_2$max under four randomly assigned double-blind conditions:

1. Control (subjects exercised after an overnight fast).
2. MCT (30 g) mixed with cereal and 240 ml (~1 cup) of skim milk (total of 621 kcal) fed 1 h before exercise.
3. LCT (30 g) mixed with cereal and 240 ml (~1 cup) of skim milk (total of 609 kcal) fed 1 h before exercise.
4. Cereal only (no additional fat added) and 240 ml (~1 cup) of skim milk (354 kcal, primarily carbohydrate) fed 1 h before exercise.

There were no differences in rate of perceived exertion among the four trials. The addition of MCT did not significantly increase the plasma fatty acid levels or the level of fat oxidation during exercise compared to the other treatments. All three experimental meals resulted in approximately 132 g of carbohydrate (CHO) and 36 g of fat being used for energy, while the control trial utilized 111 g of CHO and 45 g of fat. These authors concluded that MCT in combination with CHO was not a viable energy source during exercise since all treatments (except the control) utilized the same amounts of fat and CHO. The authors also reported that during preliminary trials, feeding either 50 or 60 g of MCT caused gastrointestinal distress in 100%

of their subjects, while 30 g caused distress in only 10% of the subjects. A subsequent study by Decombaz et al. (1983) showed similar results. In this study, 12 men consumed either 25 g MCT or 50 g carbohydrate 1 h before exercise and then exercised for 1 h at 60% $\dot{V}O_2$max. MCT did not spare muscle glycogen use but did account for 10% of total energy expenditure; however, the MCT did not appear to offer any advantages over CHO.

More recent studies have examined the effect of feeding MCT *during* exercise as part of a fluid replacement beverage. Massicotte et al. (1992) examined the effect of water, MCT (25 g), or glucose (57 g) ingested during exercise in six healthy young men exercising for 2 h at 65% $\dot{V}O_2$max. The energy provided by both MCT and glucose was similar. During exercise, MCTs and CHO were oxidized for energy at similar rates but represented only 7% and 8.5% of total energy expenditure, respectively. Neither the exogenous MCT nor glucose reduced the amount of endogenous CHO utilized. Subsequent research by Jeukendrup et al. (1995) and Jeukendrup, Saris, Brouns et al. (1996) reported similar findings. In these experiments, subjects consumed either MCT (~29 g), CHO only, or CHO + MCT during 3 h of cycling at 57% $\dot{V}O_2$max. Results showed that some MCT was oxidized for energy during exercise, but the contribution to total energy expenditure was small (3-7%). Similar to early studies, MCT did not spare muscle glycogen. Even when muscle glycogen levels were low prior to exercise, MCT contributions to total energy expenditure did not improve and remained at ~8% in the 1996 report. Although MCT can be used as a fuel source during exercise, the amount of MCT tolerated due to gastrointestinal distress is limited; feeding higher amounts is therefore not feasible.

The effect of MCT on actual exercise performance has been studied only recently. Van Zyl et al. (1996) had six endurance-trained cyclists exercise on three different occasions for 2 h at 60% peak $\dot{V}O_2$, then perform a 40-km time trial. Subjects received one of three treatments in random order: 10% glucose solution (100 g/L), 4.3% MCT solution (43 g/L), or 4.3% MCT + 10% glucose solution. Replacing glucose with MCT significantly slowed the timed trials by 5.3 min, but combining MCT and glucose in the same drink significantly improved the timed trials by 1.7 min compared to glucose alone. The authors did not measure muscle glycogen.

Jeukendrup, Thielen et al. (1998) repeated this study using seven well-trained cyclists, who again exercised for 2 h at 60% $\dot{V}O_2$max and then performed a timed trial; however, the timed trial consisted of the maximum amount of work that could be done in a 15-min period. Subjects ingested one of four treatments:

1. A 10% CHO solution (170 g glucose)
2. A 10% CHO solution with 5% MCT added (170 g glucose + 85 g MCT)
3. A 5% MCT solution (85 g MCT), or
4. A placebo containing artificially colored and flavored water

The authors compared the total amount of work done (in watts [W]) in each timed trial. When subjects consumed the glucose-only beverage (314 ± 19 W) or the glucose + MCT beverage (314 ± 13 W), their performance was similar to that of the placebo (312 ±18 W). The MCT-only treatment (263 ± 22 W) decreased performance by 17-18% compared to the placebo and the other two treatments. The MCT did not affect total carbohydrate or protein utilization during exercise, nor did it alter the amount of exogenous or endogenous carbohydrate used. In other words, MCT use did not spare muscle glycogen. The authors reported that the amount of MCT used in this study did result in some gastrointestinal distress: two subjects vomited after the MCT trial, and three complained of diarrhea. Belching and bloating were more often reported with all the treatments except the placebo. The most common complaint was gastrointestinal cramps, which occurred significantly more often when MCT was used. These two studies were similar in that neither found the use of MCT by itself to be beneficial to performance; only the Van Zyl study showed a significant improvement in performance when MCT was combined with carbohydrate. Unfortunately, Van Zyl et al. (1996) did not report data on how the subjects responded to the MCT—any benefit of MCT is negated if it causes gastrointestinal distress.

In summary, the use of MCT as a fuel source during exercise has been carefully studied in endurance exercise lasting 60 min or longer, with less research available on exercise performance (Berning 1996; Brouns and van der Vusse 1998; Jeukendrup, Saris, and Wagenmakers 1998). Although MCTs do contribute to total energy availability during exercise, the contribution to total energy expenditure appears small, ~7-8%. In addition, MCTs do not appear to significantly spare muscle glycogen or decrease the amount of endogenous or exogenous carbohydrate used. Total fat oxidation remains the same when MCTs are consumed either before or during exercise, even when glycogen levels are low prior to exercise. This suggests that MCFAs are competing with LCFAs for oxidation during exercise; hence, MCTs may be sparing endogenous fat stores (Brouns and van der Vusse 1998). It may also explain why glycogen is not spared when MCTs are fed either before or during exercise. Feeding higher amounts of MCTs might contribute to a greater proportion of total energy expenditure during exercise, but gastrointestinal distress prevents ingestion of higher doses. Although MCTs empty rapidly from the stomach and MCFAs can be quickly digested, transported, and utilized by the body for energy, use of MCTs as a fuel source during exercise appears limited due to gastrointestinal side effects. *Based on the data available, MCT ingestion either before or during exercise does not appear to spare muscle glycogen or improve exercise performance.* A final note: MCTs are very expensive!

Caffeine

Caffeine is one of the most widely used drugs in the world and has long been touted as an ergogenic substance that increases exercise performance and promotes fat burning. In the athletic world, caffeine is a "controlled or restricted drug" and is banned by the International Olympic Committee if urine levels exceed 12 µg/ml following competition. This allowable level of urinary caffeine is very liberal, and most athletes would have to consume caffeine in tablet or suppository form to reach this level (Spriet 1995). Competitive athletes usually use caffeine for its touted ability to enhance performance. For most active individuals and recreational athletes, caffeine consumption is little more than a daily habit in the form of coffee, tea, cola, or chocolate—the idea that caffeine might improve exercise performance being a "fringe benefit." For people interested in weight loss, drug companies frequently add caffeine to over-the-counter weight-loss products to speed up metabolism and increase metabolic rate. Unfortunately, many such products combine caffeine with other central nervous system stimulants such as ephedrine—products that can have serious side effects and should be avoided.

There are three major hypotheses for the ergogenic effect of caffeine during exercise, as outlined below (Graham and Spriet 1996; Spriet 1995). Various review articles have examined each of these hypotheses in detail

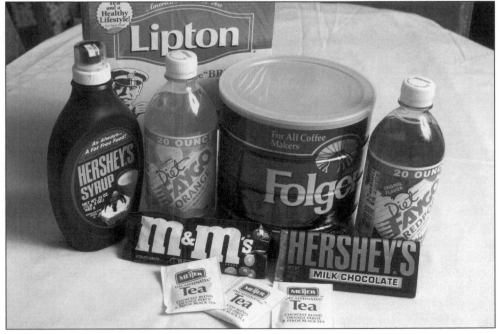

As pictured here, caffeine is found in a variety of foods and beverages.

(Clarkson 1993; Dodd et al. 1993; Graham et al. 1994; Graham and Spriet 1996; Spriet 1995). To summarize:

1. Caffeine may directly affect the central nervous system and alter one's perception of effort, or it may directly effect neural activation of muscle.

2. Caffeine may directly affect skeletal muscle by altering key enzymes or systems that regulate carbohydrate breakdown within cells.

3. Caffeine may alter metabolic factors that increase fat oxidation and decrease carbohydrate utilization. In this hypothesis it is proposed that caffeine directly increases circulating concentrations of epinephrine, which increases mobilization of FFAs from the fat or muscle cells. The increased availability of FFAs increases muscle cell oxidation of fat and improves exercise performance.

It appears that moderate doses of caffeine (3-9 mg/kg body weight) at least 1 h before exercise can enhance performance for well-trained elite or recreational athletes in endurance exercise under controlled research settings. Figure 3.16 shows the results from tests with well-trained recreational runners given caffeine (3, 6, or 9 mg/kg body weight) or a placebo (no caffeine) and asked to run to exhaustion at 85% VO_2max (Graham and Spriet 1995). Exercise performance improved with the lowest dose of caffeine, with no additional benefit from higher doses. However, attempts to repeat these results in field studies have not been successful, and extrapolation of laboratory data to actual competition may not be valid (Spriet 1995). Note that most research studies use pure caffeine, not caffeine-containing beverages such as coffee, tea, or cola. The metabolic effects of coffee may be different from those of pure caffeine since there are components in coffee that appear to moderate the effects of caffeine (Graham et al. 1998). The recreational athlete who drinks a cup of coffee and then goes out for a 10K run may not see the performance effects demonstrated in the research laboratory. There are many factors that affect both exercise performance and the physiological response to caffeine during exercise—including a person's typical or habitual caffeine intake. The metabolic and performance responses of a habitual caffeine user may be very different from those of a nonuser (Graham and Spriet 1996).

No physiological mechanism for improved endurance performance with caffeine has been identified. Caffeine appears to have its effect early in exercise (within the first 15-20 min), when it increases plasma FFA concentration and muscle triacylglycerol use, spares muscle glycogen, and decreases the respiratory exchange ratio. However, it is not clear whether increased fat oxidation spares the muscle glycogen or if there are other metabolic changes contributing to this observation. Caffeine indirectly affects muscle and adipose tissue by increasing plasma catecholamines, which in turn bind to the β-receptors of the cell membranes, increasing cAMP activity and lipolysis (Hawley et al. 1998). Stimulation of lipolysis is already high during exercise, however, and any caffeine-induced elevation of FFAs comes on top of already high plasma FFA concentrations. This may explain why the effects of caffeine on lipid oxidation are observed only in the initial stages of exercise, when lipolysis and fat oxidation are increasing, and not after 30 min when fat oxidation is high (Hawley et al. 1998). Thus, the performance-enhancing effect of caffeine is most likely related to its effect on the central nervous system rather than to significant effects on fat oxidation and glycogen sparing (Bell et al. 1998; Spriet 1996). This suggestion is supported by data from Graham and Spriet (1995) (figure 3.16), who found that a low dose of caffeine (3 mg/kg body weight) was enough to enhance exercise performance but not enough to stimulate the metabolic effects typically attributed to increased fat oxidation. At this level of caffeine, they saw no increase in plasma catecholamines, lipolysis, or plasma FFAs, all of which would have to occur if fat oxidation were enhanced and the cause for improved performance.

In summary, caffeine appears to enhance exercise performance—and it appears to increase fat oxidation at rest—but it does not increase fat oxidation after the first few minutes of exercise. According to numerous recent reviews on caffeine and exercise, use of caffeine as a significant "fat burner" is not substantiated by the research literature. Exercise is a much greater stimulant of fat oxidation than caffeine supplementation. Yet even the hint of improved fat oxidation leads many consumers to increase caffeine intake. Note, however, that high doses of caffeine can have significant side effects, especially in individuals who are not habitual users: it increases blood pressure at rest and

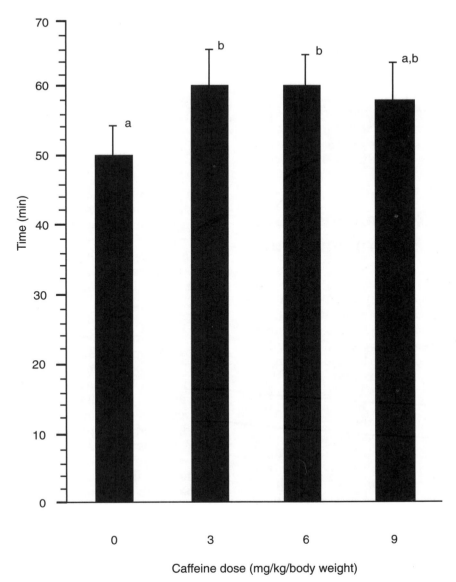

Figure 3.16 Effects of caffeine on exercise time to exhaustion. Data are means for exercise duration after placebo (0 mg/kg) or 3, 6, or 9 mg/kg caffeine. Data for histogram bars with the same letter are not significantly different from each other ($p < 0.05$). The 0 and 3 mg/kg trials were significantly different despite their exhibiting no differences in plasma epinephrine. And the 0 and 9 mg/kg times were not significantly different, although these trials had quite different plasma epinephrine data.

Reprinted from Graham and Spriet 1995.

during exercise (Daniels et al. 1998; Kaminsky et al. 1998); and high doses can cause dizziness, headache, insomnia, increased heart rate, and gastrointestinal distress.

Carnitine

Carnitine is marketed as a "fat burner" to sedentary people as well as athletes. Advertisements claim carnitine can do everything from decreasing body fat to preventing fatigue. Unlike caffeine, carnitine is an essential substance made by the body and is obtained from the diet in meat products. It is required for the transport of fatty acids into the mitochondria for β-oxidation (discussed earlier in this chapter). However, in healthy individuals the body is capable of making adequate amounts of carnitine for fatty acid transport. Although oral L-carnitine supplements increase plasma

L-carnitine concentrations, uptake by the muscles remains unchanged (Brouns and van der Vusse 1998). Chapter 16 presents more detailed information about carnitine, its role in fat metabolism, and the effect of L-carnitine supplementation on fat loss. *To date there is no consistent and convincing evidence that L-carnitine supplementation enhances fat oxidation or improves exercise performance* (Colombani et al. 1996; Kanter and Williams 1995; Trappe et al. 1994).

Dietary Fat Recommendations for Optimal Performance and Health

As you read in chapter 1, it is frequently recommended that athletes consume diets containing 60-65% of the energy from carbohydrate; but this is only part of the story. Active individuals also need adequate fat and protein. But what is the appropriate amount of fat? While we need adequate fat to meet the essential fatty acid requirements, we can meet this need with a few grams per day of flaxseed or fish oil (Ornish 1998). We also need fat as an energy source and to make our diets palatable. Finally, we want a dietary fat intake that promotes good health and prevents chronic disease. Although the optimal fat and carbohydrate intake for the prevention of chronic disease is still being debated in the research literature, we can give general guidelines to active people and athletes. These recommendations should be modified according to an individual's food preferences, training program, energy needs, and health status. Here are the guidelines:

• Carbohydrate should be 60-65% of energy intake. For diets very high in energy (>4000-5000 kcal/d), a lower carbohydrate intake (% of energy) provides adequate carbohydrate for glycogen replacement. During times of intense training or competition, carbohydrate intake can be increased, depending on individual needs. People should be encouraged to eat whole grains, fruits, vegetables, low-fat dairy products, and meats. Beans and legumes should be included whenever possible to increase fiber intake. On the day and in the hours before competition, athletes may want to eat low-fiber foods to reduce the feeling of fullness. Simple sugars should be used in moderation, representing <10% of total energy intake—except

during high training periods, or for individuals who need additional energy for weight maintenance and who are in good health.

• Fat should be 20-25% of energy intake, with <10% of energy from saturated fats and the remaining fat coming from monounsaturated (e.g., olive, canola oil) and polyunsaturated fats (e.g., canola, soy, fish, or corn oil). Athletes who prefer lower-fat diets should take care to ensure that they consume adequate essential fatty acids. People accustomed to high-fat diets can replace whole-fat foods with fat-modified foods, obtaining additional energy from increased use of complex carbohydrates or protein. People who need to reduce body fat should recognize that reduced-fat or fat-modified foods can be energy dense and should be used in moderation.

• Athletes and active people with chronic disease risk factors should modify fat and carbohydrate intake (both type and amount) based if possible on their health risk profiles and blood lipid and blood glucose profiles. For active people with family histories of diabetes, hypertension, or cardiovascular disease, more specific dietary recommendations can be made based on blood lipid and glucose profiles or on the degree of hypertension. These individuals may want to consume diets lower in saturated fats and higher in whole grains, fruits, and vegetables. In people with abnormal blood lipids or glucose levels, high simple sugar intakes and/or very-low-fat diets (which are usually high in carbohydrate) may lower LDL-cholesterol concentrations, but also increase blood triglycerides and lower HDL-cholesterol concentrations. The end result may be a blood lipid profile that does *not* improve their overall risk level! It is advisable that people with such conditions monitor their metabolic responses to any diet. People with hypertension may want to consider the DASH (Dietary Approaches to Stop Hypertension) diet outlined in table 3.6, or diet recommendations of the American Heart Association (Step 1 or 2 diet) or of the American Diabetes Association. For example, the DASH diet has been demonstrated in research settings to decrease hypertension in both normal and hypertensive individuals. It reduced blood pressure by an average of 5.5 mm Hg for systolic and 3.0 mm Hg for diastolic in 459 adults with systolic blood pressure <160 mm Hg and diastolic pressures of 80-95 mm Hg. It worked even better for individuals with high blood pressure: the systolic fell on average 11.4 mm Hg and the diastolic fell 5.5

mm Hg. Since this diet contains ≤27% of its energy from fat (depending on the food choices made), it should also improve blood lipid profiles in most individuals. Although the diet provided in table 3.6 provides only ~2000-2200 kcal/d, it can be modified to provide additional calories, based on total energy expenditure, without changing the overall meal plan. The diet provides adequate carbohydrate (55-60% of energy) for most recreational or fitness athletes, but may need to be increased for elite athletes unless their energy consumption is already high. Although the absolute amount of carbohydrate provided by this diet is ~300-320 g/d,

Table 3.6 The DASH Diet Plan

Number of servings shown is based on a 2000 kcal/d diet. Additional servings for different energy intake need to follow the basic eating plan, along with a sample 1-d menu for a 2000-kcal diet.

Food group	Daily servings	1 serving equals	Examples and notes	Significance of each food group to the DASH eating plan
Grains and grain products	7-8	1 slice bread, 1/2 cup dry cereal* 1/2 cup cooked rice, pasta, or cereal	Grains and whole wheat breads, English muffin, bagels, grits, oatmeal, pita, bread, crackers, unsalted pretzels/popcorn.	Major sources of energy and fiber
Vegetables	4-5	1 cup raw leafy vegetables 1/2 cup cooked vegetables 6 oz vegetable juice	Tomatoes, potatoes, carrots, peas, squash, broccoli, turnip greens, sweet potatoes, collards, kale, spinach, beans, artichokes.	Rich sources of potassium, magnesium, and fiber
Fruits	4-5	6 oz fruit juice 1 medium fruit 1/4 cup dried fruit 1/2 cup fresh, frozen, or canned fruit	Apricots, bananas, dates, grapes, oranges, orange juice, grapefruit, grapefruit juice, mangoes, melons, peaches, pineapples, prunes, raisins, strawberries, tangerines.	Important sources of potassium, magnesium, and fiber
Low-fat or nonfat dairy foods	2-3	8 oz milk 1 cup yogurt 1.5 oz cheese	Skim or 1% milk or low-fat buttermilk, nonfat or low-fat yogurt, part skim mozzarella cheese, nonfat cheese.	Major sources of protein and calcium
Meats, poultry, and fish	2 or less	3 oz cooked meats, poultry, or fish	Select only lean; trim away visible fats; broil, roast, or boil, instead of frying; remove skin from poultry.	Rich sources of protein and magnesium
Nuts, seeds, and dry beans	4-5 per week	1.5 oz or 1/3 cup 2 tbsp seeds 1/2 cup cooked legumes	Almonds, fibers, mixed nuts, peanuts, walnuts, sunflower seeds, kidney beans, lentils.	Rich sources of energy, magnesium, potassium, protein, and fiber
Fats and oils**	2-3	1 tsp soft margarine 1 tbsp low-fat mayonnaise 2 tbsp light salad dressing	Soft margarine, low-fat mayonnaise, light salad dressing, vegetable oil (such as olive, corn, canola, or sunflower).	DASH has ≤ 27% of energy as fat, including that in or added to foods
Sweets	5 per week	1 tbsp sugar 1 tbsp jelly or jam 1/2 oz jelly beans 8 oz lemonade	Maple syrup, sugar, jelly, jam, fruit-flavored gelatin, jelly beans, hard candy, fruit punch, sorbet, ices.	Sweets should be low in fat

*Equals 1/2-1 1/4 cup, depending on cereal type. Check the product's nutrition label.
**Fat content changes serving counts for fats and oils. For example, 1 tbsp of regular salad dressing equals 1 serving; 1 tbsp of a low-fat dressing equals 1/2 serving; 1 tbsp of a fat-free dressing equals 0 servings.

Table 3.6 *(continued)*

Additional servings for different energy intake needs follow the basic eating plan along with a sample 1-d menu for a 2000-kcal diet.

Servings/d	1600 kcal	2100 kcal	2600 kcal	3100 kcal
Grains	6.1	7.7	10.4	12.5
Fruits	3.9	5.2	5.3	6.2
Vegetables	3.6	4.4	5.2	5.8
Low-fat dairy	2.4	2.7	3.2	3.7
Meats, poultry, fish	1.4	1.6	2.0	2.3
Nuts	0.4	0.7	0.7	0.8
Fats	1.8	2.5	3.2	4.1

Sample DASH Menu

Item	Amount	Servings
Breakfast		
Orange juice	6 oz	1 fruit
1% low-fat milk	8 oz	1 dairy
Cornflakes (with 1 tsp sugar)	1 cup	2 grain
Banana	1 medium	1 fruit
Whole wheat bread (with 1 tbsp jelly)	1 slice	1 grain
Soft margarine	1 tsp	1 fat
Lunch		
Chicken salad	3/4 cup	1 poultry
Pita bread	1/2 slice, large	1 grain
Raw vegetable medley:		1 vegetable
carrot and celery sticks	3-4 sticks each	
radishes	2	
loose-leaf lettuce	2 leaves	
Part skim mozzarella cheese	1.5 slice (1.5 oz)	1 dairy
1% low-fat milk	8 oz	1 dairy
Fruit cocktail in light syrup	1/2 cup	1 fruit
Dinner		
Herbed baked cod	3 oz	1 fish
Scallion rice	1 cup	2 grains
Steamed broccoli	1/2 cup	1 vegetable
Stewed tomatoes	1/2 cup	1 vegetable
Spinach salad:		1 vegetable
raw spinach	1/2 cup	
cherry tomatoes	2	
cucumbers	2 slices	
Light Italian salad dressing	1 tbsp	1/2 fat
Whole wheat dinner roll	1 small	1 grain
Soft margarine	1 tsp	1 fat
Melon balls	1/2 cup	1 fruit
Snack		
Dried apricots	1 oz (1/4 cup)	1 fruit
Mini-pretzels	1 oz (3/4 cup)	1 grain
Mixed nuts	1.5 oz (1/3 cup)	1 nut
Diet ginger ale	12 oz	—

Reproduced from Sheps et al. 1997.

Table 3.7 **Examples of High- and Moderate-Carbohydrate Diets With Different Energy Levels for Male and Female Athletes**

Energy (kcal/d)	Male (176 lb or 80 kg) % of energy from carbohydrate									Female (121 lb or 55 kg) % of energy from carbohydrate								
	5000	5000	5000	4000	4000	4000	3000	3000	3000	3500	3500	3500	2500	2500	2500	2000	2000	2000
Carbohydrate																		
(% of energy)	70	60	55	70	60	55	70	60	55	70	60	55	70	60	55	70	60	55
g/d	875	750	688	700	600	550	525	450	413	613	525	481	548	375	344	350	300	275
g/kg BW	10.9	9.4	8.6	8.8	7.5	6.9	6.6	5.6	5.2	11.1	9.5	8.8	8.0	6.8	6.3	6.4	5.5	5.0
g/lb BW	5.0	4.3	3.9	4.0	3.4	3.1	3.0	2.6	2.3	5.1	4.3	2.7	4.5	3.1	2.8	2.9	2.5	2.3
Protein																		
(% of energy)	12	15	15	12	15	15	12	15	15	12	15	15	12	15	15	12	15	15
g/d	150	188	188	120	150	150	90	113	113	105	131	131	75	94	94	60	75	75
g/kg BW	1.9	2.4	2.4	1.5	1.9	1.9	1.1	1.4	1.4	1.9	2.4	2.4	1.4	1.7	1.7	1.1	1.4	1.4
g/lb BW	0.9	1.1	1.1	0.7	0.9	0.9	0.5	0.6	0.6	0.9	1.1	1.1	0.6	0.8	0.8	0.5	0.6	0.6
Fat																		
(% of energy)	18	25	30	18	25	30	18	25	30	18	25	30	18	25	30	18	25	30
g/d	100	139	167	80	111	133	60	83	100	70	97	117	50	69	83	40	56	67
g/kg BW	1.3	1.7	2.1	1.0	1.4	1.7	0.8	1.0	1.3	1.7	1.8	2.1	0.9	1.3	1.5	0.7	1.0	1.2
g/lb BW	0.6	0.8	0.9	0.5	0.6	0.8	0.3	0.5	0.6	1.7	0.6	1.0	0.4	0.6	0.7	0.3	0.5	0.6

BW = Body weight.

this absolute value would increase as energy intake increases. In addition, protein intake is more than adequate at ~100g/d, depending on the food selected. Finally, since the DASH diet provides only 2000 kcal/d, it may be a good dietary guide for the athletic woman who wants to lose weight, or for older active women who want to maintain weight. Energy intake would need to be increased for most male and female athletes in training, since they need more than 2000 kcal/d.

As discussed in chapter 2, making carbohydrate recommendations based on g of carbohydrate/kg body weight is probably the best approach for determining individual athletes' carbohydrate needs. Table 3.7 provides different protein, fat, and carbohydrate recommendations based on diets that contain 55-65% of energy coming from carbohydrate. Once you have selected the ideal carbohydrate recommendations for a particular person, you can use this table to make recommendations for protein and fat.

The amount of fat consumed in a diet containing 60% of its energy from carbohydrate varies dramatically with the total number of calories consumed. A 176-lb (80-kg) male athlete consuming 5000 kcal/d with 60% of the energy coming from carbohydrate would consume 750 g (3000 kcal) of carbohydrate and 139 g of fat (1250 kcal). This is equivalent to ~9.5 g of carbohydrate/kg body weight, which more than exceeds the amount of carbohydrate needed to replace glycogen at a maximum rate, and 1.7 g of fat/kg body weight. For this person, a diet with only 55% of its energy from carbohydrate would still provide 688 g of carbohydrate (8.5 g of carbohydrate/kg body weight) and 30% of its energy from fat (167 g fat). (See table 3.7 for the complete compositions of these two diets.) For many male athletes, this level of carbohydrate and fat intake would be more realistic and achievable than a diet obtaining 65% of its energy from carbohydrate—yet it would still easily replace muscle glycogen during heavy training periods. Thus, making carbohydrate and fat recommendations based solely on percentage of energy coming from carbohydrate may not be realistic or even necessary for most individuals with high energy intakes. This is especially true for athletes who are resistant to dietary changes, and who prefer diets higher in fat.

For many athletic women, who may consume only 2000-2500 kcal/d, it is almost impossible to consume the 500-600 g of carbohydrate/d frequently recommended for adequate glycogen replacement in men. A diet this high in carbohydrate would not allow for adequate fat or protein. For example, a 121-lb (55-kg) woman who consumed 6-7 g carbohydrate/kg body weight would need 330-385 g of carbohydrate/d. This is equivalent to 1320-1550 kcal from carbohydrate or 60-70% of energy coming from carbohydrate based on a 2000 kcal/d diet. For this individual the total carbohydrate intake (g/d) is below the 500-600 g/d recommendation for men, but the percentage of energy from carbohydrate is at or above the recommended level. This diet would have to be low in fat (18-25% of energy from fat). A more realistic goal might be 60-65% of energy from carbohydrate (300-325 g carbohydrate/d) and 25% of the energy from fat (similar to the DASH diet given in table 3.6). This diet would still provide adequate protein (1.4 g/kg based on a 121-lb [55-kg] woman). This level of fat intake is achievable without too many restrictions and is acceptable to most active women. It is also prudent for long-term health and weight maintenance.

Chapter in Review

Fat is an important component in the diets of active people. During weeks and months of heavy exercise training, it is recommended that the diet provide 60-65% of its energy from carbohydrate, plus adequate amounts of fat (20-25% of energy) and protein, depending on body size and dietary preferences. Fat should not be eliminated from the diet. Athletes or active individuals who limit fat intake to <15% of energy intake need to make sure that they obtain adequate levels of essential fatty acids and meet the needs for protein and energy. For active individuals who are dieting for weight loss, a lower-fat diet might be recommended (20% of energy from fat). Simple sugars should not be used to replace fat in the diet; the emphasis should rather be on whole grains, fruits, and vegetables, plus low-fat meat and dairy products (see the general DASH diet food selection in table 3.6). Beans and legumes should be included whenever possible. This type of diet assures that adequate fiber and micronutrients are consumed along with adequate protein, fat, and carbohydrate. People concerned about body weight should exercise caution when buying low-fat or reduced-fat foods. Products labeled "reduced fat" are not necessarily low in calories. It is best to use low-fat versions of whole-fat foods, which will provide the same micronutrients, protein, and carbohydrate composition of the full-fat food, but will be lower in fat and energy (kcal and fat/serving). People with risk factors for chronic disease may need to manipulate their dietary intakes based on their disease risk factors and their level of activity. A nutritionist or a registered dietitian can help make more specific dietary recommendations in these cases. Finally, it is prudent for all athletes and active people to reduce saturated fat to less than 10% of energy intake, in order to help reduce the risk of developing chronic disease.

Although a number of products are marketed to athletes to "improve fat oxidation," no scientific data support the claims of significantly improved fat oxidation. Exercise training is the only method clearly documented in the research literature to improve fat oxidation—a trained individual is a better fat oxidizer than an untrained individual. Exercise training also improves blood lipid and blood glucose profiles, and reduces blood pressure—thus reducing the risk of cardiovascular disease, hypertension, and diabetes.

KEY CONCEPTS

1. Explain the functions, classifications, and dietary sources of fat.

Dietary fat is a primary source of energy, provides the essential fatty acids and fat-soluble vitamins, and adds flavor and palatability to foods. Fat is part of the structural component of cell membranes and tissues and is the way the body stores extra energy. Dietary fats can be classified by their chain length, their level of saturation, their shape, or by the food processing methods applied to the fat (e.g., hydrogenation). Dietary fat is found primarily in the form of triacylglycerols (triglycerides), which contain saturated, monounsaturated, or polyunsaturated fatty acids. Foods with an obviously high concentration of fat, such as butter, oils, and margarine, are called visible fats. Prepared foods that are high in fat, such as cookies, cakes, and desserts, are called invisible fats. Animal foods (meats, dairy, eggs) are generally much higher in fat than plant foods (fruits, vegetables, grains).

2. Compare and contrast the current fat intake of active and inactive individuals.

The body appears to have an unlimited ability to store fat in adipose tissue. In general, active people have lower body fat stores than sedentary people, and women have higher body fat levels than men. Typical fat intake for the general population is ~34% of energy intake, which represents a decrease over the last 30 years from 45% of energy. However, absolute total fat intake (g/d) has increased slightly over the last 5-10 years due to an increase in total energy intake. Reported fat intakes of active individuals vary dramatically depending on the sport and gender, with athletes in endurance sports or who are dieting usually reporting lower fat intakes (<30% of energy).

3. Understand fat metabolism during exercise and the sources of this fat.

Exercise is a strong stimulator of fat lipolysis due to the dramatic increase in blood catecholamines that occurs with exercise. The amount of fat lipolysis, mobilization, and oxidation that occurs during exercise depends on one or more of the following factors: fitness level; the type, intensity, and duration of the exercise; availability of fat reserves in the muscle; the ability to mobilize and transport fatty acids to the muscles; the composition of the meal prior to exercise; and the availability of carbohydrate. Fat mobilized for energy during exercise comes from adipose tissue, intramuscular fat, or fat consumed in the meal before exercise. Fatty acid breakdown, mobilization, and transport from the adipose tissue to the muscle cell employ a number of metabolic pathways and transport proteins. Intramuscular fatty acids can be more readily used as an energy source by the exercising muscle (compared with those from adipose tissue) since no blood transport is required. Regulation of fat oxidation depends primarily on one's ability to mobilize fatty acids from the adipose tissue and to transport these fatty acids to the muscle for uptake, and on the mobilization of fatty acids from intramuscular fats.

4. Identify factors that can enhance or inhibit fat oxidation during exercise.

Increasing one's level of fitness is the primary factor that appears to enhance fat oxidation during exercise. Exercise training increases the body's ability to oxidize fat (1) by increasing the mitochondrial content of the muscle and by increasing the activities of various enzymes involved in fat oxidation and mobilization; (2) by increasing fatty acid uptake by the muscle; (3) by enhancing mobilization of fatty acids from adipose tissue; and (4) by improving the cardiovascular respiratory system, which augments oxygen delivery to the muscle. Other factors—e.g., high-fat diets (~60-75% of energy), long-chain fatty acids, medium-chain triacylglycerol, caffeine, and carnitine—have been examined as to their ability to improve fat oxidation during exercise. In general, none of these factors appreciably improves fat oxidation during exercise.

 5. Discuss the current dietary fat recommendations for active individuals.

Fat intakes of 20-25% of energy are generally recommended for active individuals, while extremely-low-fat diets (<15% of energy) appear to offer no health or performance benefit. Fat recommendations for individual athletes should be based on the individual's health, current dietary intake, sport, body weight and composition goals, and food preferences.

KEY TERMS

α-linolenic acid
acetyl-CoA
acylcarnitine
acyl-CoA synthetase
carnitine palmitoyl transferase I (CPT 1)
carnitine palmitoyl transferase II (CPT 2)
chylomicrons
cis fatty acid
cytoplasmic fatty acid binding protein
docosahexaenoic acid (DHA)
eicosapentaenoic acid (EPA)
epinephrine
essential fatty acid
fatty acid (FA)
fatty acid binding protein (FABP)
fatty acid translocase (FAT)
free fatty acid (FFA)
glycerol
hormone sensitive lipase (HSL)
hydrogenation

insulin
invisible fat
linoleic acid
lipolysis
lipoprotein lipase (LPL)
lipoproteins
long-chain fatty acid (LCFA)
long-chain triacylglycerol (LCT)
medium-chain fatty acid (MCFA)
medium-chain triacylglycerol (MCT)
monoglyceride lipase (MGL)
monounsaturated
polyunsaturated
re-esterification
saturated
short-chain fatty acid (SCFA)
trans fatty acid
triacylglycerols (triglycerides)
very-low-density lipoprotein (VLDL)
visible fat

References

Beals KA, Manore MM. Nutritional status of female athletes with subclinical eating disorders. J Am Diet Assoc 1998;98:419-25.

Bell DG, Jacobs I, Zamecnik J. Effects of caffeine, ephedrine and their combination on time to exhaustion during high-intensity exercise. Eur J Appl Physiol 1998;77:427-33.

Berning JR. The role of medium-chain triglycerides in exercise. Int J Sport Nutr 1996; 6:121-33.

Brouns F, van der Vusse GJ. Utilization of lipids during exercise in human subjects: metabolic and dietary constraints. Br J Nutr 1998;79:117-28.

Bulow J. Lipid mobilization and utilization. Med Sports Sci 1988;27:140-63.

Bulow J, Madsen J. Regulation of fatty acid mobilization from adipose tissue during exercise. Scand J Sports Sci 1986;8:19-26.

Callaway CW. The role of fat-modified foods in the American diet. Nutr Today 1998;33:156-63.

Calorie Control Council (CCC) National Consumer Survey. Most popular reduced-fat products. Atlanta, GA: CCC, 1998.

Carlson MG, Snead WL, Hill JO, Nurjhan N, Campbell PJ. Glucose regulation of lipid metabolism in humans. Am J Physiol 1991; 261:E815-20.

Champe PC, Harvey RA. Lippincott's Illustrated Reviews: Biochemistry. Philadelphia, PA: J. B. Lippincott Company, 1987:149-222.

Clarkson PM. Nutritional ergogenic aids: caffeine. Int J Sport Nutr 1993;3:103-11.

Colombani P, Wenk C, Kunz I, et al. Effects of L-carnitine supplementation on physical performance and energy metabolism of endurance-trained athletes: a double-blind crossover field study. Eur J Appl Physiol 1996;73:434-9.

Cortright RN, Muoio DM, Dohm GL. Skeletal muscle lipid metabolism: a frontier for new insights into fuel homeostasis. J Nutr Biochem 1997;8:228-45.

Coyle EF, Coggan AR, Hemmert MK, Ivy JL. Muscle glycogen utilization during prolonged strenuous exercise when fed carbohydrate. J Appl Physiol 1986;61(1):165-72.

Coyle EF, Jeukendrup AE, Wagenmakers AJM, Saris WHM. Fatty acid oxidation is directly regulated by carbohydrate metabolism during exercise. Am J Physiol 1997;273:E268-75.

Daniels JW, Mole PA, Shaffrath JD, Stebbins CL. Effects of caffeine on blood pressure, heart rate, and forearm blood flow during dynamic leg exercise. J Appl Physiol 1998; 85:154-9.

Decombaz J, Arnaud MJ, Milon H, et al. Energy metabolism of medium-chain triglycerides versus carbohydrates during exercise. Eur J Appl Physiol 1983;52:9-14.

Dodd SL, Herb RA, Powers SK. Caffeine and endurance performance: an update. Sports Med 1993;15:14-23.

Dreon DM, Fernstrom HA, Williams PT, Krauss RM. A very-low-fat diet is not associated with improved lipoprotein profiles in men with a predominance of large, low-density lipoproteins. Am J Clin Nutr 1999;69:411-8.

Dyck DJ, Peters SJ, Glatz J, et al. Functional differences in lipid metabolism in resting skeletal muscle of various fiber types. Am J Physiol 1997;272:E340-51.

FDA Register P99-27. FDA proposes new rules for trans fatty acids in nutrition labeling,

nutrient content claims, and health claims. Washington, DC: HHS News. **http:// www.fda.gov/bbs/topics/NEWS/ NEW00698.html**

Fogelholm M, Koskinen R, Laakso J, Rankinen T, Ruokonen I. Gradual and rapid weight loss: effects on nutrition and performance in male athletes. Med Sci Sports Exerc 1993;25:371-7.

Fogelholm M, Rehunen S, Gref C, et al. Dietary intake and thiamin, iron, and zinc status in elite Nordic skiers during different training periods. Int J Sport Nutr 1992;2:351-65.

Food Processor (software program), Version 7.01. ESHA Research, Salem, OR.

Graham TE, Hibbert E, Sathasivam P. Metabolic and exercise endurance effects of coffee and caffeine ingestion. J Appl Physiol 1998;85:883-9.

Graham TE, Rusch JWE, van Soeren MH. Caffeine and exercise: metabolism and performance. Can J Appl Physiol 1994;19:111-38.

Graham TE, Spriet LL. Caffeine and exercise performance. In: Sports Science Exchange. Barrington, IL: Gatorade Sports Science Institute, 1996;9:1-6.

Graham TE, Spriet LL. Metabolic, catecholamine, and exercise performance responses to various doses of caffeine. J Appl Physiol 1995;78:867-74.

Grundy SM. Dietary fat. In: Ziegler EE, Filer LJ, eds. Present Knowledge in Nutrition. Washington, DC: ILSI Press, 1996:44-57.

Harris WS. n-3 fatty acids and serum lipoproteins: human studies. Am J Clin Nutr 1997; 65(suppl):1645S-54S.

Hawley JA, Brouns F, Jeukendrup A. Strategies to enhance fat utilization during exercise. Sports Med 1998;25:241-67.

Hawley JA, Dennis SC, Lindsay FH, Noakes TD. Nutritional practices of athletes: are they sub-optimal? J Sport Sci 1995;13:S75-87.

Helge JW, Richter EA, Kiens B. Interaction of training and diet on metabolism and endurance during exercise in man. J Physiol 1996;292:293-306.

Helge JW, Wulff B, Kiens B. Impact of a fat-rich diet on endurance in man: role of the dietary period. Med Sci Sports Exerc 1998;30:456-61.

Horowitz JF, Mora-Rodriguez R, Byerlye LO, Coyle EF. Lipolytic suppression following carbohydrate ingestion limits fat oxidation during exercise. Am J Physiol 1997; 273:E768-75.

Hudnall MJ, Conner SJ, Conner WE. Position of the American Dietetic Association: fat replacements. J Am Diet Assoc 1991;91: 1285-8.

Hurley BF, Nemeth PM, Martin WH, Hagberg JM, Dalsky GP, Holloszy JO. Muscle triglyceride utilization during exercise: effect of training. J Appl Physiol 1986;60:562-7.

Innis SM. Essential dietary lipids. In: Ziegler EE, Filer LJ, eds. Present Knowledge in Nutrition. Washington, DC: ILSI Press, 1996: 58-66.

Ivy JL, Costill DL, Fink WJ, Maglischo E. Contribution of medium and long chain triglyceride intake to energy metabolism during prolonged exercise. Int J Sports Med 1980;1:15-20.

Jeukendrup AE, Saris WHM. Fat as a fuel during exercise. In: Berning JR, Steen SN, eds. Nutrition for Sport and Exercise. Gaithersburg, MD: Aspen Publishers, 1998:59-75.

Jeukendrup AE, Saris WHM, Brouns F, Halliday D, Wagenmakers AJM. Effects of carbohydrate (CHO) and fat supplementation on CHO metabolism during prolonged exercise. Metabolism 1996;45:915-21.

Jeukendrup AE, Saris WHM, Schrauwen P, Brouns F, Wagenmakers AJM. Metabolic availability of medium-chain triglycerides coingested with carbohydrate during prolonged exercise. J Appl Physiol 1995;79:756-62.

Jeukendrup AE, Saris WHM, Wagenmakers AJM. Fat metabolism during exercise: a review—Part I. Int J Sports Med 1998;19:231-44.

Jeukendrup AE, Saris WHM, Wagenmakers AJM. Fat metabolism during exercise: a review—Part II. Regulation of metabolism and the effects of training. Int J Sports Med 1998;19:293-302.

Jeukendrup AE, Saris WHM, Wagenmakers AJM. Fat metabolism during exercise: a review—Part III. Effects of nutritional interventions. Int J Sports Med 1998;19:371-9.

Jeukendrup AE, Thielen JJHC, Wagenmakers AJM, Brouns F, Saris WHM. Effect of medium-chain triacylglycerol and carbohydrate ingestion during exercise on substrate utilization and subsequent cycling performance. Am J Clin Nutr 1998;67:397-404.

Kaminsky LA, Martin CA, Whaley MH. Caffeine consumption habits do not influence the exercise blood pressure response following caffeine ingestion. J Sports Med Phys Fitness 1998;38:53-8.

Kanter MM, Williams MH. Antioxidants, carnitine, and choline as putative ergogenic aids. Int J Sport Nutr 1995;5:S120-31.

Kiens B, Essen-Gustavsson B, Christensen NJ, Saltin B. Skeletal muscle substrate utilization during submaximal exercise in man: effect of endurance training. J Physiol 1993;469:459-78.

Kiens B, Helge JW. Effect of high-fat diets on exercise performance. Proc Nutr Soc 1998;57:73-5.

Lambert EV, Hawley JA, Goedecke J, Noakes TD, Dennis SC. Nutritional strategies for promoting fat utilization and delaying the onset of fatigue during prolonged exercise. J Sport Sci 1997;15:315-24.

Lambert EV, Speechly DP, Dennis SC, Noakes TD. Enhanced endurance in trained cyclists during moderate intensity exercise following 2 weeks adaptation to a high-fat diet. Eur J Appl Physiol 1994;69:287-93.

Lichtenstein AH, Van Horn L. Very low-fat diets. Circulation 1998;98:935-9.

Linscheer WG, Vergroesen AJ. Lipids. In: Shils ME, Olsen JA, Shike M, eds. Modern Nutrition in Health and Disease. Philadelphia: Lea and Febiger, 1994:47-88.

Massicotte D, Peronnet F, Brisson GR, Hillaire-Marcel C. Oxidation of exogenous medium-chain free fatty acids during prolonged exercise: comparison with glucose. J Appl Physiol 1992;73:1334-9.

Odland LM, Heigenhauser GJF, Wong D, Hollidge-Horvat MG, Spriet LL. Effects of increased fat availability on fat-carbohydrate interaction during prolonged exercise in men. Am J Physiol 1998;274:R894-R904.

Okano G, Sato Y, Murata Y. Effect of elevated blood FFAs levels on endurance performance after a single fat meal ingestion. Med Sci Sports Exerc 1998;30:763-8.

Ornish D. Low-fat diets. N Engl J Med 1998; 338(2):127.

Oscai LB, Essig DA, Palmer WK. Lipase regulation of muscle triacylglycerol hydrolysis. J Appl Physiol 1990;69:1571-7.

Pathways of Nutritional Biochemistry. Carnitine and fatty acid synthesis. J Nutr Biochem 1991;2:381.

Prentice AM. Manipulation of dietary fat and energy density and subsequent effects on substrate flux and food intake. Am J Clin Nutr 1998;67(suppl):535S-41S.

Romijn JA, Coyle EF, Sidossis LS, et al. Regulation of endogenous fat and carbohydrate metabolism in relation to exercise intensity. Am J Physiol 1993;265:E380-91.

Saltin B, Åstrand PO. Free fatty acids and exercise. Am J Clin Nutr 1993; 57(suppl): 752S-8S.

Saris WHM, van Erp-Baart MA, Brouns F, Westererp KR, ten Hoor F. Study of food intake and energy expenditure during extreme sustained exercise: the Tour de France. Int J Sports Med 1989:10; S26-31.

Sheps SG, Black HR, Cohen JD, et al. The sixth report of the joint national committee on prevention, detection, and evaluation, and treatment of high blood pressure. Arch Intern Med 1997;157:2413-46.

Sherman WM, Leenders N. Fat loading: the next magic bullet? Int J Sport Nutr 1995; 5:S1-12.

Sigman-Grant M. Can you have your low-fat cake and eat it too? The role of fat-modified products. J Am Diet Assoc 1997;97(suppl): S76-81.

Simopoulos AT, Leaf A, Salem N. Essentiality of and recommended dietary intakes for omega-6 and omega-3 fatty acids. Ann Nutr Metab 1999;43:127-30.

Spriet LL. Caffeine and performance. Int J Sport Nutr 1995;5:S84-99.

Trappe SW, Costill DL, Goodpasture B, Vukovich VD, Fink WJ. The effects of L-carnitine supplementation on performance during interval swimming. Int J Sports Med 1994;15:181-5.

Turcotte LP, Richter EA, Kiens B. Lipid metabolism during exercise. In: Hargreaves M, ed. Exercise Metabolism. Champaign, IL: Human Kinetics, 1995:99-130.

USDA Center for Nutrition Policy and Promotion (CNPP). Is total fat consumption really decreasing? Nutrition Insights 1995;vol.5. Reprinted in: Nutr Today 1998;33:171-2.

Van Zyl CG, Lambert EV, Hawley JA, Noakes TD, Dennis SC. Effects of medium-chain triglyceride ingestion on fuel metabolism and cycling performance. J Appl Physiol 1996;80:2217-25.

Venkatraman JT, Pendergast D. Effects of the level of dietary fat intake and endurance exercise on plasma cytokines in runners. Med Sci Sports Exerc 1998;30:1198-204.

Vukovich MD, Costill DL, Hickey MS, Trappe SW, Cole KJ, Fink WJ. Effect of fat emulsion infusion and fat feeding on muscle glycogen utilization during cycling exercise. J Appl Physiol 1993;75:1513-8.

Whitley HA, Humphreys SM, Campbell IT, et al. Metabolic and performance responses during endurance exercise after high-fat and high-carbohydrate meals. J Appl Physiol 1998;85:418-24.

Winder WW. Malonyl CoA—regulator of fatty acid oxidation in muscle during exercise. In: Holloszy J, ed. Exercise and Sport Science Reviews. Baltimore, MD: Williams and Wilkins, 1998:117-32.

Wolfe RR. Metabolic interactions between glucose and fatty acids in humans. Am J Clin Nutr 1998;67(suppl):519S-26S.

Wolfe RR, Klein S, Carraro F, Weber JM. Role of triglyceride-fatty acid cycle in controlling fat metabolism in humans during and after exercise. Am J Physiol 1990;258:E382-9.

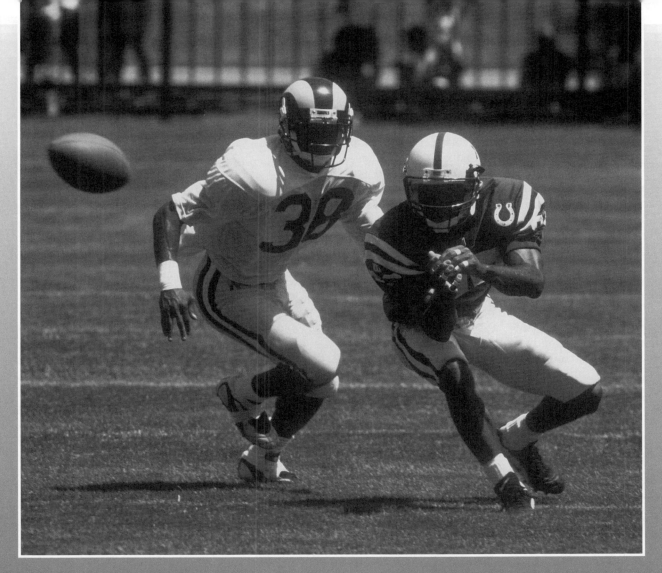

CHAPTER 4

Protein and Exercise

After reading this chapter you should be able to

- describe the functions and classifications of proteins;
- list and describe the primary methods of assessing protein status;
- discuss dietary sources of protein;
- discuss the metabolism of protein during and post-exercise; and
- describe the dietary protein recommendations for active individuals.

Protein, a required macronutrient, has played a controversial role in sport nutrition. Diets of athletes before the 20th century were typically high in protein, as protein was considered the primary energy source for exercise. In addition, many cultures believed that consuming the muscle of an animal resulted in a direct transfer of that animal's strength and prowess to the athlete.

Recent studies have indicated that, while protein is not the primary energy source fueling exercise, it does play a critical role in the health and performance of athletes. There is widespread confusion among many exercise professionals and the lay public regarding both the role that protein plays during exercise and the protein needs of active people. Here are some questions frequently posed concerning protein and exercise:

- Do athletes and active people need more protein than sedentary people need?
- Do strength athletes have a high protein requirement?
- Can a vegetarian diet provide adequate protein for athletes?
- Are there risks associated with high protein intakes or protein supplementation?

This chapter reviews the roles of protein in relation to exercise and addresses the questions listed above. Protein metabolism during exercise is still poorly understood, and many areas of study are still controversial. We will try to clarify some of the confusion, indicating where more research is needed. Finally, we provide dietary protein recommendations for active people.

Functions and Classifications

Protein is a nutrient that is critical to both the structure and function of the body. It is more appropriate to use the term "proteins" than "protein," as there are a multitude of proteins in the human body. The three-dimensional shape and sequence of amino acids determine the functional role of any particular protein within the body. Proteins have many exercise-related functions, some of which are listed below:

- Building materials for bone, ligaments, tendons, muscles, and organs.

- Enzymes that facilitate reactions associated with energy production and fuel utilization, and the building and repair of body tissues, especially muscle.
- Hormones related to energy metabolism (e.g., insulin, glucagon, epinephrine).
- Maintenance of fluid and electrolyte balance (e.g., blood albumin plays a significant role in maintaining colloidal pressure within blood vessels).
- Act as a buffer and assist with the maintenance of acid-base balance.
- Required for the synthesis of blood transport proteins that carry a number of substances such as micronutrients, drugs, and oxygen within the body (e.g., hemoglobin transports oxygen from the lungs to the working muscle; transferrin transports minerals such as iron; albumin transports micronutrients and drugs).
- Act as an energy source during and following exercise, particularly in situations of low carbohydrate and energy status.

Uniquely among the energy nutrients (fat, carbohydrate, protein, and alcohol), protein contains nitrogen (N). Proteins, both in the diet and in the body, are made up of **amino acids** that contain at least one nitrogen amine group. When body proteins are broken down, the amino acids can be oxidized for energy to CO_2 and water; the nitrogen group is eliminated in the urine, primarily as urea. The same is true when extra dietary protein is consumed: the amino acids are oxidized for energy, with the extra nitrogen eliminated as urea. The body has no way to store extra nitrogen the way it stores dietary carbohydrate as glycogen and extra dietary fat as body fat.

The amino acids found in dietary protein are typically classified as essential or nonessential (table 4.1), although the essentiality of an amino acid may depend on one's age, genetic makeup, or health status. **Essential amino acids** must be consumed in the diet, while the body can synthesize the **nonessential amino acids**. All amino acids are important for good health, growth, and the maintenance and repair of tissue. Table 4.1 lists two amino acids as **conditionally essential** since requirements for them change when synthesis becomes limited or when the diet provides inadequate amounts of precursors (Matthews 1999). For example, the body makes tyrosine from the essential amino acid phenylalanine and cysteine from the essential amino acid methionine. If the diet is low in phenylalanine or methionine, the body does not synthesize these two amino acids and their essentiality in the diet increases. Table 4.1 also lists special amino acids that are commonly found in the body—such as 3-methylhistidine, a modification of histidine after the latter is incorporated into muscle. The role of 3-methylhistidine in protein status is discussed later in this chapter.

The current Recommended Dietary Allowance (RDA) for protein, estimated for sedentary healthy adults, is 0.8 g/kg body weight (Food and Nutrition Board 1989). This value is estimated to meet the daily protein needs of most healthy adults; the unique needs of active adults were not included in this estimation. Because exercise increases oxygen transport, fuel utilization, and energy needs, and can stimulate tissue growth and repair, the current RDA may not be adequate for active people. Moreover, protein requirements may be higher than the RDA for people who are sick, injured, or recovering from illness. Before we discuss the specific protein needs of athletes and ac-

tive people, we will review the assessment techniques used to measure protein status.

Methods of Assessing Protein Status

There is a variety of ways to assess protein status. While these methods have their limitations, they have been useful in expanding our knowledge of proteins' roles in exercise. Many of the protein assessment methods are time-consuming, invasive, and require sophisticated laboratory equipment. The challenges of these procedures have limited our ability to assess the protein status of large numbers of active people.

Nitrogen Balance

Nitrogen balance involves assessing the relationship between the dietary protein intake, which contains ~16% nitrogen, and nitrogen lost from the body. When protein (or nitrogen) intake is greater than the amount lost by the body, one is said to be in **positive nitrogen**

Table 4.1 **Classifications of Common Amino Acids**

Essential amino acids		
Isoleucine	Methionine	Tryptophan
Leucine	Phenylalanine	Valine
Lysine	Threonine	Histidine[a]
Nonessential amino acids		
Alanine	Asparagine	Glycine
Arginine	Glutamic acid	Proline
Aspartic acid	Glutamine	Serine
Conditionally essential amino acids		
Cysteine	Tyrosine	
Some special amino acids		
Alloisoleucine	Hydroxylysine	3-Methylhistidine
Citrulline	Hydroxyproline	Ornithine
Homocysteine		

[a]The essentiality for histidine has been shown only for infants, but probably small amounts are needed for adults as well.

Adapted from Matthews 1999.

balance, or positive nitrogen status. This state occurs during growth and development, weight gain, pregnancy, lactation, and times of muscle healing or recovery from injury. When protein (or nitrogen) intake is less than the amount excreted, one is in a state of **negative nitrogen balance**. This state occurs during weight loss, illness, burns, or injury. When protein (or nitrogen) intake is equal to the amount excreted, one is in nitrogen balance. A state of nitrogen balance typically occurs in healthy adults during times of weight maintenance.

A number of variables must be considered when assessing nitrogen balance. Listed below are some of the key nitrogen sources that must be estimated or measured when determining nitrogen balance in an individual:

- Dietary nitrogen intake (assessed by calculating total protein intake [g/d divided by 6.25] or by directly measuring nitrogen in food).
- Total urinary nitrogen (primarily nitrogen from urea [86-90% of total urinary nitrogen], creatinine [4.5%], ammonia [2.8%], uric acid [1.7%], and other N-containing compounds [5.0%]).
- Total fecal nitrogen (primarily nitrogen from undigested proteins, sloughed off cells, and bacteria within the gut).
- Dermal and other miscellaneous nitrogen losses (primarily nitrogen in exfoliated cells and nitrogen lost in blood, sweat, nails, hair, and semen).

Total urinary nitrogen and fecal nitrogen are directly measured using the **Kjeldahl technique** (Gibson 1990). The Kjeldahl technique uses sulfuric acid to digest the material, a strong base to liberate the nitrogen as ammonia, and a colorimetric assay or titration to determine the nitrogen content. Due to the labor and time required to use this technique, total urinary and fecal nitrogen content is rarely measured outside of a research setting. Instead, urinary urea nitrogen is used to estimate total urinary nitrogen since 85% to 90% of total urinary nitrogen is accounted for by urinary urea

■ HIGHLIGHT ■

Equations Used to Calculate Nitrogen Balance

Two equations can be used to calculate nitrogen balance (Gibson 1990). The first estimates total urinary and fecal nitrogen losses. The second estimates nitrogen balance using urinary urea nitrogen and adds a constant value as a single estimate of both total fecal and dermal nitrogen losses.

Equation 1

$$\text{Nitrogen balance} = I - (U - Ue) + (F - Fe) + S$$

Where I = (protein intake in g)/6.25 (this gives an estimate of nitrogen intake); U = total urinary nitrogen; Ue = endogenous urinary nitrogen; F = fecal nitrogen; Fe = endogenous fecal nitrogen losses; S = dermal nitrogen losses (nitrogen lost in sweat and sloughed-off skin cells).

Endogenous urinary and fecal nitrogen losses refer to the nitrogen that is not excreted in urine or feces; although this nitrogen is "lost," we do not have methods to quantify these losses within the body.

Equation 2

$$\text{Nitrogen balance} = (\text{protein intake in g}/6.25 - (\text{urinary urea nitrogen [in g]} + 4^*)$$

To further simplify the estimation of nitrogen balance, a constant value of 2 g is generally used to account for fecal and dermal losses; an additional 2 g approximate the non-urea nitrogen components of urine and other miscellaneous nitrogen losses (blood, nails, hair, semen) (MacKenzie et al. 1985). This method is sometimes called crude nitrogen balance.

nitrogen (Gibson 1990). The use of urinary urea nitrogen to estimate total urinary nitrogen is controversial, and researchers disagree about the extent to which the errors associated with this estimation are clinically significant (Lee and Nieman 1996). This simple method of calculating nitrogen balance using urinary urea nitrogen is sometimes referred to as **crude nitrogen balance**. See "Equations Used to Calculate Nitrogen Balance" on page 108.

The nitrogen balance procedure involves many challenges to the volunteer being measured as well as to the researcher. The volunteer must be willing to perform multiple 24-h urine and fecal collections. The dietary protein intake is best measured if the volunteer follows a standardized diet—which means that all the food he or she eats must be measured before consumption, and duplicate meals must be made and analyzed for their nitrogen content. It is imperative that the participant eat only the foods prescribed, and that body weight is stable throughout the testing period. Compliance of the participant plays a major role in the accuracy of estimating nitrogen balance. Table 4.2 lists the advantages and limitations of the nitrogen balance method and other methods used to estimate protein status.

Tracer Method

A second method of estimating protein status uses labeled exogenous **isotopic tracers**, spe-cifically ^{13}C, ^{14}C, and ^{15}N-labeled amino acids. The procedure involves determining the enrichment or specific radioactivity of the tracer in body fluids, tissues, and excretion products such as urine and expired air. Figure 4.1 illustrates the single-pool model of whole-body protein metabolism measured with a labeled amino acid tracer (Matthews 1999). The amino acid tracer enters the free amino acid pool, which derives from dietary protein intake and amino acids released from protein breakdown. The labeled amino acid leaves the free amino acid pool via amino acid oxidation, which results in the production of urea, ammonia (NH_3), and CO_2; or it can be used for protein synthesis and incorporated into body proteins. This method provides an estimate of amino acid turnover, plus the rate at which the labeled amino acid is incorporated into body tissues. See Wolfe (1984) and Matthews (1999) for a detailed description of tracer methodology. The primary advantage of the tracer method over nitrogen balance is that the former determines the metabolic fate of an individual amino acid, resulting in an estimation of protein synthesis, oxidation, and degradation. However, the turnover of a single amino acid does not necessarily represent the turnover of all amino acids.

3-Methylhistidine Excretion

Protein status and metabolism, especially in the muscle, can also be estimated by measuring

Table 4.2 **Advantages and Limitations of Methods Used to Estimate Protein Status**

Method	Advantages	Limitations
Nitrogen balance	• Relatively accurate measure of protein status • Cost-effective means of monitoring clinical patients if crude nitrogen balance is used	• Time-consuming • Laborious • Subject compliance must be very good • Assesses only net nitrogen status
Tracer methodology	• Can estimate how protein synthesis, oxidation, and degradation contribute to overall protein status • Relatively noninvasive	• Expensive • Requires specialized gas chromatography-mass spectrometry equipment • Labeled amino acid may not respond in the same manner to exercise as non-labeled amino acids • Assumptions about certain metabolic issues may not hold true during exercise
3-Methylhistidine	• Noninvasive • Inexpensive • Can be measured in a standard laboratory	• Metabolism of contractile proteins in gut and skin can confound results • Does not indicate protein synthesis, degradation, or oxidation

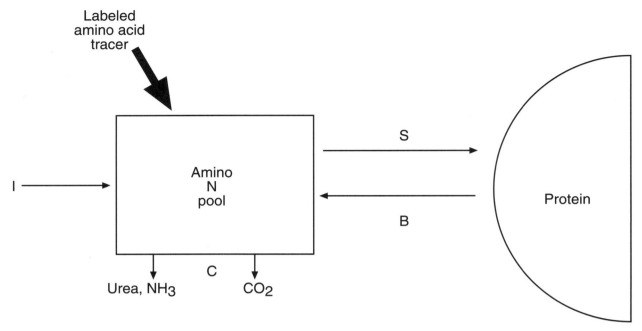

Figure 4.1 Single-pool model of whole-body protein metabolism measured with a labeled amino acid tracer. The amino acid enters the free pool from dietary intake (I) or as amino acid released from protein breakdown (B); it leaves the free pool via amino acid oxidation (C) to urea, ammonia (NH_3), and CO_2, or when used in protein synthesis (S).

Adapted from Matthews 1999.

3-methylhistidine (3-MH) (also known as N-methylhistidine) in the urine. 3-MH is formed by the methylation of histidine after it is incorporated into contractile proteins, with most of the 3-MH found in muscle tissue. Because the body cannot recycle it from degraded contractile proteins (i.e., muscle tissue), 3-MH is excreted in the urine (Dohm et al. 1987). An increased level of 3-MH in the urine may indicate increased breakdown of the contractile proteins actin and myosin. Since dietary meat confounds the measurement of 3-MH, subjects must follow a controlled diet during the measurement process.

The excretion of 3-MH is expressed as a ratio of creatinine excretion, in order to adjust for changes in renal clearance and to correct for individual differences in muscle mass. This method is controversial, the primary objection being that 3-MH is not specific to skeletal muscle breakdown (there are small amounts of contractile proteins in the gut and skin), and that the turnover of these other tissues can contribute significantly to the total 3-MH excreted in the urine (Dohm et al. 1987). Despite this limitation, many researchers value this method as a noninvasive, relatively simple, and inexpensive measurement.

Dietary Sources of Protein

Protein is abundant in the U.S. diet and in the diets of other developed countries. While meat and dairy products contain high levels of protein, a significant amount of our dietary protein comes also from cereals, grains, nuts, and legumes. Even many fruits (e.g., apricots, blueberries, and apples) and vegetables (e.g., asparagus and green beans) contain small amounts of protein. **Protein quality** is determined by both the amino acid content and the **digestibility** of the protein (Food and Nutrition Board 1989). Proteins derived from plant foods are approximately 85% digestible; those in a mixed diet of meat products and refined grains are approximately 95% digestible. Based on these differences in digestibility, it is recommended that people who eat no flesh or dairy products consume 10% more protein daily (or 0.9 g/kg body weight/d compared to the current adult RDA of 0.8 g/kg).

The term **complete protein** typically refers to proteins that contain all the essential amino acids when consumed at the recommended level of protein intake (Messina and Messina 1996). While plant proteins have been generally classified as incomplete and animal proteins as complete, all of the amino acids appear in plant proteins, but in lower amounts as compared to meat. Thus, one needs to eat more of a plant protein source in order to obtain adequate amino acids; and in some cases one must consume more than one source of plant protein in order to obtain all the amino acids. Grains tend to lack lysine, for example, and legumes tend to lack methionine. **Mutual supplementation** involves consuming plant protein sources with complementary amino acid combinations (such as soybeans and rice, wheat bread and peanut butter, pinto beans and corn tortillas) at each meal. Studies of adults have shown that it is not really necessary to consume these foods together at the same meal, as the endogenous protein levels in the gut are maintained between meals and can be used for protein synthesis at subsequent meals (Messina and Messina 1996). These findings highlight the importance of consuming high-protein sources throughout the day if one follows a vegetarian diet.

The RDA for protein for nonvegetarian adults is 0.8 g/kg body weight. Protein recommendations are also expressed as a percentage of total energy, with most nutrition professionals and organizations recommending that *protein intakes should range from 12-20% of total energy intake.* Contrary to the belief of many, most people in the United States easily meet their protein needs. Active people at risk for inadequate protein intakes are generally those who are not consuming adequate energy.

Table 4.3 reviews the protein content of common foods consumed in the United States. It is clear that individuals who eat a varied diet and consume adequate energy on a regular basis can easily meet the RDA for protein. An example: Doug weighs 180 lb (81.8 kg) and briskly walks 10 mi every week. Assuming his requirement matches the RDA, Doug needs 0.8 g of protein/kg body weight, or 65.4 g of protein per day. If he consumes 2/3 cup of oatmeal with 1/2 cup skim milk for breakfast, and a 4-oz chicken breast with no skin and 8 fl oz of skim milk for lunch, his protein intake from these foods alone is approximately 53 g, or 80% of the RDA—and his energy intake is only 417 kcal! Since Doug typically consumes 2500 to 2800 kcal per day to maintain his body weight, he easily meets his protein needs by eating other foods. This example is typical of the general population. In fact, the meat portions served in restaurants usually range from 6-15 oz, so that many people meet their RDA for protein in one meal. At least in the United States, it is easy to meet the RDA for protein when adequate energy is consumed.

Vegetarians are also quite able to meet their daily protein needs. Messina and Messina (1996) reviewed numerous studies of vegetarians and reported that protein intakes ranged between 12-14% and between 10-12% of the total energy consumed by lacto-ovo vegetarians and vegans, respectively. Beans, nuts, soy, eggs, and dairy products are excellent protein sources that can be eaten by **lacto-ovo vegetarians** (who eat eggs and dairy products), while people consuming **vegan** diets (no animal products of any kind) can obtain adequate protein from beans, nuts, soy, and other plant sources of protein. It is important that vegetarians consume a wide variety of foods; some may need supplements of micronutrients such as vitamin B_{12}, iron, and zinc. However, both sedentary and physically active vegetarians are capable of meeting their daily protein needs without requiring supplementation if they eat a variety of foods and meet their energy needs.

A common question: "Aren't the protein needs of athletes higher?" We discuss this topic in detail later in this chapter. The quick answer is "yes." The protein needs of both strength and endurance athletes are approximately 1.5 to 2.0 times higher than the present adult RDA (Lemon 1998). But, while it is true that athletes need more protein than sedentary individuals, most sedentary and active North Americans already consume over twice the adult RDA for protein with no conscious effort!

Protein Intake of the General U.S. Population

Large epidemiological surveys have estimated the dietary intake of the U.S. population. Phase 1 of the Third National Health and Nutrition Examination Survey (NHANES III), including the years 1988-1991, analyzed the energy and macronutrient intakes of persons 2 mo of age and older (McDowell et al. 1994). The average protein intake of adults over age 20 was 16% of total energy (figure 4.2). The mean protein intake was similar across ethnic groups, with men consuming 88-92 g/d and women 63-66 g/d. For males, protein intakes were highest for adolescents and young adults and declined after 29 years of age. Women consumed less protein than men, and changes in protein intake with age were similar to those in men. Table 4.4 lists

Table 4.3 **Protein Content of Foods Commonly Consumed in the United States**

Food	Serving size	Protein (g)
Beef:		
Ground, lean, baked (16% fat)	3.5 oz	24.3
Corned beef, brisket, cooked	3.5 oz	18.3
Prime rib, broiled (1/2 in. trim)	3.5 oz	20.9
Top sirloin, broiled (1/4 in. trim)	3.5 oz	27.4
Poultry:		
Chicken breast, broiled, no skin	3.0 oz	25.3
Chicken thigh, BBQ, with skin	2.2 oz	14.5
Chicken drumstick, BBQ, with skin	2.5 oz	15.8
Turkey breast meat, roasted, Louis Rich	3.5 oz	19.9
Turkey dark meat, roasted, no skin	3.5 oz	28.7
Seafood:		
Cod, steamed	3.5 oz	22.1
Salmon, Chinook, baked	3.5 oz	25.5
Shrimp, steamed	3.5 oz	20.8
Oysters, boiled	3.5 oz	18.6
Tuna, water-packed, drained	3.5 oz	29.4
Dairy:		
Whole milk (3.3% fat)	8 fl oz	8.0
1% milk	8 fl oz	8.0
Skim milk	8 fl oz	8.4
Low-fat yogurt	8 fl oz	12.9
American cheese, processed	1 oz	6.5
Swiss cheese	1 oz	6.4
Cottage cheese, low-fat (2%)	1 cup	31.0
Nuts and beans:		
Peanuts, dry roasted	1 oz	6.7
Peanut butter, creamy	2 tbsp	8.2
Almonds, blanched	1 oz	6.0
Beans, refried	1/2 cup	6.9
Kidney beans, red	1/2 cup	9.3
Grains and cereals:		
Oatmeal, quick, cooked	1 cup	6.1
Malt-O-Meal, cooked	1 cup	3.6
Cheerios	1 1/4 cup	4.3
Frosted Flakes	3/4 cup	1.1
Grape-nuts	1/4 cup	3.4
Rye bread	1 slice	2.7
Whole wheat bread	1 slice	2.7
Cheez-It crackers	12 crackers	1.2
Triscuit crackers	3 crackers	1.1
Vegetables and fruits:		
Banana	1 medium	1.2
Apple, raw, with skin	1 medium	0.3
Orange, raw, navel	1 medium	1.3
Asparagus, boiled	1/2 cup (6 spears)	2.3
Green snap beans, canned	1/2 cup	0.8
Broccoli, raw, chopped	1/2 cup	1.3
Mushrooms, raw, pieces	1/2 cup	0.7

Values from Food Processor 7.21, ESHA Research, Salem, OR.

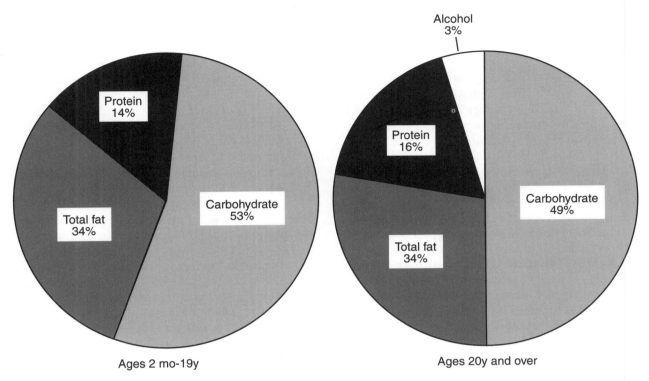

Figure 4.2 Sources of food energy: United States, 1988-91. Values expressed as % of total energy intake. Adapted from McDowell et al. 1994.

the protein intakes of the total population of adult men and women surveyed across age groups. The survey did not provide data on intake per unit of body weight.

Another large survey examining the protein intake of Americans was the randomized primary prevention trial (MRFIT—Multiple Risk Factor Intervention Trial) conducted in the

Table 4.4 **Protein Intake by Age and Sex in the United States, 1988-91**

Sex and age	Sample size	Mean intake (g/d)	Energy intake (% of total)
Male:			
20-29	844	110	14.6
30-39	735	106	15.1
40-49	626	96	15.6
50-59	473	93	16.1
60-69	546	84	16.4
70-79	444	74	16.0
80 years and older	296	69	16.0
Female:			
20-29	838	69	14.5
30-39	791	70	15.3
40-49	602	67	15.8
50-59	456	64	16.1
60-69	560	64	16.6
70-79	407	58	16.6
80 years and older	313	52	15.9

Adapted from McDowell et al. 1994

United States from 1973 through 1982. The nutrient intake of 12,847 men ages 35-57 years was determined prior to intervention (Tillotson et al. 1997). The average protein intake of this population was 16.4% of total energy intake (~99 g protein/d). The participants reported consuming 24% of their energy from meat and 11% from dairy products. Average energy intake was reported to be approximately 2420 kcal/d. Follow-up data from the NHANES I survey showed similar findings, with the average protein intake of 2580 men and 4567 women reported as 16.6% and 17.0% of total energy intake, respectively (Kant et al. 1995).

The results of these large epidemiological surveys show that the U.S. population reports eating 16-17% of total energy intake as protein. The reported energy intakes from these studies range from approximately 1800 to over 3000 kcal/d for men and approximately 1400-2000 kcal/d for women. Based on these energy intake values, the reported protein intakes are more than adequate to meet the current adult RDA.

Protein Intake of Active People

Many athletes, particularly those participating in strength- and bodybuilding-related activities, are concerned with meeting their protein needs. This concern has led many athletes to consume large amounts of protein and amino acid supplements to ensure adequate protein intakes. Are athletes and active people eating enough protein? Are supplements needed? "Protein Supplementation Practices of Athletes" (next page) addresses these questions.

Another practice popular with athletes is the use of supposedly anabolic ergogenic substances—supplements reported by manufacturers to enhance protein synthesis, resulting in significant gains in muscle size and strength. "Androstenedione: Does It Increase Protein Synthesis?" (page 116) discusses one of the most popular of these products.

Numerous scientific studies have analyzed the protein intake of athletes. Table 4.5 summarizes data from several representative reports. On average, the reported protein intakes

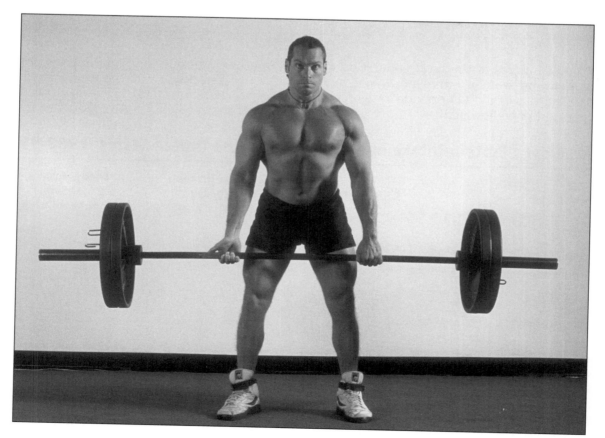

Strength athletes are often concerned with their protein intake; however, adequate protein intake is only one component of a strength-building program.

■ HIGHLIGHT ■

Protein Supplementation Practices of Athletes

Protein supplementation is popular among athletes, particularly those involved in strength and bodybuilding activities. In studying the supplementation patterns of over 300 male and female bodybuilders, Brill and Keane (1994) found that 59% of these athletes spent $25-$100/mo on supplements, while 5% spent over $150/mo. Supplementation practices involve taking protein mixtures and/or individual amino acids. Athletes use these supplements for a number of reasons, including

- to provide energy for physical performance or to replace any proteins used for energy during exercise;
- to enhance muscle growth and strength; and
- to hasten recovery from training or injury.

Is there sufficient scientific evidence to support advertising claims for protein and amino acid supplements? Kreider et al. (1993) reviewed the proposed ergogenic value of amino acid supplementation. There is some evidence that amino acids such as arginine, histidine, lysine, methionine, ornithine, and phenylalanine may enhance muscle anabolism by stimulating the release of growth hormone, insulin, and/or glucocorticoids (Carlson et al. 1989; Evain-Brion et al. 1982; Garlick and Grant 1988; Merimee et al. 1969). However, most of these studies involved intravenous infusions of individual amino acids or amino acid mixtures. Attempts to replicate these findings with oral amino acid and protein supplements have failed to show convincing evidence that these supplements enhance muscle anabolism or improve strength (Bucci et al. 1992; Fogelholm et al. 1993; Fry et al. 1993; Lambert et al. 1993).

Many endurance athletes supplement with **branched-chain amino acids (BCAAs),** since skeletal muscle metabolizes these amino acids (leucine, isoleucine, and valine) during exercise as an energy source. The BCAAs have also been linked to the **central fatigue hypothesis**—which suggests that increased concentrations of the neurotransmitter serotonin in the brain can impair function of the central nervous system during prolonged exercise, resulting in decreased performance (Newsholme et al. 1991)—and serotonin levels increase as the ratio of free tryptophan to BCAAs increases. Davis (1995) reviewed the roles of dietary carbohydrate and BCAAs in central fatigue. Although it has been theorized that supplementing with BCAAs could prevent the fall in blood BCAA levels during and following exercise, the evidence to support this claim is limited. On the other hand, carbohydrate supplementation decreases the free tryptophan:BCAA ratio, which does delay fatigue. Kreider et al. (1993) concluded that more evidence is needed before a definitive judgment can be made about the effectiveness of protein and amino acid supplementation.

are well above the adult RDA, and many even exceed recommended levels for athletes (see "Dietary Protein Recommendations for Active Individuals" later in this chapter). However, some individual athletes are at risk for low protein intakes—including female gymnasts, distance runners, figure skaters, and dieting wrestlers. These athletes sometimes compromise their protein intakes by consistently consuming too little energy.

Metabolism of Protein During and After Exercise

Dietary protein is digested into small peptides (single amino acids linked together) and single amino acids. These peptides and amino acids are absorbed by various transport mechanisms in the gut mucosal cells, where they are further digested to single amino acids. The single amino acids are

Androstenedione: Does It Increase Protein Synthesis?

Health food stores and muscle magazines are filled with ads for ergogenic products claiming to produce bigger, stronger muscles by increasing protein synthesis. Do these products work? Can you stimulate protein synthesis through supplementation? Can you really get increased performance by taking a pill? Are there any research data to support the claims made for these products?

Most ergogenic products can be classified as either (1) nutritional supplements such as proteins, amino acids, combinations of amino acids, or metabolic derivatives of amino acids; or (2) pharmacological products such as androgenic hormones or drugs. One of the most popular products in the pharmacological category is androstenedione (pronounced an-dro-STEEN-die-own). In the summer of 1998, when Mark McGwire was breaking home run records, he acknowledged using two ergogenic aids—androstenedione and creatine phosphate (see chapter 16 for critical analysis of creatine). Androstenedione catapulted into the national media, and record sales of the supplement were reported by health clubs, health food stores, mail order houses, and Internet vendors. One look at Mark McGwire's strong body and powerful baseball swing was all the evidence many athletes needed to rush to the store. They too wanted this substance that claimed to increase muscle mass and athletic performance. Does androstenedione increase protein synthesis? If so, what is the mechanism? Is it safe?

Critical Analysis of the Ergogenic Claims Made for Androstenedione

Androstenedione is one of the major androgens produced by the ovaries in females, the testes in males, and to a lesser extent the adrenal glands in both sexes. Hepatic enzymes convert the adrenal output of the hormone to either estrogens or testosterone. In men, testosterone and androstenedione are the principal androgens of the testes, with testosterone being more potent than androstenedione. Both androstenedione and testosterone are synthesized from cholesterol within the body. However, since conversion of androstenedione to testosterone is carefully regulated by luteinizing hormone (LH), supplemental androstenedione can increase endogenous testosterone levels only if LH levels are also increased.

Androstenedione supplements theoretically exert anabolic effects by being converted to testosterone in the liver (and not to estrogen). Supplement manufacturers often combine androstenedione with the herb *tribulus terrestris*, which they claim increases LH production. Together these two substances are supposed to increase testosterone production in the body, which in turn is supposed to increase protein synthesis.

Performance and Theory

Product manufacturers claim that androstenedione improves physical power and mechanical edge by increasing fat-free mass (FFM) and decreasing body fat. They also claim androstenedione can improve recovery time from exercise by decreasing the catabolic effect of weight training on muscle. Bodybuilders also use the product to increase muscle mass for a more aesthetic physical appearance.

- **How does it work?** Manufacturers of androstenedione claim that it increases protein anabolism by increasing testosterone levels by 337% (the percentage varies depending on the manufacturer). There are no published peer-reviewed research data indicating that supplemental androstenedione significantly increases blood testosterone levels.
- **Is the product effective?** There is no indication that androstenedione is effective as recommended to consumers. King et al. (1999) found that men con-

suming 300 mg/d of supplemental androstenedione had no change in testosterone after an 8-week strength training program. However, there are anecdotal reports from athletes, coaches, trainers, and physicians, who claim significant increases in muscle mass, strength, and endurance from androstenedione as well as other steroids. In acknowledgment of these anecdotal effects, the International Olympic Committee (IOC) has placed 20 anabolic steroids (including androstenedione) and related compounds on its list of banned drugs. However, no well-controlled studies have documented that these anabolic steroid drugs improve agility, skill, cardiovascular capacity, or overall athletic performance.

Safety

Androstenedione is a hormone with potential systemic physiological effects. If it does increase testosterone, one should question its long-term health effects. Studies examining excessive amounts of testosterone list effects such as increased facial and body acne, premature baldness, female-like breast enlargement in males, shrunken testicles, premature closure of growth centers in adolescents, and increased aggressiveness and violent behavior (Williams 1998). The use of androgens is especially dangerous among adolescents, in whom androgens are known to stunt growth. Finally, no independent agency regulates the product purity or contents.

Ethical and Legal Issues

There are serious ethical issues concerning the safety of androstenedione and its use as a performance enhancer. It is legal to sell in the United States, but it is banned by some sports organizations—including the National Football League (NFL), National Collegiate Athletic Association (NCAA), and the International Olympic Committee (IOC)—but not the national baseball or basketball leagues. Shot putter Randy Barnes, the 1996 Olympic gold medalist and world record holder, recently drew a lifetime ban for using androstenedione.

What We Don't Know About Androstenedione

Advertisements claim that androstenedione can improve protein synthesis, which in turn can improve muscle mass development, but no peer-reviewed data support this claim. It is important to note what *we do not know* about androstenedione:

- whether androstenedione improves athletic performance;
- how much androstenedione is converted to male or female sex steroid when it is taken by mouth or injected;
- how much androstenedione is absorbed in the body, or where in the body it goes;
- whether androstenedione shrinks testicular size like androgens do;
- whether androstenedione causes liver cancers and heart disease like some other oral androgens do; or
- how to detect androstenedione by drug testing.

What we do know is that the product is expensive, especially if one combines it with dehydroepiandrosterone (DHEA) and *tribulus terrestris* as recommended by some manufacturers. Androstenedione is not recommended by The Endocrine Society, an international research organization representing 10,000 members in 80 countries who specialize in endocrinology.

then transported to the liver via the portal vein. The liver regulates the release of amino acids into the **free amino acid pool** located in the blood and tissues (see figure 4.3). Small amounts of undigested protein may be lost in the feces. The amino acids in the free amino acid pool are either metabolized for energy or synthesized into new body tissues or other nitrogen-containing

Table 4.5   Self-Reported Protein Intakes of Athletes

Reference	Sport type	Sex	Protein intake (g per kg BW[a])	Protein intake (% total kcal)
Burke et al. 1991	Triathlon	M	2.0	13.0
	Marathon	M	2.0	14.5
	Football	M	1.5	15.0
	Weight lifting	M	1.9	18.0
Peters and Goetzsche 1997	Ultradistance running	M	1.4	16.7
Keith et al. 1996	Bodybuilding	M	2.7	22.5
Niekamp and Baer 1995	Distance running	M	1.6	12.8
Kleiner et al. 1994	Bodybuilding	M	3.1	37.7
Rico-Sanz et al. 1998	Soccer	M	2.2	14.4
Kleiner et al. 1994	Bodybuilding	F	2.7	35.8
Peters and Goetzsche 1997	Ultradistance running	F	1.2	15.1
Felder et al. 1998	Surfing	F	1.5	17.0
Wiita and Stombaugh 1996	Distance running	F	1.1	14.1
Walberg-Rankin et al. 1993	Bodybuilding	F	1.9[b]	22.6[b]

[a]BW = body weight.
[b]Average value over five time periods.

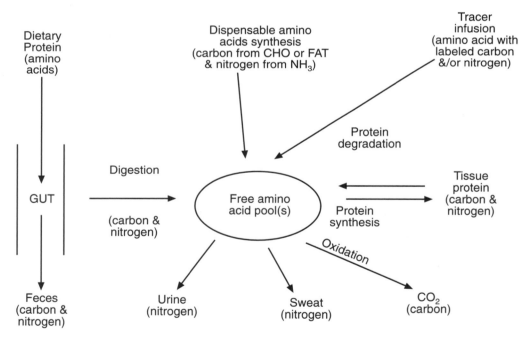

Figure 4.3   Schematic representation of protein kinetics. Shown is the movement and ultimate fate of both carbon and nitrogen from amino acids. All amino acids pass through the free amino acid pool; although only a small percentage of the body's amino acids are found there at any time (the vast majority are in tissue protein), the importance of the free amino acid pool is indicated by its large size and central location. Nitrogen balance (status) studies assess net nitrogen retention (intake minus excretion), while metabolic tracer studies assess the component processes of protein kinetics (oxidation, synthesis, degradation, etc.).

Reprinted from Lemon 1998.

compounds. Using the assessment techniques described earlier in this chapter (e.g., nitrogen balance and isotopic tracers), researchers can determine the fate of dietary proteins and individual amino acids during and after exercise.

Protein contributes to energy production during and after exercise in the following ways:

- Amino acids can become substrates for gluconeogenesis to prevent hypoglycemia.
- Amino acids can be converted to Krebs cycle intermediates to improve acetyl-CoA oxidation (see figure 4.4).
- Amino acids can be oxidized directly in the muscles for energy.
- Amino acids help build and repair tissues after exercise.

Many factors can influence protein metabolism during and following exercise—including exercise intensity, carbohydrate availability, type of exercise, energy intake, gender, training level, and age. The following sections review what we know about how the type of exercise, intensity of exercise, and training status affect protein metabolism. See Lemon (1995, 1998) for more detailed reviews of these factors and their relationship with protein metabolism.

Effect of Type of Activity on Protein Metabolism

It is a common belief that strength athletes require significantly higher protein intakes than sedentary individuals or endurance athletes. This belief is based on the assumption

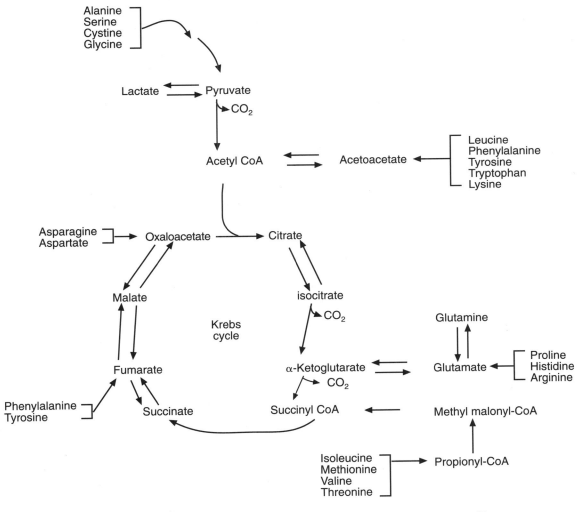

Figure 4.4 The relationship between amino acids and Krebs cycle intermediates.
Adapted from Champe and Harvey 1994.

that amino acids are used for energy during strength training or to repair muscle tissue damaged during exercise. To the contrary, Tarnopolsky et al. (1991) found that whole-body leucine oxidation did not change during strength training exercise or for 2 h following strength training. While these results seem to indicate that the protein needs of strength athletes are not increased during the actual training, nitrogen balance studies suggest that strength athletes do require higher protein intakes to maintain nitrogen balance (Lemon et al. 1992; Tarnopolsky et al. 1992; Walberg et al. 1988). Figure 4.5 illustrates the responses of novice bodybuilders to 1 mo of strength training at two levels of dietary protein. On the lower protein intake (0.99 g/kg/d), all but one subject was in negative nitrogen balance. At the higher intake (2.62 g/kg/d), all subjects achieved positive nitrogen balance. Regression analysis indicated that nitrogen balance occurred at a protein intake of 1.43 g/kg/d, while the recommended allowance (requirement +

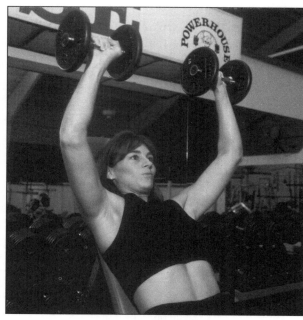

© Raymond J. Malace

Strength athletes have higher protein requirements compared to sedentary individuals.

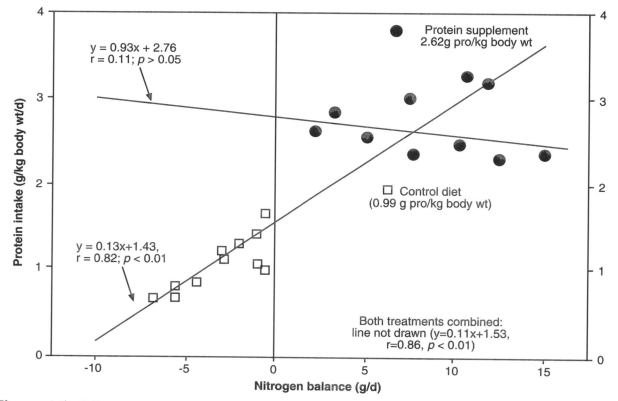

Figure 4.5 Effect of dietary protein intake on nitrogen balance (status). The strong linear relationship between these two variables is lost at high protein intakes (2.62 g/kg/d); based on the lower protein intake (0.99 g/kg/d), the protein requirement (i.e., protein intake where nitrogen balance occurs at the y-intercept) is 1.43 g/kg/d (200-212% of the current RDA).

Reprinted from Lemon et al. 1992.

2SD) for these strength athletes is 1.6 to 1.7 g/kg/d. Other evidence shows that no further increase in protein synthesis occurs at protein intakes higher than 2.0 g/kg/d (Fern et al. 1991). Lemon (1995) theorized that strength athletes need more protein in order to *accelerate* the rate of muscle protein synthesis and/or to decrease the rate of protein catabolism during and following strength training.

Studies of the effects of endurance exercise on protein metabolism indicate that moderate- to high-intensity endurance exercise stimulates the oxidation of leucine (Babij et al. 1983; Evans et al. 1983; Hagg et al. 1982). Moreover, blood urea concentrations increase during endurance exercise, resulting in increased urinary urea excretion following exercise. These findings suggest that protein oxidation increases during endurance exercise—and that protein needs of endurance athletes are probably higher than the current RDA. Additional protein may also be required to repair any muscle damage caused by intense endurance training (Lemon 1995). Nitrogen balance studies suggest that

the dietary protein intake necessary to support nitrogen balance in endurance athletes ranges from 1.2 to 1.4 g/kg/d (Brouns et al. 1989; Friedman and Lemon 1989; Meredith et al. 1989).

Effect of Exercise Intensity on Protein Metabolism

Babij et al. (1983) found that oxidation of leucine increased linearly with exercise intensity (figure 4.6)—indicating that the body increases its use of amino acids during endurance exercise and that high-intensity exercise results in greater oxidation of amino acids. And if endurance athletes are increasing their oxidation of amino acids, they clearly need to increase their intake of protein.

The mechanism responsible for this increase in leucine oxidation appears to be an increase in the activity of **branched-chain oxoacid dehydrogenase**, which is the rate-limiting enzyme in the oxidation of the BCAAs (branched-chain amino acids—leucine, isoleucine, and valine) (Kasperek and Snider 1987). Exercise

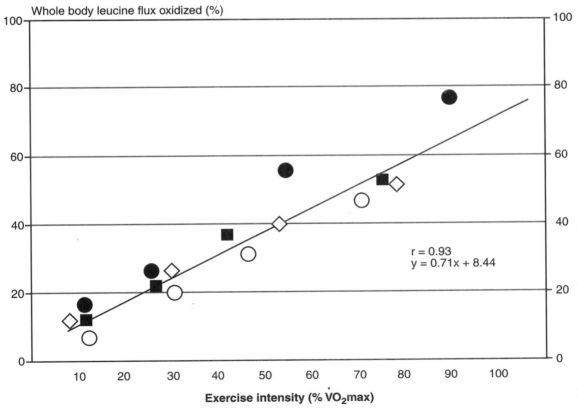

Figure 4.6 Effect of increasing exercise intensity on oxidation of the amino acid leucine. As the intensity of endurance exercise increases, there is a nearly linear increase in amino acid oxidation.
Adapted from Babij et al. 1983.

performed at less than 55-60% $\dot{V}O_2$max does not appear to stimulate amino acid oxidation (Butterfield and Calloway 1984; Todd et al. 1984).

Changes in Protein Metabolism Resulting From Training Adaptations

Although many studies show that protein utilization (and therefore protein requirements) increases with exercise, Butterfield (1987) has cautioned that the body may adapt to exercise training over time, with protein needs returning to baseline levels. Unfortunately, most researchers have measured protein metabolism only during exercise and a few days post-exercise. Butterfield (1987) suggested that the transient change in protein metabolism occurs for 12-14 d after the initiation of training, and that protein metabolism returns to baseline levels after 3-4 weeks of training. Figure 4.7 shows that individuals initiating a cycling program experienced a negative nitrogen balance with the initiation of training, but *nitrogen balance was restored after 20 d of training with no change in dietary protein intake* (Gontzea et al. 1975). Longitudinal studies need to be performed to determine if the changes in protein requirements observed with strength and endurance training are maintained over prolonged periods of training.

Dietary Protein Recommendations for Active Individuals

The following recommendations are based on current studies of protein metabolism during and following exercise:

- People who regularly engage in endurance activities need dietary protein intake of 0.55-0.64 g/lb body weight/d (1.2-1.4 g/kg body weight/d, or 1.5 to 1.75 times the current adult RDA).

- People who regularly engage in strength exercise need dietary protein intake of 0.73-0.77 g/lb body weight/d (1.6-1.7 g/kg body weight/d, or 2.0 to 2.1 times the current adult RDA).

Recently the popular press has been filled with articles suggesting that athletes need much higher protein intakes than even the recommendations given above. One popular high-protein diet for athletes is the 40-30-30 diet, or The Zone Diet, which recommends that 40% of

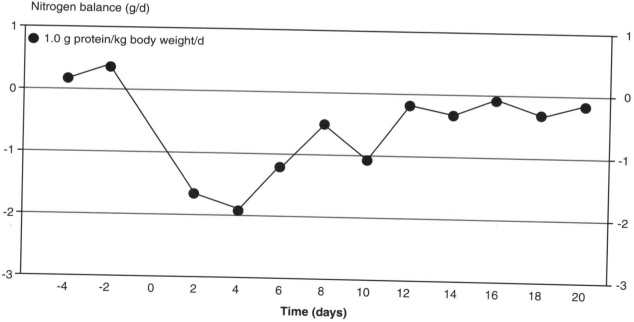

Nitrogen balance (g/d)

Figure 4.7 Effect of several weeks of endurance training on nitrogen balance. Men consumed 1 g protein/kg body weight/d for 12 d before and 20 d after initiation of a cycling program. Note that negative nitrogen balance disappeared by day 12.

Adapted from Gontzea et al. 1985.

energy come from carbohydrate, 30% from fat, and 30% from protein. "The Zone Diet: Do Athletes Need High-Protein Diets?" (see below) reviews this high-protein diet and its potential impact on weight loss and exercise performance.

Many nutrition professionals are concerned that the high protein intakes of some athletes can have adverse effects (Lemon 1998), including

- renal damage,
- increased urinary calcium excretion,
- increased serum lipoprotein levels and higher risk for heart disease,
- dehydration, and
- possible toxicity from large doses of individual amino acids.

Some of these adverse effects appear only in certain classes of people. High-protein diets are dangerous for people with kidney or liver disease, for example, but have not been shown to cause damage in healthy individuals. Protein consumption increases the excretion of urinary calcium, but its impact on the retention of calcium is debatable (Institute of Medicine, 1997). Urinary calcium loss appears to occur only in people who obtain their additional protein from purified protein supplements (vs. from foods, which also contain phosphorus). Dehydration can occur as a result of increased water loss from additional nitrogen excretion that occurs with higher protein intakes—athletes consuming higher protein diets need to increase their fluid intake to prevent dehydration. Athletes and active people should assess their current

■ HIGHLIGHT ■

The Zone Diet: Do Athletes Need High-Protein Diets?

In 1995, Barry Sears published *The Zone* (HarperCollins), a book touting the benefits of a high-protein, low-carbohydrate diet for athletes: the "40-30-30 plan." This plan recommends that 40% of energy come from carbohydrate, with the rest equally divided between fat (30% of energy) and protein (30% of energy). The Zone Diet is based on Dr. Sears's earlier Eicotec Diet, which stated that high-carbohydrate diets impair athletic performance (Sears 1993). Dr. Sears based his hypothesis on so-called "good" and "bad" eicosanoids. Eicosanoids are a class of metabolic regulators (e.g., prostaglandins, leukotrienes, and tromboxane) derived from the essential fatty acids (linoleic acid and linolenic acid) in our diet (see chapter 3). Eicosanoids help regulate a number of metabolic responses related to immune function and the cardiovascular system, such as blood pressure, blood clotting, and heart rate. They may play a role in heart disease and other diseases. Based on this fact, Dr. Sears suggested that eicosanoids are also the "underlying key to enhanced athletic performance" (Sears 1993). He was concerned about the effect high-carbohydrate diets have on blood insulin concentrations. He claimed that the insulin response to high-carbohydrate foods causes a release of "bad" eicosanoids, which alter fat metabolism. However, there are no data supporting the claim that insulin affects eicosanoid concentrations in the body (Liebman 1996). Insulin is an anabolic hormone that stimulates uptake of nutrients (protein, fat, and carbohydrate) and decreases fat mobilization from adipose tissue. High insulin levels, however, do not "make" a person fat—a high-calorie diet makes one fat (Liebman 1996).

Over the last 5-7 years, Dr. Sears has transformed his "Eicotec Diet" into "The Zone Diet" through numerous books and tapes, all of which recommend the 40-30-30 diet plan for athletic performance, weight loss, anti-aging, and super health. In addition, Dr. Sears sells various energy bars and foods that meet "The Zone" requirement of 40-30-30. Dr. Sears's recommendations are counter to what most sport nutritionists recommend for active individuals. How do we sort fact from fiction? Here we provide a brief critical analysis of The Zone Diet and some of Dr. Sears's claims. Other writers have provided more detailed reviews of this diet (Clark and Rosenbloom 1997; Coleman 1994, 1996; Liebman 1996; Cheuvront 1999).

(continued)

1. **The Zone Diet recommends a low-carbohydrate diet.** It is well established in the research literature that carbohydrate is the only substrate that can replace glycogen. A diet containing only 40% of energy from CHO is inadequate for most athletes, especially those doing endurance sports. Remember that the amount of CHO consumed (grams per day) depends on the total energy intake (kilocalories per day) (see chapter 2). For a female athlete eating 2000 kcal/d, a 40% CHO diet would provide only 800 kcal of CHO (200 g), an amount too low for any endurance athlete. If a person consumes 5000 kcal/d, a diet providing 40% of the energy from CHO would provide 2000 kcal from CHO (500 g) or 6.6 kcal/kg for a 165-lb (75-kg) athlete. This amount of CHO may be sufficient for a power athlete, but it would be inadequate for athletes in endurance sports.

2. **The Zone Diet recommends that 30% of energy come from protein.** This level of protein intake translates into 150 g of protein for someone consuming 2000 kcal/d, or 375 g/d of protein for a person consuming 5000 kcal/d (see chapter 2). General protein recommendations for active people range from 1.2 to 1.7 g/kg body weight. Thus, for a 110-lb (50-kg) female athlete consuming 2000 kcal/d, The Zone Diet would provide 3 g/kg. For a 165-lb (75-kg) male athlete consuming 5000 kcal/d, The Zone Diet would provide 5 g/kg. In both of these examples, the protein intake is much higher than recommended or needed by the body. Extra protein will be broken down and used as an energy source, and the extra nitrogen lost in the urine. Most athletes consume more than enough protein in their typical diets and do not need to add additional dietary protein. Only athletes who restrict energy intake have insufficient protein.

3. **The Zone Diet recommends that 30% of energy come from fat.** In general, it is recommended that athletes consume 20-25% of energy from fat, depending on their sport and personal food preferences. A diet providing less than 30% of energy from fat is recommended for all Americans to reduce the risk of chronic diseases and obesity (see chapter 3).

4. **The Zone Diet is too low in calories.** People who follow the Zone Diet plan as recommended may consume only 1200-1300 kcal/d. This energy intake is too low for any athlete, regardless of gender or sport. Athletes need adequate energy to maintain body weight, with approximately 60-65% of their energy from carbohydrate, 10-15% from protein (1.2-1.7 g/kg body weight), and the remainder from fat.

The Zone Diet is an energy-restricted, low-carbohydrate, high-protein diet. Yet some athletes report feeling better on this diet. For active people whose typical diets are low in protein and fat and high in carbohydrate, this dietary change may improve the way they feel because their diet was too low in protein (Clark and Rosenbloom 1997). By increasing their intake of protein, they are now providing their bodies with adequate protein for the building and repair of muscle tissue. In addition, if they are *not* following the energy restriction recommendations of the Zone Diet, they may also be increasing their energy intake (since high-protein foods typically contain some fat, which is more energy dense). For active people who already have balanced diets and adequate protein intakes, the Zone Diet can be disastrous. It provides insufficient energy and carbohydrate for highly active individuals. Thus, the response any one individual may have to the Zone Diet may depend on that person's protein intake before starting the diet. In addition, we cannot rule out a placebo response that may occur when something new is tried.

Making dietary recommendations for good health, weight loss or maintenance, and exercise performance requires *individualized* dietary changes. No one dietary plan works for everyone—especially for active people who need diets tailored to their energy needs and their sport. Active individuals cannot perform long on a diet providing only 1200-1300 kcal/d, as recommended by the Zone Diet. They will lose weight and deplete their glycogen stores. Under these conditions, following the Zone Diet can actually be detrimental to performance.

protein intake to determine if an increase is warranted. Although no one should exceed the recommendations listed previously, there is no evidence to suggest that protein intake of 1.2-2.0 times the RDA is hazardous for basically healthy people.

Chapter in Review

This chapter has reviewed the important role of protein in supporting exercise and ensuring adequate recovery from exercise. Studies of nitrogen balance and metabolic tracers show that strength athletes and endurance athletes need more protein than most people—but only about 1.2-2.0 times the current adult RDA, which is lower than the protein level many athletes already consume. By consuming adequate energy and a varied diet, most athletes—including vegetarians—can obtain adequate dietary protein without the need for supplements. People following higher protein diets should drink extra fluids to avoid becoming dehydrated; people at risk for heart or kidney disease or for bone loss should avoid excessive protein.

KEY CONCEPTS

 1. Describe the functions and classifications of proteins.

Proteins serve as critical components of building materials for bone, ligaments, tendons, muscles, and organs. Proteins are also enzymes and hormones; they assist with maintaining fluid and acid-base balance; and they are an important energy source during and following exercise. Amino acids are classified as essential or nonessential, with both classes being critical for health, growth, and maintenance/repair of tissue.

 2. List and describe the primary methods of assessing protein status.

The three primary assessment methods are nitrogen balance, isotopic tracers, and 3-methylhistidine excretion. Each method has advantages and limitations. While nitrogen balance gives a good indication of whole-body nitrogen balance, it cannot estimate protein synthesis, oxidation, or degradation. Tracer methods can estimate these variables, but they are expensive and do not accurately indicate the activity of all amino acids. The 3-methylhistidine method indicates excretion levels of contractile proteins but is confounded by dietary meat intake and by excretion of contractile proteins from the gut and skin.

 3. Discuss dietary sources of protein.

Protein is abundant in the U.S. diet, with meat and dairy products containing high amounts of protein. Adequate protein can also be obtained in the vegetarian diet: cereals, grains, nuts, and legumes contain significant amounts of protein, and mutual supplementation can be used to obtain complete protein. The U.S. population generally consumes adequate dietary protein, but athletes with low energy intakes are vulnerable to inadequate protein intakes.

 4. Discuss the metabolism of protein during and post-exercise.

Protein plays many roles during and after exercise. Amino acids are used as substrates for gluconeogenesis and as Krebs cycle intermediates; they also are used for energy in the muscle and for building and repair of tissues following exercise. Protein oxidation is increased during and following both endurance and strength training exercise, raising the protein requirements for active people. Although rigorous training can temporarily cause a negative nitrogen balance, nitrogen balance can be restored once the body has adapted to the training.

 5. Describe the dietary protein recommendations for active individuals.

The protein intake for people regularly participating in endurance activities should be about 0.55-0.64 g/lb/d (or 1.2-1.4 g/kg/d, 1.5-1.75 times the current adult RDA). The protein intake of people regularly engaging in strength exercise should be about 0.73-0.77 g/lb/d (or 1.6-1.7 g/kg/d, 2.0-2.1 times the current adult RDA).

KEY TERMS

3-methylhistidine
amino acid
branched-chain amino acid (BCAA)
branched-chain oxoacid dehydrogenase
central fatigue hypothesis
complete protein
conditionally essential amino acid
crude nitrogen balance
digestibility
essential amino acid
free amino acid pool

isotopic tracers
Kjeldahl technique
lacto-ovo vegetarian
mutual supplementation
negative nitrogen balance
nitrogen balance
nonessential amino acid
positive nitrogen balance
protein quality
vegan

References

Babij P, Matthews SM, Rennie MJ. Changes in blood ammonia, lactate and amino acids in relation to workload during bicycle ergometer exercise in man. Eur J Appl Physiol 1983;50:405-11.

Brill JB, Keane MW. Supplementation patterns of competitive male and female bodybuilders. Int J Sport Nutr 1994;4:398-412.

Brouns F, Saris WHM, Beckers E, et al. Metabolic changes induced by sustained exhaustive cycling and diet manipulation. Int J Sports Med 1989;10(suppl. 1):S49-S62.

Bucci LR, Hickson JF, Wolinsky I, Pivarnik JM. Ornithine supplementation and insulin release in bodybuilders. Int J Sport Nutr 1992;2:287-91.

Burke LM, Gollan RA, Read RSD. Dietary intakes and food use of groups of elite Australian male athletes. Int J Sport Nutr 1991;1:378-94.

Butterfield GE. Whole-body protein utilization in humans. Med Sci Sports Exerc 1987; 19:S157-S165.

Butterfield GE, Calloway DH. Physical activity improves protein utilization in young men. Brit J Nutr 1984;51:171-84.

Carlson HE, Miglietta JT, Roginsky MS, Stegink LD. Stimulation of pituitary hormone secretion by neurotransmitter amino acids in humans. Metabolism 1989;28:1179-82.

Champe PC, Harvey RA. Lippincott's Illustrated Reviews: Biochemistry. 2nd ed. Philadelphia: J.B. Lippincott Company, 1994:244.

Cheuvront SN. The Zone Diet and athletic performance. Sports Med 1999;27(4):213-28.

Clark N, Rosenbloom C. To Zone or not to Zone: people respond to the Zone Diet plan. SCAN Pulse 1997;16(3):5-7.

Coleman E. Debunking the "Eicotec" myth. SCAN Pulse 1994;13(1):7-8.

Coleman EJ. The biozone nutrition system: a dietary panacea? Int J Sport Nutr 1996;6:69-71.

Davis JM. Carbohydrates, branched-chain amino acids, and endurance: the Central Fatigue Hypothesis. Int J Sport Nutr 1995; 5(Suppl.):S29-S38.

Dohm GL, Tapscott EB, Kasperek GJ. Protein degradation during endurance exercise and recovery. Med Sci Sports Exerc 1987; 19(5):S166-S171.

Evain-Brion D, Donnadieu M, Roger M, Job JC. Simultaneous study of somatotrophic and corticotrophic pituitary secretion during ornithine infusion test. Clin Endocrinol 1982;17:119-22.

Evans WJ, Fisher EC, Hoerr RA, Young VR. Protein metabolism and endurance exercise. Phys Sportsmed 1983;11:63-72.

Felder JM, Burke LM, Lowdon BJ, Cameron-Smith D, Collier GR. Nutritional practices of elite female surfers during training and competition. Int J Sport Nutr 1998; 8:36-48.

Fern EB, Bielinski RN, Schutz Y. Effects of exaggerated amino acid and protein supply in man. Experientia 1991;47:168-72.

Fogelholm GM, Näveri HK, Kiilavuori KTK, Härkönen MHA. Low-dose amino acid supplementation: no effects on serum human growth hormone and insulin in male weightlifters. Int J Sport Nutr 1993; 3:290-7.

Food and Nutrition Board, Institute of Medicine. Recommended Dietary Allowances, 10th ed. Washington, DC: National Academy Press, 1989.

Food Processor (software program), Version 7.21. ESHA Research, Salem, OR.

Friedman JE, Lemon PWR. Effect of chronic endurance exercise on the retention of dietary protein. Int J Sports Med 1989;10:118-23.

Fry AC, Kraemer WJ, Stone MH, Warren BJ, et al. Endocrine and performance responses to high volume training and amino acid supplementation in elite junior weightlifters. Int J Sport Nutr 1993;3:306-22.

Garlick PJ, Grant I. Amino acid infusion increases the sensitivity of muscle protein synthesis in vivo to insulin. Biochem J 1988;254:579-84.

Gibson RS. Principles of Nutritional Assessment. New York: Oxford University Press, 1990.

Gontzea I, Sutzescu P, Dumitrache S. The influence of adaptation of physical effort on nitrogen balance in man. Nutr Rep Int 1975;11:231-4.

Hagg SA, Morse EL, Adibi SA. Effect of exercise on rates of oxidation, turnover, and clearance of leucine in human subjects. Am J Physiol 1982;242:E407-E410.

Institute of Medicine. Dietary reference intake. Calcium, phosphorus, magnesium, vitamin D, and fluoride. Washington, DC: National Academy Press, 1997.

Kant AK, Graubard BI, Schatzkin A, Ballard-Barbash R. Proportion of energy intake from fat and subsequent weight change in the NHANES I epidemiologic follow-up study. Am J Clin Nutr 1995;61:11-7.

Kasperek GJ, Snider RD. Effect of exercise intensity and starvation on the activation of branched-chain keto acid dehydrogenase by exercise. Am J Physiol 1987;252:E33-E37.

Keith RE, Stone MH, Carson RE, Lefavi RG, Fleck SJ. Nutritional status and lipid profiles of trained steroid-using bodybuilders. Int J Sport Nutr 1996;6:247-54.

King DS, Sharp RL, Vukovich MD, et al. Effect of oral androstenedione on serum testosterone and adaptations to resistance training in young men: a randomized controlled trial. JAMA 1999;281(21):2020-8.

Kleiner SM, Bazzarre TL, Ainsworth BE. Nutritional status of nationally ranked elite bodybuilders. Int J Sport Nutr 1994;4:54-69.

Kreider RB, Miriel V, Bertun E. Amino acid supplementation and exercise performance. Sports Med 1993;16(3):190-209.

Lambert MI, Hefer JA, Millar RP, MacFarlane PW. Failure of commercial oral amino acid supplements to increase serum growth hormone concentrations in male body-builders. Int J Sport Nutr 1993;3:298-305.

Lee RD, Nieman DC. Nutritional Assessment. 2nd ed. St. Louis: Mosby, 1996.

Lemon PWR. Do athletes need more dietary protein and amino acids? Int J Sport Nutr 1995;5:S39-S61.

Lemon PWR. Effects of exercise on dietary protein requirements. Int J Sport Nutr 1998;8:426-47.

Lemon PWR, Tarnopolsky MA, MacDougall JD, Atkinson SA. Protein requirements and muscle mass/strength changes during intensive training in novice bodybuilders. J Appl Physiol 1992;73:767-75.

Liebman B. Carbo-phobia: Zoning out on the new diet books. Nutrition Action HealthLetter 1996;July:3-5.

MacKenzie TA, Clark NG, Bistrian BR, Flatt JP, Hallowell EM, Blackburn GL. A simple method for estimating nitrogen balance in hospitalized patients: a review and supporting data for a previously proposed technique. J Am Coll Nutr 1985;4:575-81.

Matthews DE. Proteins and Amino Acids. In: Shils ME, Olson JA, Shike M, Ross AC, eds. Modern Nutrition in Health and Disease 9th ed. Williams & Wilkins, 1999.

McDowell MA, Briefel RR, Alaimo K, et al. Energy and macronutrient intakes of persons ages 2 months and over in the United States: Third National Health and Nutrition Examination Survey, Phase 1 1988-1991. Advance Data, 1994;255:1-24.

Meredith CN, Zackin MJ, Frontera WR, Evans WJ. Dietary protein requirements and protein metabolism in endurance-trained men. J Appl Physiol 1989;66:2850-6.

Merimee TJ, Rabinowitz D, Fineberg SE. Arginine-initiated release of human growth hormone. N Engl J Med 1969;280:1434-8.

Messina M, Messina V. The Dietitian's Guide to Vegetarian Diets. Gaithersburg, MD: Aspen Publishers, 1996.

Newsholme EA, Parry-Billings M, McAndrew N, Budgett R. A biochemical mechanism to explain some characteristics of overtraining. In: Brouns F, ed. Medical Sports Science, Vol. 32, Advance in Nutrition and Top Sport. Basel: Karger, 1991:79-93.

Niekamp RA, Baer JT. In-season dietary adequacy of trained male cross-country runners. Int J Sport Nutr 1995;5:45-55.

Peters EM, Goetzsche JM. Dietary practices of South African ultradistance runners. Int J Sport Nutr 1997;7:80-103.

Rico-Sanz J, Frontera WR, Molé PA, Rivera MA, Rivera-Brown A, Meredith CN. Dietary and performance assessment of elite soccer players during a period of intense training. Int J Sport Nutr 1998;8:230-40.

Sears B. The Mythology of High Carbohydrate Diets. Marblehead, MA: Eicotec Foods, 1993.

Tarnopolsky MA, Atkinson SA, MacDougall JD, Chesley A, Phillips S, Schwarcz HP. Evaluation of protein requirements for trained strength athletes. J Appl Physiol 1992;73:1986-95.

Tarnopolsky MA, Atkinson SA, MacDougall JD, Senor BB, Lemon PWR, Schwarcz HP. Whole body leucine metabolism during and after resistance exercise in fed humans. Med Sci Sports Exerc 1991;23:326-33.

Tillotson JL, Bartsch GE, Gorder D, Grandits GA, Stamler J. Chapter 5. Food group and nutrient intakes at baseline in the Multiple Risk Factor Intervention Trial. Am J Clin Nutr 1997;65(suppl.):228S-57S.

Todd KS, Butterfield GE, Calloway DH. Nitrogen balance in men with adequate and deficient energy intake at three levels of work. Br J Nutr 1984;114:2107-18.

Walberg JL, Leidy MK, Sturgill DJ, Hinkle DE, Ritchey SJ, Sebolt DR. Macronutrient content of a hypoenergy diet affects nitrogen retention and muscle function in weight lifters. Int J Sports Med 1988;9:261-6.

Walberg-Rankin J, Eckstein Edmonds C, Gwazdauskas FC. Diet and weight changes of female bodybuilders before and after competition. Int J Sport Nutr 1993;3:87-102.

Wiita BG, Stombaugh IA. Nutrition knowledge, eating practices, and health of adolescent female runners: a 3-year longitudinal study. Int J Sport Nutr 1996;6:414-25.

Williams MH. The Ergogenic Edge: Pushing the Limits of Sports Performance. Champaign, IL: Human Kinetics, 1998.

Wolfe RR. Tracers in Metabolic Research: Radio-isotope and Stable Isotope/Mass Spectrometry Methods. New York: Liss, 1984.

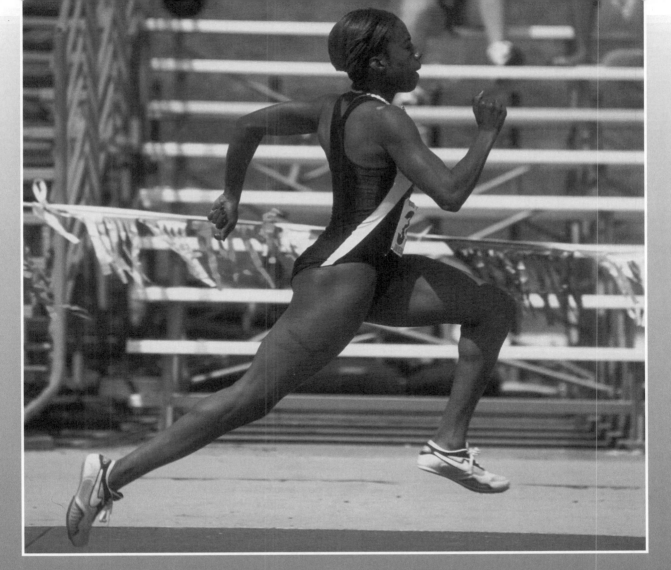

CHAPTER 5

Energy and Nutrient Balance

After reading this chapter you should be able to

- explain the energy and nutrient balance equations;
- understand the concept of nutrient balance and the contributions of carbohydrate, protein, fat, and alcohol to energy balance;
- identify the various components of energy expenditure, how they are measured, and the contribution of energy expenditure to the energy balance equation; and
- understand the role of energy intake in the energy balance equation.

129

Most individuals maintain a stable body weight over time. Think about your own body weight—how much has it fluctuated over the last year? Over the last 5 years? Unless you diet frequently or have dramatically changed your activity level, your body weight has probably been relatively stable. What factors play a role in weight stability? How can our bodies maintain body weight within such a narrow range, especially when we pay little attention to the amount of energy we consume or expend each day? This chapter addresses these questions. First we present the energy balance equations and discuss the concept of energy and macronutrient balance. To understand energy balance and why a person gains, loses, or maintains weight, you must know the factors that influence energy intake and expenditure.

Energy and Macronutrient Balance Equations

The classic energy balance equation states that if energy intake (total kcal consumed) equals energy expenditure (total kcal expended), then weight is maintained. However, this equation does not allow for changes in body composition and energy stores, nor does it help us understand the many factors associated with weight change, especially weight gain. We now know that *maintenance of body weight and body composition over time requires not only that energy intake equals energy expenditure—but also that intakes of protein, carbohydrate, fat, and alcohol equal their oxidation rates.* People who meet these criteria are in **energy balance** and will maintain their weight and body composition. A number of factors affect these components of energy balance. Some of them may be further modified by socioeconomic and psychological

influences (Flatt 1993). These factors, which are listed below, vary among individuals in their importance and influence:

- Genetic makeup
- Dietary intake and habits
- Environmental conditions
- Lifestyle

Maintenance of body weight and composition depends on how these factors influence the energy balance principles in table 5.1.

The equations given in table 5.1 are both dynamic and time-dependent, allowing for the effect of changing energy stores on energy expenditure over time. Swinburn and Ravussin (1993) illustrate this point with the following example. What would happen if you consumed an extra chocolate chip cookie (~100 kcal each) every day for 40 years? The amount of extra energy would equal 1.5 million kcal. If we assume that there are ~3500 kcal/lb (7700 kcal/kg) of adipose tissue, your weight gain would be about 417 lb (190 kg) over this 40-year period. Yet this clearly does not happen. If you really ate these extra kilocalories every day for 40 years, you would probably gain only about 6 lb (2.7 kg). After a short period of positive energy balance, the extra kcal would cause you to gain weight (both fat and lean tissues), and *your larger body size would increase energy expenditure sufficiently to balance the extra kilocalories consumed.* Of course, the amount of weight you gain will depend on the number of extra kilocalories you eat, the composition of those kilocalories (i.e., the amount of fat, carbohydrate, protein, or alcohol), and your energy expenditure. Thus, weight gain can result from an initial positive energy balance, but also can eventually restore energy balance (see "Example of Weight Stability," next page).

Table 5.1 **Energy and Nutrient Balance Equations Required for Weight to be Maintained Over an Extended Period of Time**

1. Energy balance:
   - Rate of energy input (dietary energy + stored energy) = Rate of energy expenditure

2. Nutrient balance:
   - Rate of protein intake = Rate of protein oxidation
   - Rate of fat intake = Rate of fat oxidation
   - Rate of carbohydrate intake = Rate of carbohydrate oxidation
   - Rate of alcohol intake = Rate of alcohol oxidation

■ HIGHLIGHT ■

Example of Weight Stability

To illustrate how weight stable we appear to be, here is an example from research done in Germany in 1902 (as reported by Keesey 1980). A researcher reported being weight-stable while ingesting 1766 kcal/d for 1 year. The next year he increased his energy intake to 2199 kcal/d, and then to 2403 kcal/d for the third year. Thus, he consumed nearly 160,000 more kcal/d in the second year than the first, and approximately 230,000 more kcal the third year compared to year one. The researcher's weight changed little over this time (he reported gaining only several pounds), although energy intake increased 26%.

Macronutrient Balance

Alternations of energy intake or expenditure are just one part of the energy balance picture. Changes in the type and amount of macronutrients consumed (protein, fat, carbohydrate, alcohol) and the oxidation of these nutrients within the body must also be considered. In fact, it is difficult to separate these two factors when explaining energy balance. Under normal physiological conditions, carbohydrate, protein, and alcohol are not easily converted to body fat (Swinburn and Ravussin 1993); *increases in the intake of nonfat nutrients stimulate their oxidation rates proportionally.* Fat is different. Increased fat intake does *not* immediately stimulate fat oxidation, increasing the probability that dietary fat will be stored as adipose tissue (Abbott et al. 1988; Westerterp 1993). The type of food consumed therefore plays a major role in the amount of energy consumed and expended each day (Acheson, Ravussin et al. 1984; Swinburn and Ravussin 1993). The following section reviews each of these nutrients and the role it plays in energy balance.

Carbohydrate Balance

Carbohydrate balance is precisely regulated by the body (Acheson, Schutz et al. 1984; Flatt 1988; Jebb et al. 1996). Ingestion of carbohydrate stimulates both glycogen storage and glucose oxidation and inhibits fat oxidation. Glucose not stored as glycogen is thought to be oxidized directly in almost equal balance to that consumed (Flatt et al. 1985). Conversion of excess dietary carbohydrate and protein to triacylglycerides (de novo lipogenesis) apparently does not occur to a significant extent in normal-weight people ex-

cept in nonphysiolo-gical conditions (Hellerstein et al. 1991): only when very large amounts of carbohydrate (85% of total energy) are consumed over several consecutive days, *and* dietary energy is in excess of need, does the body appear to convert the excess carbohydrate to fat in the form of triacylglyceride (Acheson et al. 1988). As figure 5.1 illustrates, consumption of carbohydrate promotes the oxidation of carbohydrate—and any excess energy stored appears to come directly from dietary fat made available by inhibition of fat oxidation. Jebb et al. (1996) overfed three lean men for 12 d and measured changes in energy expenditure and changes in protein, fat, and carbohydrate oxidation in a metabolic chamber (figure 5.2). The diet provided 15% of its energy as protein, 35% as fat, and 50% as carbohydrate, while energy intake was 33% higher than required to maintain energy balance. Carbohydrate and protein oxidation matched intake, while fat oxidation was not sensitive to fat intake. The subjects consumed 150 g of fat/d but oxidized only 59 g. The result was a 6.5-lb (2.9-kg) weight gain during the 12 d period. The researchers verified the inability of fat oxidation to match dietary fat intake when they underfed three lean men for 12 d using the same mixed diet. Energy intake was 67% less than required to maintain energy balance. Again, carbohydrate and protein oxidation matched dietary intakes, but fat did not. The subjects consumed 20 g of fat but oxidized 59 g. The subjects lost on average 7 lb (3.2 kg) in 12 d. Changes in fat balance explained 74% of the energy imbalance during the overfeeding period and 84% of the imbalance during the underfeeding period.

The metabolic consequences of the preferential storage of dietary fat are significant. The

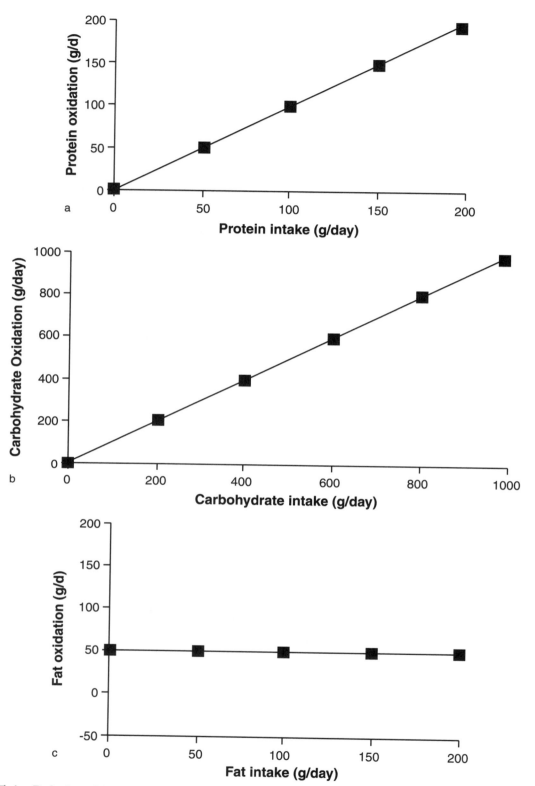

Figure 5.1 Relationship between intake and oxidation of protein, carbohydrate, and fat in 21 weight-stable men (n = 11) and women (n = 10) after 7 d of consuming a diet that contained 62% of energy from carbohydrate and 26% of energy from fat.

Reprinted from Thomas et al. 1992.

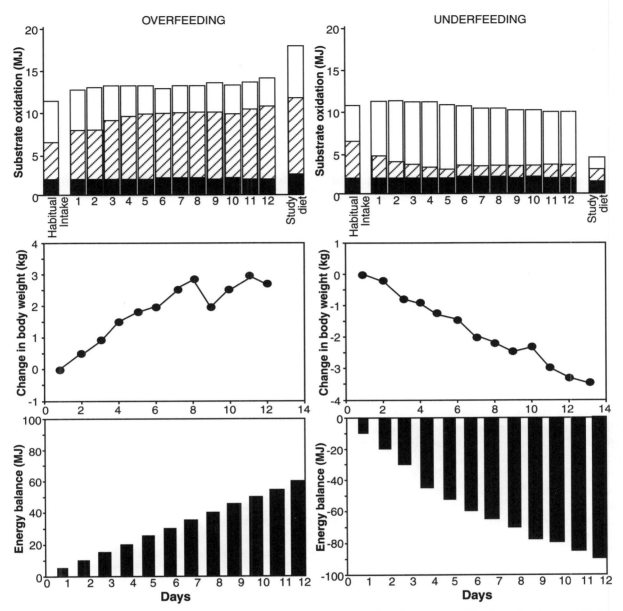

Figure 5.2 Changes in energy balance, body weight, and substrate oxidation during a 12-d period of overfeeding or underfeeding. Overfeeding consisted of a mixed diet (15% of energy from protein, 35% from fat, 50% from carbohydrate) that was 33% higher in energy than that required to maintain energy balance. Underfeeding consisted of the same mixed diet, which was 67% lower in energy than required to maintain energy balance. Top graphs show changes in energy expenditure with over- and underfeeding and the contributions from separate macronutrinets. Solid bar = protein; hatched bar = carbohydrate; open bar = fat. To convert MJ (Megajoules) to kcals: MJ × 1000/4.12 = kcal.

Reprinted from Jebb et al. 1996.

energy required to digest, absorb, and convert carbohydrate energy to adenosine triphosphate (ATP) is greater than that lost in converting dietary fat to ATP—leaving only about 80% of the carbohydrate energy available for work, whereas 94% of the fat energy is available. Thus, when dietary fat is stored as adipose tissue, it may represent a greater relative fuel reservoir than had previously been considered.

The body's glycogen storage capacity is

limited to 1.1-1.8 lb (~500-800 g) in the liver and skeletal muscle combined, a capacity much smaller than that for protein or fat. Exercise training can increase the storage capacity, but even then it cannot be enlarged much past ~4.4 lb (2 kg). Glycogen storage fluctuates greatly in response to feeding and exercise: feeding increases and exercise decreases glycogen stores. Flatt (1988) proposed that a carbohydrate "appetite" drives people to replenish glycogen stores, and that satiety occurs when this replenishment is complete. Researchers at Laval University in Quebec (Tremblay et al. 1991) have shown that people on a high-fat diet (i.e., a diet low in carbohydrate) may overconsume energy to satisfy the drive for carbohydrate. The overconsumption results in a positive energy balance, which can increase amounts of adipose tissue. Some researchers feel this approach is too simplistic, and that control of carbohydrate appetite may result from relative rates of breakdown and synthesis (flux) of both carbohydrate and fat (Friedman and Tordoff 1986). Other investigators have been unable to show such a drive for maintenance of carbohydrate stores. Stubbs et al. (1993) found that men given diets of varying carbohydrate content did not change energy intake on days after being fed either a diet providing 3% of energy from carbohydrate (depletion diet) or 47% (control diet). However, the study lasted only 1 d, and the diet provided during the control phase may have been sufficient to replenish any glycogen stores used by these inactive individuals over the 1 d of testing. These investigators also found that carbohydrate oxidation decreased with the lower carbohydrate intake and increased with the higher carbohydrate intake.

Protein Balance

The concept of protein or nitrogen balance (see chapter 4) is essential to the discussion of energy balance. The body adjusts to a wide range of protein intakes by altering the oxidation rate of dietary protein. After all anabolic needs are met, the carbon skeletons of any excess amino acids are diverted into the energy substrate pool where they are used for energy production. The adequacy of total energy intake, and carbohydrate intake in particular, appears to dramatically affect this process. Inadequate intakes of either energy or carbohydrate result in negative protein balance and may adversely affect the balances of individual amino acids (Krempf et al. 1993). Conversely, excess intake of either energy or carbohydrate will spare protein, which is then available to support brief periods of protein accumulation until the protein pool is expanded to a new balance point. At this point, the degradation of endogenous protein matches the available exogenous protein. Excess protein consumed or protein made available through protein sparing may contribute *indirectly* to fat storage by sparing dietary fat, as was seen with the consumption of excess carbohydrate energy. However, excess dietary protein is not made *directly* into triacylglycerides (or triglycerides) and stored as fat.

Fat Balance

Fat balance is not as precisely regulated as protein and carbohydrate balance. Figure 5.1 shows that as fat intake increases, fat oxidation does not increase proportionately. In marked contrast to carbohydrate, body adipose tissue stores are large, and most evidence shows that the acute intake of fat has little influence on fat oxidation (Thomas et al. 1992). Because most research shows that fat intake does not directly promote fat oxidation, it is now commonly accepted that excess energy eaten as dietary fat is stored as triacylglyceride in adipose tissue, with little energy being consumed in the storage process.

Over the long term, a positive fat balance due to excess energy intake leads to a progressive increase in total body fat stores in an attempt to achieve energy balance. These expanded stores also increase the free fatty acid concentrations in the blood. This increase in circulation of free fatty acids may slightly increase fat oxidation and probably promote recycling. Thus, the larger adipose tissue mass promotes increased fat oxidation. When the new rate of fat oxidation equals the rate of fat intake, a person again achieves fat balance (and hence energy balance)—but at a significantly higher body weight (figure 5.3).

If increasing fat stores allow fat oxidation to match fat intake, then obesity may be viewed as a compensatory mechanism to reestablish energy balance at a new steady state in response to the chronic ingestion of excess energy. For example, Astrup et al. (1994) found a higher rate of fat oxidation in obese women (40%) as compared to nonobese women (36%)

Long-term changes in fat oxidation and body fat stores when excess dietary fat in consumed with no change in energy expenditure

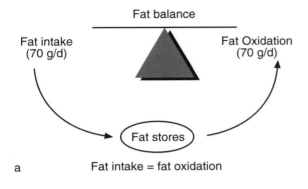

a

Fat intake = fat oxidation

Long-term changes in fat oxidation and body fat stores when exercise is added to increase total daily energy expenditure, with no change in energy or fat intake.

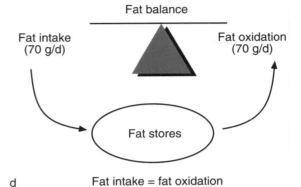

d

Fat intake = fat oxidation

Fat overfeeding

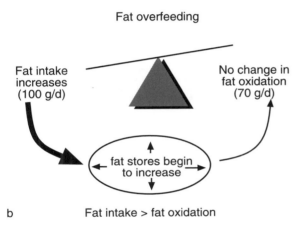

b

Fat intake > fat oxidation

Exercise is added (300 kcal/d)

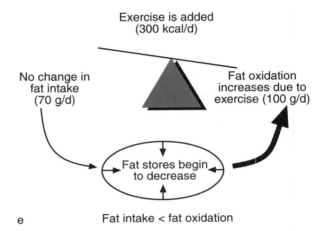

e

Fat intake < fat oxidation

Post-overfeeding fat balance

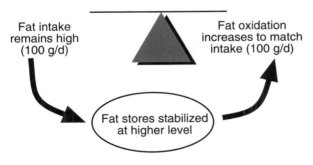

c

Fat intake = fat oxidation
(Body weight and fat stores are stable at higher levels.)

Long-term changes in fat oxidation and body fat stores when exercise is added.

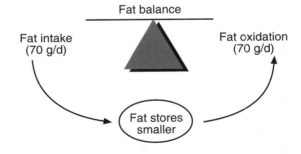

f

Fat intake = fat oxidation
(Body weight and fat stores are stable at lower levels.)

Figure 5.3 Schematic illustration of the proposed long-term adaptations in fat oxidation and body fat storage induced by *(a-c)* excess dietary fat over a prolonged period and *(d-f)* exercise. Reprinted from Schutz et al. 1992 *(a-c)*; redrawn from Butterfield and Tremblay 1994 *(d-f)*.

after adjusting for their percentage of energy from dietary fat, age, and 24-h energy balance. Percentage of fat oxidation also increased with fat mass—the higher the fat mass, the greater an individual's fat oxidation rate. Schutz et al. (1992) reported that an excess fat intake of 20 g/d (180 kcal/d) would lead to an increase in body fat of 22 lb (10 kg) before fat balance would be achieved with a corresponding increase in fat oxidation. Thus, in susceptible sedentary individuals, the expansion of fat stores is a prerequisite to increase fat oxidation to match a high percentage of dietary fat energy. Schutz et al. (1992) found a decrease in fat oxidation in obese women losing weight.

Alcohol Balance

Alcohol is a "priority fuel," which means alcohol oxidation rises quickly after ingestion of alcohol until all the alcohol is cleared from the body. Alcohol can suppress the oxidation of fat and to a lesser degree that of protein and carbohydrate (Shelmet et al. 1988). Alcohol is not converted to triacylglycerides and stored as fat, nor can it contribute to the formation of muscle or liver glycogen. *It may, however, indirectly divert fat to storage by providing an alternative and preferred energy source for the body* (Sonko et al. 1994). Thus, at ~7 kcal/g, alcohol can contribute significantly to total daily energy intake; individuals who consume alcohol may have to reduce their consumption of energy from other dietary components to maintain energy balance.

Energy Expenditure

Energy expenditure is one side of the energy balance equation. Any alteration in energy expenditure can result in weight gain/loss, if energy intake and composition are held constant. In this section, we review the various components of energy expenditure and how these components are measured; we also discuss how being physically active can influence these components. Because direct assessment of energy expenditure is difficult, we present methods for predicting energy expenditure based on age, gender, and anthropometric measurements.

Components of Energy Expenditure

The components of total daily energy expenditure are generally divided into three main categories: (1) **resting metabolic rate (RMR),**

basal metabolic rate (BMR), or **resting energy expenditure (REE)** (see "What Are the Differences Between RMR, BMR, REE, and SMR?", page 138); (2) thermic effect of food; and (3) energy expended in physical activity, or as it is frequently called, the thermic effect of activity (see figure 5.4). The RMR is the energy required to maintain the systems of the body and to regulate body temperature at rest. RMR is measured in the morning after an overnight fast (12 h) while the individual is resting in a bed. The person must be comfortable and free from stress, medications, or any other stimulation that would increase metabolic activity. The room where RMR is measured should be quiet, temperature-controlled, and free of distractions. RMR accounts for approximately 60-80% of total daily energy expenditure in most sedentary healthy adults (Ravussin et al. 1986; Ravussin and Bogardus 1989). In active individuals this percentage will vary greatly—it is not unusual for some athletes to expend 1000-2000 kcal/d just in sport-related activities. When Thompson et al. (1993) determined energy balance in 24 elite male endurance athletes over 3-7 d, they found that RMR represented only 38-47% of total daily energy expenditure. Beidleman et al. (1995) reported similar figures for active women. During days of repetitive heavy competition, such as ultramara-thons, RMR may represent <20% of total energy expenditure (Rontoyannis et al. 1989).

The **thermic effect of food (TEF)** represents the increase in energy expenditure above RMR that results from the consumption of food throughout the day. Although TEF is frequently used interchangeably with the thermic effect of a meal, the terms are not synonymous. The **thermic effect of a meal (TEM)** represents the increase in metabolic rate above RMR after eating a meal. It is easier to measure TEM than TEF because of the difficulties in trying to assess the cumulative energy cost of all foods consumed within a day. Most research literature that examines the energy costs of active individuals reports TEM, unless the researchers are able to use a metabolic chamber. Figure 5.4 illustrates the TEM concept by showing the increase in metabolic rate above RMR over a 3-h period on two different occasions in male triathletes fed a meal containing approximately 750 kcal.

The TEF includes the energy cost of food digestion, absorption, transport, metabolism, and storage within the body. TEF usually accounts

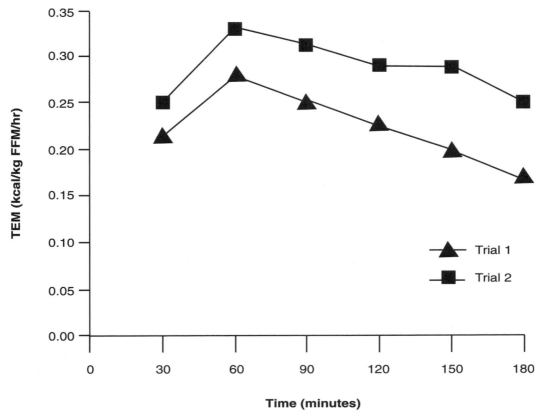

Figure 5.4 Thermic effect of a meal (TEM) on two different occasions in male triathletes consuming 12 kcal/kg of fat free mass (FFM) (~750 kcal). TEM was calculated as the difference between resting metabolic rate (RMR) and the thermic response to the test meal. The liquid meal provided 60% of energy from carbohydrate, 25% from fat, and 15% from protein.

Adapted from Thompson et al. 1993.

for approximately 6-10% of total daily energy expenditure, with women usually having a lower value (~6-7%) (Poehlman 1989). This value varies depending on the total number of kilocalories in the meal, types of foods consumed, and the degree of obesity. TEF has two general components: obligatory and facultative thermogenesis. **Obligatory thermogenesis** is the energy cost associated with digestion, absorption, and transport of nutrients, and with the synthesis of protein, fat (triacylglycerides), and carbohydrate (glycogen). Approximately 50-75% of the TEF can be attributed to the obligatory component (Flatt 1992). Research has shown that the measured TEF is higher than the theoretical cost of nutrient digestion, absorption, and storage (Acheson, Ravussin et al. 1984). The energy expended above obligatory thermogenesis is termed **facultative thermogenesis** and is due primarily to sympathetic nervous system activity. For example, after eating a meal or after the infusion of glucose,

plasma levels of norepinephrine increase. If medication blocks this release of norepinephrine, the TEF of food declines (Acheson, Ravussin et al. 1984). Thus, the TEF is a combination of the energy required to digest and metabolize the food we eat, and the energy expended due to sympathetic nervous system activity brought about by seeing, smelling, and eating food.

The **thermic effect of activity (TEA)** is the most variable component of energy expenditure. It includes the energy cost of daily activities above RMR and TEF, such as purposeful activities of daily living (making dinner, dressing, cleaning house) or planned exercise events (running, weight training, walking). It also includes the energy cost of involuntary muscular activity such as shivering, fidgeting, and maintenance of posture. This type of movement is called **spontaneous physical activity (SPA)** or **nonexercise activity thermogenesis (NEAT)** (Levine et al. 1999; Ravussin and

■ HIGHLIGHT ■

What Are the Differences Between RMR, BMR, REE, and SMR?

In research literature, the terms RMR, BMR, and REE are often used interchangeably; you may also see references to **sleeping metabolic rate (SMR)**. If BMR is used, it usually means that the measurements are taken after the subject has stayed overnight in a metabolic chamber or research ward and has not eaten in the last 12 h. If RMR or REE is used, it usually means the subject slept at home and drove or was driven to the research lab for testing. RMR and BMR usually differ by less than 10%. If SMR is reported, it means the subject slept in a metabolic chamber where technicians measured the metabolic rate during sleep (usually the period of fewest movements). SMR is usually 5-10% lower than BMR. Read the research methods carefully to know which technique was used for data collection. In general, BMR may better represent the energy required at rest because the subject does not have to get up, dress, and drive to a research site. However, some researchers now report that BMR and RMR are similar *if* strict research protocols are followed during data collection (Bullough and Melby 1993; Thompson et al. 1995; Turley et al. 1993).

Swinburn 1993). TEA may be only 10-15% of total daily energy expenditure in sedentary persons but may be as high as 50% in active people. The addition of RMR, TEF, and TEA should account for 100% of total energy expenditure (figure 5.5). A number of factors can increase energy expenditure above normal baseline levels (e.g., cold, fear, stress, and various medications). The thermic effect of these factors is frequently referred to as **adaptive thermogenesis (AT)**. AT represents a temporary increase in thermogenesis that may last for hours or even days, depending on the duration and magnitude of the stimulus (e.g., a serious physical injury, the stress associated with an upcoming event, going to a higher altitude, or the use of certain medications) (table 5.2).

Biological Factors That Influence Resting Metabolic Rate

A variety of factors can influence RMR for a given individual on any given day. Table 5.2 briefly outlines these factors, which should be considered when measuring or predicting an individual's RMR. This section reviews the most common influences on RMR and discusses how they may be altered in active individuals.

Effects of Age, Sex, and Body Size on Resting Metabolic Rate

It is well documented that RMR is influenced by age, sex, and body size, including fat-free mass (FFM) and fat mass. Three of these variables (FFM, age, and sex) generally explain about 80% of the variability in RMR (Bogardus et al. 1986). Since FFM is very metabolically active tissue, any change in FFM dramatically influences RMR. Figure 5.6 shows the strong linear relationship between FFM and RMR. This relationship appears to be true for all individuals regardless of sex or race. In general, men have larger RMRs than women simply because they usually weigh more and have more FFM, but other factors may contribute to the male/female differences in RMR. Ferraro et al. (1992) found lower RMRs in women than in men (~100 kcal/d less) even after controlling for differences in FFM, fat mass, and age.

Age also influences RMR, which declines ~1-2% per decade from the second through the seventh decade of life (Keys et al. 1987). Part of the decrease is attributed to the decline in FFM that frequently occurs with aging, especially as people lead more sedentary lifestyles (Poehlman et al. 1992; Poehlman et al. 1993). Yet not all the decline in RMR that occurs with aging is attributed to decreases in FFM. A study by Vaughan et al. (1991) found a small but significant negative impact of age on metabolic rate independent of FFM, fat mass, and sex. These researchers used a metabolic chamber to measure metabolic rates of 39 elderly and 64 young men and women. After adjusting for differences in FFM, fat mass, and sex, the researchers found significantly lower BMRs (~100 kcal/d) in the elderly versus the younger subjects. Conversely, Poehlman et al. (1992)

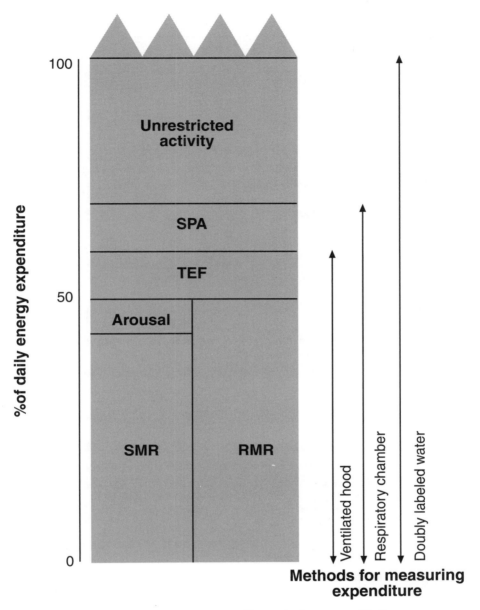

Figure 5.5 Components of daily energy expenditure in humans. Daily energy expenditure can be divided into three major components: the resting metabolic rate (RMR) (sum of the sleeping metabolic rate [SMR] and the energy cost of arousal), which usually represents 50-70% of daily energy expenditure; the thermic effect of food (TEF), which represents ~10% of daily energy expenditure; and the energy cost of physical activity (sum of spontaneous physical activity [SPA] and unrestricted/voluntary physical activity), which represents 20-40% of daily energy expenditure.

Reprinted from Ravussin and Swinburn 1993.

found no difference in RMR between males aged 17-39 years, as compared with males aged 40-78 years even after adjusting for FFM, fat mass, and $\dot{V}O_2$max. Their data suggest that age alone does not independently influence RMR. Although the exact effect of age on RMR has not yet been determined, it seems clear that the decrease in RMR with age will be mini-

mized for people who stay physically active throughout their lives.

Effect of Genetics on Resting Metabolic Rate

It is now known that RMR has a genetic component: individuals within families tend to have similar RMRs. After measuring RMR in 130 nondiabetic adult Southwestern

Table 5.2 Factors That Influence Resting Metabolic Rate (RMR)

Factor	Effect on RMR
Age	↓ <1-2% per decade between second and seventh decades (Keys et al. 1987)
Weight	↑ RMR with ↑ weight (Bray and Atkinson 1977)
Fat-free mass (FFM)	↑ RMR with ↑ FFM
Fat mass	↑ RMR with ↑ fat mass
Sex	↑ RMR in males versus females (Ferraro et al. 1992)
Genetics	RMR shows familial relationship (Bouchard et al. 1989; Bogardus et al. 1986)
Body temperature	12% ↑ RMR with each 1°C ↑ body temperature
Severe dieting/starvation	↓ RMR
Feasting/overeating	↑ RMR
Illness/catabolic conditions/injury	↑ RMR
Menstrual cycle (variable responses reported)	RMR ↑ in luteal phase (100-300 kcal/d) versus follicular phase (Ferraro et al. 1992; Bisdee et al. 1989; Solomon et al. 1982)
Growth/pregnancy	↑ RMR with ↑ body weight
Fitness level (trained vs. untrained)	Variable responses reported, may depend on level of training and amount of training done daily
Acute exercise	Variable responses reported, may depend on the intensity and duration of the exercise (see figure 5.10)
Thyroid hormones	↓ RMR if below normal levels; ↑ RMR if abnormally high
Catecholamines (epinephrine and norepinephrine)	↑ RMR
Cortisol	↑ RMR
Growth hormone	↑ RMR
Alcohol	↑ RMR (Klesges et al. 1994)
Smoking	Four cigarettes ↑ RMR by 3% over 3 h (Collins et al. 1994)
Caffeine	Single dose of 100 mg oral caffeine ↑ RMR by 3-4% over 150 min (Dulloo et al. 1989); single-dose of 200 mg oral caffeine ↑ RMR by 5-8% (Collins et al. 1994); 4 mg/kg dose ↑ RMR by 13-15% over 30 min (Yoshida et al. 1994)

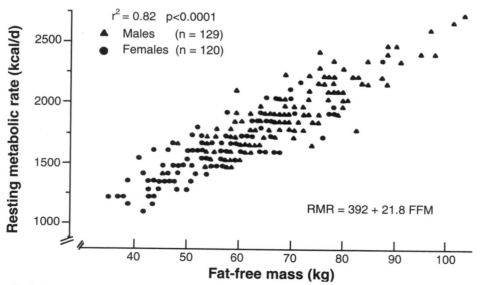

Figure 5.6 Relationship between resting metabolic rate (RMR) and fat-free body mass (FFM). Reprinted from Ravussin and Bogardus 1989.

American Indians from 54 families (figure 5.7), Bogardus et al. (1986) found that family membership explained 11% of the variability in RMR ($p < 0.0001$). In studies of twins and parent-child pairs, Bouchard et al. (1989) reported that heritability explained approximately 40% of the variability in RMR after adjustments were made for age, gender, and FFM.

Effect of Body Temperature on Resting Metabolic Rate

Although we know that RMR increases as body temperature increases above normal, such as in febrile diseases (see table 5.2), until recently it was not known whether a relationship existed between RMR and body temperature within normal temperature ranges. After adjusting for differences in body size, body composition, and age, Rising et al. (1992) found a strong positive correlation ($r = 0.80; p < 0.0001$) between metabolic rate and body temperature within the range 95.0-97.7°F (35.0-36.5°C). The question remains whether lower body temperatures are inherited, thus predisposing one to a lower RMR and an increased risk for obesity.

Effect of Reproductive Hormones on Resting Metabolic Rate

Research has not clearly determined whether RMR fluctuates over the phases of the menstrual cycle. Some studies report that RMR values are lowest during the follicular phase of the cycle and highest during the luteal phase (Bisdee et al. 1989; Solomon et al. 1982). Figure 5.8 illustrates this change in RMR over the menstrual cycle. The difference in RMR between these two phases is estimated to be approximately 100-300 kcal/d; however, adaptations in energy intake appear to mimic the changes in RMR. Barr et al. (1995) reported that women consume approximately 300 kcal/d more during the luteal phase of the menstrual cycle (end of the cycle) as compared with the follicular phase (beginning of the cycle). Thus, the increased energy expenditure, due to a higher RMR during the luteal phase, is compensated for by an increase in energy intake during this period. Conversely, Weststrate (1993) showed no effect of menstrual cycle on RMR, and Piers et al. (1995) showed no effect of menstrual cycle phase on RMR or energy intake. Until these issues are resolved, the phase of the menstrual cycle should be recorded when measuring RMR or energy intake in females. Ideally, if repeated measures of energy intake or RMR are being recorded, they should be taken at the same time during the menstrual cycle. Lebenstedt et al. (1999) found that RMR was significantly lower in female athletes with menstrual dysfunction (nine periods within the last 12 mo) compared to athletes with normal menstrual function (~111 kcal/d lower; $p < 0.02$). If a female is amenorrheic (not menstruating) or postmenopausal, these

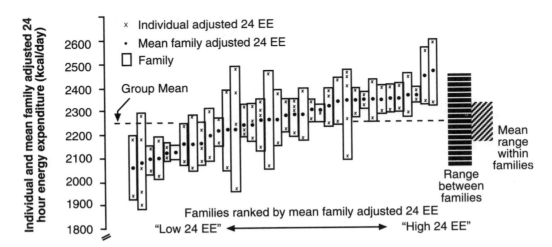

Figure 5.7 Individual and mean family 24-h energy expenditure (24 EE) adjusted for fat-free mass, fat mass, age, and sex. Intrafamily correlation coefficient was 0.26. Families are ranked according to adjusted resting metabolic rate (RMR). The range of the mean family adjusted RMR and the mean range within families are depicted by the hatched bars on the right.

Reprinted from Ravussin and Bogardus 1986.

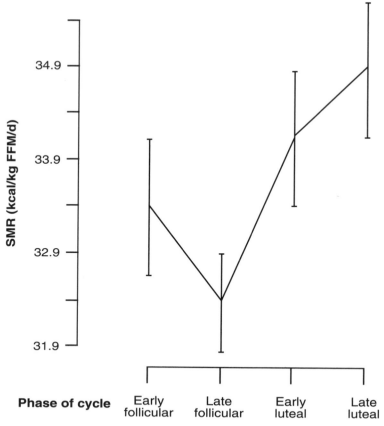

Figure 5.8 Mean sleep metabolic rate (SMR) at four phases of the menstrual cycle. Values are means with standard errors represented by vertical bars.

Reprinted from Bisbee et al. 1989.

changes in RMR and energy intake do not occur.

Effect of Exercise on Resting Metabolic Rate

Exercise can affect energy expenditure both directly and indirectly. Metabolism increases during exercise, directly increasing the amount of energy expended. Exercise can also increase energy expenditure indirectly by increasing a person's amount of FFM, which in turn elevates RMR. Researchers have asked the following questions:

1. Within the general population, do aerobically trained people have higher RMRs than untrained individuals?

2. For a given individual, does becoming more aerobically trained increase RMR?

3. Does metabolic rate stay elevated for a time after exercise is over?

Within the General Population, Do Aerobically Trained People Have Higher Resting Metabolic Rates Than Untrained Individuals?

Researchers have addressed this question by comparing the RMRs of aerobically trained and untrained people. Figure 5.9 summarizes some of the current studies in this area. Results have been mixed. Poehlman et al. (1990) found that active men had RMRs significantly (~5%) higher than untrained men of similar size and FFM but Broeder et al. (1992) found no significant difference in RMR between active and inactive men—mean RMR was only 3.4% higher in the trained group. As yet there is no consensus in this area of research (see "Why Is the Research Literature Inconsistent Regarding the Effect of Exercise on Metabolism?", page 146). As figure 5.9 demonstrates, researchers have reported a wide range of differences in RMR (~3-16%). The discrepancies in these data may be due to a number of factors, including the subjects' levels of fitness, types of training program, methods used

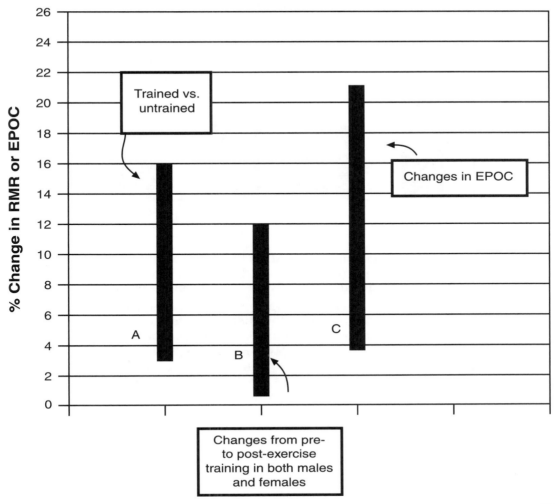

Figure 5.9 Effect of exercise on RMR and excess post-exercise oxygen consumption (EPOC). *(a)* Effect of exercise on RMR in young trained vs. untrained men. *(b)* Effect of exercise training on posttraining RMR in previously untrained men and women. *(c)* Effect of exercise and exercise intensity on changes in EPOC (see page 144). In each case, bar represents range of changes reported in the literature.

Adapted from Bullough et al. 1995.

when measuring RMR, and levels of **energy flux** (a factor that includes kilocalories expended in exercise compared with kilocalories consumed each day, and also the amount of time between exercise sessions). Concerning the last point: RMR values may be influenced by acute changes in exercise energy expenditure and/or energy intake. Bullough et al. (1995), for example, found that athletes' RMRs measured after 3 d of high-intensity exercise (90 min of cycling at 75% $\dot{V}O_2max$) were significantly higher than when measured after 3 d of no exercise. During each of these periods, energy intake was fed to match energy expenditure. The authors also compared the RMRs of the trained group with those of an untrained control group and found no differences in RMR between groups, if the trained group was measured after 3 d of no exercise. However, there were significant differences (~16%) between the trained and untrained groups when RMR was measured in the trained group after 3 d of high-intensity exercise. The researchers also found that, if energy intake was low on high-exercise days, RMR was not elevated as compared to RMR on high-exercise days when energy intake was adequate (see figure 5.10).

Another factor that influences RMR is the timing of the RMR measurement. Herring et al. (1992) examined RMR 15, 39, 63, and 87 h after the last exercise bout in nine long-distance female runners. By 39 h post-exercise, RMR declined by 8%. This lower RMR was maintained

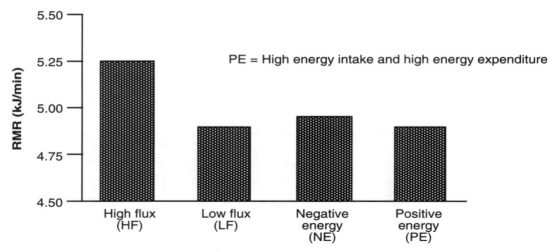

Figure 5.10 Average resting metabolic rates (RMRs) for each of four different energy balance/flux conditions in eight highly trained men (mean ± SEM). High flux was significantly different from all other conditions ($p < 0.05$). Trained male athletes were used for the following four conditions:

- High flux (HF) = Subjects were in a state of high energy flux, exercising at 75% $\dot{V}O_2$max for 90 min on each of 3 d while consuming a controlled diet adequate to maintain energy balance. HF turnover is characterized by high intake and exercise energy expenditure.
- Low flux (LF) = Subjects were in a state of low energy flux, abstaining from exercise for 3 d while consuming a controlled diet adequate to maintain energy balance.
- Negative energy (NE) balance = Subjects were in NE balance, exercising at 75% $\dot{V}O_2$max for 90 min on each of 3 d while consuming the controlled diet designed to maintain energy balance during LF.
- Positive energy (PE) balance = Subjects were in PE balance, abstaining from exercise for 2 d while consuming the controlled diet designed to maintain energy balance during HF.

Adapted from Bullough et al. 1995.

up to 87 h post-exercise. Thus, if RMR is measured within 24 h of the last exercise bout, it may be higher than if measured 35-48 h afterward. However, since most active people exercise 5-7 d per week, there is rarely a time when no exercise occurs for a 48-h period. In fact, many athletes actually train twice a day, so they rarely have even a 24-h period in which they do not exercise. Choosing the exact time to measure RMR post-exercise in active individuals can be difficult!

For a Given Individual, Does Becoming More Aerobically Trained Increase Resting Metabolic Rate?

Researchers have examined pre- and post-training RMRs in sedentary individuals who participated in exercise training programs (see figure 5.9b). Published data on change in RMR with exercise training range from <1% to 12%. For example, Wilmore et al. (1998) saw no change in RMR in 74 men and women (17-63 years) who participated in a 20-week endurance training program (cycle exercise) that in-

creased $\dot{V}O_2$max by 17.9%. But Poehlman and Danforth (1991) reported an 11.8% increase in RMR in 19 older subjects (64 ± 1.6 years) participating in an 8-week endurance training program (cycle exercise). Again, the mixed results presumably depend on a number of variables such as age, gender, level of obesity, type of training program used, and levels of fitness achieved. Although there appears to be no consensus in this area, we do know that becoming more physically active can increase or preserve FFM. This increased activity may in turn help to stabilize or increase RMR.

Does Metabolic Rate Stay Elevated After Exercise Is Over?

Oxygen consumption remains elevated for a short time after exercise has stopped (Gaesser and Brooks 1984). During this cool-down period, heart rate and metabolic processes usually return to normal within a short time. How quickly the return to homeostasis occurs depends on a number of factors including level of training, age, environmental conditions, and intensity and duration of the exercise. Can exercise significantly increase oxygen consumption after exercise (the term generally used is **excess post-exercise oxygen consumption** or **EPOC**)? Figure 5.11 illustrates the change in EPOC with different exercise intensities and durations in 10 trained male triathletes. In this study, EPOC appears to be greater after high-intensity exercise, although the duration is short (20 min).

How long and to what magnitude does EPOC increase after an exercise bout? Does a strenuous exercise session on one day significantly increase oxygen consumption on subsequent days? Figure 5.9 gives the range of changes in EPOC (~4-21%) reported in the research literature. It appears that to produce a significant increase in EPOC, exercise intensity must be high or the duration of exercise must be long. A normal exercise bout of 30-60 min of moderate intensity (50-65% $\dot{V}O_2$max) does not appear to significantly elevate EPOC for any appreciable length of time after the exercise ends—oxygen levels usually return to normal within 1 h. However, if exercise is of high intensity or of long duration, EPOC appears to be elevated for hours after exercise. In some cases, oxygen consumption is even elevated on subsequent days after strenuous exercise.

The type of exercise performed (aerobic vs. strength training) may also influence EPOC. Most research examining the effect of exercise on EPOC uses aerobic activity as the mode of exercise. However, Melby et al. (1993) observed a significant EPOC in trained males lifting weights for 90 min. On the morning after the exercise session, oxygen consumption was elevated by 5-10% over baseline levels. Thus, although it is well documented that O_2 consumption is elevated after exercise, the magnitude and duration of the elevation appears to depend on the intensity and duration of the exercise bout as well as the type of exercise.

Factors That Influence the Thermic Effect of Food

A number of factors can influence how our bodies respond metabolically when we consume food. Some of these factors are associated with the physiological characteristics of an individual such as genetic background, age, level of physical fitness, sensitivity to insulin, or level of obesity. Other factors are associated with the meal—such as its size, composition, palatability, and timing.

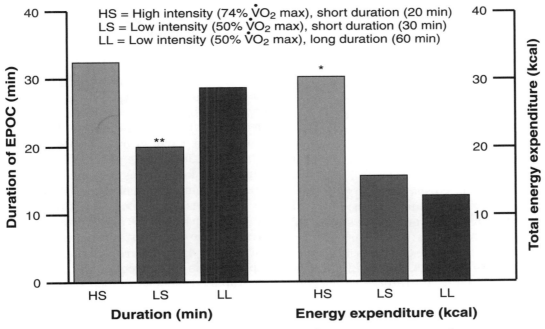

Figure 5.11 Duration and total energy expenditure for excess post-exercise oxygen consumption (EPOC) in 10 trained male triathletes performing three cycle ergometer exercises. ** Significantly different ($p < 0.05$) from HS and LL for duration. * Significantly different ($p < 0.05$) from LS and LL for energy expenditure.

Adapted from Sedlock et al. 1989.

■ HIGHLIGHT ■

Why Is the Research Literature Inconsistent Regarding the Effect of Exercise on Metabolism?

A variety of factors may contribute to the inconsistency of published data on the effect of exercise on metabolism (especially on RMR):

- Some experiments used only a small number of subjects, and some have great variability in the subjects' characteristics (level of training, FFM, body size, age, diet behaviors).

- The time of the RMR measurements after the last exercise bout has not been standardized.

- Methods for measuring oxygen consumption vary (no repeated measures, no standardization of protocol), making comparisons between studies difficult.

- There often is variability in repeated measurements on the same individual due to prior dietary practices, exercise patterns, or other uncontrolled variables.

- Experimental subjects have variable levels of training (minutes exercised per week) and fitness (level of $\dot{V}O_2max$).

Effect of Food Composition and Meal Size on the Thermic Effect of Food

The TEF can last for several hours after a meal, and depends on the size of the meal consumed (number of kilocalories) and its composition (percentage of kilocalories from protein, fat, carbohydrate) (Stock 1999). In general, the thermic effect of a mixed diet is about 6-10% of total daily energy intake; however, the total TEF also depends on the macronutrient composition of the diet. For example, the thermogenic effect of glucose is 5-10%; the figures are 3-5% for fat and 20-30% for protein (Flatt 1992). The lower thermic responses for carbohydrate and fat are due to the lower energy requirement to store carbohydrate as glycogen and fat as triacylgly-cerides, as compared to the energy-expensive synthesis of proteins from amino acids. The TEF also depends on how the body uses the energy it consumes: Is the body going to use the food for immediate energy or will the energy be stored? If the energy will be stored, in what form will it be stored? Table 5.3 reviews the energy costs of storing various macronutrients. For example, the amount of energy required to store dietary carbohydrate as glycogen is much lower than when dietary carbohydrate is converted to endogenous fat and stored. In general, converting dietary carbohydrate or protein to stored fat requires more energy than converting dietary fat to stored fat. In weight-stable, normal-weight people who consume a mixed diet, however, synthesis of fat from carbohyrate appears to be negligible. Under normal physiological conditions, excess protein and carbohydrate consumed are preferentially used for energy, while fat is stored. Diets higher in fat generally have a lower TEF than diets that contain more carbohydrate or protein—and a meal higher in kilocalories will have a higher TEF compared to a low-calorie meal, which has fewer calories and less food to be digested, transported, and stored. For example, the TEF of a person who consumes 3000 kcal/d would be approximately 180-300 kcal/d, while someone consuming only 1500 kcal/d would have a TEF of 90-150 kcal/d. The total TEF for a day does not appear to be influenced by meal size or number, as long as the same number of kilocalories are consumed throughout the day (Belko and Barbieri 1987). Thus, the TEF depends on the number of kilocalories consumed during the day and the composition of those kilocalories.

In the research laboratory, it is time-consuming to measure TEF and TEM; and these parameters are the least reproducible components of energy expenditure. Of the two measures, the TEM is more frequently used to measure metabolic response to food because it is more reproducible and less expensive than measuring TEF in a metabolic chamber (Tataranni et al. 1995). The TEM represents the metabolic response to a single meal (usually over a 6-h period), while the TEF represents the metabolic response to all the food consumed during the day. As mentioned earlier, these terms are frequently used interchangeably in the research

146

Table 5.3 Calculated Cost of Nutrient Thermogenesis and Energy Stored in Humans

Nutrient	Storage form	Thermogenesis[a]	Cost of nutrient storage[b]
Glucose	glycogen (liver)	6-8%	5-10%
	glycogen (muscle)	—	5-10%
	fat (adipose)	—	24-28%[c]
Fat	fat (adipose)	2-3%	4-7%
Protein	protein	25-40%	25-40%

[a]Percent of the energy content of the infused nutrient.

[b]Percent of the energy content of the stored nutrient.

[c]In humans under normal physiological conditions, little de novo synthesis of triglycerides (fat) occurs from excess protein or carbohydrate.

Adapted from Jequier 1992; Flatt 1978.

literature, so you need to read the methods carefully to determine what was being measured. To determine the reproducibility of these measurements, one can measure an individual's day-to-day variability for TEM as well as the variability among individuals. A recent study by Houde-Nadeau et al. (1993) reported the within-subject coefficient of variation for TEM to be 10.7%, while the between-subject variability was twice as high at 24%. This study measured TEM in four men and four women on three different occasions for 6 h. The subjects ate a standardized meal of 792 kcal (44% carbohydrate, 16% protein, 40% fat). The measured TEM was 7% after 6 h, but since the increase in energy expenditure due to the meal had not returned to baseline, the total TEM was actually higher. This study found no significant difference between men and women for TEM when values were expressed as kilocalories/hour. However, when the values were expressed as a percentage of RMR, the response was 10.7% for the women and 5% for the men after 6 h.

Effect of Exercise on the Thermic Effect of Food

In general, it appears that aerobically trained males have a lower TEF than sedentary males, while studies in trained women do not support a lower TEF (Poehlman 1989). These gender differences might be attributed to researchers' not controlling for the time of the menstrual cycle (Li et al. 1999) or menstrual status in studies measuring the TEF in active women.

The effect of acute exercise on TEF appears to depend on a number of factors, including the level of obesity, the timing of the meal and of the exercise session, the intensity and duration of the exercise, and the level of fitness. Segal et al. (1992) reported that exercise before a meal had no significant effect on TEM in lean subjects but increased TEM in obese subjects by 40%. However, the absolute increase in total kilocalories was small (10-15 kcal/3 h). Few data are available on the effect of exercise before and after a meal in exercise-trained subjects. A study by Nichols et al. (1988) reported that, in trained swimmers (both men and women), 45 min of swimming significantly increased the metabolic response to a meal when the meal preceded the exercise (24.8 kcal/h) compared with no exercise (20.2 kcal/h). However, this is a difference of only 18 kcal over the 4-h measurement period: the long-term significance of this tiny difference may be small, especially considering the high variability in the TEM measurement between individuals.

Measurement of Total Daily Energy Expenditure

Total daily energy expenditure or its components can be measured in the laboratory or can be estimated with prediction equations. We will discuss the most commonly used laboratory techniques as well as prediction equations that can be used to estimate energy expenditure when laboratory facilities are not available.

Calorimetry

Energy expenditure in humans can be assessed by either direct or indirect calorimetry. **Direct calorimetry** measures the amount of heat given off by the body through radiation, convection, and evaporation. Since neither oxygen nor carbon dioxide is stored in the body under normal physiological conditions, **indirect calorimetry** estimates the heat released through oxidative processes by measuring rates of oxygen consumption and carbon dioxide production. Under basal conditions, both methods give identical results; but due to cyclical changes in body temperature throughout the day, direct calorimetry cannot be used to assess heat production for periods less than 24 h (Jequier and Shultz 1983). Direct calorimetry uses an airtight calorimetric chamber in which the heat produced by the body warms the water surrounding the chamber (figure 5.12). Research-

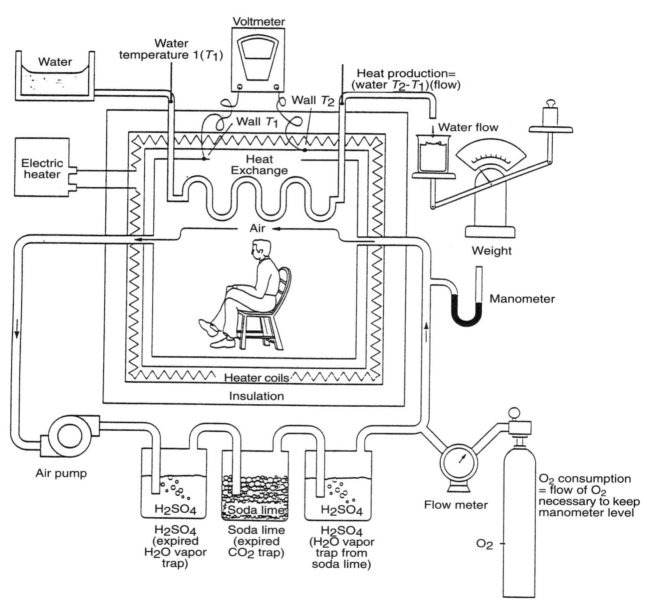

Figure 5.12 A direct calorimetry chamber suitable to accommodate a resting human and simultaneously determine that individual's O_2 consumption and CO_2 production. This device permits correlation of direct and indirect calorimetry. O_2 consumption is equal to the volume of O_2 added to keep the internal (manometer) pressure constant. In the calorimeter, heat loss through the walls is prevented by heating the middle wall (wall T_2) to the temperature of the inner wall (wall T_1). Metabolic heat production is then picked up in the water-heat exchanger.

Reprinted from Brooks et al. 1999.

ers calculate the amount of energy expended from the recorded changes in water temperature. This method is very expensive and is not currently used. Indirect calorimetry is much less expensive, and is the method of choice for many researchers. Indirect calorimetry either uses a metabolic chamber or a mask, hood, or mouthpiece in which gases are collected and analyzed for a specified period of time.

Indirect calorimetry assumes that metabolic rate can be estimated by measuring the rate of transformation of chemical energy into heat. It involves measuring the oxygen consumed, the carbon dioxide produced, and, if possible, the amount of urinary nitrogen excreted (to provide an estimate of protein oxidation). The amounts of oxygen and carbon dioxide exchanged in the lungs closely represent the use and release of these substances by the body tissues. Indirect calorimetry measures the amounts of oxygen consumed and carbon dioxide produced during various activities, in order to estimate the amount of energy being expended by those activities. The ratio between the volume of carbon dioxide produced and the volume of oxygen consumed (VCO_2:VO_2) is termed the nonprotein **respiratory quotient (RQ)** and represents the ratio between oxidation of carbohydrates and lipids (see the following discussion of RER). Various published formulas permit estimation of total energy expenditure, using data on the amount of each energy substrate oxidized and the amounts of oxygen consumed and carbon dioxide produced. Appendix C.1 provides some of the most frequently used formulas. Figure 5.13 shows the equipment used in indirect calorimetry. Consuming 1 L of oxygen typically results in the expenditure of approximately 4.81 kcal, if the fuels oxidized represent a mixture of protein, fat, and carbohydrate.

One must also know the types of foods being oxidized in order to estimate the amount of energy used by the body because fat, protein, and carbohydrate differ dramatically in their energy content and in their content of carbon and oxygen. The amount of oxygen used during exercise depends on the types of fuels being burned, and can be estimated by calculating the **respiratory exchange ratio (RER)**. This ratio is calculated the same way RQ is calculated. As mentioned in "What Is the Difference Between Respiratory Quotient (RQ) and Respiratory Exchange Ratio (RER)?" (page 150), the two terms are frequently used inter-

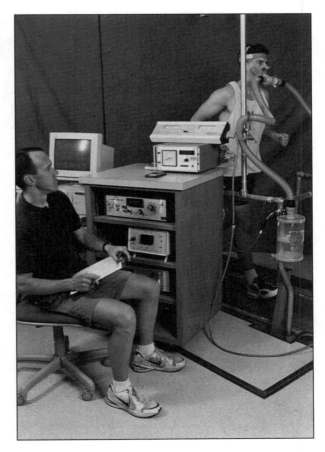

Figure 5.13 Indirect calorimetry.

changeably even though their definitions differ. True RQ is the exchange of oxygen and carbon dioxide at the *cellular level*, but since this parameter cannot be easily measured, RER is used to represent the ratio between carbon dioxide and oxygen that can be measured from expired gases using indirect calorimetry. The assumption is that RER adequately represents what is occurring metabolically at the cellular level under steady-state conditions.

RER indicates the types of fuels being oxidized for energy at any particular time. RER values range from 1.0 to 0.7, with pure carbohydrate having a value of 1.0 and pure fat having a value of 0.7. *When a molecule of glucose is oxidized completely, equal amounts of oxygen and carbon dioxide are used and released—thus the RQ or RER for glucose is 1.0. If fat is oxidized completely, the RQ or RER is 0.7.* Most people consuming a mixed diet of protein, fat, and carbohydrate will have an RER value between 0.82 and 0.87. During times of high exercise intensity, RER will move closer to 1.0;

■ HIGHLIGHT ■

What Is the Difference Between Respiratory Quotient (RQ) and Respiratory Exchange Ratio (RER)?

As the ratio between CO_2 produced and O_2 consumed (VCO_2:VO_2), RQ is an indication of the types of fuels being burned for energy at the cellular level. Since we cannot easily measure what is occurring at the cellular level, we measure RER. RER is also calculated, using indirect calorimetry, as the ratio between CO_2 production and O_2 from expired gases (it thus represents the CO_2 released and the O_2 retained in lung tissue). Because RQ and RER are calculated using the same equation, the terms are often used interchangeably. However, it is appropriate to use RQ only when calculations are made to estimate *cellular metabolism*. When expired gases are measured and used to estimate *fuel utilization*, the term RER should be used. Nutrition research literature more frequently uses the term RQ, while exercise scientists tend to use the term RER. Here is an example of *glucose oxidation* and the resulting RER value:

$$6\ O_2 + C_6H_{12}O_6 \rightarrow 6\ CO_2 + 6\ H_2O + 38\ ATP$$

Thus, the RER = 6 CO_2/6 O_2 = 1

Here is an example of *fat oxidation* and the resulting RER, using a theoretical triacylglycerol containing two molecules of stearic acid and one of palmitic acid:

$$C_{55}H_{106}O_6 + 76.5\ O_2 \rightarrow 55\ CO_2 + 53\ H_2O$$

Thus, the RER = 55 CO_2/76.5 O_2 = 0.719

during times of fasting or low energy intake, RER will be closer to 0.7. Thus, RER depends on the composition of the foods consumed, the energy demands placed on the body, and whether weight is being maintained. Yet there are times when RER does not reflect what is occurring metabolically (e.g., hyperventilation can artificially elevate RER during exercise).

Doubly Labeled Water

Because calorimetry requires that a subject be confined to a laboratory setting or a metabolic chamber, it is difficult to measure a person's free-living or habitual activity. Several field methods for determining energy expenditure have been tested, ranging from factorial methods (described later in this chapter) to heart rate monitors and pedometers. Unfortunately, these methods have disadvantages that frequently make them unacceptable for use with certain groups, or they can be too time-consuming to use with large populations (Schoeller and Racette 1990). Recently the **doubly labeled water (DLW)** technique has been validated as a field method for determining total daily energy expenditure (figure 5.4).

The DLW ($^2H_2^{18}O$) method has become a valuable tool for determining free-living energy expenditures. This method was first developed for use in animals (Lifson et al. 1955) but eventually was applied to humans (Schoeller et al. 1986). The DLW method is a form of indirect calorimetry based on the differential elimination of ^2H (deuterium) and ^{18}O from body water following a dose of water labeled with these two stable isotopes. The deuterium is eliminated as water, while the ^{18}O is eliminated as both water and carbon dioxide. The difference between the two elimination rates is a measure of carbon dioxide production (Coward and Cole 1991; Prentice et al. 1991). The method differs from traditional indirect calorimetry in that it measures only CO_2 production and not oxygen consumption. One advantage to the method is that it can measure energy expenditure in free-living subjects for 3 d to 3 weeks and requires only periodic collection of urine for measurement of the isotope elimination rates. Another advantage is that it is free of bias, and subjects can engage in normal daily activities without the interruption of writing down activities or wearing a heart rate monitor. Today the DLW method has been validated and used to measure energy expenditure in a number of populations, including athletes (Sjodin et al. 1994; Westerterp et al. 1986), lean (Seale et al. 1993) and obese individuals (Prentice et al. 1986; Ravussin et al. 1991), and children (Kaskoun et al. 1994). It has become a valuable tool for validating other less expensive field methods of measuring energy expenditure, such as accelerometers (Schoeller and Racette 1990). The major disadvantages of the technique are that (1) it is too expensive for large population-based studies; (2) it has a five times greater potential error on the energy expenditure calculation because it uses only the caloric equivalent of carbon dioxide instead of the caloric equivalent of oxygen (Jequier et al. 1987); (3) its experimental variability appears to be high (±8.5%), both when repeating the technique in the same individual and between individuals (Goran et al. 1994).

Predicting Energy Expenditure

How can we estimate or predict total energy expenditure outside the laboratory setting? As mentioned earlier, total energy expenditure comprises RMR, TEF, and TEA. One of the most common ways to estimate total energy expenditure is to first estimate RMR using a prediction equation and then multiply RMR by an appropriate activity factor. A number of prediction equations have been developed using populations that differ in age, gender, level of obesity, and activity level. In general, it is best to use the prediction equation most representative of the population with whom you are working. For example, if you want to predict the RMR of young active women, employ an equation developed using that population. Table 5.4 gives some of the commonly used RMR prediction equations and the populations from which they were predicted. For RMR prediction equations for obese individuals, see appendix C.6 (page 481). Most of these prediction equations were developed using sedentary individuals. In an effort to determine which of the equations works best for active individuals, Thompson and Manore (1996) compared actual RMR values measured in the laboratory with RMR values predicted by equations listed in table 5.4. They found that for both active men and women the Cunningham equation best predicted RMR, with the Harris-Benedict equation being the next best predictor. Figure 5.14 shows how closely these equations predicted RMR in a group of endurance-trained men and women.

Because the Cunningham equation requires the measurement of lean body mass (LBM), the Harris-Benedict equation is easier to use when LBM cannot be directly measured.

Once a value for RMR has been obtained, total daily energy expenditure can be estimated by a variety of factorial methods, which vary in labor-intensiveness and in the level of respondent burden. Appendix C.2 describes these methods in detail. The easiest methods multiply RMR by an appropriate **activity factor (AF)** to estimate total daily energy expenditure. This factor may be as low as 10-20% of RMR for a bedridden person to >100% for a very active individual. Although many laboratories establish unique activity factors for their particular research setting, factors of 1.3-1.6 are commonly used with sedentary people or those doing only light activity. One activity factor can be applied to the whole day, or a weighted activity factor can be determined. This activity factor is then multiplied by the RMR to provide a total daily energy expenditure value in kilocalories/day. For example, if an individual has an RMR of 1500 kcal/d and an activity factor of 1.3, then the daily energy expenditure would be 30% above RMR or 1950 kcal/d (1500 × 1.3 = 1950). A third method estimates a **general activity factor (GAF)** and a **specific activity factor (SAF)**. GAF represents energy expended for everyday activities like walking about, driving, watching TV, going to class, and so on (table 5.5); SAF is activity expended in planned or purposeful activity like running, swimming, cycling, or weight training for a designated amount of time at a specific level of intensity. GAF is calculated as indicated earlier, while SAF is obtained by multiplying the amount of time spent in a specific activity by the energy required for that activity in kilocalories/kilogram body weight/minute (see appendix E.4 for tables giving these values). The GAF and SAF are then added together to get the total amount of energy expended per day in activity. This value is added to the estimated RMR value to give a subtotal for energy expenditure; an additional 6-10% is then added to this value to represent TEF. The final number then represents the total energy expended in a day or **total daily energy expenditure (TDEE)** (see appendix C.2 for an example). This method is relatively easy to use with active individuals who have specific training or exercise programs they follow and who already keep training logs. A final method of estimating total energy expenditure is to record all activities

Table 5.4 Equations for Estimating Resting Metabolic Rate (RMR) in Healthy Individuals

Harris-Benedict 1919:[a]	Males: RMR = 66.47 + 13.75 (wt) + 5 (ht) − 6.76 (age) Females: RMR = 655.1 + 9.56 (wt) + 1.85 (ht) − 4.68 (age)
Owen et al 1986:[b]	Active females: RMR = 50.4 + 21.1 (wt) Inactive females: RMR = 795 + 7.18 (wt)
Owen et al. 1987:[c]	Males: RMR = 290 + 22.3 (LBM) Males: RMR = 879 + 10.2 (wt)
Mifflin et al. 1990:[d]	RMR = 9.99 (wt) + 6.25 (ht) − 4.92 (age) + 166 (sex: male = 1, female = 0) − 161
Cunningham 1980:[e]	RMR = 500 + 22 (LBM)

	Sex	Age range (y)	Equation to derive RMR in kcal/d
World Health Organization (WHO) 1985:[f]	Males	0-3	(60.9 × wt) − 54
		3-10	(22.7 × wt) + 495
		10-18	(17.5 × wt) + 651
		18-30	(15.3 × wt) + 679
		30-60	(11.6 × wt) + 879
		60	(13.5 × wt) + 487
	Females	0-3	(61.0 × wt) − 51
		3-10	(22.5 × wt) + 499
		10-18	(12.2 × wt) + 746
		18-30	(14.7 × wt) + 496
		30-60	(8.7 × wt) + 829
		>60	(10.5 × wt) + 596

wt = weight (kg), ht = height (cm), age = age (years), and LBM = lean body mass (kg).

[a]Harris-Benedict equation was published in 1919, based on 136 men (mean age 27 ± 9 years; mean wt 64 ± 10 kg) and 103 women (mean age 33.1 ± 14; mean wt 56.5 ± 11.5 kg). Included trained male athletes. The derived equations for men and women included weight, height, and age as variables. Researchers frequently report that Harris-Benedict equation overpredicts RMR by >15%.

[b]Owen et al. (1986) equation used 44 lean and obese women, 8 of whom were trained athletes (ages 18-65 years; 48-143 kg). No women were menstruating during the study; all were wt stable for at least 1 mo.

[c]Owen et al. (1987) equation used 60 lean and obese men (ages 18-82 years; 60-171 kg). All were wt stable for at least 1 mo. No athletes were included in this study.

[d]Mifflin et al. (1990) equation used 498 healthy lean and obese subjects (247 women and 251 men), ages 18-78 years. Weight ranged from 46-120 kg for the women and 58-143 kg for the men. No mention was made of physical activity level.

[e]Cunningham (1980) used 223 subjects (120 men and 103 women) from the 1919 Harris and Benedict database. They eliminated 16 males who were identified as trained athletes. In this study, LBM accounted for 70% of the variability of basal metabolic rate (BMR). Age variable did not add much because group age range was narrow. LBM was not calculated in the Harris-Benedict equation, so Cunningham established LBM based on body mass (kg) and age.

[f]WHO (1985) derived these equations from BMR data.

over a 24-h period, then to calculate (using energy expenditure tables) the total energy expended in each of these activities (kilocalories/kilogram body weight/minute). The number of kcal expended in each activity is then added to represent the total amount of energy expended for that day (appendix C.2). Many computer programs allow you to calculate energy expenditure in this way. See appendix E.2 for a sample 24-h energy expenditure form. Regardless of which method is used, keep in mind that all values are estimates. The accuracy of these values depends on how carefully activity is re-corded and how accurate the database is that is used to generate the energy estimates.

Energy Intake

Since energy intake is one side of the energy balance equation, knowing total energy intake gives some indication of total energy expenditure *if* body weight is stable. Collection and assessment of dietary intake are the most frequently used procedures for monitoring energy and nutrient intakes in active individuals.

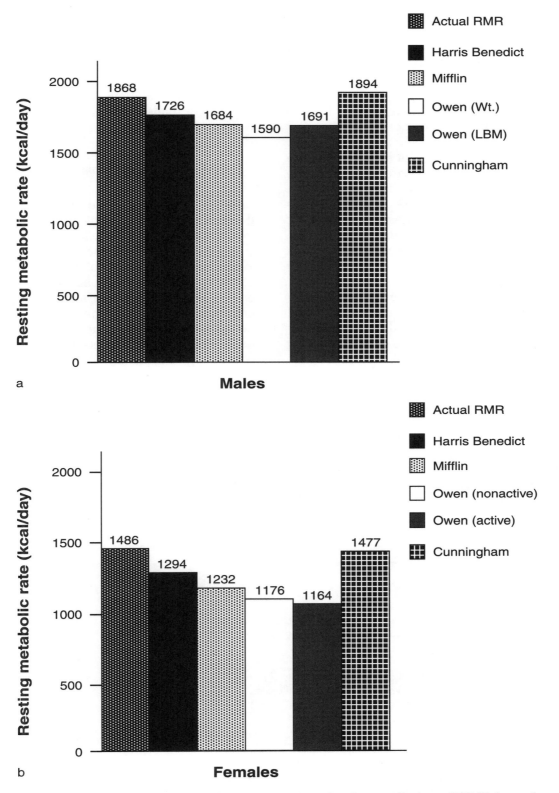

Figure 5.14 (a) Comparison of five different equations for the prediction of RMR in endurance-trained men, compared to actual measured RMR. (b) Comparison of five different equations (see tabel 5.4) for the prediction of RMR in endurance-trained women, compared to actual measured RMR.

Adapted from Thompson and Manore 1996.

The goal is to achieve the most accurate possible description of a person's typical food intake, then to use that information (1) to assess mean energy and nutrient intakes, (2) to make recommendations for changing or improving food habits, (3) to determine the need for micronutrient supplements, or (4) to help the person achieve his or her dietary and/or weight goal.

Collecting dietary data is only part of the assessment process. The data then must be analyzed using a computerized nutrient analysis program, with the results compared to nutrient standards or goals. Energy intakes must be compared to estimated energy expenditure values. To avoid introducing additional error into the process of dietary assessment, care should be taken in choosing and using a computerized nutrient analysis program; the program should allow you to enter additional food data, such as specific sport foods or food supplements, that may not be in the database.

Once diet data are analyzed, results are usually compared to some type of dietary standard. Although a variety of standards are available, the most commonly used standards are the Recommended Dietary Allowances (RDAs) (Food and Nutrition Board 1989), Dietary Reference Intakes (DRIs) (Institute of Medicine 1997, 1998), the Dietary Guidelines for Americans (USDA 1994), and the Food Guide Pyramid (USDA 1992) (all discussed in chapter 1). Additional recommendations for nutrient intakes are frequently made for active individuals, especially female athletes (see chapter 15).

Chapter in Review

This chapter has discussed the components that determine energy balance—both energy input (dietary energy plus the contribution of energy stores within the body) and energy expenditure. We have covered how the various components of energy expenditure can be measured. For any one individual, the factors that influence energy balance may be numerous, including gender, age, family history, dietary choices, level of daily activity, and stress level. If a person wishes to permanently change body size, then one or more of the components of energy balance must be altered over an extended time. The following chapter presents methods for doing this.

Table 5.5 **Approximate Energy Expenditure for Various Activities in Relation to Resting Needs for Men and Women of Average Size**

Activity category*	Representative values for activity factor per unit of time of activity	kcal/min
Resting Sleeping, reclining	RMR × 1.0	1.0-1.2
Very light Seated and standing activities, painting trades, driving, laboratory work, typing, sewing, ironing, cooking, playing cards, playing a musical instrument	RMR × 1.5	up to 2.5
Light Walking on a level surface at 2.5 or 3 mph, garage work, electrical trades, carpentry, restaurant trades, house cleaning, child care, golf, sailing, table tennis	RMR × 2.5	2.5-4.9
Moderate Walking 3.5 to 4 mph, weeding and hoeing, carrying a load, cycling, skiing, tennis, dancing	RMR × 5.0	5.0-7.4
Heavy Walking with a load uphill, tree felling, heavy manual digging, basketball, climbing, football, soccer	RMR × 7.0	7.5-12.0

*When reported as multiples of basal needs, the expenditures of men and women are similar.
Adapted from FNB 1989.

KEY CONCEPTS

1. Explain the energy and nutrient balance equations.

Energy balance, or long-term weight maintenance, requires that the amount and composition of energy input (both from dietary sources and stored energy in the body) equal energy expended. It also requires that the oxidation of protein, fat, and carbohydrate must equal the proportion in which they are consumed within the diet. Thus, energy balance depends not only on the balance between energy intake and energy expenditure but also on the oxidation rate of the energy consumed (carbohydrate, protein, fat, and alcohol).

2. Understand the concept of nutrient balance and the contributions of carbohydrate, protein, fat, and alcohol to energy balance.

Nutrient balance means that oxidation rates of dietary protein, fat, carbohydrate, and alcohol are equal to their intake. Oxidation of protein and carbohydrate closely match their dietary intake—as protein or carbohydrate intake increases, so does its oxidation within the body. Fat oxidation is less sensitive to change in dietary fat intake: an excess of dietary fat results in increased fat storage. Since in humans there is little synthesis of endogenous fat from excess dietary carbohydrate or protein, increased intakes of these nutrients increase their oxidation rates, resulting in dietary fat being stored in adipose tissue. Alcohol is a priority fuel that is oxidized rapidly, while suppressing the oxidation of other substrates, especially fat.

3. Identify the various components of energy expenditure, how they are measured, and the contribution of energy expenditure to the energy balance equation.

Total daily energy expenditure includes RMR, TEF, TEA (daily activities, exercise, SPA, and AT). Of these factors, TEA can vary the most and is most susceptible to lifestyle changes, while TEF or TEM are the most difficult to measure and have a greater degree of variability. A variety of factors can influence resting metabolic rate. Some are fixed and cannot be changed (e.g., age, sex, heredity), while others may be influenced by lifestyle (e.g., level of fitness and FFM). Energy expenditure is generally measured in the laboratory using indirect calorimetry or estimated using 24-h activity logs.

4. Understand the role of energy intake in the energy balance equation.

Total daily energy intake is one side of the energy balance equation. If a person is in energy balance, energy intake equals energy expenditure. Knowing total energy intake provides some indication of total energy expenditure if weight is stable. It is difficult and time-consuming to record accurate total daily energy intakes that represent typical dietary patterns.

KEY TERMS

activity factor (AF)
adaptive thermogenesis (AT)
basal metabolic rate (BMR)
direct calorimetry
doubly labeled water (DLW)
energy balance
energy flux
excess post-exercise oxygen consumption (EPOC)

facultative thermogenesis
general activity factor (GAF)
indirect calorimetry
nonexercise activity thermogenesis (NEAT)
obligatory thermogenesis
respiratory exchange ratio (RER)
respiratory quotient (RQ)
resting energy expenditure (REE)
resting metabolic rate (RMR)

(continued)

sleeping metabolic rate (SMR)
specific activity factor (SAF)
spontaneous physical activity (SPA)
thermic effect of activity (TEA)

thermic effect of a meal (TEM)
thermic effect of food (TEF)
total daily energy expenditure (TDEE)

References

Abbott WGH, Howard BV, Christin L, et al. Short-term energy balance: relationship with protein, carbohydrate, and fat balances. Am J Physiol 1988;255:E332-7.

Acheson KJ, Ravussin E, Wahren J, Jequier E. Thermic effect of glucose in man. Obligatory and facultative thermogenesis. J Clin Invest 1984;74:1572-80.

Acheson KJ, Schutz Y, Bessard T, Anantharaman K, Flatt JP, Jequier E. Glycogen storage capacity and de novo lipogenesis during massive carbohydrate overfeeding in man. Am J Clin Nutr 1988;48:240-7.

Acheson KJ, Schutz Y, Bessard T, Ravussin E, Jequier E, Flatt JP. Nutritional influences on lipogenesis and thermogenesis after a carbohydrate meal. Am J Physiol 1984; 246:E62-E70.

Astrup A, Buemann B, Western P, Toubro S, Raben A, Christensen NJ. Obesity as an adaptation to a high-fat diet: evidence from a cross-sectional study. Am J Clin Nutr 1994;59:350-5.

Bahr R, Sejersted OM. Effect of intensity of exercise on exercise post-exercise O_2 consumption. Metabolism 1991;40:836-41.

Barr SI, Janelle KC, Prior JC. Energy intakes are higher during the luteal phase of ovulatory menstrual cycles. Am J Clin Nutr 1995; 61:39-43.

Beidleman BA, Pahl JL, De Souza MJ. Energy balance in female distance runners. Am J Clin Nutr 1995;61:303-11.

Belko AZ, Barbieri TF. Effect of meal size and frequency on the thermic effect of food. Nutr Res 1987;7:237-42.

Bisbee JT, James WPT, Shaw MA. Changes in energy expenditure during the menstrual cycle. Br J Nutr 1989;61:187-99.

Bjorntorp P, Brodoff BN. Obesity. New York: JB Lippincott Company, 1992.

Bogardus C, Lillioja S, Ravussin E, et al. Familial dependence of the resting metabolic rate. N Engl J Med 1986;315:96-100.

Bouchard C, Tremblay A, Nadeau A, et al. Genetic effect in resting and exercise metabolic rates. Metabolism 1989;38:364-70.

Bray AB, Atkinson RL. Factors affecting basal metabolic rate. Prog Food Nutr Sci 1977;2:395-403.

Broeder CE, Burrhus KA, Svanevik LS, Wilmore JH. The effect of aerobic fitness on resting metabolic rate. Am J Clin Nutr 1992;55:795-801.

Bullough RC, Gillette CA, Harris MA, Melby CL. Interaction of acute changes in exercise energy expenditure and energy intake on resting metabolic rate. Am J Clin Nutr 1995; 61:473-81.

Bullough RC, Melby CL. Effect of inpatient versus outpatient measurement protocol on resting metabolic rate and respiratory exchange ratio. Ann Nutr Metab 1993;27:24-32.

Butterfield G, Trembley A. Physical activity and nutrition in the context of fitness and health. In: Bouchard C, Shephard RJ, Stevens S, eds. Physical Activity, Fitness and Health. International proceedings and consensus statement. Champaign, IL: Human Kinetics, 1994:257-69.

Collins LC, Cornelius MF, Vogel RL, Walker JF, Stamford BA. Effect of caffeine and/or cigarette smoking on resting energy expenditure. Int J Obesity 1994;18:551-6.

Coward WA, Cole TJ. The doubly labeled water method for the measurement of energy expenditure in humans: risks and benefits. In: Whitehead RG, Prentice A, eds. New Techniques in Nutritional Research. New York: Academic Press, 1991:39-176.

Cunningham JJ. A reanalysis of the factors influencing basal metabolic rate in normal adults. Am J Clin Nutr 1980;33:2372-4.

Dulloo AG, Geissler CA, Horton T, Collins A, Miller DS. Normal caffeine consumption: influence on thermogenesis and daily energy expenditure in lean and postobese human volunteers. Am J Clin Nutr 1989;49:44-50.

Ferraro R, Lillioja S, Fontvieille AM, Rising R, Bogardus C, Ravussin E. Lower sedentary metabolic rate in women compared to men. J Clin Invest 1992;90:780-4.

Flatt JP. The biochemistry of energy expenditure. In: Bray G, ed. Recent advances in obesity research II. London: John Libbey, 1978:211-28.

Flatt JP. Importance of nutrient balance in body weight regulation. Diabetes Metab Rev 1988;4:571-81.

Flatt JP. Dietary fat, carbohydrate balance, and weight maintenance. Ann NY Acad Sci 1993;683:122-40.

Flatt JP. The biochemistry of energy expenditure. In: Bjornthrop P, Brodoff BN, eds. Obesity. New York: J.B. Lippincott, 1992:100-16.

Flatt JP, Ravussin E, Acheson KJ, Jequier E. Effects of dietary fat on postprandial substrate oxidation and on carbohydrate and fat balance. J Clin Invest 1985;76:1019-24.

Fleisch A. Le metabolisme basal stand et sa determination au moyen du "metabocalculator". Helv Med Acta 1951;1:23-44.

Food and Nutrition Board. Recommended Dietary Allowances, 10th ed. National Research Council. Washingtion, DC: National Academy Press, 1989.

Friedman MI, Tordoff MG. Fatty acid oxidation and glucose utilization interact to control food intake in rats. Am J Physiol 1986; 251:R840-R845.

Gaesser GA, Brooks GA. Metabolic bases of excess post-exercise oxygen consumption: a review. Med Sci Sports Exerc 1984;16:29-43.

Goran MI, Poehlman ET, Danforth E. Experimental reliability of the doubly labeled water technique. Am J Physiol 1994;266:E510-E515.

Harris JA, Benedict FG. A biometric study of basal metabolism in man. Carnegie Inst Wash Pub No. 279. Philadelphia: F.B. Lippincott Co., 1919:227.

Hellerstein MK, Christiansen M, Kaempfer S. Measurement of de novo hepatic lipogenesis in humans using stable isotopes. J Clin Invest 1991;87:1841-52.

Herring JL, Mole PA, Meredith CN, Stern JS. Effect of suspending exercise training on resting metabolic rate in women. Med Sci Sports Exerc 1992;24:59-65.

Houde-Nadeau M, de Jonge L, Garrel DR. Thermogenic response to food: intra-individual variability and measurement reliability. J Am Coll Nutr 1993;12:511-6.

Institute of Medicine. Dietary reference intakes. Calcium, phosphorus, magnesium, vitamin D, and fluoride. Washington, DC: National Academy Press, 1997.

Institute of Medicine. Dietary reference intakes. Thiamin, riboflavin, niacin, vitamin B-6, folate, vitamin B-12, pantothenic acid, biotin, and choline. Washington, DC: National Academy Press, 1998.

Jebb SA, Prentice AM, Goldberg GR, Murgatroyd PR, Black AE, Coward WA. Changes in macronutrient balance during over- and underfeeding assessed by 12-d continuous whole-body calorimetry. Am J Clin Nutr 1996;64:259-66.

Jequier E. Regulation of thermogenesis and nutrient metabolism in the human: relevance for obesity. In: Bjorntorp P, Brodoff BN, eds. Obesity. Philadelphia: Lippincott, 1992:130-5.

Jequier E, Acheson K, Schultz Y. Assessment of energy expenditure and fuel utilization in man. Ann Rev Nutr 1987;7187-208.

Jequier E, Shultz Y. Long-term measurement of energy expenditure in humans using a respiration chamber. Am J Clin Nutr 1983;38:989-98.

Kaskoun MC, Johnson RK, Goran MI. Comparison of energy intake by semiquantitative food-frequency questionnaire with total energy expenditure by the doubly labeled water method in young children. Am J Clin Nutr 1994;60:43-7.

Keesey RE. The set-point analysis of the regulation of body weight. In: Stunkard AJ, ed. Obesity. Philadelphia: W.B. Saunders Company, 1980:144-65.

Keys A, Taylor HL, Grande F. Basal metabolism and age of adult man. Metabolism 1987;22:5979-87.

Klesges RC, Mealer CA, Klesges LM. Effects of alcohol intake on resting energy expenditure in young women social drinkers. Am J Clin Nutr 1994;59:805-9.

Krempf M, Hoerr RA, Pelletier VA, Marks LA, Gleason R, Young VR. An isotopic study of the effect of dietary carbohydrate on the metabolic fate of dietary leucine and phenylalanine. Am J Clin Nutr 1993;57:161-9.

Lebenstedt M, Platte P, Pirke K. Reduced resting metabolic rate in athletes with menstrual disorders. Med Sci Sports Exerc 1999; 31:1240-56.

Levine JA, Eberhardt NL, Jensen MD. Role of nonexercise activity thermogenesis in resistance to fat gain in humans. Science 1999; 283:212-4.

Li ETS, Tsand LBY, Lui SSH. Resting metabolic rate and thermic effects of a sucrose-sweetened soft drink during the menstrual cycle in young Chinese women. Can J Physiol Pharma 1999;77:544-50.

Lifson N, Gordon GB, McClintock R. Measurement of total carbon dioxide productioin by means of doubly labeled water. J Appl Physiol 1955;7:704-10.

Melby C, Scholl C, Edwards G, Bullough R. Effect of acute resistance exercise on post-exercise energy expenditure and resting metabolic rate. J Appl Physiol 1993;75:1847-53.

Mifflin MD, St. Jeor ST, Hill LA, Scott BJ, Daugherty SA, Koh YO. A new predictive equation for resting energy expenditure in healthy individuals. Am J Clin Nutr 1990;51:241-7.

Nichols J, Ross S, Patterson P. Thermic effect of food at rest and following swim exercise in trained college men and women. Ann Nutr Metab 1988;32:215-9.

Owen OE, Holup JL, D'Alessio DA, et al. A reappraisal of the caloric requirements of men. Am J Clin Nutr 1987;46:875-85

Owen OE, Kavle E, Owen RS, et al. A reappraisal of caloric requirements in healthy women. Am J Clin Nutr 1986;44:1-19.

Piers LS, Diggavi SN, Rijskamp J, van Raaij JMA, Shetty PS, Hautvast JGAJ. Resting metabolic rate and thermic effect of a meal in the follicular and luteal phases of the menstrual cycle in well-nourished Indian women. Am J Clin Nutr 1995;61:296-302.

Poehlman ET. A review: exercise and its influence on resting energy metabolism in man. Med Sci Sports Exerc 1989;21:515-25.

Poehlman ET, Berke EM, Joseph JR, Gardner AW, Katzman-Rooks SM, Goran MI. Influence of aerobic capacity, body composition, and thyroid hormones on the age-related decline in resting metabolic rate. Metabolism 1992;41:915-21.

Poehlman ET, Danforth E. Endurance training increases metabolic rate and norepinephrine appearance rate in older individuals. Am J Physiol 1991;261:E233-E239.

Poehlman ET, Goran MI, Gardner AW, et al. Determinants of decline in resting metabolic rate in aging females. Am J Physiol 1993; 264:E450-E455.

Poehlman ET, McAuliffe TL, Van Houten DR, Danforth E. Influence of age and endurance training on metabolic rate and hormones in healthy men. Am J Physiol 1990;259:E66-E72.

Prentice AM, Black AE, Coward WA, et al. High levels of energy expenditure in obese women. Br Med J 1986;292:983-7.

Prentice AM, Diaz EO, Murgatroyd PR, Goldberg GR, Sonko BJ, Black AE, Coward WA. Doubly labeled water measurements and calorimetry in practice. In: Whitehead RG, Prentice A, eds. New Techniques in Nutritional Research. New York: Academic Press, 1991:177-207.

Ravussin E, Bogardus C. Relationship of genetics, age and physical fitness to daily energy expenditure and fuel utilization. Am J Clin Nutr 1989;49:968-75.

Ravussin E, Harper IT, Rising R, Bogardus C. Energy expenditure by doubly labeled water: validation in lean and obese subjects. Am J Physiol 1991;261:E402-E409.

Ravussin E, Lillioja S, Anderson TE, Christin L, Bogardus C. Determinants of 24-hour energy expenditure in man: methods and results using a respiratory chamber. J Clin Invest 1986;78:1568-78.

Ravussin E, Swinburn BA. Energy metabolism. In: Stunkard JA, Wadden TA, eds. Obesity: Theory and Therapy. New York: Raven Press Ltd, 1993:97-123.

Rising R, Keys A, Ravussin E, Bogardus C. Concomitant interindividual variation in body temperature and metabolic rate. Am J Physiol 1992;263:E730-E734.

Robertson JD, Reid DD. Standards for the basal metabolism of normal people in Britain. Lancet 1952;1:943.

Rontoyannis GP, Skoulis T, Pavlou KN. Energy balance in ultramarathon running. Am J Clin Nutr 1989;49:976-9.

Schoeller DA, Racette SB. A review of field techniques for the assessment of energy expenditure. J Nutr 1990;120:1492-5.

Schoeller DA, Ravussin E, Schutz Y, Acheson KJ, Baertschi P, Jequier E. Energy expenditure by doubly labeled water: validation in humans and proposed calculations. Am J Physiol 1986;250:823-30.

Schutz S, Flatt JP, Jequier E. Failure of dietary fat intake to promote fat oxidation: a factor favoring the development of obesity. Am J Clin Nutr 1989;50:307-14.

Schutz Y, Tremblay A, Weinsier RL, Nelson KM. Role of fat oxidation in the long-term stabilization of body weight in obese women. Am J Clin Nutr 1992;55:670-4.

Seale JL, Conway JM, Canary JJ. Seven-day validation of doubly labeled water method using indirect room calorimetry. J Appl Physiol 1993;74(1):402-9.

Sedlock DA, Fissinger JA, Melby CL. Effect of exercise intensity and duration on post-exercise energy expenditure. Med Sci Sports Exerc 1989;21:662-6.

Segal KR, Chun A, Coronel P, Valdez V. Effects of exercise mode and intensity on postprandial thermogenesis in lean and obese men. J Appl Physiol 1992;72(5):1754-63.

Shelmet JJ, Reichard GA, Skutches CL, Hoeldtke RD, Owen OE, Boden G. Ethanol causes acute inhibition of carbohydrate, fat, and protein oxidation and insulin resistance. J Clin Invest 1988;81:1137-45.

Sjodin AM, Andersson AB, Hogberg JM, Westerterp KR. Energy balance in cross-country skiers: a study using doubly labeled water. Med Sci Sports Exerc 1994;26:720-4.

Solomon SJ, Kurzer MS, Calloway DH. Menstrual cycle and basal metabolic rate in women. Am J Clin Nutr 1982;36:611-6.

Sonko BJ, Prentice AM, Murgatroyd PR, Goldberg GR, van de Ven MLHM, Coward WA. Effect of alcohol on postmeal fat storage. Am J Clin Nutr 1994;59:619-25.

Stock MJ. Gluttony and thermogenesis revisited. Int J Obesity 1999;23:1105-17.

Stubbs RJ, Murgatroyd PR, Goldberg GR, Prentice AM. Carbohydrate balance and the regulation of day-to-day food intake in humans. Am J Clin Nutr 1993;57:897-903.

Swinburn B, Ravussin E. Energy balance or fat balance? Am J Clin Nutr 1993;57(suppl):766S-71S.

Tataranni PA, Larson DE, Snitker S, Ravussin E. Thermic effect of food in humans: methods and results from use of a respiratory chamber. Am J Clin Nutr 1995;61:1013-9.

Thomas CD, Peters JC, Reed WG, Abumrad NN, Sun M, Hill JO. Nutrient balance and energy expenditure during ad libitum feeding of high-fat and high-carbohydrate diets in humans. Am J Clin Nutr 1992;55:934-42.

Thompson JL, Manore MM. Predicted and measured resting metabolic rate of male and female endurance athletes. J Am Diet Assoc 1996;96:30-4.

Thompson J, Manore MM, Skinner JS. Resting metabolic rate and thermic effect of a meal in low- and adequate-energy intake male endurance athletes. Int J Sport Nutr 1993;3:194-206.

Thompson JL, Manore MM, Skinner JS, Ravussin E, Spraul M. Daily energy expenditure in male endurance athletes with differing energy intakes. Med Sci Sports Exerc 1995;27:347-54.

Tremblay A, Lavallee N, Almeras N, Allard L, Despres JP, Bouchard C. Nutritional determinants of the increase in energy intake associated with a high-fat diet. Am J Clin Nutr 1991;53:1134-7.

Turley KR, McBride PJ, Wilmore JH. Resting metabolic rate measured after subjects spent the night at home vs at a clinic. Am J Clin Nutr 1993;58:141-4.

United States Department of Agriculture (USDA). The Food Guide Pyramid. Washington, DC: Human Nutrition Information Service, Home and Garden Bulletin Number 252, 1992.

United States Department of Agriculture (USDA) and United States Department of Health and Human Services (USDHHS). Nutrition and your health: Dietary Guidelines for Americans. 4th Edition, Dec. 1994, Home and Garden Bulletin No. 232.

Vaughan L, Zurlo F, Ravussin E. Aging and energy expenditure. Am J Clin Nutr 1991;53:821-5.

Westerterp KR. Food quotient, respiratory quotient, and energy balance. Am J Clin Nutr 1993;57(suppl):759S-65S.

Westerterp KR, Sarris WHM, van Es M, ten Hoor F. Use of doubly labeled water technique in humans during heavy sustained exercise. J Appl Physiol 1986;61:2162-7.

Weststrate JA. Resting metabolic rate and diet-induced thermogenesis: a methodological reappraisal. Am J Clin Nutr 1993;58:592-601.

Wilmore JH, Costill DL. Physiology of sport and exercise. Champaign, IL: Human Kinetics, 1999.

Wilmore JH, Stanforth PR, Hudspeth LA, et al. Alterations in resting metabolic rate as a consequence of 20 wk of endurance training: the HERITAGE Family Study. Am J Clin Nutr 1998;68:66-71.

Yoshida T, Sakane N, Umekawa T, Kondo M. Relationship between basal metabolic rate, thermogenic response to caffeine, and body weight loss following combined low calorie and exercise treatment in obese women. Int J Obesity 1994;18:345-50.

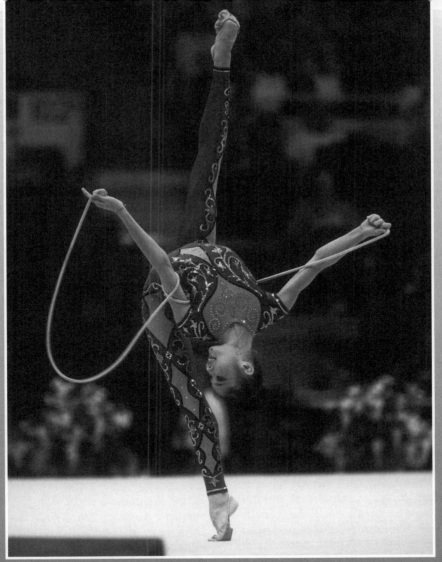

© Photo Run

CHAPTER 6

Achieving Healthy Body Weight

After reading this chapter you should be able to

- discuss the role of diet and exercise in achieving healthy body weight;
- describe the recommendations for maintaining a healthy body weight;
- discuss the weight concerns of athletes; and
- define the recommendations for weight gain.

Katie is a soccer player faced with the challenge of losing body weight in order to regain her competitive edge. She recently gained 20 lb (9.1 kg) during her recovery from knee surgery. Her body fat has increased from 17% to 27%, and she knows that in order to compete at her best, she needs to lose body fat and weight and gain fat-free mass (FFM). While her physician and family recommend that she achieve this weight loss slowly, Katie feels pressure to lose the weight quickly, using whatever means possible. She feels the quicker she can lose the weight, the sooner she can rejoin the team and feel better about herself.

The need or desire to lose weight is common among competitive athletes; however, it is also common among many recreational athletes and sedentary individuals who wish to alter their physical appearances. Individuals throughout the United States appear to be obsessed with body weight and an aesthetically pleasing body shape. It has been estimated that, at any one time, at least 38-40% of the women and 23-24% of the men in our population are dieting (Horm and Anderson 1993; Serdula et al. 1993). Ironically, it appears that many individuals who are dieting are either underweight or of normal weight. While weight loss would be recommended in Katie's case, many people are inappropriately concerned with weight loss. Why do people who are normal or underweight diet? Many feel that they are still not thin enough for society's standards or for the image they wish to portray. Unfortunately, concerns with body weight are not limited to adults. Research has shown that U.S. girls as young as 12-14 years of age express concerns about body weight and actually restrict energy intake (The National Adolescent Student Health Survey 1989). These data certainly indicate that the obsession with body weight and shape can begin at a young age.

With the widespread anxiety in our society about weight, one might guess that the prevalence of obesity is on the decline. On the contrary, the U.S. population is becoming more obese, with an estimated 97 million adults either overweight or obese (National Heart, Lung and Blood Institute [NHLBI] 1998). A paradox exists: those who need to lose weight are not dieting, but those who do not need to lose weight are dieting. Why aren't overweight people dieting? There are probably many answers to this question. One answer is that people have tried numerous diets, have been unsuccessful, and are unwilling to try again. Statistics of dieters who successfully maintain weight loss are not very impressive. Depending on the sources quoted, it is estimated that most dieters regain over 70% of the weight lost during the first year after the diet is over and gain all or more of the remaining 30% lost over the next 5 years (Kramer et al. 1989; Thomas 1995).

Being overweight (or incorrectly viewing oneself as overweight) is very stressful. Overweight individuals are often portrayed as being lazy, stupid, and unsuccessful, and are targets of ridicule. The media constantly suggest that the only way to be desirable and adorable is to be thin and perfectly proportioned. Defining optimal body weights and educating people about healthy ways to achieve and maintain optimal body weight appear to be critical to the emotional and physical health of athletes and other members of our society.

Role of Diet and Exercise in Achieving Optimal Body Weight

What is optimal body weight? How do you determine your optimal body weight? Although it is very difficult to determine because no charts or tables provide the answer, the following criteria are frequently used to help determine a person's optimal body weight:

- Weight that can be maintained without constant dieting or restraining food intake
- Weight in which health risks are minimized and good health promoted
- Weight that promotes good eating habits
- Weight that allows one to participate in some type of physical activity
- Weight that can be accepted by the individual
- Weight that allows optimal performance in the sport of one's choice
- Weight that takes into consideration one's genetic makeup and family history of body weight and body shape
- Weight appropriate for one's age and level of physical development

Thus, optimal body weight should promote good health and be "reasonable" in terms of whether or not it can be achieved and maintained. If people are constantly dieting or are repeatedly gaining and losing weight, they may be trying to achieve or maintain an unrealistic (or non-ideal) body weight.

Determination of Body Size, Percentage of Body Fat, and Fat Distribution

There are a variety of methods for determining body size, percentage of body fat, and body fat distribution. All are used somewhat in determining if a person is at risk for developing health problems related to being overfat. In addition, change in body size is often used to determine whether a weight-loss program has been successful. Although weight loss should not be the only criterion for success, it is often a major component measured in any weight-loss effort.

Body Mass Index (BMI)

One way of expressing body size is to determine the body mass index. The **body mass index (BMI)** is defined as a ratio of weight (in kilograms) to the square of height (in meters squared), that is, kg/m^2. To estimate BMI using pounds and inches, multiply $(lb/in.^2) \times 703$. **Overweight** is usually defined as a BMI between 25-29.9, and **obesity** is usually defined as a BMI ≥ 30 (NHLBI 1998). Although BMI is relatively easy and inexpensive to measure, it has some major disadvantages. It gives no information about a person's percentage of body fat, fat distribution, or amount of FFM; and it does not account for differences in frame size, age, activity level, or gender. For example, a male bodybuilder who weighs 210 lb (95.3 kg), has a height of 68 in. (1.72 m), and has 6-8% body fat would have a BMI of 32. According to our previous definition, this individual would be considered obese from his BMI value, although his actual body fat percentage is very low. This person is very active, moreover, and his risk for chronic diseases is low. "The Relationship Between Weight and BMI" (page 164) demonstrates how changes in body weight affect BMI.

The National Heart, Lung and Blood Institute (NHLBI) of the National Institutes of Health (NIH) has developed a risk assessment table for use with BMI and waist circumference measurements. Table 6.1 shows this table, which helps classify individuals based on both their BMI and body fat distribution. For example, an individual with a small waist and a BMI of 28 would be classified as having increased risk. However, if this same person had a large waist circumference, he or she would be classified as high risk. It is important to remember that this table has limited application to people who have disproportionately greater FFM for a given height (weight lifters, bodybuilders).

Percentage Body Fat

Most determinations of body fat percentage involve estimating the ratio of body fat to FFM. Chapter 7 describes the techniques in detail. While knowing an individual's body fat is useful in both clinical and sport settings, it does not give an indication of the distribution of body fat and FFM, or whether the body fat is found predominantly subcutaneously or within the tissues. Please refer to chapter 7 for more details regarding body composition assessments.

Body Fat Distribution

Body fat distribution is assessed to determine whether body fat deposits are located mainly in the upper part of the body (abdomen and trunk regions—referred to as android or "apple-shaped") or in the lower part of the body (buttocks, hips, and thigh regions—referred to as gynoid or "pear-shaped"). Upper body obesity appears to increase risks for elevated blood lipids, glucose, and insulin—changes that may eventually lead to cardiovascular disease (CVD), diabetes, and hypertension. In general, men tend to have a higher incidence of upper body obesity, while women have a higher incidence of lower body obesity. Body fat distribution may be one of the factors that contributes to men having a higher incidence of CVD than premenopausal women.

Determination of body fat distribution is usually done by measuring the **waist-to-hip ratio (WHR)**, by measuring only the waist circumference, or by measuring the actual ratio of abdominal visceral fat (the fat around the internal organs) to subcutaneous fat (fat located directly under the skin) using **computerized tomography (CT).** Both the WHR and the waist circumference are simple and inexpensive field measurements for determining body fat distribution; however, they cannot distinguish between visceral and subcutaneous fat. Visceral abdominal fat is more closely associated than subcutaneous fat with increased risk of disease. Figure 6.1 represents CT scans of two different individuals—a young man with a lower amount of abdominal visceral fat *(a),* and a middle-aged man with a higher amount of intra-abdominal visceral fat *(b).* Because determining body fat distribution by the use of CT scans is very expensive and predominantly used for research

The Relationship Between Weight and BMI

Body mass index is one of the most frequently reported measures of body size in the research literature. To better understand the concept of BMI and how it changes as weight changes, do the following exercise using your own weight and height. First, determine your own BMI [using English measures, calculate weight/height^2 using the units ([lb/in.^{2}] × 703); then calculate how your BMI would change as you repeatedly add 10 lb (4.5 kg) to your weight. Keep adding 10 lb (4.5 kg) until you have reached a BMI of 40. If you started with a BMI > 20, subtract 10 lb (4.5 kg) from your current weight until you have reached a BMI of less than 20. Now using table 6.1, determine your health risk classification based upon the ranges of BMI you calculated. The following example is given for a woman who is 60 in. (1.52 m) tall and weighs 110 lb (50 kg):

Weight (lb)	Weight (kg)	BMI (kg/m²)	Health risk classification
100	45.5	19.6	—
110	50.0	21.5	—
120	54.5	23.5	—
130	59.0	25.4	Increased or high
140	63.6	27.4	Increased or high
150	68.2	29.4	Increased or high
160	72.7	31.3	High or very high
170	77.3	33.3	High or very high
180	81.8	35.2	Very high
190	86.4	37.2	Very high
200	90.9	39.1	Very high
210	95.5	41.0	Extremely high

Table 6.1 **Classification of Overweight and Obesity by Body Mass Index (BMI), Waist Circumference, and Associated Disease Risk**

	BMI kg/m²	Obesity class	Disease risk* relative to normal weight and waist circumference	
			Men ≤102 cm (≤40 in.) Women ≤88 cm (≤35 in.)	>102 cm (>40 in.) >88 cm (>35 in.)
Underweight	<18.5		—	—
Normal⁺	18.5-24.9		—	—
Overweight	25.0-29.9		Increased	High
Obesity	30.0-34.9	I	High	Very high
	35.0-39.9	II	Very high	Very high
Extreme obesity	≥40	III	Extremely high	Extremely high

*Disease risk for type II diabetes, hypertension, and cardiovascular disease.
⁺Increased waist circumference can be a marker for increased risk even in persons of normal weight.

Reprinted from NHLBI 1998.

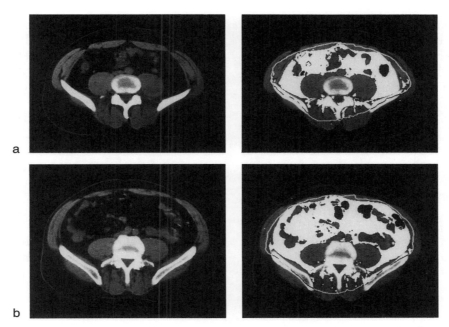

Figure 6.1   Cross-sectional images of the abdomen obtained by computerized tomography (CT) at L4-L5 in *(a)* a young man with excess intra-abdominal visceral fat; and *(b)* a middle-aged man matched for total body fat mass (19.8 kg). The visceral adipose tissue area (96 cm² for the young man and 155 cm² for the middle-aged man), which is delineated by drawing a line within the muscle wall surrounding the abdominal cavity, is highlighted in the images on the right.
Reprinted from Després, Ross, and Lemieux 1996.

purposes, the WHR and the waist circumference are the more frequently used techniques for determining body fat distribution.

The WHR is fairly easy to measure; but the specific measurement sites have not been standardized, making comparisons between research studies difficult. Bray (1989) has suggested the following method as a standard:

1. Measure the waist circumference at the level of the natural waist (or the narrowest part of the torso as observed from the front).

2. Measure the hip at the maximal circumference of the hips (including the maximum width of the buttocks as observed from the side).

All measurements should be done with a flexible tape and recorded in centimeters (cm). Increased health risks are associated with a WHR >0.90 for men and >0.80 for women.

Another way of estimating body fat distribution or abdominal body fat is to measure only waist circumference, which may be easier to measure in a clinical setting than the WHR and has been positively correlated with abdominal fat (NHLBI 1998). As table 6.1 indicates, once

waist circumference increases above 102 cm (>40 in.) for men and above 88 cm (>35 in.) for women, risks increase for hypertension, heart disease, and diabetes. Thus, if a person has a BMI of 28 and increased abdominal fat (waist circumference above the cut-off), this person's relative risk for disease is higher than someone with the same BMI but a smaller waist. This general risk assessment assumes that other disease risk factors are similar.

The exact mechanism linking higher levels of abdominal visceral body fat with an increased risk for high blood lipids, glucose, and insulin has not been determined, but the following hypothesis has been proposed (Reaven 1994). Visceral fat appears to be more responsive to catecholamines (epinephrine and norepinephrine) than subcutaneous fat, leading to increased breakdown and release of free fatty acids (FFAs) from the visceral fat into the blood. Visceral fat is located close to the body's internal organs, from which venous blood drains directly into the portal vein, which in turn flows to the liver. High levels of FFAs in the portal vein result in high levels of FFAs entering the liver, which can decrease insulin clearance from the blood and increase very-low-density lipoprotein (VLDL) production by the

165

liver. Decreased insulin clearance by the liver increases blood insulin levels and can lead to hyperinsulinemia and abnormal glucose control. Hyperinsulinemia can also increase sodium retention by the kidneys, which can contribute to higher risk of hypertension. Increased VLDL production by the liver can lead to elevated blood levels of VLDL-cholesterol and low-density lipoprotein (LDL)-cholesterol, which are both risk factors for cardiovascular disease. Figure 6.2 is a schematic diagram of this proposed mechanism linking high visceral body fat with increased disease risk.

Thus, abdominal obesity is more highly correlated with abnormal biochemical profiles (high blood lipids, insulin, and glucose) as compared to lower-body obesity, which is often considered relatively "benign." It is not, however, truly benign: lower-body obesity can stress the weightbearing joints, contribute to varicose veins and osteoarthritis, and discourage participation in regular physical activity due to the discomfort associated with carrying excess body weight.

Health Problems Associated With Obesity

Uncomplicated obesity is seldom fatal; once body size (or BMI) reaches a certain critical point, however, mortality increases. The J-shaped curve in figure 6.3 shows the relation-

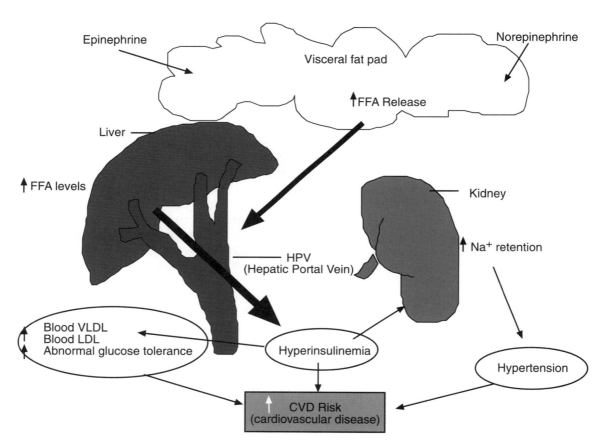

Figure 6.2 A proposed mechanism linking high visceral body fat with increased disease risk. Epinephrine and norepinephrine stimulate visceral fat to increase the production of free fatty acids (FFAs). This results in an increased transport of FFAs to the liver through the hepatic portal vein (HPV). The increased uptake of FFAs by the liver leads to decreased insulin clearance by the liver, resulting in hyperinsulinemia; and increased production of very-low-density lipoproteins (VLDL). The hyperinsulinemia and increased VLDL production are linked to an increase in cardiovascular disease (CVD) risk by increased levels of VLDL and low-density lipoproteins (LDL) in the blood; abnormal glucose tolerance; and hypertension (resulting from increased sodium or Na^+ retention by the kidneys).

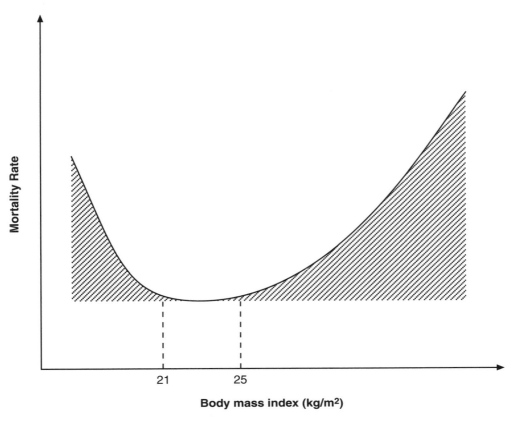

Figure 6.3 Generic J- or U-shaped curve describing the relationship of body mass index (BMI) to mortality ratio.

Reprinted from Van Itallie 1992.

ship between BMI and mortality: mortality increases as BMI increases above 25, with the sharpest risk associated with a BMI >30. From this curve, one would also conclude that the risk of mortality increases at a BMI <20.

Yet there are some problems with the data used to generate the curve in figure 6.3. First, women have a curve different than men—women have a lower mortality risk than men at similar weights. This difference may be related to the fact that women exhibit predominantly lower-body obesity, while men exhibit more upper-body obesity. Second, individuals who may have had low body weights (and BMI) due to illness or cigarette smoking were not eliminated from the analyses. If these data are eliminated from the analyses, the curve of the relationship between BMI and risk of mortality changes, with no increased risk of mortality observed at a lower BMI. In a 14-year epidemiological study of more than 1 million men and women, Calle et al. (1999) found that white men and women in all age groups had a higher risk of death from all causes—but especially cardiovascular disease and cancer—as their BMI increased. The lowest death rates occurred at a BMI of about 24 for men and 23 for women. Mortality risks for black men and women, however, were not strongly associated with BMI. A study of nurses in the United States found that the BMI associated with the lowest risk of mortality was less than 20, which represents body weights at least 15% less than the U.S. average for women of similar age to those studied (Manson et al. 1995). These data suggest that the lowest mortality is associated with very low BMI values. However, this is an area of heated controversy, as others argue that higher BMI values are associated with increased mortality only in individuals who lead a sedentary lifestyle *and* consume a high-fat, low-fiber diet (Gaesser 1999). For a recent, detailed discussion of these issues, see Willett et al. (1999).

Obesity may play a role in morbidity by either causing or exacerbating certain diseases. Figure 6.4 illustrates how obesity may exacerbate an existing health problem (Bray 1992).

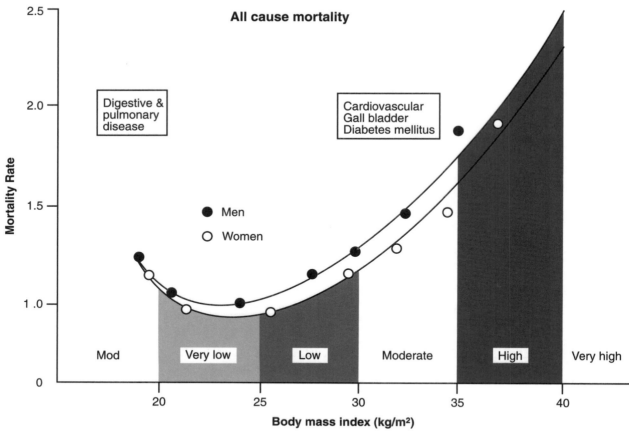

Figure 6.4 Relationship of BMI to risk.
Reprinted from Bray 1992.

An individual with a BMI of 37 has twice the risk of all-cause mortality than someone with a BMI of 23. Results from the Second National Health and Nutrition Examination Survey (NHANES II) (Van Itallie 1985) showed a 2.9 times greater risk of developing diabetes in obese as compared to nonobese people. Thus, obesity may increase the risk of developing certain diseases, as well as increase the risk of dying from obesity-related diseases. Note that health risks related to obesity are also risks associated with a sedentary lifestyle. It can be quite difficult to separate the health effects of excess body fat from those of inactivity. In fact, Wei et al. (1997) showed that regular exercise improved the lipid profiles of men, and the improvement was similar for both overweight and normal-weight men. And Lee et al. (1999) found that unfit lean men had a significantly higher risk of all-cause and cardiovascular disease mortality than fit obese men. Table 6.2 outlines a number of health disorders thought to be caused or exacerbated by obesity (Van Itallie 1979).

Weight Loss Interventions

Over the last 20 years, numerous approaches have been used for weight loss. Highly trained athletes and individuals participating in regular physical activity possess the greatest potential for combining energy restriction with physical activity when appropriate. It is important for any person attempting to lose weight to include regular exercise in his or her weight-loss program. *The primary goal of a weight-loss program is to improve health by lowering body fat, while maintaining or increasing the proportion of FFM or muscle tissue.* If FFM can be increased or maintained during weight loss, it is easier to sustain resting metabolic rate (RMR) and the reduced level of body fat. Preserving FFM is also important to increase muscle strength and the ability to perform physical activity. Since many people not currently involved in regular physical activity are attempting to lose weight using only energy restriction, it is important to understand the role that diet alone plays in the scheme of weight loss.

Table 6.2 Some Health Disorders and Other Problems Thought To Be Caused or Exacerbated by Obesity

Heart
Premature coronary heart disease
Angina pectoris
Congestive heart failure

Vascular system
Hypertension
Stroke
Venous stasis (with lower extremity edema, varicose veins)

Respiratory system
Obstructive sleep apnea
Right ventricular hypertrophy

Hormonal and metabolic functions
Diabetes mellitus (type II diabetes)
Gout
Hyperlipidemia (hypertriglyceridemia and hyper-cholesterolemia)

Joints, muscles, and connective tissue
Osteoarthritis of the knees and hips
Bone spurs of the heel

Cancer
Increased risk of endometrial cancer
Possible increased risk of breast cancer

Reproductive function
Impaired obstetric performance (increased risk of toxemia, hypertension, and gestational diabetes)
Irregular menstruation and frequent anovulatory cycles
Reduced fertility

Psychosocial function
Reduced self-image or feelings of inferiority
Social isolation
Subject to social, economic, and other types of discrimination
Loss of mobility and reduced ability to do physical activity

Adapted from Van Itallie 1979.

Before we discuss the various diets used for weight loss, we need to first set the ground rules for weight loss. Here are some basic facts about dieting that should be remembered, regardless of what diet is used:

• Kilocalories or calories are important! Decreasing energy intake below the level of energy expenditure can reduce body weight. The amount of weight lost for a given energy deficit is difficult to predict for any one person, however, since the energy deficit needed to bring about weight loss appears to be highly individualized. Thus, we cannot expect everyone to respond the same to any given dietary treatment—many people report eating very few kilocalories without experiencing weight loss, and feel they are truly "resistant" to weight loss. However, Bray and Gray (1988) have reported that no healthy adult has ever been studied in a metabolic chamber who required less than 1200 kcal/d to maintain body weight. Note also that the lowest-energy diets do not always bring about the best weight-loss results. Because severely restricted diets result in loss of FFM and subsequent decrease in RMR, they are rarely successful.

• Composition of the diet is important. A dieting person needs to know the amount of energy consumed each day, and also the percentages of energy that come from carbohydrate, fat, protein, and alcohol. Diets that vary in nutrient composition can impact weight loss and changes in body composition.

• Protein intake is important, especially the ratio of nitrogen (or protein) intake to energy intake. When a low-kilocalorie diet is consumed, a higher nitrogen:kilocalorie ratio is required than normally recommended in a weight maintenance diet. Higher quality protein is also required to maintain FFM. Because people on reduced-energy diets use some dietary protein for energy instead of for the building and repair of body tissues, a higher intake of protein is necessary to meet their needs. This is especially true for people who exercise while reducing energy intake.

• Frequency of meals is important. It may be better for dieters to consume numerous small meals throughout the day instead of eating all of the day's kilocalories in one large meal. Frequent feedings may help improve regulation of blood glucose and insulin, improve nitrogen retention, and increase the ability to maintain self-control. People who become too hungry have a greater tendency to overconsume when food is finally available. There is some evidence that people who eat more frequent, smaller meals ($\geq$5/d) have lower skinfold thicknesses than those eating $\leq$3/d (Fábry et al. 1964).

All of the commonly used diets can produce weight loss because they restrict energy intake.

Unfortunately, few promote good eating habits, long-term weight maintenance strategies, exercise, and good health. Understanding these diets will help you make better weight-loss recommendations to your clients and help you evaluate the next fad diet that comes along.

Starvation Diets

Starvation, or fasting, is often used as a quick method to lose unwanted pounds. **Starvation diets** are usually defined as those providing <200 kcal/d (Bray and Gray 1988). The primary advantage of a starvation diet is the very rapid weight loss that occurs. There are a number of serious problems, however:

- There are major protein losses, including from muscle and organ tissues.
- There are major fluid and electrolyte losses, which can also lead to problems with hypotension and dehydration.
- Malnutrition often develops, including nutrient deficiencies and bone loss—especially if the diet is done without medical supervision and for an extended period of time.
- Refeeding needs to be done slowly, and accumulation of fat can occur even on the consumption of moderately few kilocalories.
- Long-term success is poor, with individuals usually regaining most or all of the weight lost.
- Resting metabolic rate is blunted, which reduces the number of kilocalories one can consume to maintain body weight.

The severity of these problems depends on how long people are on the diet and whether or not they are exercising while they are consuming little or no food. Starvation dieting is never recommended for weight loss, especially for active individuals.

Very-Low-Calorie Diets

Very-low-calorie diets (VLCDs) are usually defined as diets providing between 200 and 800 kcal/d. They have been in existence since the 1930s but did not become popular until the 1970s. Interest in VLCDs as an effective weight-loss treatment stemmed from the success of complete starvation in achieving spectacular weight loss. The negative side effects associated with starvation diets, including large losses of lean body tissue (especially from muscles and organs) and even death, made them unpopular with patients and professionals.

These limitations of starvation diets led to the development of the **protein-sparing modified fast (PSMF)** in the early 1970s. The PSMF consisted of a high-protein (usually 1.5 g/kg body weight) and low-kilocalorie (200-400 kcal/d) meal plan, with all of the protein and energy being derived from lean meat (high-quality protein sources). This diet was modestly successful because it resulted in improved nitrogen balance while still producing rapid weight loss. VLCDs also can improve many comorbid conditions by decreasing elevated blood pressure, improving blood lipid profiles and glucose tolerance, and improving breathing in individuals with pulmonary problems.

In the late 1970s, VLCDs made from low-quality protein sources (hydrolyzed gelatin and collagen) became extremely popular. By 1977, approximately 98,000 Americans were using liquid-protein VLCDs as their sole source of food for at least 1 mo, with 37,000 Americans using it as their sole source of food for 2 mo or more (Van Itallie and Yang 1984). During 1977-1978, 58 deaths were reported in obese adults who had recently been on or were currently using these diets. Many of these otherwise healthy people died of cardiac arrhythmias due to catabolism of cardiac tissue during the dietary period (Van Itallie and Yang 1984). A significant positive correlation was found between BMI before initiating the VLCD and months of survival while on the VLCD. VLCDs should be supervised by physicians and are appropriate only for severely overweight people; a limit should be placed on the length of time a person consumes a VLCD.

There is disagreement as to whether some carbohydrate should be included in the VLCD. VLCDs containing little or no carbohydrate are termed **ketogenic diets**, as they stimulate production of ketones to provide an alternative source of energy for the central nervous system. *However, increased ketone production can be toxic (via increased acidity), which can be dangerous if maintained for prolonged periods of time.* VLCDs containing carbohydrates are termed nonketogenic diets. Support for ketogenic VLCDs stems from the fact that these diets produce more rapid weight loss due to increased diuresis, and they suppress insulin levels, which can increase fat utilization and spare protein breakdown (Blackburn et al. 1986). Others argue that inclusion of some carbohydrate (nonketogenic diet) is important to prevent excess fluid and electrolyte losses and the hypotension that may accompany these losses.

Low-Kilocalorie Diets

Low-kilocalorie diets are those that provide 800 to 1200 kcal/d and may comprise regular foods, specially formulated foods, or a combination. These diets typically provide less than 30% of total energy from fat, enough carbohydrate to avoid **ketosis** (abnormal increase of "ketone bodies"—i.e., acetoacetate, acetone, or β-hydroxybutyrate), and usually involve vitamin and mineral supplementation. Commercial programs in this category include those from Weight Watchers, Diet Center, and Jenny Craig. Slim Fast is an example of a specially formulated over-the-counter food designed as a meal replacement in this type of diet program. Although weight loss on these diets—averaging 1-3 lb/week (0.5 to 1.5 kg/week)—is not as rapid as with VLCDs, long-term compliance may be improved, and there are fewer side effects. Low-kilocalorie diets are relatively safe, and healthy obese individuals can initiate them without physician supervision. It is important to investigate the nutritional adequacy of these diets, however, as they can range from low-fat, high-carbohydrate, nutritionally balanced plans to diets void of nutritional value.

Note that the diets just reviewed are too low in energy and carbohydrate for most women and for all men, regardless of activity level (they cannot replace the glycogen necessary for engaging in exercise). The diets were designed to help obese people lose weight, and were not intended for use by moderately overweight active individuals. While many people follow these types of diets, their long-term mainte-nance of weight loss is very poor. None of these diets is recommended for physically active people who are trying to decrease body fat.

Popular or Fad Diets

Fad diets are those that enjoy short-lived success and popularity and are based on a marketing gimmick. Athletes can be particularly vulnerable to fad dieting because of their intense desire to optimize body composition and performance. Celebrities or other well-known persons endorse these diets in an attempt to give credibility to the diet (see "The Zone Diet: Do Athletes Need High-Protein Diets?" in chapter 4). Justification for these diets is typically based on a scientific or biochemical claim that may be speculative and unproven. Consumers must remember that if the diets were true to their claims, there would be no need for people to continue dieting or for the next fad diet! For example, if the Dr. Atkins's Diet, popular in the 1970s, had worked, there would be no need for the "new and improved" Dr. Atkins's New Diet Revolution in the 1990s.

The criteria listed below will help you recognize a potential fad diet or nutrition program. If the diet either you or your clients are considering contains one of the claims listed below, it is probably just another fad diet:

1. Claims to be new, modern, improved, or recently discovered, yet no scientific data are available to back up the claim.
2. Claims rapid loss of weight or fat, usually more than 2 lb (0.9 kg) per week.

■ HIGHLIGHT ■

Evaluation of a Fad Diet

Fad diets are widely publicized in the popular media. A recent search on the Internet brought to our attention the ConQuest System for Ultimate Weight Control. The ConQuest System includes the PrimeQuest program, whose marketing included many of the claims that are common to fad diets and programs. It claimed that many athletes around the world used this diet (e.g., Dan O'Brien, U.S. decathlete and Olympic gold medal winner), which resulted in their endorsing the diet and the products marketed with it. The marketers claim that these products were developed from previously secretive research done in the Soviet Union by a world-renowned pharmacologist. These products contain "adaptogens," which are the proposed miracle ingredients of these products. The PrimeQuest products supposedly do the following:

- Stop the "stress eating" syndrome (i.e., prevent users from overeating in response to stress).
- Reprogram the way your body deals with food by providing the body with "metabolic potentiators" that assist it in using nutrients and calories more efficiently.

(continued)

- Cause you to lose fat and maintain lean tissue (the ads also claim that losing lean tissue is what causes wrinkles and loose skin—thus using this product will help you look as if you stopped the aging process).
- Result in the maintenance of permanent weight control by satisfying hunger and preventing snacking and nervous eating.
- Result in a "more desirable" metabolic rate by maintaining muscle mass with weight loss.
- Make you feel better than ever due to the regular intake of these unique herbal supplements and food formulas.

Table 6.3 lists the ingredients of the ConQuest Starter Kit, which includes the Prime 1 herbal supplement and the Prime Perfect weight control meals.

Table 6.3 Prime 1 Herbal Supplement and Prime Perfect Weight Control Meals: Ingredients and Nutrition Facts

Prime 1 Liquid Herbal Supplement Ingredients (31 oz total):

Distilled water, M.A. complex brand of biologically active golden molasses in combination with herbal blend *(Eleutherococcus senticosus, Rhaponticum carthamoides, Glycyrrhiza uralensis, Rhodiola rosea, Schizandra chinensis, Rosa majalis, Aralia mandshurica),* natural flavors, lactic acid, citric acid, and potassium benzoate and potassium sorbate to protect freshness.

Prime Perfect Food Formula—Powder, Weight Control Meals (48 g each packet, 14 packets [meals] per box):

Ingredients: Myo-Pro (protein blend including partially hydrolyzed proteins from total milk protein, fresh curd, calcium caseinate, whey protein hydrolysate, soy proteins, and egg protein from dried egg albumin. Prime Vigor (a blend of carbohydrates including fructose, glucose polymers, adaptogenic molasses, and fructooligosaccharides or FOS), *Garcinia camgogia, Ginkgo biloba* extract, and xylitol. Prime Fiber (a blend of fiber sources including soy fiber, vegetable gum, oat fiber, and corn bran). Flavor Blend (including cocoa powder, natural and artificial flavors, carob powder, and acesulfame K). Prima Vita (a vitamin and mineral blend including sodium citrate, potassium chloride, potassium phosphate, calcium phosphate, choline dihydrogen citrate, magnesium oxide, calcium carbonate, ascorbic acid, vitamin E acetate, ferrous fumarate, creatine monohydrate, niacinamide, zinc oxide, calcium pantothenate, vitamin A [palmitate, beta carotene], copper sulfate, manganese sulfate, vitamin D, pyridoxine iodide, sodium selenite, vitamin K, and cyanocobalamin). Myo-Statin (including L-glutamine, acetyl-L-carnitine, *Eleutherococcus senticosus* extract and chromium picolinate). Lipids (medium-chain triglycerides [MCT] and soy lecithin).

Prime Perfect Weight Control Meals—Nutrition Facts:

Serving size: 1 packet (48 g)
Servings per carton: 14

	Amount per serving (mix with water)
Energy (kcal)	170
Calories from fat	10
Total fat	1 g
Saturated fat	0 g
Cholesterol	0 g
Sodium	240 mg
Potassium	660 mg
Total carbohydrates	23 g
Dietary fiber	4 g
Sugars	14 g
Protein	18 g

Includes 50% of Daily Values based on 2000 kcal/d of the following: vitamins A, C, D, E, B_6, B_{12}, thiamine, niacin, riboflavin, biotin, pantothenic acid, iron, iodine, zinc, and copper. Includes 35% of Daily Values (based on 2000 kcal/d) of calcium, folate, phosphorus, and magnesium.

3. Claims weight loss success with no or little physical exercise.

4. Includes special foods that are expensive and difficult to find; suggests consuming foods in a particular order or "combination;" suggests avoiding consumption of certain "bad" foods; or includes "magic" or "miracle" foods that claim to burn fat.

5. Includes a rigid menu that must be followed daily; or the dieter can eat only from a limited list of foods (these diets frequently require adherents to eat the same foods day after day).

6. Includes supplemental meals, foods, or nutrient supplements that claim to cure disease or a variety of ailments.

"Evaluation of a Fad Diet," page 171, reviews a fad supplement/diet program aimed at athletes and the public. Thousands of similar products or programs exist, and it is important for nutrition and fitness professionals to educate consumers about the limitations of these products. While many products may be physically harmless (albeit expensive!), others can cause illness or even death. It is very important to consider the safety and efficacy of any fad diet before recommending it to a client.

Moderate Energy Restriction Diets

VLCDs and low-kilocalorie diets can result in substantial weight loss but are also associated with large losses of fat-free mass and decreases in resting metabolic rate. These changes make long-term weight maintenance very difficult. It is becoming increasingly common to recommend moderate energy restriction combined with physical activity in an attempt to prevent the loss of metabolically active tissues.

Moderate energy restriction diets have an energy content of more than 1200 kcal/d, with the recommended energy intake usually based on an individual's current energy requirements for weight maintenance. For instance, Belko et al. (1987) and Fox et al. (1996) reported significant weight loss over 3-6 mo by prescribing energy intakes of 500 and 700 kcal/d less than estimated energy needs for moderately overweight premenopausal and postmenopausal women, respectively. These women also performed moderate-intensity aerobic exercise alone or in combination with strength training.

While weight loss is less rapid with moderate energy restriction as compared to diets employing more severe energy reductions, FFM

and RMR do not appear to be compromised. In addition, healthy dietary practices can be stressed with moderate energy restriction, thereby assisting people with long-term maintenance of healthy body weight.

High-Carbohydrate Diets

Recent studies have shown that people can successfully lose weight on diets comprising mainly unprocessed carbohydrates (e.g., whole grains, legumes, beans, fruits, and vegetables). A **high-carbohydrate diet** is defined as one containing 60%, 25%, and 15% of energy from carbohydrate, fat, and protein, respectively. Weight loss occurs even in those who are allowed ad libitum consumption of complex, unprocessed high-carbohydrate foods. These findings are encouraging for individuals who find it difficult to restrict energy, as weight loss may be possible without experiencing the deprivation and sacrifice associated with dieting.

Two mechanisms may explain the ability to lose weight on ad libitum, unprocessed high-carbohydrate diets. First, there is growing evidence that people consuming such diets consume significantly less energy than those consuming an ad libitum high-fat diet (Duncan et al. 1983; Lissner et al. 1987; Schutz et al. 1989; Tremblay et al. 1989). The lower energy intake is probably due to the higher fiber and lower fat content of a high-carbohydrate diet as compared to diets higher in fat. The increased bulk leads to feeling more full after eating foods that are much less energy dense, which prevents overeating. In addition, it appears that eating a high-carbohydrate diet causes a person to feel less hungry between meals (Duncan et al. 1983). *It is important to note that these high-carbohydrate diets have a low energy density* per gram of food: one can eat large amounts of whole grains, fruits, and vegetables while consuming relatively few kilocalories. Note, however, that it is possible to eat a high-carbohydrate diet that has a *high* energy density per gram of food (e.g., fat-free cookies, fat-free frozen yogurt or ice cream) and *not* lose weight—you might even gain weight. Such diets comprise highly processed carbohydrate foods, which are energy dense and contain few vitamins and minerals. "Diets Varying in Carbohydrate and Dietary Fiber Content" (page 175) includes examples of high-carbohydrate diets with both low and high energy densities, plus a high-fat diet. In addition, figure 6.5 illustrates that a significant increase in body

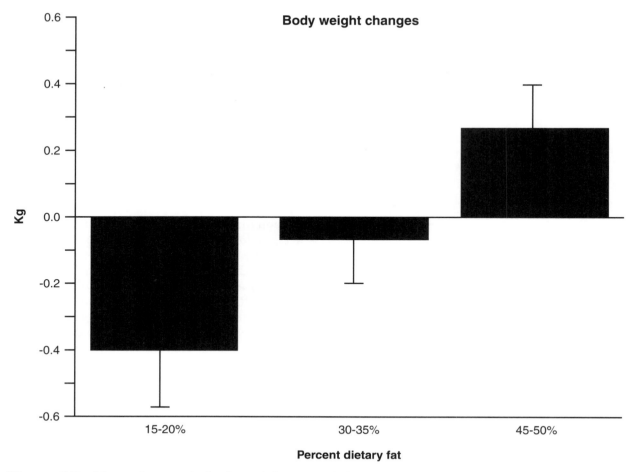

Figure 6.5 Mean changes in body weight over 14-d treatment periods, calculated as day 14 minus day 1. Differences in diet effect significant at $p < 0.001$.
Reprinted from Lissner et al. 1987.

weight over a 14-d period has been observed in humans consuming a high-fat diet as compared to diets of relatively low or moderate fat content (Lissner et al. 1987).

A second mechanism contributing to weight loss on high-carbohydrate diets is the relationship between the energy composition of the diet (termed the **food quotient**, or **FQ**) and the oxidation of fuels by the body (the **respiratory quotient**). Flatt (1992) has proposed that in order for weight maintenance to occur, energy intake must be equal to energy expenditure, *and* the average FQ must be equal to the average respiratory quotient (RQ) (i.e., the body is oxidizing the fuels it consumes). It appears that a high carbohydrate intake promotes oxidation of carbohydrate by the body, but that high fat intake does not promote fat oxidation (Flatt 1992). This means that a person who consumes a high-energy, high-carbohydrate diet is more

likely to oxidize the excess carbohydrate consumed; but someone consuming a high-energy, high-fat diet will not oxidize the excess fat consumed, instead storing it in the adipose tissue. Chapter 5 describes in detail these concepts, which help explain how body fat levels can steadily increase on an ad libitum high-fat diet, but not on an ad libitum high-carbohydrate diet. Note that a high-carbohydrate diet does not refer to a diet composed *exclusively* of carbohydrate; foods with fat and protein should also be included in a high-carbohydrate diet.

In summary, weight loss can be accomplished if energy intake is lower than energy expenditure (due to either decreased energy intake or increased energy expenditure). Starvation and VLCDs result in rapid weight loss but are associated with dehydration, loss of FFM, a decrease in RMR, and potential death if not accompanied by appropriate medical supervision.

174

Diets Varying in Carbohydrate and Dietary Fiber Content

High-carbohydrate diet (low energy density, high fiber)

Breakfast

    1 1/2 cups Cheerios

    1 cup skim milk

    2 slices whole wheat toast with 1 tbsp light margarine

    1 medium banana

    8 fl oz fresh orange juice

Lunch

    8 fl oz low-fat blueberry yogurt

    tuna sandwich (2 slices whole wheat bread; 1/4 cup tuna packed in water, drained; 1 tsp Dijon mustard; 2 tsp low-calorie mayonnaise)

    2 carrots, raw, with peel

    1 cup raw cauliflower

    1 tbsp. peppercorn ranch salad dressing

Dinner

    1/2 chicken breast, roasted

    1 cup brown rice, cooked

    1 tbsp shredded parmesan cheese

    1 cup cooked broccoli

    spinach salad (1 cup chopped spinach, 1 whole egg white, 2 slices turkey bacon, 3 cherry tomatoes, and 2 tbsp creamy bacon salad dressing)

    2 baked apples—no added sugar

Nutrient analysis: 2150 kcal; 60% of energy from carbohydrate, 22% from fat, 18% from protein; 38 g dietary fiber, 13 g soluble fiber

High-carbohydrate diet (high energy density, low fiber)

Breakfast

    1 1/2 cups Fruit Loops cereal

    1 cup skim milk

    2 slices white bread (toast) with 1 tbsp light margarine

    8 fl oz fresh orange juice

Lunch

    McDonald's Quarter Pounder—1 sandwich

    large order French fries

    16 fl oz cola beverage

    30 jelly beans

Snack

    1 cinnamon raisin bagel (3 1/2 in.)

    2 tbsp cream cheese

    8 fl oz low-fat strawberry yogurt

(continued)

Dinner

    1 whole chicken breast, roasted

    2 cups mixed green salad

    2 tbsp ranch dressing

    1 serving macaroni and cheese

    12 fl oz cola beverage

    cheesecake (1/9th of cake)

Late-night snack

    2 cups gelatin dessert—cherry

    3 raspberry oatmeal no-fat cookies

Nutrient analysis: 4012 kcal; 60% of energy from carbohydrate, 25% from fat, 15% from protein; 18.5 g dietary fiber, 2 g soluble fiber

High-fat diet (high energy density, moderately high fiber)

Breakfast

    2 slices whole wheat toast with 1 tbsp regular margarine

    2 large eggs, fried in butter

    8 fl oz fresh orange juice

Lunch

    bacon double cheeseburger—1 sandwich

    1 large order French fries with 3 tbsp ketchup

    1 medium apple

    16 fl oz cola beverage

Dinner

    fried chicken—1 drumstick and 1 thigh

    2 buttermilk biscuits with 2 tbsp regular margarine

    2 cups mixed green salad

    1 cup broccoli with cheese sauce

    1 medium baked potato with 3 tbsp margarine and 3 tbsp sour cream

    8 fl oz 2% milk

Nutrient analysis: 3983 kcal; 35% of energy from carbohydrate, 51% from fat, 13% from protein; 28.5 g dietary fiber, 6 g soluble fiber

All diets were analyzed using Food Processor 7.21 (ESHA Research, Salem, OR).

The changes in FFM and RMR are detrimental to the maintenance of body weight when a standard diet is reintroduced. Moderate energy restriction and high-carbohydrate diets (60% of total energy as carbohydrate) result in slower weight loss than that observed with more severe energy restriction but with fewer detrimental effects on FFM and RMR. Active individuals needing to lose weight can safely incorporate moderate energy restriction or high-carbohydrate diets into their program. In addition, these types of diets can be used as models for a healthy lifetime meal plan, which may allow for long-term weight maintenance and compliance.

Effect of Exercise Alone on Weight Loss

It is well established that diet alone and diet combined with exercise can result in weight loss. Exercise plays a number of important roles in regard to body weight and health (Blair 1993). Many active people consume more energy than sedentary obese individuals but maintain a lean physique. Active people also have a healthier WHR than do sedentary

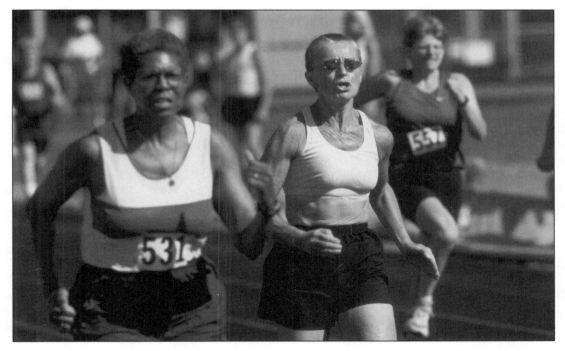

Energy expenditure during exercise depends on body size, type of exercise, environmental conditions, and exercise intensity.

people. Furthermore, active lifestyles may prevent or minimize the weight gain observed with aging. Among those who are active and overweight, the risk of morbidity and mortality is much lower than for sedentary overweight and lean individuals.

Weight loss occurs when energy intake is less than energy expenditure. Exercise alone can be used to increase energy expenditure, resulting in weight loss if energy intake is not increased to compensate for the higher energy expenditure.

Table 6.4 lists energy expenditures for various activities. The energy expended for any given activity is usually expressed per kilogram body weight or as a multiple of RMR. Although these energy values are useful as a guide, they may not be exact. A number of errors are inherent in the estimation of energy expenditure (see chapter 14 for detailed discussion). Appendix E.4 provides a more complete table of energy expenditure values.

Exercise-induced weight loss depends on both the total amount of energy expended and the type of fuels used for energy during the activity. Exercising is an ideal way to increase fat oxidation since skeletal muscle readily uses fat for energy. Fat oxidation is also proportionately greater during prolonged exercise of low to moderate intensity as compared to exercise performed at a higher intensity (Flatt 1992). Activities causing the greatest energy expenditure are those that are endurance related and use large muscle groups (e.g., running) (table 6.4). Remember also that fat oxidation is maximized at activities of low to moderate intensity (figure 6.6). This means that performing activities such as walking, swimming, aerobics, and bicycling at low to moderate intensities increases relative fat oxidation as compared to activities of greater intensity (i.e., the majority of the energy will come from fat). However, the *total* energy expenditure over a given period of time for low- to moderate-intensity activities is less than that for more intense activities such as running. A critical point to remember is that the *relative* contribution of fat as a fuel is greater during moderate exercise than during intense exercise, when carbohydrate contributes proportionately more energy (figure 6.6). However, it is the *total* energy and nutrient balance over an entire day that determines the absolute amount of fat used as a fuel.

Results of a study by Tremblay et al. (1994) challenge this theory. These results indicate that high-intensity intermittent training may result in greater fat loss than moderate-intensity endurance training. The subjects in this

Table 6.4 Energy Expenditure for Various Physical Activities

Activity	Energy expenditure (kcal/min/kg)	Energy expenditure for selected body weights (kcal/min)			
		110 lb (50 kg)	130 lb (59 kg)	150 lb (68 kg)	170 lb (77 kg)
Cycling:					
Leisure (5.5 mph)	0.064	3.2	3.8	4.4	4.9
Leisure (9.4 mph)	0.100	5.0	5.9	6.8	7.7
Racing	0.169	8.5	10.0	11.5	13.0
Dancing:					
Aerobic (medium)	0.103	5.2	6.1	7.0	7.9
Aerobic (intense)	0.135	6.7	7.9	9.2	10.4
Ballroom	0.051	2.6	3.0	3.5	3.9
Walking (normal pace):					
Asphalt road	0.080	4.0	4.7	5.4	6.2
Fields and hillsides	0.082	4.1	4.8	5.6	6.3
Running (horizontal):					
11 min, 30 s per mile	0.135	6.8	8.0	9.2	10.5
8 min per mile	0.208	10.8	12.5	14.2	16.0
6 min per mile	0.252	13.9	15.6	17.3	19.1
Swimming:					
Backstroke	0.169	8.5	10.0	11.5	13.0
Breaststroke	0.162	8.1	9.6	11.0	12.5
Crawl, fast	0.156	7.8	9.2	10.6	12.0
Crawl, slow	0.128	6.4	7.6	8.7	9.9

Adapted from Ainsworth et al. 1993.

study performed either 20 weeks of continuous cycling (four times/week for 30-45 min at 60-85% of maximal heart rate reserve) or 15 weeks of high-intensity intermittent training (19 short- and 16 long-interval workouts, accompanied by 25 30-min sessions of continuous cycling). The high-intensity exercisers showed a significantly greater reduction in skinfold thickness as compared to the endurance exercisers, despite the fact that the energy cost of the high-intensity program was less than half of the energy cost of the endurance program. One mechanism to explain these findings was the significant increase in muscle **3-hydroxyacyl coenzyme A dehydrogenase (HADH)** enzyme activity with high-intensity training. HADH is a marker of β-oxidation, and increased activity of this enzyme indicates an increase in fat oxidation. Other factors that were not measured may also explain these findings, including an increased excess post-exercise oxygen consumption (EPOC), suppression of food intake, and/or increased metabolic cost of tissue

damage related to the high-intensity exercise. It is important to emphasize that many people are not physically capable of performing high-intensity exercise due to their low fitness level, age, or other health problems. For these people, participation in low- to moderate-intensity endurance-type activities will still be effective for weight loss. However, many athletes and active people are capable of participating in high-intensity activities, and those needing to lose body fat may benefit from incorporating more of these types of activities into their regimen.

Resistance training also plays a critical role in weight loss. It may not significantly increase energy expenditure, and fat is not the predominant fuel source for resistance training—but increasing one's FFM, which is a result of resistance training (but not of endurance training), increases RMR (Ballor et al. 1988; Broeder et al. 1992; Tremblay et al. 1986). Resistance training can also help reshape the body by toning and/or adding FFM—a goal often sought by those who are trying to lose weight.

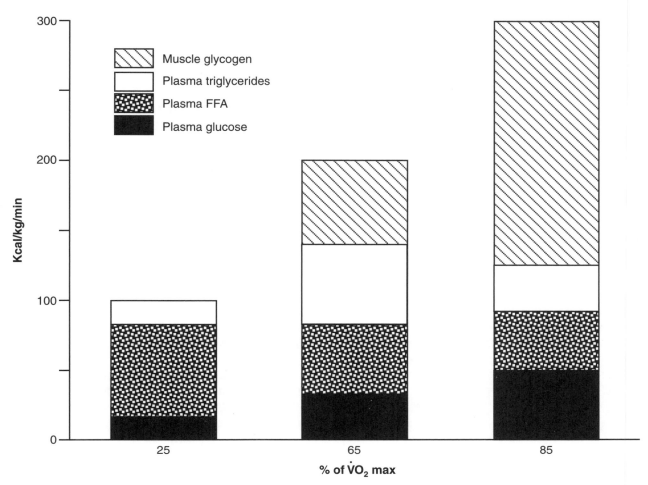

Figure 6.6 Illustration of the crossover from lipid to carbohydrate dependency as exercise intensity increases from mild (25% $\dot{V}O_2$max) to hard (85% $\dot{V}O_2$max).

Reprinted from Romijn et al. 1993.

What Is a Meta-Analysis?

Meta-analysis is a research method that combines the results of many studies into an overall result, or "effect," of a given intervention (or interventions). This form of research is usually conducted in research areas that are controversial and/or that report copious equivocal findings. For example, meta-analyses have been conducted to determine the effects of weight reduction on serum lipoproteins (Datillo and Kris-Etherton 1992), the effect of diet or diet plus exercise on RMR (Thompson et al. 1996), and to assess the effectiveness of diet plus exercise on body composition changes (Garrow and Summerbell 1995). Proponents of meta-analytical research claim that it is an accurate, unbiased research process that can combine numerous research findings from a variety of settings to determine treatment effectiveness. Those opposed to meta-analysis believe that it is fraught with bias and is akin to comparing "apples and oranges." Regardless of one's stance on the use of meta-analyses, it is important to remember that the meta-analysis is only as good as the original studies used.

Surprisingly, many studies do not support the contention that exercise alone results in significant weight loss (Lawson et al. 1987; Meredith et al. 1989). Epstein and Wing (1980) performed a **meta-analysis** (see "What Is a Meta-Analysis?" on page 179) of studies that prescribed either exercise alone or no exercise, and found that the average weight loss due to exercise alone was approximately 0.2 lb/week (0.09 kg/week). The nonexercising control groups exhibited no change in weight. A more recent meta-analysis by Garrow and Summerbell (1995) found that endurance exercise resulted in similar weight loss (~0.09 kg/week) for men and women. Most subjects participating in these studies did not lose as much weight as expected from their increased energy expenditure. Since energy intake was not controlled, presumably either a compensatory increase in energy intake occurred with the increase in energy expenditure, or the subjects decreased the duration or intensity of activities associated with daily living. These changes would result in relatively small perturbations in body weight.

For exercise alone to be effective in weight loss, energy intake must be maintained at a level lower than that of total daily energy expenditure. Exercising women lost significant amounts of weight when their energy intake was held constant at sedentary maintenance levels (Keim et al. 1990). These women lost approximately 1.1 lb/week (0.5 kg/week) when walking on a treadmill 6 d/week at a level equal to 25% of their energy intake. These women lost weight because they were not allowed to compensate for their increased energy expenditure. Note, however, the results of research by Woo et al. (1982): subjects allowed an ad libitum diet did not compensate for the excess energy expended in daily walking, leading to an average weight loss of 1.8 lb/week (0.8 kg/week). It has been suggested that lean individuals increase their energy intake in response to exercise, but obese individuals do not (Durrant et al. 1982; Woo et al. 1982). *For some obese individuals trying to lose weight, exercise apparently can both increase energy expenditure and prevent an increase in energy intake.*

For exercise to assist in maintaining healthy body weight, it is important not only to practice some form of regular exercise training but also to increase the activities of daily living.

Methods for Increasing Total Daily Energy Expenditure

Here are a few suggestions for increasing total energy expenditure. Please keep in mind that the list is by no means exhaustive:

- Leave your desk frequently at work, and take the stairs between floors.
- Skip the escalators and elevators at the mall or at work, and take the stairs instead.
- Park farther away from your destination (or walk instead).
- Walk to lunch when the weather permits.
- Play with your children, grandchildren, and/or pet(s) on a regular basis.
- Clean the house a little every day. Not only will you expend energy, but cleaning will not seem like such an overwhelming chore.
- Replace some of your television viewing time with gardening, fixing up your home, or some other active hobby.
- Do stretching and resistance training activities while watching television.
- Take a 10-min walk during your break or lunch time or after dinner.

Not only can performing these activities help increase total daily energy expenditure, but recent studies have shown that they can be just as effective as structured exercise in improving fitness and health (Andersen et al. 1999; Dunn et al. 1999).

See "Methods for Increasing Total Daily Energy Expenditure" for suggestions on ways to increase your daily activity levels (in addition to your organized exercise session).

When trying to lose weight, an individual must not increase energy intake to compensate for the energy expended during exercise. From the information presented in this chapter, it appears that consuming a diet high in complex carbohydrates (e.g., whole grains, legumes, beans, fruits, and vegetables) and increasing one's activity should result in weight loss over time. Combining moderate-intensity (or even high-intensity) exercise with a diet high in complex carbohydrates, moreover, can promote fat oxidation. Consumption of a high-carbohydrate diet also supports participation in exercise, as it ensures adequate glycogen stores and helps maintain a person's endurance (Bogardus et al. 1981).

Diet and Exercise in Weight Loss

Research data clearly show that energy restriction results in weight loss, and that exercise alone without compensatory increases in energy intake can also lead to gradual losses of body weight. It has been suggested throughout this chapter that *the most effective regimen for weight loss is combining diet with exercise.* This section addresses the validity of the following claims of combining energy restriction with exercise:

* Exercise prevents the decrease in RMR seen with dieting.

* Exercise added to dieting increases the amount of weight lost.

* Exercise added to dieting helps preserve FFM.

Does Exercise Prevent the Decrease in RMR Seen With Dieting? Numerous studies have attempted to answer this question. Yet there appears to be no clear understanding of the additive effects of exercise and diet on RMR. Some studies have suggested that exercise can prevent the decrease in RMR observed with dieting (Hammer et al. 1989; Hill et al. 1987, 1989; Svendsen et al. 1993; Thompson et al. 1997); others either show no effect of exercise or find that RMR can decline even further when exercise is added to dietary restriction (Donnelly et al. 1991, 1994; Heymsfield et al. 1989; Phinney et al. 1988; van Dale et al. 1990). A number of factors can contribute to these discrepancies. For example, level of energy restriction, intensity and type of prescribed exercise, duration of the diet and exercise programs, and the char-

acteristics of the subjects studied can all influence the results reported in the literature.

A meta-analysis of the effects of diet alone and diet-plus-exercise regimens on RMR has attempted to answer this question by reviewing all of the available studies to determine the overall effect of diet alone or diet plus exercise on changes in RMR (Thompson et al. 1996). In this analysis, exercise (predominantly endurance exercise) was found to prevent some of the decrease in RMR observed with dieting. However, there were a number of unique factors in these studies that may limit the widespread application of this analysis:

* Very few studies were available on men or postmenopausal women.

* The majority of studies prescribed energy intakes less than 800 kcal/d.

* The endurance exercise prescribed in most studies was moderate in intensity (50-70% of $\dot{V}O_2$max).

* Only half of the studies combined strength training with endurance exercise.

* No studies employed only strength training.

* The average duration of the studies was 9 weeks.

The results of this meta-analysis suggest that adding moderate-intensity endurance exercise can prevent some of the RMR decrease when obese, premenopausal women diet. Additional studies need to be conducted to see if other types of people benefit from exercise while dieting and if other forms of exercise can prevent some or even the entire decline in RMR.

Does Exercise Increase the Amount of Weight Lost and Help Preserve FFM Over Dieting Alone? One would assume that adding exercise to dietary restriction would result in a greater energy deficit, and hence lead to greater weight loss. However, the plethora of studies addressing the effectiveness of diet alone or diet plus exercise regimens on weight loss and changes in body composition do not overwhelmingly support this assumption. Most studies show little or no difference in weight loss between individuals who diet and those who participate in diet plus exercise. When the combination of diet and exercise does result in added weight loss compared with diet alone, the added weight loss is less than that expected for the prescribed energy deficit (Pavlou, Krey, and Steffee 1989).

This lack of greater weight loss with the addition of exercise to a diet program is most likely due to a decrease in the total amount of energy expended over the day and/or to an increase in energy intake that compensates for the energy expended during exercise. There is evidence that exercisers compensate for their increased energy expended by increasing the time spent sleeping, sitting, and lying during the day. Dieters, on the other hand, appear to spend more time in sedentary activities because their lack of energy intake makes them feel "more tired." Note that most studies of diet and exercise are "outpatient" in nature, which increases the probability that subjects may be consuming more kilocalories/day than what is prescribed on the diet. These additional kilocalories consumed would explain why most people participating in diet and exercise studies do not lose as much weight as predicted from the prescribed energy deficit.

While adding exercise to dieting may not lead to substantially greater weight loss, it does appear to increase the amount of body fat lost. Endurance exercise not only results in the oxidation of fat—it increases the potential to sustain FFM in a way not observed with dieting alone (Donnelly et al. 1991; Garrow and Summerbell 1995). Adding exercise to dietary restriction can enhance fat loss and maintain or slow the loss of FFM that consistently occurs with dieting alone. It is important to emphasize that the studies reporting significant losses of FFM involved relatively low energy intakes (<1000 kcal/d). Less restrictive diets may have much less impact of loss of FFM.

The most critical role exercise may play is in maintaining weight loss after the diet is over. Figure 6.7 shows how individuals who continued their exercise program were able to sus-

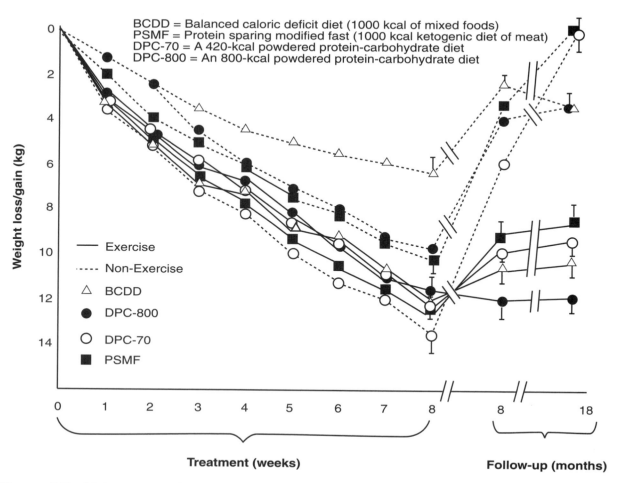

BCDD = Balanced caloric deficit diet (1000 kcal of mixed foods)
PSMF = Protein sparing modified fast (1000 kcal ketogenic diet of meat)
DPC-70 = A 420-kcal powdered protein-carbohydrate diet
DPC-800 = An 800-kcal powdered protein-carbohydrate diet

Exercise
Non-Exercise
△ BCDD
● DPC-800
○ DPC-70
■ PSMF

Treatment (weeks)

Follow-up (months)

Figure 6.7 Maintenance of weight loss after dieting with or without exercise.
Reproduced from Pavlou, Krey, and Steffee 1989.

tain virtually all of their weight loss, while those who did not exercise regained over 90% of the weight they lost within 18 mo following participation in a diet-only program (Pavlou, Krey, and Steffee 1989). Experts in the area of weight loss consistently stress the importance of regular exercise to achieve both weight loss and the long-term maintenance of weight loss.

Recommendations for Maintenance of Healthy Body Weight

Maintaining a healthy or optimal body weight appears to be linked to a person successfully addressing three lifestyle issues on a daily basis:

- Consuming a diet low in fat and high in complex carbohydrate (e.g., high in fruits, vegetables, whole grains, legumes, and beans)
- Performing regular exercise
- Making appropriate behavioral modifications related to dietary intake and exercise ("Components of a Behavior Modification Program for Weight Loss or Weight Maintenance" reviews the components of a behavior modification program.)

Reports of those who have shown success with long-term maintenance of weight loss

■ HIGHLIGHT ■

Components of a Behavior Modification Program for Weight Loss or Weight Maintenance

Brownell and Kramer (1994) thoroughly review the components of behavioral management of obesity. The following is a brief synopsis of the important components of any behavior modification program aimed at weight loss or weight maintenance. Note that these programs address nutrition and exercise, reinforcing the important interactions among diet, exercise, and behavior on weight loss and weight maintenance.

- **Self-monitoring:** Involves completing regular records on amount, location, and circumstances surrounding food intake to assess initial patterns of eating and exercise behavior. Also used to track motivation and document positive changes in behavior.

- **Stimulus control:** Involves controlling the environment in which one consumes food, such as keeping food out of sight, avoiding the purchase of problematic foods, eating at specific times and places, and breaking habitual eating routines.

- **Reinforcement:** Involves applying techniques that reward achievement of goals, such as reinforcement by self, family, and friends. Should also involve rewards that provide pleasures other than eating (e.g., buying new clothes).

- **Nutrition:** Requires going beyond just counting calories (kilocalories). Involves understanding the nutrient composition of foods and setting specific dietary goals, such as decreasing energy and fat intake or eating more nutrient-dense foods (e.g., carrots instead of jelly beans). Also includes educating oneself on the importance of healthy eating regardless of energy intake.

- **Exercise:** Involves learning how to increase activities of daily living, including the gradual introduction of a regular exercise program into one's lifestyle. Requires committing to a lifetime of exercise.

- **Social support:** Involves receiving positive support from fellow dieters, family members, and friends. Also involves preventing the undermining of the dieting effort by spouse or family members and avoiding ridicule of efforts by peers.

- **Cognitive change:** Involves improving attitudes about one's body, life, and chances of success for weight loss and long-term maintenance.

■ HIGHLIGHT ■

Case Study: Weight Loss in an Overweight Active Woman

Margaret is 5 ft 5 in. tall, 35 years old, and weighs 160 lb (72.6 kg). Her BMI is 26.7, and she recently had her body fat measured at 33%. Margaret was a competitive athlete in college and has remained active. She has always struggled with her weight, which has ranged from 135 lb (62 kg) to 170 lb (77 kg) throughout her adult life. She currently walks/runs an average of 25 mi/week and attends a 90-min yoga class once a week. While Margaret considers herself fit, she would like to decrease her body fat since she has had consistently elevated serum low-density lipoprotein (LDL)-cholesterol levels for the past 3 years. Her doctor recommended that she lose 15 lb (6.8 kg).

Margaret's diet and activity logs show that she requires approximately 2500 kcal/d to maintain her current body weight and activity level. While individuals certainly differ, a universal rule of thumb is that one must have an energy deficit of 3500 kcal in order to lose 1 lb of fat. Margaret would like to lose her excess body fat rapidly but knows from her previous dieting experiences that she is more likely to maintain weight loss with a more gradual program. She has decided to maintain her current activity level (increasing her activity level exacerbates her chronic lower leg pain), reminding herself that she should perform some sort of physical activity at least 4 d/week. She has decided to decrease her energy intake by 500 kcal/d, which should result in a loss of 1 lb (0.45 kg) of weight per week. Her goal is to maximize fat loss and minimize loss of muscle tissue. Margaret feels this is a realistic goal, as she can skip the chocolate bar she eats every afternoon (220 kcal), give up the two light beers she drinks every night after work (180 kcal), and eat one less piece of toast for breakfast in the morning (100 kcal). In addition, she plans to pay close attention to the amount of saturated fat in her diet, eating less than 10% of her total fat intake as saturated fat in an attempt to lower her LDL-cholesterol levels. By reducing her daily energy intake in this manner, it should take approximately 15 weeks for Margaret to reach her weight goal of 145 lb (66 kg). It is important for Margaret to remember that as she gets closer to her goal weight, the rate of weight loss will be slower than at the beginning of her program. This response is primarily due to her lower body weight (since she weighs less, the energy deficit will be less than the original 500 kcal/d) and may also be due to the potential reduction in RMR that occurs with dietary restriction and weight loss.

clearly state that incorporating healthy lifestyle modifications into daily life is critical to that success. Moreover, it is essential that people accept the fact that *maintenance of healthy body weight is a life-long process.* (See "Case Study: Weight Loss in an Overweight Active Woman," above.)

Weight Concerns of Athletes

The casual observer of athletic events sees young, healthy individuals with lean and muscular bodies. Many noncompetitive people give little thought to the rigorous training it takes for an athlete to achieve and maintain the body that is necessary for optimal performance.

While it may appear "easy" for athletes to maintain their lean physiques due to their high levels of training, there are a number of sports where body weight and percentage of body fat are major concerns. The pressures to achieve and maintain a low body weight and low body fat can lead to unhealthy—and many times dangerous—behaviors by athletes.

Lean-Build Sports

Several sports could be classified as "lean-build sports," meaning that a lean build is associated with successful performance (e.g., diving, track and field, dance, swimming, gymnastics, cross-country skiing, and bodybuilding). In addition to increasing the athlete's individual performance, lean bodies may also facilitate the scoring of the athlete in sports such as diving, gymnastics, and bodybuilding. In diving and gymnastics, judgments on the "look" of an individual are incorporated into performance evaluations, and, in bodybuilding, the "look" of the individual is the sole criterion of competing. The weight concerns of athletes in these sports can lead to unhealthy behaviors that threaten not only athletic performance but also the athlete's health. Consequences of competing in lean-build sports can include the following:

- ***Poor eating habits:*** Result from concerns about keeping body weight and fat low and inattention to healthy eating due to heavy training schedules and a busy lifestyle.

- ***Increased risk for eating disorders:*** Results from a combination of poor eating habits; pressure from self, peers, and coaches to maintain low body weight; and psychosocial stressors within family and social environments.

- ***Increased risk for injury:*** Results from poor eating habits, disordered eating, failure to take adequate rest periods to allow for recovery, or poor nutritional status.

Muscular injuries and stress fractures in these types of sports have been linked to poor diet, eating disorders, and failure to rest. Stress fractures and increased risk for premature osteoporosis are major concerns for female athletes in these sports (Warren 1980). Chapters 13 and 15 provide more detailed discussion of nutrition, bone health, and eating disorders.

It is widely believed that people for whom physical appearance is a major concern are more at risk for eating disorders. The incidence of disordered eating is higher for female than for male athletes. This difference could possibly be due to male athletes being more concerned with losing weight to enhance performance, while female athletes are more concerned with achieving the "ideal" body image and appearance (Fogelholm 1994). Between 15% and 60% of female athletes may employ pathogenic techniques for weight loss (including fasting, self-induced vomiting, laxatives, and diuretics) (Rosen et al. 1986; Rosen and Hough 1988; Sundgot-Borgen 1993). Of female athletes considered at high risk for eating disorders, the incidence of using **pathogenic weight-loss techniques** can be very high (80%). Athletes more likely to use these techniques are those in aesthetic, weight-dependent, and endurance sports (Sundgot-Borgen 1993). It is well known that using diuretics and laxatives can lead to cardiac disorders and gastrointestinal damage. Athletes should avoid these products except under medical supervision.

Research with elite gymnasts demonstrates how poor nutrition is related to menstrual dysfunction and increased incidence of eating disorders and injuries. Sundgot-Borgen (1996) compared 12 females (age range 13-20 years) on the Norwegian National Rhythmic Gymnastics Team with an age-matched control group for incidence of eating disorders and menstrual dysfunction. Only one-third of the gymnasts had reached menarche, compared with 100% of the controls. Of the athletes who had reached menarche, all reported either irregular menstrual cycles or amenorrhea. Eight of the twelve athletes reported overuse injuries; all were dieting, the primary motivation being improved performance. While both athletes and controls self-defined their ideal weight at a value lower than their present weight, the athletes had much higher scores on the eating disorder inventory. Four of the twelve athletes had either overt or subclinical eating disorders. When the athletes were interviewed regarding dietary practices, it became apparent that both athletes and coaches could benefit from nutritional education. The athletes reported following nutritional myths such as those listed below:

- Never eat after 5 P.M.
- Rhythmic gymnasts need only 800 kcal/d.
- Eat only cold food.
- Do not eat meat, bread, or potatoes.
- Drinking during training will destroy your practice.

Some of the preoccupation with weight and body image may change for female athletes after they discontinue competing. For example, O'Conner et al. (1996) found that former college gymnasts (mean age 36.6 ± 3.8 years) were more preoccupied with thinness during their collegiate gymnastics career, but were more satisfied years later with their bodies, than were a nonathletic matched control group. Interestingly, the former gymnasts were leaner and closer to their self-reported ideal body weight after college than the control group.

Bodybuilding has also been associated with many behaviors that could be viewed as unhealthy:

Case Study: Weight Loss in a Bodybuilder

A unique case of a drug-free world-class bodybuilder illustrates how healthy dietary practices and a rigorous training regimen can achieve favorable changes in body composition. This athlete was following a program designed to maintain FFM and decrease body fat. He performed weight training to maintain FFM and increased his amount of endurance exercise to reduce body fat. He made no attempt to decrease energy intake. He performed 2 h of endurance exercise daily, consisting of 1 h of stationary cycling and 1 h of StairMaster (at ~60% $\dot{V}O_2$ max). He performed 3 h of strength training. Table 6.5 outlines his strength training program.

Table 6.6 reviews this bodybuilder's dietary regimen. It was self-imposed, not recommended by a nutritionist. Note his minimal use of protein supplements and his use of **medium-chain triglyceride (MCT) supplements** (fatty acids with 6 to 12 carbons) (see chapter 3 for more information on MCTs). This man's dietary fat intake was extremely low (5% of total energy), and the MCTs provided energy during training. MCTs are absorbed directly into the circulation and transported to the liver, and are rapidly used for energy, with minimal potential for storage in adipose tissue (Bach and Babayan 1982; Johnson et al. 1990; Swift et al. 1990). This diet and exercise regimen is unique since many bodybuilders report consuming high-protein, low-carbohydrate, low-energy diets.

Table 6.5 Three-Day Rotating Weight Training Routine Using a Light, Medium, and Heavy Weight Regimen

Muscle group worked	Number of sets (repetitions/set)		
	Light weights	Medium weights	Heavy weights
Morning workout			
Chest	5 (15)	5 (12)	5 (6-10)
Number of exercises*	6	4	3
Calves	5 (20)	5 (15-20)	5 (15)
Number of exercises	4	2	2
Shoulders	5 (15)	4 (12)	5 (6-10)
Number of exercises	4	6	4
Legs	5 (20)	4-6 (12)	3-5 (10)
Number of exercises	5	3	3
Back	5 (15)	5 (12)	5 (6-10)
Number of exercises	5	4	6
Evening workout			
Triceps	5 (15)	5 (12)	5 (6)
Number of exercises	4	3	3
Hamstrings	5 (20)	5 (15)	5 (6)
Number of exercises	3	5	3
Biceps	5 (15-21)	5 (12)	5 (6)
Number of exercises	3	3	3
Abdomen	5 (20-50)	5 (20)	4-5 (20)
Number of exercises	3	3	3

*Indicates the number of exercises done for each muscle group. For example, for light weights there were six exercises done (incline dumbbell press, incline dumbbell fly, supine barbell bench press, pectoral deck flys, dips, cable crossover) for the chest.

Reprinted from Manore 1993.

Table 6.6 **Mean Nutrient Intakes, From Diets With and Without Medium-Chain Triglyceride (MCT), of a Male Bodybuilder Over an 8-Week Precompetition Training Period**

Nutrient intake	Diet without MCT*	Diet + MCT**
Energy (kcal/d)	3674 ± 279	4952 ± 279
Protein (g/d)*	175 ± 17	175 ± 17
% of kcal/d	19	14
g/kg body wt/d	1.9	1.9
Carbohydrate (g/d)	696 ± 63	696 ± 63
% of kcal/d	76	56
g/kg body wt/d	7.5	7.5
Fat (g/d)	22 ± 4	176 ± 4
% of kcal/d	5	30
Cholesterol (mg/d)	182 ± 61	182 ± 61

*Diet includes carbohydrate (CHO)-containing sport beverage (Exceed, Ross Lab., Columbus, OH): subject consumed 24-36 oz/d; 1 oz = 7.1 g CHO and 28.4 kcal. An additional 12.8 g/d of protein were consumed each day in amino acid supplements; thus, protein intake from diet alone was 162 g/d or 1.75 g/kg body wt.

**MCT = medium-chain triglyceride; MCT provides 8.3 kcal/g; 1 tbsp (15 ml) weighs 14 g. Mean MCT consumed per day was 154 g, which represented 26% of the energy consumed.

Reprinted from Manore 1993.

- Consuming low-kilocalorie diets to decrease body weight and fat
- Use of diuretics and practice of extreme fluid restriction to achieve a more "cut" look
- Use of multiple drugs (including anabolic steroids) and heavy consumption of protein and amino acid supplements in an attempt to achieve large, rapid gains of muscle mass

The incidence of amenorrhea in female bodybuilders has been reported to range from 25-81%. Unhealthy practices, however, are not necessary for success in bodybuilding. Results of a case study of a drug-free bodybuilder illustrate how one athlete was able to achieve desirable changes in body composition by employing healthy recommendations (see "Case Study: Weight Loss in a Bodybuilder," previous page) (Manore et al. 1993).

Sports That Require "Making Weight"

A number of sports require "making weight," or achieving a weight goal within a strictly defined weight class. These sports include horse racing (jockeys), wrestling, boxing, and crew (rowers). Athletes in these sports commonly seek to compete in a weight class lower than their typical body weight to give them an advantage over people who are naturally smaller, and/or to minimize weight that must be carried during an event.

There are two primary concerns about athletes who must make weight: (1) They frequently "weight cycle," a term defined as engaging in repeated cycles of weight loss and weight gain. Some researchers suspect that weight cycling results in a permanent decrease in RMR, which in turn could increase an athlete's risk of obesity and make future attempts at weight loss very difficult. Weight cycling may also increase a person's risk of early mortality. (2) Weight cycling may increase the risk of eating disorders. Weight-cycling sports are associated with an increased incidence of bingeing and purging behaviors, in addition to the abuse of diuretics. Does the scientific literature support these theories?

The well-controlled studies of weight cycling in humans do not show any evidence that weight cycling results in a permanent decrease in RMR (McCargar and Crawford 1992; McCargar et al. 1993; McCargar et al. 1996; Wadden et al. 1996). While the RMR of weight-cycling athletes has been shown to decrease during the competitive season, it increases back to preseason levels once the athletes resume normal eating behaviors (Melby et al. 1990). Whether weight cycling can lead to early death is still controversial. Epidemiological studies suggest that people who experience large fluctuations in weight have increased mortality risk (Hamm et al. 1989). Data from the Framingham Study (Ashley and Kannel 1974) suggest that blood pressure declines with weight loss, while weight gain is associated with a disproportionate increase in blood pressure. Thus, weight cycling could lead to hypertension. Renal ischemia has also been reported in weight-cycling wrestlers (Tcheng and Tipton 1973; Zambraski et al. 1976), which could lead to future problems with hypertension. Others argue that these findings are misleading, as only one longitudinal study of obese individuals participating in weight-cycling behaviors has been done, and found no adverse effects on RMR, body composition, or body fat distribution (Wadden et al. 1996). In addition, there have been no studies of weight cycling and mortality in athletes. As with individuals participating in lean-build sports, athletes attempting to make weight are at an increased risk of eating disorders or of exhibiting disordered eating behaviors. Many of these athletes have very low energy intakes, use diuretics, exercise in extremely warm environments to dehydrate themselves, and even purge themselves to avoid gaining weight after an episode of bingeing. These practices are dangerous to bone health and to fluid and electrolyte balance, and prove detrimental to athletic performance.

Regardless of the sport in which one participates, rapid and extreme weight loss is associated with many detrimental consequences. Table 6.7 lists negative consequences associated with weight loss in athletes and includes healthy recommendations for athletes concerned with body weight (Brownell et al. 1987; Fogelholm 1994; Hoffman and Coleman 1991). It is critical that athletes and coaches understand that there is no single ideal body weight or percentage body fat for an athlete. While many people believe that having a woman decrease her body fat from

14% to 11% will dramatically increase her speed, her performance may actually suffer because of the extreme practices she employs to reach this very low level of body fat. Appendix D provides a table of body fat percentages reported in the literature for a variety of athletes. We have included this table to give coaches, athletes, and sports nutrition professionals an idea of the range of body fat values reported within many sports. Also included in the list are the ranges of body fat percentages reported for amenorrheic female athletes.

Recommendations for Weight Gain

Weight gain is also a concern for many athletes. The ideal would be to achieve maximal gains in lean tissue and minimal gains in fat tissue. It may be unrealistic, however, to expect to gain exclusively lean tissue on a weight-gain program. The key to gaining weight is to consume more energy than one expends. Consuming a high-carbohydrate, low-fat (and high-kilocalorie) diet should result in gaining extra weight that comprises very little body fat.

To have a successful weight-gain program, an athlete should do the following:

- Set realistic weight-gain goals.
- Allow adequate time to reach your goals.
- Assess energy and nutrient levels required for weight maintenance.
- Assess daily energy expenditure.
- Increase energy intake, emphasizing a high-carbohydrate diet.
- Incorporate strength training into the exercise regimen.

Just as it is unrealistic to expect to lose significant amounts of body fat in a short period, gaining weight cannot be accomplished overnight. Realistic weight gains of 0.5-2.0 lb/week (0.2-0.9 kg/week) can be expected based on reasonable increases in energy intake. It is important to document the energy intake, expenditure, and diet composition being consumed at the level of weight maintenance. Once these levels have been established, appropriate recommendations for increases in energy intake can be made. Carbohydrate intake should be maintained at approximately 60% of total daily energy intake, with fat at 20-25%. Increased carbohy-

Table 6.7 Detrimental Consequences of Weight Loss in Athletes, and Recommendations for Avoiding These Consequences

Detrimental consequences of weight loss:
- Decreased aerobic and anaerobic performance
- Glycogen depletion
- Dehydration
- Impaired thermoregulation
- Impaired oxygen and nutrient exchange
- Impaired buffering capacity
- Increased loss of fat-free mass

Recommendations for weight-conscious athletes:
- Initiate weight-control program well in advance of competitive season.
- Determine body fat levels so that realistic weight goals can be set.
- Establish a range of acceptable body fat and weight values, and monitor health and performance within this range.
- Determine specific target level for body weight associated with optimal performance.

■ HIGHLIGHT ■

Gaining Muscle Mass: How Much Energy Is Required?

The exact number of kilocalories needed to gain 1 lb of muscle tissue is not known. One pound of muscle is equal to 454 g (~0.45 kg), but muscle tissue contains mostly water (70-75%), with protein, fat, carbohydrate, and minerals constituting the remaining components. Thus, in 1 lb (454 g) of muscle tissue, only approximately 113.5-136.2 g (assuming 25-30% as protein-containing tissue) is actually protein tissue. To gain 1 lb of muscle/protein tissue, one could suggest an excess intake of 454-545 kcal (assuming 4 kcal/g of protein). However, Bouchard et al. (1990) have shown that consuming excess energy results in a highly variable thermic effect of food. Thus, it is important to keep in mind that the amount of excess weight one can gain will be influenced by the thermic response to overfeeding. It has been suggested that 8 kcal/g are required to support weight gain in adults (Forbes et al. 1986). Considering the above information, a reasonable recommendation for excess energy intake necessary to result in gaining 1 lb (or 454 g) of muscle mass ranges from 1000-3500 kcal.

The following is a brief illustration of recommendations for weight gain. The individual who wishes to gain weight is a 25-year-old man. His body weight is 135 lb (61.4 kg), his height 67 in. (170.2 cm). He wants to weigh 150 lb (68.2 kg), which equals a gain of 15 lb, or 6.8 kg. Analysis of this individual's diet and activity records indicates that he requires approximately 3000 kcal/d to maintain his current weight.

According to the recommendations previously mentioned, this person would need to consume an excess of 1000-3500 kcal to gain 1 lb of lean tissue. Assuming a gain of 1 lb (454 g) per week, this would translate into consuming an excess of 143-500 kcal/d over a 15-week period. Consuming 16 fl oz of 1% or 2% milk (200-240 kcal); one can of a sports supplement drink (360 kcal); or a large bagel, banana, and 1 tbsp of low-fat peanut butter (420 kcal), could easily accomplish this level of energy intake.

In addition to consuming excess energy, this person could also manipulate his energy expenditure to achieve increased FFM. He could perform more strength training and limit endurance exercise to three times/week for 30 min per session (enough to maintain cardiovascular health without burning excessive energy).

drate drives carbohydrate oxidation, but increased fat intake does not drive fat oxidation. Consumption of a high-carbohydrate diet should prevent excessive gains in body fat, and protein intake of 12-15% (or 1-2 g/kg body weight) should be adequate to assist with lean tissue accretion. "Gaining Muscle Mass: How Much Energy Is Required?" (above) discusses some of the issues associated with making energy recommendations for weight gain.

For athletes who are already consuming 4000-5000 kcal/d, weight gain can be quite challenging. These athletes must consume excess energy even if they feel no hunger. Consuming excess solid food can lead to gastrointestinal distress in these athletes, and many find they do not have enough time during the day to consume extra food. For these people, sport supplement drinks or bars between meals may increase energy intake to levels sufficient to cause weight gain.

Ergogenic Aids and Weight Gain— Chromium Supplements

Numerous over-the-counter supplements purport to increase body weight and lean tissue. Chapter 16 describes in detail the use of ergogenic aids in sports. Chapter 4 discusses some of the anabolic supplements athletes might use for weight gain. Following, we briefly discuss three supplements that supposedly result in substantial gains in muscle mass: chromium, amino acids, and creatine.

Some people believe that chromium, via its relationship to the glucose tolerance factor, can enhance the action of insulin, which is critical for the uptake of carbohydrate, fat, and protein into muscle. The glucose tolerance factor is a compound that binds with chromium and contains nicotinic acid, glutamic acid, glycine, and cysteine (Stoecker 1996). Thus, it is theorized that taking chromium (in the form of chromium picolinate) may enhance the muscle's uptake of amino acids (Clarkson 1991; Lefavi et al. 1992), thereby increasing muscle mass and strength. It has also been suggested that athletes may be at an increased risk for chromium deficiency due to inadequate intake and poor absorption of dietary chromium (Lefavi et al. 1992).

Clarkson (1991) reviewed the few published studies of chromium supplementation's effect on body composition in exercising humans. Two studies found that, combined with strength training, chromium supplementation increased FFM and decreased fat mass in men; only one study found these effects in women. There are major limitations in the methodological designs of these studies, however:

- Failure to document chromium status prior to study initiation
- Lack of control for chromium status and dietary intake during the study period
- Measurement of body composition using skinfold calipers

It is possible that the subjects were deficient in chromium, meaning that the supplementation may have normalized levels of chromium and of lean tissue. Unfortunately, the intake of other sources of chromium during the study period was not controlled or documented. Skinfold measures are not considered as accurate in determining body composition as other methods, such as hydrostatic weighing. In addition, the increases in lean tissue and decreases in fat mass reported in these studies were within the margin of error for the method of measurement. Even with the reported changes in body composition, no additional increases in strength were measured because of chromium supplementation. These limitations make it difficult to state with confidence that chromium supplementation results in increases in lean tissue and muscle strength.

Two research groups attempted to address the limitations of the other studies. Clancy et al. (1994) measured body composition using hydrostatic weighing, asked subjects to record dietary

intake, and measured chromium excretion. Chromium supplementation increased chromium excretion but had no effect on body composition (FFM or fat mass) or changes in muscle strength with resistance training. Lukaski et al. (1996) had subjects perform strength training exercise and take one of two forms of chromium supplements (chloride or picolinate) or a placebo. Body composition was assessed using dual-energy X-ray absorptiometry (DXA). Dietary intake was reported before and following training, and chromium status was assessed at baseline and throughout the study. While strength training increased muscle strength and FFM, fat mass was unchanged, and chromium supplements did not enhance strength or FFM. From these findings it appears that chromium supplementation does not increase strength or FFM or reduce body fat in individuals with normal chromium status.

Ergogenic Aids and Weight Gain—Amino Acid Supplements

Amino acid supplementation is widespread among strength athletes and bodybuilders, who believe supplementation of certain amino acids increases secretion of human growth hormone (Evain-Brion et al. 1982; Fogelholm et al. 1993), which is critical for increasing muscle mass and strength. Certain amino acids also increase circulating insulin levels (Bucci et al. 1992; Floyd et al 1966), and, since insulin increases the uptake of amino acids into muscle, the proposed result is increased FFM. Available research data, however, show that *elevation of growth hormone and insulin levels occurs only with certain amino acids infused at supraphysiological doses.* Studies have shown no effects of taking tolerable doses of oral amino acids (doses prescribed by the manufacturer) on growth hormone levels, insulin levels, or muscle strength in humans (Bucci et al. 1992; Fogelholm et al. 1993; Fry et al. 1993; Lambert et al. 1993).

Ergogenic Aids and Weight Gain—Creatine Supplements

Supplementation with creatine (in the form of creatine monohydrate or monophosphate) has been suggested to increase body weight and/or FFM. Creatine supplementation does increase intramuscular levels of creatine, which conceivably could enhance performance by allowing for faster recovery from sprints and explosive-type activities (Maughan 1995). Whether creatine supplementation actually results in improved performance is still controversial. Some studies have shown improvements in performance of high-intensity and sprint exercises with creatine supplementation (Harris et al. 1993; Soderlund et al. 1994), while others have found no benefit (Burke et al. 1996; Redondo et al. 1996).

Creatine may, however, have beneficial effects on body mass and muscle strength. A recent study by Kreider et al. (1996) compared the effects of consuming a carbohydrate supplement, Gainers Fuel 1000 or Phosphagain, on changes in body composition in a group of resistance-trained men. Gainers Fuel 1000 is a supplemental formula that, when taken as directed, supplies 1400 kcal, 290 g carbohydrate, and 60 g protein per day; it also contains chromium picolinate and boron. Phosphagain supplies 570 kcal, 64 g carbohydrate, 67 g protein, and 5 g fat per day, and contains creatine, taurine, and glutamine. After 28 d of treatment, all groups showed significant gains in body weight. However, only the individuals taking the Phosphagain experienced a significant increase in lean tissue (approximately 4.1 lb, or 1.9 kg, in 28 d). The Gainers Fuel 1000 group gained a significant amount of fat weight (1.6 lb or 0.7 kg). No one experienced any change in total body water. All groups trained at similar levels, were asked to maintain their regular diets, and avoided any additional supplements other than those prescribed. Interestingly, the people taking Phosphagain significantly increased lean tissue but reported consuming only 287 kcal/d above initial baseline levels. The Gainers Fuel group reported consuming 1100 kcal/d above baseline by the end of the study period and gained significant levels of body fat. Volek et al. (1999) found that resistance-trained men increased FFM and muscle strength, and changed muscle morphology with creatine supplementation combined with heavy resistance training.

These findings suggest that supplemental formulas containing creatine may result in increases in body weight and lean tissue, and that creatine supplements can impact body composition, muscle strength, and muscle morphology. For anyone trying to gain weight, it is important to avoid any supplements that may result in significant gains in fat mass.

Chapter in Review

The incidence of obesity is rising in developed countries, including the United States. Many people in the United States are attempting to lose weight, including both obese and nonobese individuals who view their body weight as unacceptable. How do we determine the optimal, or healthy, body weight for each individual? *Optimal body weight should be a weight that can be maintained without constant dieting, one that allows physical activity and promotes healthy eating habits, and one for which genetic history of body weight and shape are considered.*

Although the market is flooded with weight-loss programs, sorting fact from fiction can be difficult. Very-low-calorie and starvation diets result in rapid weight loss but also can cause dangerous dehydration and loss of body protein. In addition, few people maintain the weight lost on these diets. Safer and less rapid weight loss can be achieved through low-kilocalorie and moderately low-kilocalorie diets. The key to weight loss and maintenance of optimal body weight is participation in regular physical activity. Athletes can achieve healthy and successful weight loss by avoiding use of pathogenic weight-loss techniques, setting appropriate body composition goals, and avoiding weight loss during the competitive season. When the desire is to gain weight, it is important to maximize lean tissue by (1) increasing total energy intake above daily energy expenditure; (2) eating a diet high in energy and high in complex carbohydrate; and (3) incorporating strength training into the exercise program. Some weight-gain supplements may also be effective in increasing body weight. However, one must be careful when using these products, as some or all of the weight gain may be in body fat.

KEY CONCEPTS

 1. Discuss the role of diet and exercise in achieving healthy body weight.

Both diet and exercise play a critical role in achieving healthy body weight. Energy expenditure must be greater than energy intake for weight loss to occur. Sound weight-loss programs include consumption of a moderately low-energy/fat and high-complex carbohydrate diet (e.g., whole grains, legumes, beans, fruits, and vegetables) plus regular physical activity. Regular physical activity can also help prevent some of the decrease in RMR that occurs with a decrease in energy intake. Maintaining a healthy body weight can decrease the risk of morbidity and mortality from cardiovascular disease, diabetes, and certain forms of cancer.

2. Describe the recommendations for maintaining a healthy body weight.

The recommendations for achieving and maintaining a healthy body weight are similar. Consuming a moderate- to low-fat, high-complex carbohydrate diet, performing regular exercise, and making appropriate behavioral modifications related to dietary intake and exercise are keys to success in maintaining a healthy body weight.

3. Discuss the weight concerns of athletes.

Athletes that compete in lean-build sports such as diving, track and field, dance, swimming, gymnastics, and bodybuilding, and those needing to make weight (e.g., wrestlers and jockeys) are generally quite concerned about their weight. Unfortunately, this intense concern can lead to increased risk for eating disorders and injuries and can threaten athletes' physical, mental, and emotional health. There is no evidence that weight cycling permanently decreases RMR or increases one's risk of mortality. However, rapid and extreme weight loss can lead to dehydration, reduced performance, and even death.

4. Define the recommendations for weight gain.

Weight gain can be achieved safely by setting realistic goals, increasing energy intake (and emphasizing a high-carbohydrate diet that supplies adequate protein), and incorporating strength training into one's exercise regimen. Using sport supplement drinks and bars between meals can help athletes increase energy intake, and creatine supplements can help increase lean mass and muscle strength. Other supplements (e.g., chromium and amino acids) do not appear effective in increasing lean mass, and supplementation can lead to a gain of body fat.

KEY TERMS

3-hydroxyacyl coenzyme A dehydrogenase (HADH)
body mass index (BMI)
computerized tomography (CT)
fad diet
food quotient (FQ)
high-carbohydrate diet
high-fat diet
ketogenic diet
ketosis
low-kilocalorie diet

medium-chain triglyceride (MCT) supplement
meta-analysis
moderate energy restriction diet
obesity
overweight
pathogenic weight-loss technique
protein-sparing modified fast (PSMF)
respiratory quotient (RQ)
starvation diet (or fasting)
very-low-calorie diet (VLCD)
waist-to-hip ratio (WHR)

References

Ainsworth BE, Haskell WL, Leon AS, Jacobs Jr. DS, Montoye HJ, Sallis JF, Paffenbarger Jr. RS. Compendium of physical activities: classification by energy costs of human physical activities. Med Sci Sport Exerc 1993;25:71-80.

Andersen RE, Wadden TA, Bartlett SJ, Zemel B, Verde TJ, Franckowiak BS. Effects of lifestyle activity vs structured aerobic exercise in obese women: a randomized trial. JAMA 1999;281:335-40.

Ashley FW, Kannel WB. Relation of weight change to changes in atherogenic traits. J Chronic Diseases 1974;27:103-14.

Bach AC, Babayan VK. Medium-chain triglycerides: an update. Am J Clin Nutr 982;36:950-62.

Ballor DL, Katch VL, Becque MD, Marks CR. Resistance weight training during caloric restriction enhances lean body weight maintenance. Am J Clin Nutr 1988;47:19-25.

Belko AZ, VanLoan M, Barbieri TF, Mayclin P. Diet, exercise, weight loss, and energy expenditure in moderately overweight women. Int J Obesity 1987;11:93-104.

Blackburn GL, Lynch ME, Wong SL. The very-low-calorie diet: a weight-reduction technique. In: Brownell KD, Foreyt JP, eds. Handbook of Eating Disorders: Physiology, Psychology, and Treatment of Obesity, Anorexia, and Bulemia. New York: Basic Books, 1986:198-212.

Blair SN. Evidence for success of exercise in weight loss and control. Ann Internal Med 1993;119:702-6.

Bogardus C, LaGrange BM, Horton ES, Sims EA. Comparison of carbohydrate-containing and carbohydrate-restricted hypocaloric diets in the treatment of obesity. J Clin Invest 1981;68:399-404.

Bouchard C, Tremblay A, Després J-P, et al. The response to long-term overfeeding in identical twins. N Engl J Med 1990;322:1477-82.

Bray GA. Classification and evaluation of the obesities. Med J North Am 1989;73:161-84.

Bray GA. Pathophysiology of obesity. Am J Clin Nutr 1992;55:488S-94S.

Bray GA, Gray DS. Obesity. Part II—Treatment. West J Med 1988;149:555-71.

Broeder CE, Burrhus KA, Svanevik LS, Wilmore JH. The effects of either high-intensity resistance or endurance training on resting metabolic rate. Am J Clin Nutr 1992;55:802-10.

Brooks GA, Fahey TD, White TP. Exercise Physiology: Human Bioenergetics and Its Applications. 2nd ed. Mountain View, CA: Mayfield, 1996.

Brownell KD, Kramer FM. Behavioral management of obesity. In: Blackburn GL, Kanders BS, eds. Obesity. Pathophysiology, Psychology, and Treatment. New York: Chapman and Hall, 1994.

Brownell KD, Steen SN, Wilmore J. Weight regulation practices in athletes: analysis of metabolic and health effects. Med Sci Sports Exerc 1987;19:546-56.

Bucci LR, Hickson JF, Wolinsky I, Pivarnik JM. Ornithine supplementation and insulin release in bodybuilders. Int J Sport Nutr 1992;2:287-91.

Burke LM, Pyne DB, Telford RD. Effect of oral creatine supplementation on single-effort sprint performance in elite swimmers. Int J Sport Nutr 1996;6:222-33.

Calle EE, Thun MJ, Petrelli JM, Rodriguez C, Heath CW, Jr. Body-mass index and mortality in a prospective cohort of U.S. adults. N Engl J Med 1999;341:1097-105.

Clancy SP, Clarkson PM, DeCheke ME, Nosaka K, Freedson PS, Cunningham JJ, Valentine B. Effects of chromium picolinate supplementation on body composition, strength, and urinary chromium loss in football players. Int J Sport Nutr 1994;4:142-53.

Clarkson PM. Nutritional ergogenic aids: chromium, exercise, and muscle mass. Int J Sport Nutr 1991;1:289-93.

Datillo AM, Kris-Etherton PM. Effects of weight reduction on blood lipids and lipoproteins: a meta-analysis. Am J Clin Nutr 1992;56:320-8.

Deprés J-P, Ross R, Lemieux S. Imaging techniques applied to the measurement of human body composition. In: Roche AF, Heymsfield SB, Lohman TG, eds. Human Body Composition. Champaign, IL: Human Kinetics, 1996.

Donnelly JE, Jacobsen DJ, Jakicic JM, Whatley JE. Very low calorie diet with concurrent versus delayed and sequential exercise. Int J Obesity 1994;18:469-75.

Donnelly JE, Pronk NP, Jacobsen DJ, Pronk SJ, Jakicic JM. Effects of a very-low-calorie diet and physical-training regimens on body composition and resting metabolic rate in obese females. Am J Clin Nutr 1991;54:56-61.

Duncan KH, Bacon JA, Weinsier RL. The effects of high and low energy density diets on satiety, energy intake, and eating time of obese and nonobese subjects. Am J Clin Nutr 1983;37:763-7.

Dunn AL, Marcus BH, Kampert JB, Garcia ME, Kohl HW, Blair SN. Comparison of lifestyle and structured interventions to increase physical activity and cardiorespiratory fitness: a randomized trial. JAMA 999;281:327-34.

Durrant ML, Royston JP, Wloch RT. Effect of exercise on energy intake and eating patterns in lean and obese humans. Physiol Behav 1982;29:449-54.

Epstein LH, Wing RR. Aerobic exercise and weight. Addictive Behav 1980;5:371-88.

Evain-Brion D, Donnadieu M, Roger M, Job JC. Simultaneous study of somatotrophic and corticotrophic pituitary secretions during ornithine infusion test. Clin Endocrinol 1982;17:119-22.

Fábry P, Fodor J, Hejl Z. The frequency of meals: its relationship to overweight, hypercholesterolemia, and decreased glucose-tolerance. Lancet 1964;2:614-5.

Flatt JP. The biochemistry of energy expenditure. In: Bjorntorp P, Brodoff BN, eds. Obesity. Philadelphia: Lippincott Co., 1992:100-16.

Floyd JC, Fajans SS, Conn JW, Knopf RF, Rull J. Stimulation of insulin secretion by amino acids. J Clin Invest 1966;45:1487-1502.

Fogelholm M. Effects of bodyweight reduction on sports performance. Sports Med 1994;18:249-67.

Fogelholm GM, Näveri HK, Kiilavuori KTK, Härkönen MHA. Low-dose amino acid supplementation: no effects on serum human growth hormone and insulin in male weightlifters. Int J Sport Nutr 1993;3:290-7.

Food Processor (software program), Version 7.21. ESHA Research, Salem, OR.

Forbes GB, Brown MR, Welle SL, Lipinski BA. Deliberate overfeeding in women and men: energy cost and composition of the weight gain. Br J Nutr 1986;56(1):1-9.

Fox AA, Thompson JL, Butterfield GE, Gylfadottir U, Moynihan S, Spiller G. Effects of diet and exercise on common cardiovascular disease risk factors in moderately obese older women. Am J Clin Nutr 1996;63:225-33.

Fry AC, Kraemer WJ, Stone MH, et al. Endocrine and performance responses to high volume training and amino acid supplementation in elite junior weightlifters. Int J Sport Nutr 1993;3:306-22.

Garrow JS, Summerbell CD. Meta-analysis: effect of exercise, with or without dieting, on the body composition of overweight subjects. Eur J Clin Nutr 1995;49:1-10.

Gaesser G. Thinness and weight loss: beneficial or detrimental to longevity? Med Sci Sports Exerc 1999;1118-28.

Hamm P, Shekelle RB, Stamler J. Large fluctuations in body weight during young adulthood and twenty-five-year risk of coronary death in men. Am J Epidemiol 1989;129:312-8.

Hammer RL, Barrier CA, Roundy ES, Bradford JM, Fisher AG. Calorie-restricted low-fat diet and exercise in obese women. Am J Clin Nutr 1989;49:77-85.

Harris RC, Viru M, Greenhaff PL, Hultman E. The effect of oral creatine supplementation on running performance during maximal short term exercise in man. J Physiol 1993;467:74P.

Heymsfield SB, Casper K, Hearn J, Guy D. Rate of weight loss during underfeeding: relation to level of physical activity. Metabolism 1989;38:215-23.

Hill JO, Schlundt DG, Sbrocco T, et al. Evaluation of an alternating-calorie diet with and without exercise in the treatment of obesity. Am J Clin Nutr 1989;50:248-54.

Hill JO, Sparling PB, Shields TW, Heller PA. Effects of exercise and food restriction on body composition and metabolic rate in obese women. Am J Clin Nutr 1987;46:622-30.

Hoffman CJ, Coleman E. An eating plan and update on recommended dietary practices for the endurance athlete. J Am Diet Assoc 1991;91:325-30.

Horm J, Anderson K. Who in America is trying to lose weight? Ann Intern Med 1993;119:672-6.

Johnson RC, Young SK, Cotter R, Lin L, Rowe WB. Medium-chain-triglyceride lipid emulsion: metabolism and tissue distribution. Am J Clin Nutr 1990;52:502-8.

Keim NL, Barbieri TF, VanLoan MD, Anderson BL. Energy expenditure and physical performance in overweight women: response to training with and without caloric restriction. Metabolism 1990;39:651-8.

Kramer FM, Jeffery RW, Forster JL, Snell MK. Long-term follow-up of behavioral treatment for obesity: patterns of weight regain among men and women. Int J Obesity 1989;13:123-36.

Kreider RB, Klesges R, Harmon K, et al. Effects of ingesting supplements designed to promote lean tissue accretions on body composition during resistance training. Int J Sport Nutr 1996;6:234-46.

Lambert MI, Hefer JA, Millar RP, Macfarlane PW. Failure of commercial oral amino acid supplements to increase serum growth hormone concentrations in male body-builders. Int J Sport Nutr 1993;3:298-305.

Lawson S, Webster JD, Pacy PJ, Garrow JS. Effect of a 10-week aerobic exercise programme on metabolic rate, body composition and fitness in lean sedentary females. Br J Clin Prac 1987;41:684-8.

Lee CD, Blair SN, Jackson AS. Cardiorespiratory fitness, body composition, and all-cause and cardiovascular disease mortality in men. Am J Clin Nutr 1999;69:373-80.

Lefavi RG, Anderson RA, Keith RE, Wilson GD, McMillan JL, Stone MH. Efficacy of chromium supplementation in athletes: emphasis on anabolism. Int J Sport Nutr 1992;2:111-22.

Lissner L, Levitsky DA, Strupp BJ, Kalkwarf HJ, Roe DA. Dietary fat and the regulation of energy intake in human subjects. Am J Clin Nutr 1987;46:886-92.

Lukaski HC, Bolonchuk WW, Siders WA, Milne DB. Chromium supplementation and resistance training: effects on body composition, strength, and trace element status of men. Am J Clin Nutr 1996;63:954-65.

Manore MM, Thompson JL, Russo M. Diet and exercise strategies of a drug-free world class bodybuilder. Int J Sport Nutr 1993;3:76-86.

Manson JE, Willett WC, Stampfer MJ, et al. Body weight and mortality among women. N Engl J Med 1995;333:677-85.

Maughan RJ. Creatine supplementation and exercise performance. Int J Sport Nutr 1995;5:94-101.

McCargar LJ, Crawford SM. Metabolic and anthropometric changes with weight cycling in wrestlers. Med Sci Sports Exerc 1992;24:1270-5.

McCargar LJ, Sale J, Crawford SM. Chronic dieting does not result in a sustained reduction in resting metabolic rate in overweight women. J Am Diet Assoc 1996;96:1175-7.

McCargar L, Taunton J, Laird Birmingham C, Paré S, Simmons D. Metabolic and anthropometric changes in female weight cyclers and controls over a 1-year period. J Am Diet Assoc 1993;93:1025-30.

Melby CL, Schmidt WD, Corrigan D. Resting metabolic rate in weight-cycling collegiate wrestlers compared with physically active, noncycling control subjects. Am J Clin Nutr 1990;52:409-14.

Meredith CN, Frontera WR, Fisher EC, Hughes VA, Herland JC. Peripheral effects of endurance training in young and old subjects. J Appl Physiol 1989;66:2844-9.

The National Adolescent Student Health Survey. The National Adolescent Student Health Survey: A Report on the Health of America's Youth. Oakland, CA: Third Party Publishing, 1989.

National Heart, Lung and Blood Institute (NHLBI). Clinical Guidelines on the Identification, Evaluation, and Treatment of Overweight and Obesity in Adults. The Evidence Report. National Institutes of Health, U.S. Dept. of Health and Human Services, June 1998.

O'Conner PJ, Lewis RD, Kirchner EM, Cook DB. Eating disorder symptoms in former female college gymnasts: relations with body composition. Am J Clin Nutr 1996;64:840-3.

Pavlou KN, Krey S, Steffee WP. Exercise as an adjunct to weight loss and maintenance in moderately obese subjects. Am J Clin Nutr 1989;49:1115-23.

Pavlou KN, Whatley JE, Jannace PW, DiBartolomeo JJ, Burrows BA, Duthie EAM, Lerman RH. Physical activity as a supplement to a weight-loss dietary regimen. Am J Clin Nutr 1989;49:1110-4.

Phinney SD, LaGrange BM, O'Conner M, Danforth EJ. Effects of aerobic exercise on energy expenditure and nitrogen balance during very low calorie dieting. Metabolism 1988;37:758-65.

Reaven GM. Syndrome X: 6 years later. J Int Med 1994;236(suppl. 736):13-22.

Redondo DR, Dowling EA, Graham BL, Almada AL, Williams MH. The effect of oral creatine monohydrate supplementation on running velocity. Int J Sport Nutr 1996;6:213-21.

Rosen LW, Hough DO. Pathogenic weight-control behaviors of female college gymnasts. Phys Sportsmed 1988;16:141-4.

Rosen LW, McKeag DB, Hough DO, Curley V. Pathogenic weight-control behaviors in female athletes. Phys Sportsmed 1986;14:79-86.

Schutz Y, Flatt JP, Jéquier E. Failure of dietary fat intake to promote fat oxidation: a factor favoring the development of obesity. Am J Clin Nutr 1989;50:307-14.

Serdula MK, Collins ME, Williamson DF, Anda RF, Pamuk E, Byers TE. Weight control practices of U.S. adolescents and adults. Ann Intern Med 1993;119:667-71.

Soderlund K, Balsom PD, Ekblom B. Creatine supplementation and high intensity exercise: Influence on performance and muscle metabolism. Clin Sci 1994;87(suppl.):120-1.

Stoecker BJ. Chromium. In: Ziegler EE, Filer LJ, eds. Present Knowledge in Nutrition, 7th ed. Washington, DC: ILSI Press, 1996.

Sundgot-Borgen J. Prevalence of eating disorders in elite female athletes. Int J Sport Nutr 1993;3:29-40.

Sundgot-Borgen J. Eating disorders, energy intake, training volume, and menstrual function in high-level modern rhythmic gymnasts. Int J Sport Nutr 1996;6:100-9.

Svendsen OL, Hassager C, Christiansen C. Effect of an energy-restrictive diet, with or without exercise, on lean tissue mass, resting metabolic rate, and cardiovascular risk factors, and bone in overweight postmenopausal women. Am J Med 1993;95:131-40.

Swift LL, Hill JO, Peters JC, Greene HL. Medium-chain fatty acids: evidence of incorporation into chylomicron triglycerides in humans. Am J Clin Nutr 1990;52:834-6.

Tcheng TK, Tipton CM. Iowa Wrestling Study: anthropometric measurements and the prediction of a minimal body weight. Med Sci Sports 1973;5:1-10.

Thomas PR, ed. Weighing the Options. Food and Nutrition Board, Institute of Medicine. Washington, DC: National Academy Press, 1995.

Thompson JL, Gylfadottir UK, Moynihan S, Jensen CD, Butterfield GE. Effects of diet and exercise on energy expenditure in postmenopausal women. Am J Clin Nutr 1997;66:867-73.

Thompson JL, Manore MM, Thomas JR. Effects of diet and diet-plus-exercise programs on resting metabolic rate: a meta-analysis. Int J Sport Nutr 1996;6:41-61.

Tremblay A, Plourde G, Després J-P, Bouchard C. Impact of dietary fat content and fat oxidation on energy intake in humans. Am J Clin Nutr 1989;49:799-805.

Tremblay A, Simoneau JA, Bouchard C. Impact of exercise intensity on body fatness and skeletal muscle metabolism. Metabolism 1994;43(7);814-8.

Tremblay A, Fontaine E, Poehlman ET, Mitchell D, Perron L, Bouchard C. The effect of exercise-training on resting metabolic rate in lean and moderately obese individuals. Int J Obesity 1986;10:511-7.

van Dale D, Beckers E, Schoffelen PFM, ten Hoor F, Saris WHM. Changes in sleeping metabolic rate and glucose induced thermogenesis during a diet or a diet/exercise treatment. Nutr Res 1990;10:615-26.

Van Itallie TB. Obesity: adverse effects on health and longevity. Am J Clin Nutr 1979;32:2723.

Van Itallie TB. Health implications of overweight and obesity in the United States. Ann Inter Med 1985;103:983-8.

Van Itallie TB. Body weight, morbidity, and longevity. In: Bjorntorp B, Brodoff BN, eds. Obesity. Philadelphia: Lippincott Co., 1992.

Van Itallie TB, Yang M-U. Cardiac dysfunction in obese dieters: a potentially lethal complication of rapid, massive weight loss. Am J Clin Nutr 1984;39:695-702.

Volek JS, Duncan ND, Mazzetti SA, et al. Performance and muscle fiber adaptations to creatine supplementation and heavy resistance training. Med Sci Sports Exerc 1999; 31:1147-56.

Wadden TA, Foster GD, Stunkard AJ, Conill AM. Effects of weight cycling on the resting energy expenditure and body composition of obese women. Int J Eating Disorders. 1996;19:5-12.

Warren MP. The effects of exercise on pubertal progression and reproductive function in girls. J Clin Endocrinol Metab 1980;51: 1150.

Willett WC, Dietz WH, Colditz GA. Guidelines for healthy weight. New Engl J Med 1999;341:427-34.

Woo R, Garrow JS, Pi-Sunyer FX. Voluntary food intake during prolonged exercise in obese women. Am J Clin Nutr 1982;36:478-84.

Wei M, Macera CA, Hornung CA, and Blair SN. Changes in lipids associated with change in regular exercise in free-living men. J Clin Epidemiol 1997;50:1137-42.

Zambraski EJ, Foster DT, Gross PM, Tipton CM. Iowa Wrestling Study: weight loss and urinary profile of collegiate wrestlers. Med Sci Sports 1976;8:105-8.

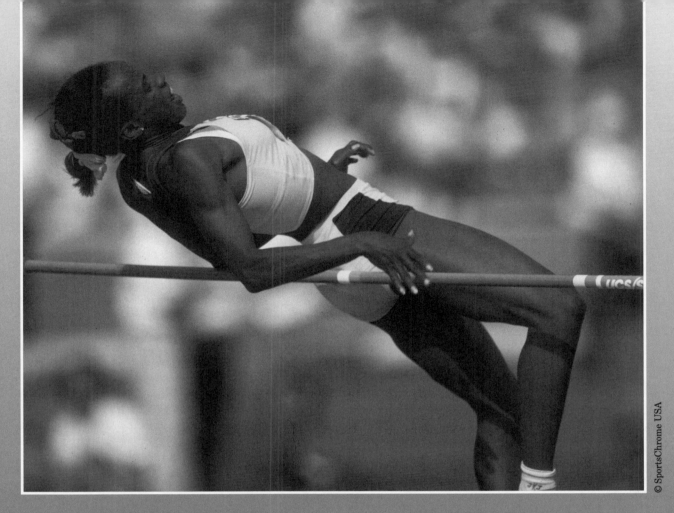

© SportsChrome USA

CHAPTER 7

Body Composition

After reading this chapter you will be able to

- understand the relationship between body composition and health;
- describe the relationship between body composition and sport performance;
- compare body composition assessment models and methods;
- understand the accuracy of body composition assessment;
- identify selection criteria for field methods;
- discuss body composition status of athletes; and
- explain the relationship between body composition standards and health.

What is the ideal level of body fat? How do my weight and body fat level affect my athletic performance or health? What is the best way to measure body composition? These are questions frequently asked by athletes and fitness enthusiasts. To answer their questions, you must understand how body composition relates to health and athletic performance and how to accurately and reliably measure body composition.

Although a scale can accurately measure body weight, mere weight provides no information about the body's composition. For example: a male bodybuilder or football player may weigh more for his height than standard weight tables recommend simply because he is very muscular, and not because he has excess body fat. Measuring body composition provides information on the absolute and relative amounts of the components that make up the human body. Direct measurement of body composition in living humans is not feasible, since it requires the dissection and chemical analysis of the body. Scientists have therefore developed various models and methods for indirect estimation of body components.

This chapter briefly summarizes the relationships among body composition, health, and athletic performance; reviews the strengths and limitations of body composition assessment models and methods; and presents guidelines

for making and interpreting body composition measurements.

Body Composition and Health

The human body contains more than 30 major components at the elemental (atomic), molecular, cellular, and tissue-system levels (Wang et al. 1992). Chemical components of body composition that can be estimated include relative fat mass (FM), fat-free mass (FFM), and the major components of FFM—water, mineral, and protein. Although FM is the component of body composition most often assessed, FFM and its components have an equal, if not more important, relationship to health and athletic performance (see "Body Fat and Health," below). FFM includes the organs, soft tissues, and skeletal tissues. Low levels of FFM and loss of FFM are related to impaired functional capacity and decreased physical activity/energy expenditure—and thus to increased risk for gain of FM. Muscle wasting that occurs with certain diseases and with aging not only decreases muscle strength and the capacity to perform even routine activities, but it is also strongly related to mortality (Going and Davis 1998). Low bone mineral mass and density are key predictors of osteoporotic fracture risk.

■ HIGHLIGHT ■

Body Fat and Health

There is a strong association between excess body fat—especially excess intra-abdominal (visceral) fat—and increased risk of coronary artery disease, non-insulin dependent diabetes, hypertension, and certain types of cancers (Going and Davis 1998). This means that obese people with android, or central-body, fat distribution (apple shape), who store excess fat in their trunk region, are at greater risk for certain diseases than those with a gynoid fat distribution in which excess fat is stored in hips and thighs (pear shape).

The ratio between waist circumference and hip circumference is often used as an index of the distribution of adipose tissues. An elevated waist:hip ratio (WHR) is usually considered to be an indication of proportionally more abdominal adipose tissue and is associated with an increased risk for some cardiovascular diseases and diabetes. The usefulness of WHR as an indicator of relative adipose tissue distribution has been established in adults but not in children and youth (Malina 1996). Additional research is needed to separate effects of fat distribution from those of total body fat and to assess fat distribution as an independent factor for health risks.

Body Composition and Sport Performance

Although various researchers have reported ranges of relative body fat (%BF) for successful athletes within specific sports, body composition by itself cannot accurately predict athletic performance. All the components of physique—body size, structure, and composition—are significant determinants of athletic success. Each is related to performance in a logical and predictable way. More massive individuals, for example, have an advantage over their lighter counterparts when an activity demands that the inertia of another body or an external object must be overcome (e.g., tackling a runner in football). People with less body mass have the advantage when the goal is to move the body, especially over moderate to long distances (e.g., marathon runner). Taller people, with longer levers (limbs) and a higher center of gravity, have the advantage in jumping and throwing events (e.g., javelin throw or long jump), whereas shorter persons have the advantage when the body must be rotated around an axis (e.g., diving and tumbling).

Fat Mass and Performance

There generally appears to be an inverse relationship between FM and performance of physical activities requiring movement of the body either vertically (such as in jumping) or horizontally (as in running) (Boileau and Lohman 1977; Malina 1992; Pate et al. 1989). Excess fatness is detrimental to these types of activities because it adds non-force-producing mass to the body. Since acceleration is proportional to force but inversely proportional to mass, excess fat at a given level of force can result in slower changes in velocity and direction (Boileau and Lohman 1977; Harman and Frykman 1992). Excess fat also increases the metabolic cost of physical activities requiring movement of the total body mass (Buskirk and Taylor 1957). In most activities involving movement of the body mass, therefore, a relatively low %BF should be advantageous both mechanically and metabolically (Boileau and Lohman 1977).

Cross-sectional data indicate that %BF is inversely related both to aerobic capacity ($\dot{V}O_2$max) expressed relative to body weight and to distance running performance (Cureton 1992). Only a few experimental studies have investigated the effects of altered body composition on physical performance. Running performance of fit, normal-weight people in these studies decreased with increasing weight added by a weight belt and shoulder harness (Cureton and Sparling 1980; Cureton et al. 1978; Sparling and Cureton 1983). Their performances were similar to those of obese individuals with similar FFM but greater body weight.

In contrast, in some sports for which absorbing force or momentum is important (such as contact sports), adequate amounts of appropriately distributed FM are advantageous. Long-distance swimmers also benefit from a relatively high FM compared to other athletic groups because of the role fat plays in thermal insulation and its contribution to buoyancy (Sinning 1985).

Fat-Free Mass and Performance

Performance of activities that require application of force, particularly against external objects (e.g., throwing, pushing, and weight lifting), is positively related to the absolute amount of FFM and therefore to body size (Boileau and Lohman 1977; Harman and Frykman 1992). On the other hand, a large absolute amount of FFM and large body size can negatively affect performance that requires translocation of body weight—such as running, jumping, or rotation of the body about an axis (as in gymnastics or diving). It is obvious that an elite gymnast would not perform well as an offensive lineman in football, or vice versa.

The best positive correlations of physical performance for military-related physical tasks are with FFM rather than %BF. In investigations of the relationship of body composition to performance of military tasks, FFM was the best predictor of performance as assessed by maximal aerobic capacity; treadmill run time; 12-min run distance; and the ability to push, carry, and exert torque (Harman and Frykman 1992). *For most sports, high FFM:FM ratios at a given body weight are associated with better performance, although too little body fat results in deterioration of both health and performance* (Houtkooper 1998; Sinning 1985; Wilmore 1992).

Problems of Extreme Leanness

Athletes in sports such as gymnastics, dancing, diving, bodybuilding, distance running, and track are typically very lean. They follow rigorous training programs and often restrict their dietary intake in order to control their weight. Male athletes most desirous of low fat mass are in sports for which participants must make weight (e.g., wrestling, boxing, horse racing, lightweight rowing, or football). The potential advantage of a low %BF for successful performance of athletes in these types of sports is evident. However, there are negative health and performance implications related to extreme weight loss (Sinning 1996). Minimal levels of %BF considered compatible with good health are 5% for males and 12% for females (Lohman 1992b).

Athletes whose weight drops below a certain desirable level are likely to experience decrements in performance and increases in both minor and major illnesses and injuries (Sinning 1996; Wilmore 1992). Severe weight cutting, secondary to severe short-term starvation and dehydration, can reduce isometric and dynamic strength; over the long term, it can contribute to abnormal kidney function (Sinning 1985).

Athletes who constantly strive to reach or maintain an inappropriate weight or %BF are at risk for developing eating disorders. At the elite or world-class level of several sports, the prevalence of eating disorders in females is approximately 50% (Houtkooper 1998; Wilmore 1992). Female athletes prone to eating disorders are also at high risk of developing a triad of interrelated disorders that includes anorexia nervosa or bulimia nervosa, menstrual dysfunction, and bone demineralization (Houtkooper 1998; Wilmore 1992).

Body Composition Assessment Models and Methods

Methods of assessing body composition can be categorized as direct, indirect, or double indirect. **Direct methods** such as dissection and chemical analysis of tissues or of whole cadavers are obviously not feasible for living humans. However, they are critical because they provide the basic data that are the foundation from which indirect assessment techniques are developed. **Indirect methods** can be either property- or component-based (Heymsfield et al. 1996). **Property-based methods** measure specific properties such as body volume, decay properties of specific atomic isotopes, or bioelectrical resistance. For example, neutron activation analysis of living humans (Ellis 1996) has made possible nondestructive chemical analysis of the human body by measuring radiation given off during decay of excited atoms. A more common property-based

method is estimation of **total body water (TBW)** from deuterium dilution, which involves measuring the dilution in the body of a known dose of deuterium isotope using a sample of body fluid.

Component-based methods depend on well-established models that usually represent ratios of measurable quantities of body components that are assumed constant both within and between individuals. With component-based methods, the measured quantity of one component is first estimated by a property-based method, and then another body component is estimated using a body composition model. For example, FFM can be estimated using deuterium dilution to measure the TBW component—the observed TBW value is converted to FFM based on the assumed constant relationship between TBW and FFM. Since this ratio in healthy adults is about 0.74 (74% of FFM is TBW), FFM = TBW × 1.35 (Brozek 1963). While it is known that the ratio is higher in healthy infants, children, and youths, studies to determine values in aging adults are currently being conducted.

Two types of mathematical functions are used to estimate body composition using property- and component-based methods (Going and Davis 1998). The **model approach,** which depends on a known ratio between a specific constituent and the component of interest, was illustrated above. In the other approach, **regression analysis** of experimental data provides a prediction equation that relates a measured property or component to an "unknown" (estimated) component. Usually, the prediction equation is developed by measuring the unknown component using a reference method in a defined group of subjects. For example, you can use **densitometry (underwater weighing)** as a reference method to measure body volume (see figure 7.1) and a weight scale to measure body mass on land—then you calculate body density using the simple equation body density = mass/volume. The property of a known component related to body composition is also measured in these same subjects. For example, the known component can be skinfold thicknesses. Regression analysis then provides equations relating the known component (in this case skinfold thicknesses) to the unknown component (body density). This approach has yielded equations for estimating body fat from skinfolds, circumferences, or bioelectrical resistance. Because they generally depend on a combination of both property-based and component-based methods and are then used to estimate an unknown component, these assessment methods are considered to be "doubly indirect."

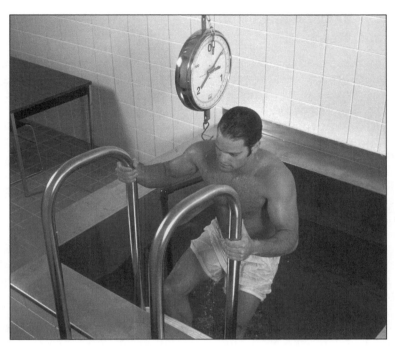

Figure 7.1 Underwater weighing (UWW) is a two-component body composition model (FFM and FM) that uses the principle of densitometry. It is considered one of the criterion methods for body composition assessment.

Two-Component Models and Methods

The two-component chemical model has been the primary one used to study the relationship between body composition and physical performance. This model divides the body into fat mass and fat-free mass. Fat is a molecular-level chemical component, not to be confused with fat cells or adipose tissue, which are cellular and tissue-system components of body composition. The terms fat and lipid are often confused and inappropriately interchanged (Heymsfield and Wang 1993). Fat refers to the family of chemical compounds called triacylglycerols (triglycerides), whereas lipid is the more general term that includes triacylglycerols and many other compounds (Gurr and Harwood 1991). In the two-component chemical model, the fat component historically has included all lipids; all other body constituents are included in the FFM. The **fat mass (FM)** is the *weight of all the lipids in the body that can be chemically extracted, using ether as the solvent. FFM is the weight of all tissues in the body minus the FM.* In more complex three- or four-component chemical models, the FFM is subdivided into its major constituents water, mineral, and protein (Boileau and Lohman 1977).

This two-component model is based on the assumptions that FFM and FM each have a constant density and a constant composition of constituents for all individuals in a given population (Siri 1961). The density of adult human fat is relatively constant within and among individuals at 0.900 g/cm³ (Lohman 1986). Considerable data demonstrate that the density and composition of FFM are not constant in growing children, and studies are in progress to assess changes in FFM in adults during aging. Chemical maturity of FFM in humans (i.e., chemical stability in the constituents of FFM) does not occur until after puberty (Lohman 1986, 1989). A person is considered to be **chemically mature** when FFM composition reaches the reference values for a chemically mature adult male: 73.8% water, 6.8% mineral, and 19.4% protein, with a density of 1.100 g/cm³ (Brozek et al. 1963); this usually happens between 16 and 18 years of age, with girls maturing earlier than boys (Lohman et al. 1984). Prepubescent and pubescent children deviate considerably from adults in FFM composition and density—generally having relatively higher water content and lower mineral and protein contents, which together result in an FFM density lower than the 1.100 g/cm³ of chemically mature adults (Boileau et al. 1984; Hewitt et al. 1993; Lohman 1986).

201

Multiple-Component Body Composition Criterion Models and Methods

In theory, the more constituents of the FFM (water, mineral, protein) that can be accurately measured, the more accurate the FFM and FM estimates. This theory has been the basis for development of multiple-component "criterion" methods for estimating body composition in youths. Such methods, which are considered the "gold standard" of methods, are referred to as **criterion methods** because they provide more accurate estimates of body composition—especially of chemically immature youths—than those based on two-component models (Lohman 1992b; Siri 1961). (See "Criterion Methods of Assessing Body Composition," below.)

Multiple-component models minimize potential errors in estimates of %BF associated with variability in FFM composition. The ideal laboratory procedure is to combine measures of **whole-body density (D_b)** with measures of body water and bone mineral and to estimate body composition using an equation based on a four-component model. This approach eliminates the need for assumptions about the proportions of FFM constituents and provides the best estimate of body composition against which to validate field methods of body composition assessment.

Alternatively, D_b can be combined with measures of body water or bone mineral, and equations based on three-component models can be derived. Although more accurate than the two-component equations, these equations assume a constant protein:mineral or protein:water ratio—and individual deviations from the assumed ratios introduce error, albeit less than in the two-component model.

A concern about multi-component models has been the increased potential for measurement error when measuring individual components of the FFM. Several investigators have assessed the extent to which measurement errors for individual techniques in the multi-component model are passed on (propagated) in the assessment of body composition (Friedl et al. 1992; Fuller et al. 1992; Lohman 1992b). The data suggest that the improved accuracy of three-component and four-component models is not compromised by errors arising from individual techniques *if measurements are carefully made.*

Validation of Body Composition Assessment Methods

A new or existing method is considered to be valid if it provides an estimate of body composition that is close to the value obtained using a criterion method described previously and if the estimate is reproducible (Lohman 1992b). The relative *accuracy* of the method being tested is determined by the size of the prediction error (standard error of the estimate, or root-mean-square error). *Reliability* (also referred to as *precision)* is assessed by the magnitude of the standard deviation for repeated measurements, or magnitude of the coefficient of variation for the measurements.

Cross-validation is the final aspect of validating a new or existing assessment method. In the cross-validation process, the assessment method being evaluated is used to estimate body composition in an independent group to determine how closely the method predicts body composition compared to the criterion method. An independent group ideally comprises a new, representative sample of individuals. In the most rigorous cross-validation studies, the tests are done in a laboratory run by investigators other than the ones who conducted the original validation study but using the same techniques employed in the original study. Alternative cross-validation stud-

■ HIGHLIGHT ■

Criterion Methods of Assessing Body Composition

There are many different ways to assess body composition. Those methods that to date are considered the most accurate are called "criterion methods" or "gold standards." Since the measurement of body composition can involve different models (two-, three-, and four-component models), each model has its own criterion method(s). For example, densitometry (underwater weighing) is considered a criterion method for the two-component model of assessing body composition. Thus, it has been used as the criterion method to develop another two-component model of assessing body composition, the skinfold method.

ies are conducted in the same laboratory that developed the new method or equation, using either a separate sample of subjects or the subjects in the original study but with statistical adjustments. The body composition assessment method being tested is considered accurate and reliable or precise if the results of the cross-validation study indicate that the prediction errors and reliability estimates for the body composition variables are within acceptable ranges. A later section of this chapter presents the criteria for acceptable ranges of prediction errors.

Criterion Methods of Body Composition Assessment

The four most widely applied criterion methods or "gold standard" methods of measuring body composition are densitometry, hydrometry, ^{40}K spectroscopy, and dual-energy X-ray absorptiometry (DXA) (see figure 7.2). Each of these methods has been described in detail by others and will be briefly reviewed in this chapter (Brozek et al. 1963; Ellis 1996; Going 1996; Lohman 1986, 1996; Lukaski 1987; Siri 1961).

Densitometry The densitometry approach to body composition assessment is based on the relationship between whole-body density (D_b) and the respective densities of the body compartments, regardless of how they are defined. The general principle is that D_b varies inversely with FM:

Equation 1 $F = f(1/D_b)$

where F is the ether-extractable lipid fraction of body mass (FM), and f is the function describing the relationship between FM and D_b.

To derive simple, useful solutions of equation 1, one must assume that the densities of the two compartments (FM and FFM) are constant. Siri's well-known equation for predicting %BF (Siri 1961) represents the simplest solution of equation 1. In these equations, %BF is calculated from D_b, and fat and fat-free constituents, respectively, are assumed to have densities of 0.900 g/cm^3 and 1.100 g/cm^3:

Equation 2 $1/D_b = F/d_F + FFM/d_{FFM}$

where $1/D_b$ is body mass; D_b is whole-body density; and F/d_F and FFM/d_{FFM} are the fractions of body mass that are fat and fat-free devided by their respective densities (Brozek et al. 1963; Fidanza et al. 1953).

In the simplest chemical model, FFM comprises primarily water (W), protein (P), and mineral (M) components, and d_{FFM} is derived from the proportions of W, P, and M divided by constant values for their densities (Lohman 1992b; Siri 1956, 1961):

Equation 3 $d_{FFM} = W/d_W + P/d_P + M/d_M$

Thus, for d_{FFM} to be constant, the proportions of W, P, and M must be constant—or they must vary in such a way that d_{FFM} does not change.

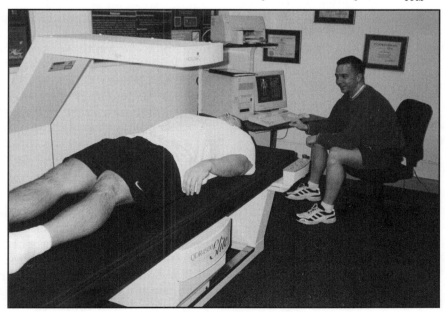

Figure 7.2 Dual-energy x-ray absorptiometry (DXA) is a three-component body composition model (FFM, FM, and bone mineral). It is considered one of the criterion methods for body composition assessment.
Reprinted from Heyward 1998.

In the adult two-component densitometric approach, any deviation of D_b from the d_{FFM} of 1.100 g/cm³ is assumed to be due to the addition of body fat. Thus, %BF may be overestimated in people with lower than average bone mineral mass and underestimated in people with more than average bone mass. These errors in the densitometric criterion method for fat estimation are then passed on to other body composition assessment methods when they are validated against this two-component criterion method.

When densitometry is used to assess body composition, underwater weighing is typically used to measure body volume, and D_b is then estimated using the following equation:

Equation 4 $D_b = BM/V$

where D_b is whole-body density, BM is body mass (weight) measured on a scale, and V is body volume.

The usefulness of densitometry as a criterion method for children is limited because of the changes in relative water and bone mineral content of FFM that occur during growth and development. These differences between children and adults result in overestimation of body fatness in children when %BF estimates are made using adult two-component models (e.g., the Siri [1961] and Brozek [1963] equations). These equations can be problematic even for estimating %BF in adults—they can be even more invalid for younger youths and those who mature especially late. The Siri equation is

Equation 5 $\%BF = \left[\dfrac{4.95}{D_b} - 4.50\right]100$

where D_b is whole-body density. This equation was derived from the following equation, using the density constants of 1.100 g/cm³ for d_{FFM} and 0.900 g/cm³ for d_{FM}.

Siri (1961) has published the complete derivation of equation 6.

Equation 6

$$\%BF = \left[\frac{1}{D_b}\left(\frac{d_{FFM}d_{FM}}{d_{FFM} - d_{FM}}\right) - \frac{d_{FM}}{d_{FFM} - d_{FM}}\right]100$$

In youths, %BF can be estimated more accurately from measured D_b by using modified versions of the Siri equation, which are derived from estimates of FFM composition in youths at different ages. In the same way that the Siri

equation was derived based on the adult reference male constants for fractions and densities of components of FFM and FM, Lohman (1989) derived equations for youths for predicting %BF from D_b, using constants based on average measured values for fractions of the water and mineral components of FFM. The result was a set of average FFM density values for boys and girls in nine age groups. For example, the equation for 9- to 11-year-old boys is

Equation 7 $\%BF = \left[\dfrac{5.30}{D_b} - 4.89\right]100$

The terms in this equation came from solving equation 6, substituting 1.084 for d_{FFM} (the average FFM density for 9- to 11-year-old boys), and using 0.900 g/cm³ for d_{FM} (the same density of the FM for adults). Using Lohman's (1989) gender- and age-specific constants instead of the constants in the Siri equation (equation 5) permits one to use D_b (measured using underwater weighing or skinfolds) to estimate %BF values for youths more accurately than is possible with the Siri equation.

There are limitations to this approach because youths of the same gender differ to some extent from the average measured water and mineral fraction of the FFM. These deviations lead to increased errors in %BF estimation when these gender- and age-group specific average values for constants are used in prediction equations (Lohman 1989; Lohman 1992a). Unfortunately, there has been no systematic attempt to define these constants in different ethnic groups of physically active youths or older adults—and estimation of %BF from density can be confounded by variability in FFM composition and density in youths and adults. A better description of these parameters in different groups of youths, adults, and older adults, including athletes, is an important focus for future research.

Anthropometry—Skinfolds Many prediction equations have been developed for estimating whole-body density (D_b) from relatively simple anthropometric measurements such as skinfolds. Although these skinfold-based prediction equations may give accurate estimates of D_b, substantial errors in the estimation of body composition values can occur when D_b is converted to %BF using prediction equations based on adult two-component models such as the Siri or Brozek equations. An alternative approach is to directly predict %BF using skinfold equations that were developed specifically for the group or individual you are measuring, using a multi-component approach (Lohman 1989; Heyward and Stolarczyk 1996; Roche 1996). Heyward and Stolarczyk (1996) have provided "decision trees" to help quickly locate the most appropriate skinfold equations for estimating body composition in different populations.

Hydrometry and Spectroscopy In some research and clinical situations, hydrometry or ^{40}K spectroscopy are the criterion methods used to measure body composition. The validity of both methods depends largely on the appropriateness of the identified conversion constants for the individual to which they are applied. FFM can be estimated using hydrometry, by first estimating total body water using isotopically labeled water dilution techniques. FFM is then calculated from TBW on the basis of the average hydration of FFM, which is assumed to be about 73.8% in the chemically mature reference adult male (Brozek et al. 1963). Once TBW is known, one can calculate FFM using the equation FFM = TBW/(constant for water fraction of FFM). For example, in adults the equation is FFM = TBW/0.738.

Since the average relative hydration of FFM in children is higher than in adults, use of the adult constant for the fraction of water in the FFM (73.8%) leads to underestimates of FFM and overestimates of %BF in children. Clearly, the predicted %BF values for youths using hydrometry are more accurate if prediction equations are based on data from youths rather than adults (Lohman 1989). For example, the average values for the water fraction of FFM range from 77% at 7-10 years of age to 74% for youths 15-17 years old.

FFM can also be calculated from total body potassium (TBK), which is measured using ^{40}K spectroscopy (Forbes 1987). Once TBK is determined, FFM is calculated from the average concentration of potassium (K) in FFM. In adult males, with TBK expressed in grams, FFM = TBK/2.66 g K/kg FFM; and in adult females, FFM = TBK/2.55 g K/kg FFM (Forbes 1987). TBK concentration constants for girls and boys respectively range from 2.32-2.40 g K/kg FFM at 7-9 years of age to 2.40-2.61 g K/kg FFM at 15-17 years.

Dual-Energy X-Ray Absorptiometry Computer-assisted tomography (CAT) scans offer an accurate way to directly measure body composition. Because of high costs and radiation exposure, however, this approach is limited. An alternative to CAT scans is dual-energy X-ray absorptiometry (DXA), which can assess regional and total bone mineral content as well as regional and total fat and fat-free content of soft body tissues. To date there has been limited but promising research validating DXA as an approach for assessing body composition (Lohman 1996).

Field Methods of Body Composition Assessment

Field methods are relatively simple techniques for estimating body composition. The techniques are validated and cross-validated using one or more criterion methods. Field methods include anthropometry, bioelectrical impedance, and near-infrared reactance. The anthropometric measures of height, weight, and body mass index have been the most common means of evaluating relative body weight (Deurenberg et al. 1991; Guo et al. 1994; Lohman 1992b; Roche 1996). Skinfolds and circumferences have been used to assess body composition and fat distribution (Guo et al. 1989; Kaplowitz et al. 1989; Lohman 1992b; Malina 1996; Mueller and Kaplowitz 1994; Thorland et al. 1983). More recently, bioelectrical impedance has been validated as a method of assessing body composition (Houtkooper et al. 1996).

Anthropometry Body mass index (BMI) is less accurate than skinfolds for assessing %BF (Lohman 1992b) because body weight (the numerator) is influenced by the amount of muscle, organs, and skeleton as well as FM in the body. A person with a large musculoskeletal system in relation to height can have a high-percentile BMI, without having a high %BF level. Conversely, people with a small musculoskeletal mass relative to height can have a low-percentile BMI even if their %BF is not extremely low.

Interpreting BMI across age ranges in children is particularly difficult because growth of the musculoskeletal system is adding weight relative to height as well as fat weight. For example, the 50th percentile for BMI in boys changes from 15.4 at 6 years of age to 21.5 in 17-year-olds—but the sum of two skinfolds (triceps plus subscapular) only increases on average from 12 mm to 15 mm (Lohman 1992b).

Anthropometric measurements—including skinfold thicknesses, bone dimensions, and limb circumferences—can be used in equations to directly predict %BF or to predict D_b, which in turn can be used to estimate %BF (Lohman 1992b; Roche 1996). The skinfold method is the most commonly used anthropometric method for estimating %BF (figure 7.3). It is based on the assumptions that (1) the thickness of the subcutaneous adipose tissue reflects a constant proportion of the total FM, and (2) the sites selected for measurement represent the average thickness of the subcutaneous adipose tissue (Lukaski 1987).

Accurate estimation of %BF from skinfolds depends on several factors. A key factor is the selection of a prediction equation appropriate for the individual being assessed. The skinfold sites used in the prediction equation should reflect the expected location of most subcutaneous fat deposits for the individual. It is also important to use the same type of skinfold caliper used to develop the prediction equation: different calipers yield systematic differences in skinfold thickness measurements (Heyward and Stolarczyk 1996). Finally, it is critical to measure accurately the same skinfold sites used in developing the pre-

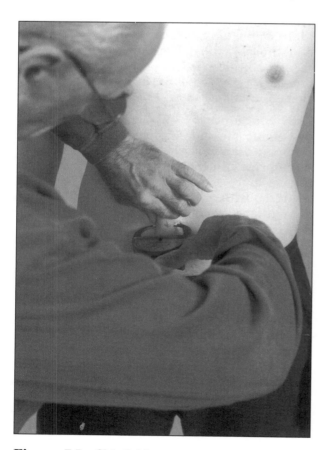

Figure 7.3 Skinfold measurements are an example of a field method of body composition assessment.

diction equation (Lohman 1992b). The preferred skinfold prediction equations are those used to estimate %BF directly from anthropometric measurements and those that have been validated using three- or four-component criterion models. Unfortunately, few such equations have been published and cross-validated for youths (Janz et al. 1993; Slaughter et al. 1988). Heyward and Stolarczyk (1996) provide "decision trees" for selecting the most appropriate skinfold equations for different populations.

One can also track changes in body fat by measuring skinfold thicknesses without conversion to %BF. Careful measurement of skinfolds at specific body sites at regular intervals can indicate if the thicknesses of subcutaneous body fat levels are changing. A limitation of this technique in children and youths is that skinfold thicknesses increase with normal growth, independent of changes in relative body fatness.

Bioelectrical Impedance Bioelectrical impedance analysis (BIA) is based on the relationship between the volume of a conductor (in this case the body), the conductor's length (an individual's height in this case), and its impedance (i.e., the resistance to the flow of an electric current). Impedance measurements are made with an individual lying flat on a nonconducting surface (figure 7.4). With electrodes attached to specific sites on the wrist and ankle of the right side of the body, a technician measures resistance while passing a low-dose (800 μamp), single-frequency (50-KHz) current through the individual. FFM is estimated using a prediction equation that includes measurements of both impedance and height squared as well as other variables including body weight and age. Validity of BIA values is significantly compromised if measurements are not made using standard technique and if appropriate prediction equations are not used (Houtkooper et al. 1996). Standard technique includes having the subject recline on a nonconducting surface; restricting the subject's food intake 3-4 h prior to measurements; assuring the subject's normal hydration status; and placing electrodes at standard locations.

One can improve the accuracy of FFM prediction equations derived from BIA by using population-specific equations that have been validated and cross-validated with multi-component criterion methods (Houtkooper et al. 1996; Lohman 1992b). Heyward and Stolarczyk (1996) provide "decision trees" for selecting the most appropriate BIA equations for different populations.

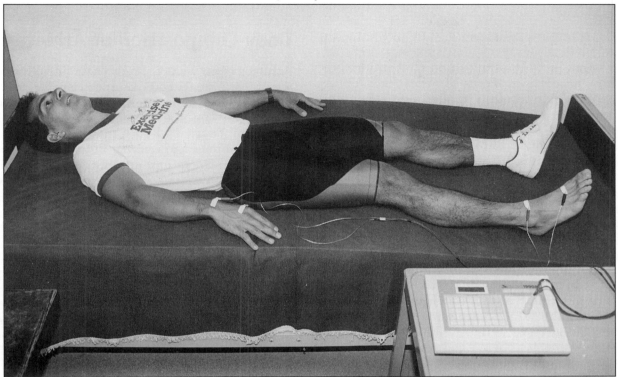

Figure 7.4 Bioelectrical impedance (BIA) is a field method for assessing body composition. Impedance measurements are made while a person lies flat on a non-conducting surface; electrodes are attached to specific sites on the wrist and ankle.

Near Infrared Reactance This method is based on the principles of light absorption and reflection. A fiber optic probe positioned at midbiceps emits an infrared light beam; the beam penetrates subcutaneous fat and muscle, is reflected off the bone, and is finally conducted to the probe's optical detector. Limited validation research with youths or adults has been conducted using this method. More well-designed studies are needed to validate and cross-validate this technique in order to determine if it can accurately and reliably estimate body composition in youths and adults (Cassady et al. 1993; Heyward and Stolarczyk 1996).

Accuracy of Body Composition Assessment Methods

The size of errors from prediction equations represents a compounding of errors from variations in FFM composition and from the measurement errors within criterion and field methods. For example, when D_b is estimated from skinfolds, the total prediction error includes (1) deviations of the individual's body water and minerals from the standards assumed in the criterion model, and (2) the technical errors of measuring skinfolds. Additional errors are possible if the measured skinfold sites are not representative of the subject's fat distribution and if the ratio of external to internal fat is different from that of the group in which the equation was developed. The magnitude of errors can be minimized by selecting a prediction equation developed and cross-validated using an appropriate multi-component criterion model for the group whose body composition is being estimated, and by carefully following standardized techniques when making all measurements.

Using D_b as the criterion variable for determining FFM, Lohman (1992b) published guidelines for evaluating the magnitude of the standard errors of estimates in young adult men and women. Prediction errors (standard errors of estimate [SEE]) for FFM of 4.4-7.7 lb (2.0-3.5 kg) for men and 4.0-6.2 lb (1.8-2.8 kg) for women are rated from ideal to good. Standard errors of estimate between 2.0-3.5% are rated as ideal to good for %BF. For example, an estimate of 15% BF could be accurate anywhere from 8 to 22% BF (±2SEE).

It is possible to determine %BF or FFM with sufficient accuracy to monitor exercise-induced changes in body composition that are larger than prediction errors for the assessment method. With carefully applied skinfold or bioelectrical impedance measurements, one can estimate %BF with an error of approximately 3% and estimate FFM with an error of 5.5 lb (2.5 kg) (Lohman 1992b; Lukaski 1987). This means that if %BF is actually 15%, predicted values may be as high as 18% or as low as 12%; and if the actual FFM value is 66 lb (30 kg), predicted values could range from 60.6-71.6 lb (27.5-32.5 kg). With inappropriate prediction equations and poor measurement technique, prediction errors will be much larger.

If you are recommending body composition goals to a client, always consider the potential errors in the data you are using. Recommend a range of goals for %BF or FFM rather than a single value. If a client's body composition falls at the low or high end of the recommended %BF range, perform additional assessments in order to confirm the %BF values by more than one method.

Selection Criteria for Field Methods

Skinfolds and bioelectrical impedance analysis (BIA) provide similar estimates of %BF that can be within 3% to 4% of criterion values, *if* the measurements are made using established techniques and the appropriate prediction equations are used. Obtaining accurate and reliable skinfold measurements requires more skill than measuring impedance—but the cost of equipment for BIA is much greater than for skinfold measurements. The choice of whether to use skinfolds or BIA depends in part on available funds and available expertise—including the potential cost of training to develop adequate technical skills for measuring skinfolds.

Several authors have recommended equations for estimating body composition using anthropometry and BIA (Heyward and Stolarczyk 1996; Houtkooper and Going 1994; Lohman 1992b) and also have summarized the reasons for selecting these equations (Going and Davis, 1998; Heyward and Stolarczyk 1996). Heyward and Stolarczyk's (1996) "decision trees" simplify the selection of equations for different field methods as well as for people of different gender, age, ethnicity, and activity level.

Body Composition of Athletes

Athletes often want to know their "ideal" body weight or "ideal" body composition for peak performance—implying the existence of some "universal," optimal combination of body FM and FFM. There is no such thing. It is difficult even to define ideal *relative* FM or FFM for a particular athlete in a specific sport since all aspects of physique, plus many other factors, contribute to successful performance. Recommendations for athletes' body weight and body composition are usually based on average %BF and FFM values obtained from representative athletes in a given sport (Sinning 1985; Wilmore 1992). In other words, they are best guesses within a reasonable range.

Figures 7.5 and 7.6 summarize reported %BF values of elite female and male athletes in various sports (Berg et al. 1990; Clarkson et al. 1985; DeGaray et al. 1974; Fleck 1983; Hirata 1966; Houtkooper et al. 1992; Thorland et al. 1983; Wilmore 1992).

Few data have been published on the body composition of athletes less than 18 years of age. Malina and Bouchard (1991) and Fleck (1983) reported %BF values for young athletes and nonathletes based on two-component densitometric estimates. The data indicated that young athletes have lower %BF levels than nonathletes of the same age and gender. These studies included swimmers, runners, gymnasts, football players, and wrestlers. The range of %BF was 13-23% for girls and 4-15% for boys. Remember always to consider errors inherent in the measurement methods when you interpret such values.

Body Composition Standards and Health

There are no accepted %BF standards for all ages (Going and Davis 1998). Most body composition studies use small groups of volunteers (convenience samples) who are usually healthy young adults. These studies have shown that body fat levels typically range between 10-20% for men and 20-30% for women. Based on these studies, past recommendations for desirable levels of body fat have been 15% for men and 25% for women (Lohman et al. 1997). These "standards" represent no more than the average percent fat values for relatively small samples of young, healthy adults—their usefulness in other age groups has not been established.

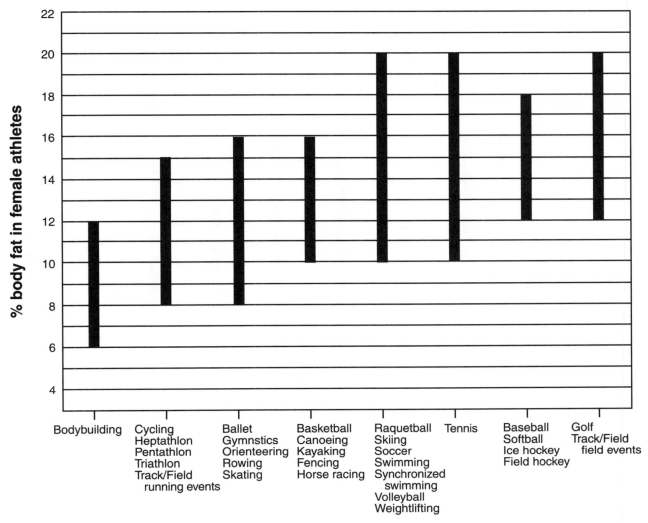

Figure 7.5 Reported ranges of % body fat of female athletes from various sports.
Adapted from Houtkooper and Going 1994.

Adult Standards

The National Health and Nutrition Examination Survey (NHANES II) performed skinfold measurements on a large (20,000) representative sample of U.S. men and women. Despite the limitations of skinfolds, these data provide a better basis for developing body fatness standards than data from convenience samples of young adults (Lohman et al. 1997). Conversion of the NHANES skinfold data (triceps and subscapular skinfolds) to percent body fat using the equations from Jackson and Pollock (1978) and Jackson et al. (1980) shows that median (50th percentile) %BF values for men and women 20-34 years old are 12% and 28%, respectively. The %BF values corresponding to the 15th (considered low) and 85th (consid-

ered high) percentiles are 5% and 22%, respectively, for young men, and 22% and 39% for young women. All of the values clearly vary with age as well as gender—and although it reasonably follows that standards should also vary with age, young adult values typically (and unfortunately) have been applied to all age groups.

Proposed new standards include some increase in %BF with age rather than imposing the current young adult standard on all age groups (Lohman et al. 1997). For example, a young adult male at 24% fat would be encouraged to lower his %BF, while a middle-aged man at 24% would be in the healthy range (table 7.1). Future testing of these proposed standards will lead to their further refinement. The recommended adjustments of these fat

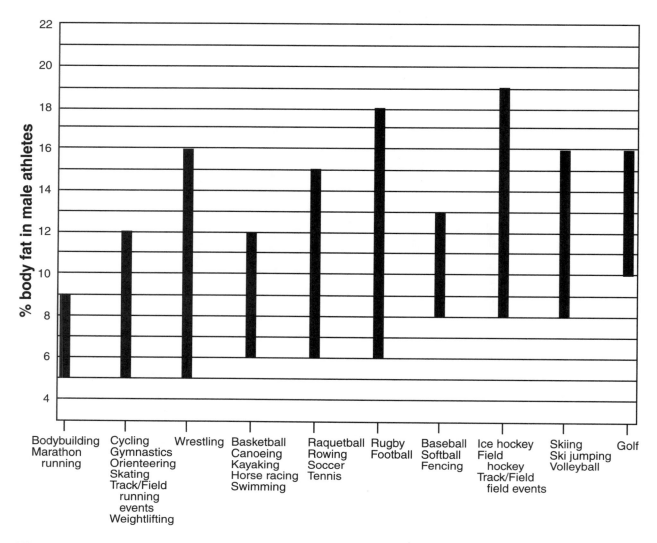

Figure 7.6 Reported ranges of % body fat of male athletes from various sports.
Adapted from Houtkooper and Going 1994.

standards with age are based on studies showing that, in middle age, a lower level of body fat or decreasing body fat is associated with lower bone mineral content—which puts a person at greater risk for osteoporosis and bone fractures (Lohman et al. 1997). Thus, the emphasis on lower levels of %BF to prevent heart disease, especially in women, must be balanced against the increased risk of bone fractures—particularly if bone mineral content is already low.

New standards have also been proposed for %BF in physically active men and women (table 7.2). Although the lower values may not improve health, they may be associated with improved physical performance.

Standards for Children and Youths

Because it is difficult to estimate body composition in young people, definitions of obesity and extreme leanness in this population typically depend on ratios of weight to height or on percentiles of skinfold measurements. For example, when triceps skinfolds are used to assess body composition, children have typically been considered obese if they are in the 85th-95th percentiles (Dietz and Gortmaker 1984; Gortmaker et al. 1987). Dietz and Gortmaker (1984), who used the 85th percentile to define obesity, observed that more children 6-11 years old and 12-17 years old were above the 85th percentile in 1971-1974 and

Table 7.1 Health Standards for Percent Body Fat

	Not rec.	Low	Mid	Upper	Obesity
	Recommended body fat levels				
Men					
Young adult	<8	8	13	22	→
Middle adult	<10	10	18	25	→
Elderly	<10	10	16	23	→
Women					
Young adult	<20	20	28	35	→
Middle adult	<25	25	32	38	→
Elderly	<25	25	30	25	→

Reprinted from Lohman et al. 1997.

Table 7.2 New Fat Fitness Standards for Percent Body Fat in Active Men and Women

	Low	Mid	Upper
	Recommended body fat levels		
Men			
Young adult	5	10	15
Middle adult	7	11	18
Elderly	9	12	18
Women			
Young adult	16	23	28
Middle adult	20	27	33
Elderly	20	27	33

Reprinted from Lohman et al. 1997.

1976-1980 as compared to 1963-1965. The authors concluded that the prevalence of obesity increased for boys and girls 6-11 years old by 61% and 46%, respectively. For youths 12-17 years old, the reported increase in the prevalence of obesity was 18% for boys and 58% for girls. When the 95th percentile was used as the definition of obesity, an even greater increase in the prevalence of obesity for children was reported.

Clear interpretation of these data requires determination of %BF values, for a given age group, that correspond to the 85th and 95th percentiles (Dietz and Gortmaker 1984; Gortmaker et al. 1987). Lohman (1992b) developed such tables, calculating %BF from the sum of two skinfolds using equations of Slaughter et al. (1988) that were developed specifically for youths using a multi-component criterion model (table 7.3).

Table 7.3 Percent Fat Corresponding to the 50th, 85th, and 95th Percentiles for Triceps Plus Subscapular Skinfolds (SK)

	Males Percentiles						Females Percentiles					
	50th		85th		95th		50th		85th		95th	
Age, years	$\Sigma 2SK$	% Fat	$\Sigma 2SK$	% Fat	$\Sigma 2SK$	% Fat	$\Sigma 2SK$	% Fat	$\Sigma 2SK$	% Fat	$\Sigma 2SK$	% Fat
6	12	11.7	16	15.6	20	19.6	14	13.5	19	18.1	27	23.9
8	13	12.7	19	18.4	28	25.9	16	15.5	25	22.6	36	29.4
10	14	12.7	24	21.9	33	28.8	18	17.2	31.6	26.5	43	33.2
12	14.5	12.5	27	23.6	44	35.0	19.5	18.5	34	27.7	47.3	35.5
14	14	11.0	26.5	22.0	39	30.5	23.5	21.6	37.5	30.2	52.6	38.4
16	14	9.0	24	18.9	39	29.3	25.5	23.0	42	32.6	58	41.4

Males: For 6- and 8-year-olds, the intercept was –1.7; for 10-year-olds, –2.5; for 12-year-olds, –3.4; for 14-year-olds, –4.4; for 16-year-olds, –5.5; and the equation is % fat = 1.21 ($\Sigma 2SK$) – 0.008 ($\Sigma 2SK$) 2 + 1. For males with skinfolds greater than 35 mm, % fat = 0.783 ($\Sigma 2SK$) + 2.2 (6- to 8-year-olds), 0.6 (10- to 12-year-olds), and –1.2 (14- to 16-year-olds).

Females: % fat = 1.33 ($\Sigma 2SK$) – 0.013 ($\Sigma 2SK$) 2 – 2.5 (one intercept for all ages). For females with skinfolds greater than 35 mm, % fat = 0.546 ($\Sigma 2SK$) + 9.7, all ages.

Note. Calculations were derived using National Health Examination Survey (NHES) norms (1963-1965), computed from data obtained from the NHES (1973).

■ HIGHLIGHT ■

A Universal Body Fat Standard for Boys and Girls?

Some researchers have proposed using a single %BF standard for defining obesity in boys and girls of all ages (Hoerr et al. 1992; Lohman 1992b). Current availability of equations for predicting %BF for children using skinfolds makes it possible to use a %BF value as a guideline to define obesity for boys and girls of all ages (Janz et al. 1993; Slaughter et al. 1988).

Instead of using percentile-referenced standards to derive %BF standards for children and youths, Williams et al. (1992) used criterion-referenced standards. They assessed the risks for high levels of blood pressure, total cholesterol, and low-density lipoprotein (LDL)-cholesterol and for low levels of high-density lipoprotein (HDL)-cholesterol in males and females aged 6-18 years at different levels of body fatness. They found no excess risk until %BF values exceeded 25% in males and 30% in females. Age and ethnicity were not significant predictors of risk in this age group. Thus, they have proposed >25% BF in males and >30% BF in females as useful health standards for black and white girls and boys aged 6-18 years. A similar criterion-referenced approach would be useful in adults to determine whether "risk" varies with age and %BF, or whether one %BF standard is valid for all ages and ethnic groups.

Table 7.4 Guidelines for Interpreting % Body Fat Values for Children

Ratings	% Body fat	
	Boys	Girls
Very low	<5	<12
Low	5-10	12-15
Optimal	11-20	16-25
Moderately high	21-25	26-30
High	26-31	31-36
Very high	>31	>36

Reprinted from Lohman et al. 1987.

The data in these tables show that boys at the 85th percentile for the triceps plus subscapular skinfolds have equivalent %BF values that range from a low of only 15.6% at 6 years of age to a high of 23.6% at 12 years. For girls, the equivalent %BF values for the 85th percentile in skinfolds range from a low of only 18.1% at 6 years to 32.6% at 16 years (Lohman 1992b). Note that the same skinfold percentile at a given age varies considerably in equivalent %BF value. If the 85th percentile defines obesity in children, a 6-year-old boy would be classified as obese if his %BF was only 15.6%,

and a 16-year-old girl would not be classified as obese until she had a %BF value of 32.6%. This large variation in the equivalent %BF values for a given skinfold percentile demonstrates the limitation of using such data to assess body composition or as criteria for defining obesity in children (Going and Williams 1989).

Lohman (1992b) has published guidelines for evaluating the estimated %BF values for youths. Table 7.4 summarizes these guidelines for girls and boys. These guidelines offer a new approach to interpreting estimated %BF values in youths.

In this approach, obesity for boys is defined as a %BF >25%; for girls it is >32%. The concept supporting this approach is sound, but the classifications for the actual %BF levels need further research to determine what levels of body fatness are related to increase risks for diseases. See "A Universal Body Fat Standard For Boys and Girls?" for more on this approach. Future research that helps more clearly define the relation between body fatness and health status or sport performance will improve the interpretation of body composition status.

Chapter in Review

Over the last 30 years, much research has focused on the development of body composition methods that more accurately and reliably measure %BF and FFM. Yet, there is little research on the relationship between body composition and athletic performance. We know that excess body fat negatively influences performance in some sports, and that a high ratio of FFM to FM at a given body weight is generally positively related to sport performance. However, very low levels of body fat can negatively impact health and exercise performance.

Practitioners working with athletes need to be aware of the inherent errors associated with body composition assessment and should not attempt to define an exact level of optimal %BF or FFM for an individual athlete. It is reasonable, however, to define a %BF or FFM *range* associated with athletes who are top performers in their sports. These ranges can then be used to establish reasonable training goals for weight, %BF, and FFM, as long as the goals are realistic and are compatible with good health for an individual athlete. More emphasis needs to be placed on defining optimal ratios of FFM and FM for various sports to replace the body weight goals currently used in many sports.

KEY CONCEPTS

 **1. Understand the relationship between body composition and health.**

There is a strong association between excess body fat—especially excess intra-abdominal fat—and increased risk of coronary artery disease, non-insulin dependent diabetes, hypertension, and certain types of cancers. Low levels of FFM and loss of FFM are related to impaired functional capacity and decreased physical activity/energy expenditure, and increase the risk of gaining fat mass.

 2. Describe the relationship between body composition and sport performance.

High ratios of FFM to FM at a given body weight are generally positively related to physical performance, but too little body fat results in deterioration in health and performance. The ideal relative FM or FFM for an athlete in a specific sport is difficult to define—body size and structure as well as many other factors also contribute to successful athletic performance.

 3. Compare body composition assessment models and methods.

Body composition refers to the amounts of constituents in the body at atomic, molecular, cellular, tissue-system, and whole-body levels. The simplest and most common model of body composition partitions the body into two major components (compartments)—fat mass and fat-free mass.

 4. Understand the accuracy of body composition assessment.

Accuracy of field methods for estimation of athletes' body composition depends upon selection of appropriate models and measurement methods, the skill of individuals taking the measurements, and use of appropriate gender- and age-specific prediction equations.

 5. Identify selection criteria for field methods.

Appropriate field methods and careful measurements make it possible to estimate relative body fat with an error of approximately 3% fat, and fat-free mass with an error of about 5.5 lb (2.5 kg).

 6. Discuss body composition status of athletes.

The relative body fat ranges of top athletes vary by sport and by gender within a sport. Excess body fat negatively influences physical performance.

 7. Explain the relationship between body composition standards and health.

There are no universally acceptable percent body fat standards for adults or children, nor is there a universally accepted upper or lower limit of percent body fat at which health problems will occur. In general, a high %BF is associated with diabetes, hypertension, and heart disease, while a low %BF is associated with osteoporosis, bone fractures, menstrual dysfunction, eating disorders, and muscle wasting. Future research will help to more clearly define the relationship between body fatness and health.

KEY TERMS

bioelectrical impedance analysis (BIA)
body mass index (BMI)
chemically mature
criterion methods
densitometry (underwater weighing)
direct method
fat mass (FM)

indirect method
model approach
property-based methods
regression analysis
total body water (TBW)
whole-body density (D_b)

References

Berg K, Latin RW, Baechle T. Physical and performance characteristics of NCAA Division I football players. Res Q Exerc Sport 1990;61(4):395-401.

Boileau RA, Lohman TG. The measurement of human physique and its effect on physical performance. Orthop Clin North Am 1977;8:563-81.

Boileau RA, Lohman TG, Slaughter MH, Ball TE, Going SB, Hendrix MK. Hydration of the fat-free body in children during maturation. Hum Biol 1984;56:651-66.

Brozek JF, Grande F, Anderson JT, Keys A. Densitometric analysis of body composition: revision of some quantitative assumptions. Ann NY Acad Sci 1963;110:113-40.

Buskirk E, Taylor HL. Maximal oxygen intake and its relation to body composition with special reference to chronic physical activity and obesity. J Appl Physiol 1957;11:72-8.

Cassady SL, Nielsen DH, Janz KF, Wu WT, Cook JS, Hansen JR. Validity of near infrared body composition analysis in children and adolescents. Med Sci Sports Exerc 1993;25:1185-91.

Clarkson PM, Freedson PS, Keller S, Carney D, Skrinar M. Maximal oxygen uptake, nutritional patterns and body composition of adolescent female ballet dancers. Res Q Exerc Sport 1985;56(2):180-4.

Cureton KJ. Effects of experimental alterations in excess weight on physiological responses to exercise and physical performance. In: Marriott BM, Grumstrup-Scott J, eds. Body Composition and Physical Performance: Applications for the Military Services. Washington, DC: National Academy Press, 1992:71-88.

Cureton KJ, Sparling PB. Distance running performance and metabolic responses to running in men and women with excess weight experimentally equated. Med Sci Sports Exerc 1980;12:288-94.

Cureton KJ, Sparling PB, Evans PW, Johnson SM, Kong UD, Purvis JW. Effect of experimental alterations in excess weight on aerobic capacity and distance running performance. Med Sci Sports Exerc 1978;15:218-23.

DeGaray AL, Levine L, Carter JEL. Genetic and Anthropological Studies of Olympic Athletes. New York: Academic Press, 1974.

Deurenberg P, Westrate JA, Seidell JC. Body mass index as a measure of body fitness: age- and sex-specific prediction formulas. Br J Nutr 1991;65:105-14.

Dietz WH, Gortmaker SL. Factors within the physical environment associated with childhood obesity. Am J Clin Nutr 1984;39:619-24.

Ellis KJ. Whole-body counting and neutron activation analysis. In: Roche AF, Heymsfield SB, Lohman TG, eds. Human Body Composition. Champaign, IL: Human Kinetics, 1996:45-62.

Fidanza FA, Keys A, Anderson JT. Density of body fat in man and other animals. J Appl Physiol 1953;6:252-6.

Fleck SJ. Body composition of elite American athletes. Am J Sports Med 1983;11:398-403.

Forbes GB. Human Body Composition: Growth, Aging, Nutrition and Activity. New York: Springer-Verlag, 1987.

Friedl KE, DeLuca JP, Marchitelli LS, Vogel JA. Reliability of body-fat estimations from a four-component model by using density, body water, and bone mineral measurements. Am J Clin Nutr 1992;55:764-70.

Fuller NJ, Jebb SA, Laskey MA, Coward WA, Elia M. Four-component model for the assessment of body composition in humans: comparison with alternative methods, and evaluation of the density and hydration of fat-free mass. Clin Sci 1992;82:687-93.

Going SB. Densitometry. In: Roche AF, Heymsfield SB, Lohman TG, eds. Human Body Composition. Champaign, IL: Human Kinetics, 1996:3-23.

Going SB, Davis R. Body Composition. In: Roitman JL, ed. ACSM's Resource Manual for Guidelines for Exercise and Testing Prescription. American College of Sports Medicine. Baltimore, MD: Williams and Wilkins, 1998.

Going SB, Williams D. Understanding fitness standards. J Phy Ed Rec Dance 1989;60:34-8.

Gortmaker SL, Dietz WH, Sobal AM, Wehler CA. Increasing pediatric obesity in the United States. Am J Dis Child 1987;141:535-40.

Guo SS, Roche AF, Chumlea WC, Gardner JD, Siervogel RM. The predictive value of childhood body mass index values for overweight at age 35 y. Am J Clin Nutr 1994;59:810-9.

Guo SS, Roche WC, Houtkooper L. Fat-free mass in children and young adults predicted from bioelectric impedance and anthropometric variables. Am J Clin Nutr 1989;50:435-43.

Gurr MI, Harwood JL. Lipid Biochemistry. London: Chapman and Hall, 1991.

Harman EA, Frykman PN. The relationship of body size and composition to the performance of physically demanding military tasks. In: Marriott BM, Grumstrup-Scott J, eds. Body Composition and Physical Performance: Applications for the Military Services. Washington, DC: National Academy Press, 1992:105-18.

Hewitt MJ, Going SB, Williams DP, Lohman TG. Hydration of the fat-free body mass in children and adults: implications for body composition assessment. Am J Physiol 1993;265:E88-E95.

Heymsfield SB, Wang Z. Measurement of total-body fat by underwater weighing: new insights and uses for old method. Nutrition 1993;9:472-3.

Heymsfield SB, Wang ZM, Withers RT. Multi-component molecular level models of body composition. In: Roche AF, Heymsfield SB, Lohman TG, eds. Human Body Composition. Champaign, IL: Human Kinetics, 1996:129-47.

Heyward VH, Stolarczyk LM. Applied Body Composition Assessment. Champaign, IL: Human Kinetics, 1996.

Hirata K. Physique and age of Tokyo Olympic champions. J Sports Med Phys Fitness 1966;6:207-22.

Hoerr SL, Nelson RA, Lohman TG. Discrepancies among predictors of desirable weight for black and white obese adolescent girls. J Am Diet Assoc 1992;92:450-3.

Houtkooper LB. Exercise and Eating Disorders. In: Lamb D, Murray R, eds. Perspectives in Exercise Science and Sports Medicine. Exercise, Nutrition, and Control of Body Weight. Carmel, IN: Cooper Publishing Group, 1998.

Houtkooper LB, Going SB. Body composition: how should it be measured? Does it affect sport performance? Sports Sci Exchange 1994;7:1-8.

Houtkooper LB, Going SB, Lohman TG, Roche AF, VanLoan M. Bioelectric impedance estimation of fat-free body mass in children and youth: a cross-validation study. J Appl Physiol 1992;72:366-73.

Houtkooper LB, Lohman TG, Going SB, Howell WH. Why bioelectrical impedance analysis should be used for estimating adiposity. Am J Clin Nutr 1996;64:436S-48S.

Jackson AS, Pollock ML. Generalized equations for predicting body density in men. Br J Nutr 1978;40:497-504.

Jackson AS, Pollock ML, Ward A. Generalized equations for predicting body density of women. Med Sci Sports Exerc 1980;12:175-82.

Janz KF, Nielsen DH, Cassady SL, Cook JR, Wu YT, Hansen JR. Cross-validation of the Slaughter skinfold equations for children and adolescents. Med Sci Sports Exerc 1993;25:1070-6.

Kaplowitz H, Martorell R, Mendoza FS. Fatness and fat distribution in Mexican-American children and youths from the Hispanic health and nutrition examination survey. Am J Hum Biol 1989;1:631-48.

Lohman TG. Applicability of body composition techniques and constants for children and youth. In: Pandolf KB, ed. Exercise and Sports Science Reviews. New York: Macmillan, 1986:325-57.

Lohman TG. Assessment of body composition in children. Pediatr Exerc Sci 1989;1:19-30.

Lohman TG. Exercise training and body composition in childhood. Can J Sports Sci 1992a;17:284-7.

Lohman TG. Basic concepts in body composition assessment (pp. 1-5); Body density, body water, and bone mineral: controversies and limitations of the two-component system (pp. 7-24); Estimating body composition in children and the elderly (pp. 65-78); The prevalence of obesity in children in the United States (pp. 79-90). In: Roche AF, Heymsfield SB, Lohman TG, eds. Advances in Body Composition Assessment. Champaign, IL: Human Kinetics, 1992b.

Lohman TG. Dual-energy x-ray absorptiometry. In: Roche AF, Heymsfield SB, Lohman TG, eds. Human Body Composition. Champaign, IL: Human Kinetics, 1996:63-78.

Lohman TG. Measuring Body Fat Using Skinfolds (videotape). Champaign, IL: Human Kinetics, 1987.

Lohman TG, Houtkooper L, Going SB. Body fat measurement goes high-tech: not all are created equal. ACSM's Health Fit J 1997;7:30-5.

Lohman TG, Slaughter MH, Boileau RA, Bunt J, Lussier L. Bone mineral measurements and their relation to body density in children, youth, and adults. Hum Biol 1984;56:667-9.

Lukaski HC. Methods for the assessment of human body composition: traditional and new. Am J Clin Nutr 1987;46:537-56.

Malina RM. Physique and body composition: effects on performance and effects on training, semistarvation, and overtraining. In: Brownell KD, Rodin J, Wilmore JH, eds. Eating, Body Weight, and Performance in Athletes. Philadelphia: Lea & Febiger, 1992:94-114.

Malina RM. Regional body composition: age, sex, and ethnic variation. In: Roche AF, Heymsfield SB, Lohman TG, eds. Human Body Composition. Champaign, IL: Human Kinetics, 1996:217-26.

Malina RM, Bouchard C. Characteristics of young athletes. In: Malina RM, Bouchard C, eds. Growth, Maturation and Physical Activity. Champaign, IL: Human Kinetic Books, 1991:443-463.

Mueller WH, Kaplowitz HJ. The precision of anthropometric assessment of body fat distribution in children. Ann Hum Biol 1994;21:267-74.

National Health Examination Survey (NHES). Sample design and estimation procedures for a national health examination survey of children. National Center for Health Statistics Publication No. HRA 74-1005. Rockville, MD: Health Resource Administration, 1973.

Pate RR, Slentz CA, Katz DP. Relationships between skinfold thickness and performance of health related fitness test items. Res Q Exerc Sport 1989;60(2):183-9.

Roche AF. Anthropometry and ultrasound. In: Roche AF, Heymsfield SB, Lohman TG, eds. Human Body Composition. Champaign, IL: Human Kinetics, 1996:167-89.

Sinning WE. Body composition and athletic performance. In: Clark DH, Eckert HM, eds. Limits of Human Performance. American Academy of Physical Education Papers, No. 18, 1985:45-56.

Sinning WE. Body composition in athletes. In: Roche AF, Heymsfield SB, Lohman TG, eds. Human Body Composition. Champaign, IL: Human Kinetics, 1996:257-74.

Siri WE. The gross composition of the body. Adv Biol Med Physiol 1956;4:239-80.

Siri WE. Body composition from fluid spaces and density: analysis of methods. In: Brozek J, Henschel A, eds. Techniques for Measuring Body Composition. Washington, DC: National Academy of Science, 1961:223-44.

Slaughter MH, Lohman TG, Boileau RA, et al. Skinfold equations for estimation of body fatness in children and youth. Hum Biol 1988;60:709-23.

Sparling PB, Cureton KJ. Biological determinants of sex difference in 12 min run performance. Med Sci Sports Exerc 1983;15:218-22.

Thorland WG, Johnston GO, Housh TJ, Refsell MJ. Anthropometric characteristics of elite adolescent competitive swimmers. Hum Biol 1983;55:735-48.

Wang Z, Pierson Jr RN, Heymsfield SB. The five-level model: a new approach to organizing body-composition research. Am J Clin Nutr 1992;56:19-28.

Williams DP, Going SB, Lohman TG, Hewitt MJ, Haber AE. Estimation of body fat from skinfold thicknesses in middle-aged and older men: a multiple component approach. Am J Human Biol 1992;4:595-605.

Wilmore JH. Body weight standards and athletic performance. In: Brownell KD, Rodin J, Wilmore JH, eds. Eating, Body Weight, and Performance in Athletes. Philadelphia: Lea & Febiger, 1992:315-29.

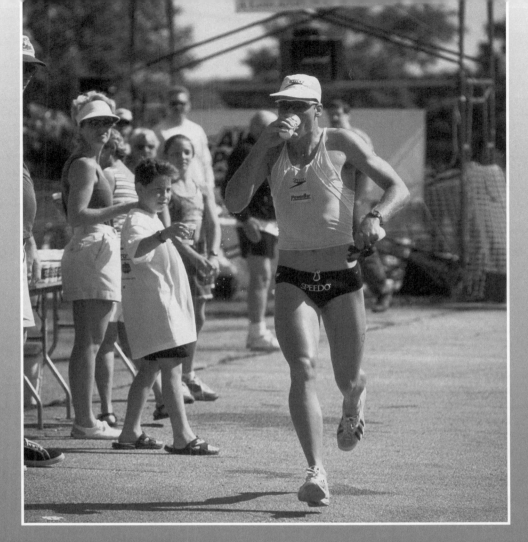

CHAPTER 8

Fluid and Electrolyte Balance

After reading this chapter you will be able to

- understand the function and regulation of water and electrolyte balance within the body, and the adverse health effects of dehydration, hypohydration, and hyponatremia;

- identify the fluid and electrolyte recommendations for exercise; and

- understand the role of sport drinks in preventing and maintaining fluid balance before, during, and after exercise.

Although we often do not think of water as an essential nutrient, it is! It is the most abundant constituent of the body. Abnormal decreases in body water (dehydration) can cause death more quickly than the removal of any other essential nutrient from the diet. One can go weeks without eating food, while death from dehydration can occur within 3 to 4 d. Water provides more than just fluid to bathe our cells. Most of the water we drink, depending on its source, also contains numerous electrolytes and minerals, including sodium, chloride, magnesium, potassium, fluoride, and calcium. Thus, the water we drink can contribute to our intake of these important nutrients.

Because exercise increases the loss of body water and electrolytes, and because these losses can impair exercise performance and the ability and desire to perform work, it is important to understand how to maintain water and electrolyte balance during exercise. This is especially true for exercise in a hot environment. In sports where dehydration is used to reduce body weight before competition or "weigh-in," the effect on health and performance can be extremely detrimental or even deadly. This was tragically demonstrated late in 1997 when three collegiate wrestlers died trying to make weight through dehydration (Remick et al. 1998). In this chapter, we provide background information on water and electrolyte balance, outline body water and electrolyte losses, and discuss the factors influencing fluid uptake at rest and during exercise. Then we review the importance of consuming adequate fluids before, during, and after exercise, along with recommendations for fluid consumption in different types of exercises/sports and environmental conditions, and for fluid consumption in children and adolescents. Finally, we discuss the composition and role of various commercial fluid replacement beverages and sport drinks.

Water and Electrolyte Balance

Total body weight comprises about 60% (range 45-70%) water (Sawka and Pandolf 1990). People with more muscle mass have a higher percentage of body water than those with more body fat since water comprises ~74% of muscle and organ weight but only ~20-30% of adipose tissue. Because men generally have a higher percentage of lean body mass than women, they generally have a higher percentage of water in their total body weight. For example, men less than 40 years of age average ~60-65% water, while women of the same age average ~50-55% (Kleinman and Lorenz 1996). Thus, as a percentage of total body weight, a very lean male may have a body water content of 70%, while an obese man may have only 50%. As people age, muscle mass usually declines, decreasing total body water content.

Function of Water

Water serves a number of functions within the body:

- Water acts as a lubricant that bathes every tissue and cell of the body. It is a transport medium in which many compounds (e.g., nutrients, drugs, hormones, and peptides) can be transported to the cells. It is the medium in which waste materials are removed from the body via the kidneys, and the medium in which many body solutes, both organic and inorganic, are dissolved.

- Water is necessary for numerous chemical reactions within the body, especially metabolic reactions involved in energy production.

- Water is a structural part of body tissues such as proteins and glycogen.

- Water is extremely important in the regulation of body temperature. If the body is not cooled properly through sweating, severe metabolic consequences can occur, including death.

Body Water Compartments and Composition

Total body water can generally be divided into intracellular and extracellular components (Kleinman and Lorenz 1996). **Intracellular water** includes all the water enclosed within cell membranes, while **extracellular water** is all the water outside cells. Some of the extracellular water compartments include the water in the plasma (**intravascular water**); water around the cells (**interstitial fluid**); and water normally present in the gastrointestinal and urinary tracts, the humor of the eye, and the cerebrospinal fluid (**transcellular water**) (Kleinman and Lorenz 1996). Extracellular water constitutes the medium through which all metabolic exchanges occur, while intracellular water constitutes the medium in which all chemical reactions of cellular metabolism occur. Table 8.1 indicates the compartment volumes in liters for each of the major body water pools. As you can see from this table, a 154-lb (70-kg) man must maintain ~42 L of body water in order to achieve optimal fluid balance.

To maintain fluid balance, the body needs more than just water. Electrolytes such as sodium, chloride, potassium, calcium, and magnesium ions, as well as many small molecules, play an important role in fluid balance. We must consume electrolytes in food and beverages in order to maintain fluid balance. Since water can easily diffuse across cell membranes, it is the chemical activity and concentrations of the ions and small molecules (e.g., glucose, albumin) that determine body water distribution within the various compartments. The more concentrated the solutes are within a particular compartment, the greater their osmotic pressure (and hence the greater their ability to attract water). If more sodium is found in one compartment than in an adjacent compartment, for example, the sodium will attract water into the first compartment. **Osmotic pressure** is defined as the force necessary to exactly oppose osmosis (movement) of water into a solution across a semipermeable membrane. Another way to view osmotic pressure is to think of it as the force that tends to move water from dilute solutions to concentrated solutions. If a membrane is permeable to a solute, then the solute exerts no osmotic pressure across the membrane. The effective osmotic pressure of a solution depends on (1) the total number of solute particles in the solution, and on (2) the permeability characteristics of the membrane through which the solute must pass (Kleinman and Lorenz 1996).

The **osmolarity** of a fluid or solution is a measure of the total number of solute particles (moles) per unit volume. The more solutes found in a fluid, the greater its osmolarity or concentration. Thus, electrolytes help maintain fluid balance within the body by keeping water within a particular body water compartment. If excess loss of electrolytes occurs, the body loses its ability to maintain fluid balance. For example, sodium attracts water; therefore, sodium intake can increase fluid retention within the body. The effect of sodium on water retention may be beneficial for some people and detrimental for others. For someone who wants to rehydrate after strenuous exercise, moderate amounts of sodium in post-exercise drinks or foods will be beneficial. But for a person who retains body fluid due to salt sensitivity, additional dietary sodium may not be beneficial. Therefore, in addition to adequate water intake, a proper electrolyte balance is necessary to insure proper fluid balance within the body. **Osmolality** refers to the number of moles or particles per kilogram of water (1 L of water weighs 1 kg). This term is used when measuring the osmotic characteristics of a beverage, such as a sport drink (Horswill 1998).

Body Water and Electrolyte Losses

Under normal conditions, daily body water losses come from urine, feces, sweat, and respiration, with the greatest losses coming from urine (~1-2 L/d depending on fluid intake and environmental conditions). Blood losses also decrease total body water since blood is 80% water by weight. For example, donating 1 pint of blood (473 ml) depletes the body of 378 ml of fluid. Table 8.2 outlines normal fluid losses under various conditions. Note that under

Table 8.1 **Distribution of Body Water Volume Into Various Compartments**

	Percentage of body weight	Percentage of total body water	Volume in 70-kg man
Total body water	60%	—	42 L
Extracellular water	20%	33%	14 L
Plasma	5%	8%	3.5 L
Interstitial fluid	15%	25%	10.5 L
Intracellular water	40%	67%	28 L

Reprinted from Kleinman and Lorenz 1996.

Table 8.2 **Water Balance in Average Adult Under Various Conditions**

	Normal	Hot environment	Strenuous work
Fluid intake (ml/d)			
Drinking water	1200	2200	3400
Water from food	1000	1000	1150
Water of oxidation	300	300	450
Total	2500	3500	5000
Fluid output (ml/d)			
Urine	1400	1200	500
Insensible water			
Skins	400	400	400
Lungs	400	300	600
Sweat	100	1400	3300
Stool (feces)	200	200	200
Total	2500	3500	5000

Reprinted from Kleinman and Lorenz 1996.

exercise conditions, especially in the heat, the amount of water lost in sweat can dramatically increase to 1-2 L/h, compared to the 100-200 ml/d typically lost on nonexercise days in a cool or temperate environment.

Exercise increases total body metabolism by 5 to 20 times above resting conditions, depending on the exercise intensity and a person's level of physical conditioning. Much of this increase in metabolic rate, anywhere from 70-100%, results in heat that must be dissipated from the body in order to maintain normal body temperature. The amount of sweat produced depends on (1) environmental conditions—air temperature, humidity, wind speed, and radiant load (heat given off by sun and surrounding objects); (2) clothing (insulation and moisture permeability); (3) exercise intensity; (4) level of physical conditioning; and (5) acclimation to the environment (Sawka and Pandolf 1990). Figure 8.1 shows hourly sweat rates in liters/hour when a person runs at various speeds in different types of environmental conditions. Sweat rate increases as metabolism increases (i.e., a person is running faster) and as the environment becomes more hot and humid. If this fluid is not replaced, the body becomes dehydrated. Since the body cannot adapt to dehydration, the loss of body water can severely affect physiological function, the ability to do work, and overall health.

Electrolyte losses in sweat appear to be highly variable, depending on when the sweat sample is taken during exercise, the subject's state of acclimation, and even on physiological differences between individuals. Research methods for collecting sweat during exercise and estimating total electrolyte losses are very cumbersome and time-consuming. It is not surprising that values for sweat electrolyte concentrations in the research literature vary dramatically. Although many minerals are lost in sweat, including sodium, chloride, potassium, magnesium, calcium, and iron, the primary electrolytes lost are sodium and potassium. In general, typical values for sweat sodium concentrations range from 20-80 mmol/L, with potassium values about 4-8 mmol/L (Maughan and Shirreffs 1997). It is difficult to determine the amount of electrolytes lost in sweat for any one individual without directly measuring it since the amount lost depends on many variables. We must therefore rely on estimates of electrolyte losses in sweat, determined under various laboratory conditions, to predict sweat losses of people performing a wide range of exercises in various environmental conditions.

Regulation of Water and Electrolyte Balance

How does the body know it needs water? What triggers the thirst response? How does the body know when fluid and electrolyte needs have been met? The body has an intricate way of regulating body water—through the stimulation of thirst and through regulation of fluid losses through the kidneys (e.g., increasing or

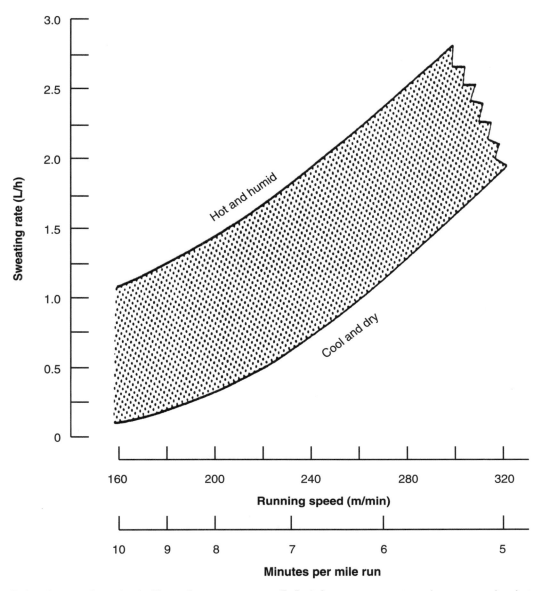

Figure 8.1 Approximation of hourly sweat rates (L/hr) for runners at various exercise intensities. Reprinted from Sawka and Pandolf 1990.

decreasing output as necessary). The body is constantly assessing fluid balance and adjusting both intake and output to maintain total body water at an optimal level. For example, if blood volume decreases due to increased fluid losses in sweat, the body responds by constricting the blood vessels to increase blood pressure, reducing fluid losses via the kidney, and stimulating the thirst mechanism. All these responses help increase blood pressure and restore fluid balance by decreasing the total vascular space, reducing the probability of continued fluid losses in the urine, and increasing fluid intake. The details of fluid and sodium regulation, in-

cluding the endocrine and neurological control mechanisms, are reviewed in detail elsewhere (Greenleaf 1992; Pivarnik and Palmer 1994; Senay 1998; Wade 1996; Zambraski 1996).

Gastric Emptying and Intestinal Absorption

Optimal fluid balance, especially during exercise, depends on the effectiveness of oral rehydration to maintain plasma volume and electrolyte balance—which in turn depends on the rates of fluid ingestion, gastric emptying, and intestinal fluid absorption (Puhl and Buskirk

1998; Schedl et al. 1994). Since little water or nutrients are absorbed in the stomach, these substances must enter the small intestine for absorption. Water is absorbed readily in the small intestine, while other nutrients (glucose, fructose, and sodium) are absorbed at different rates. Therefore, the rate that water and nutrients empty into the small intestine from the stomach is an important limiting factor to absorption and determines to a great extent the benefit derived from drinking a particular beverage. A good oral rehydration fluid or sport drink should empty rapidly from the stomach, enhance intestinal absorption, and promote fluid retention (Gisolfi et al. 1995). These issues have prompted a number of research questions related to fluid replacement before, during, and after exercise.

- What type of fluid is absorbed most rapidly?
- What is the optimal composition of this fluid?
- Do warm fluids absorb more quickly than cold fluids?
- Is sodium required for fluid absorption and retention? If so, how much?
- What effect do different types of sugars and carbohydrates have on fluid absorption?
- Are sport drinks absorbed more quickly than water or fruit juices?

A number of factors influence the rate of gastric emptying and the subsequent absorption of fluid from the small intestine. Figure 8.2 shows some of the factors known to affect gastric emptying. The primary factors are fluid

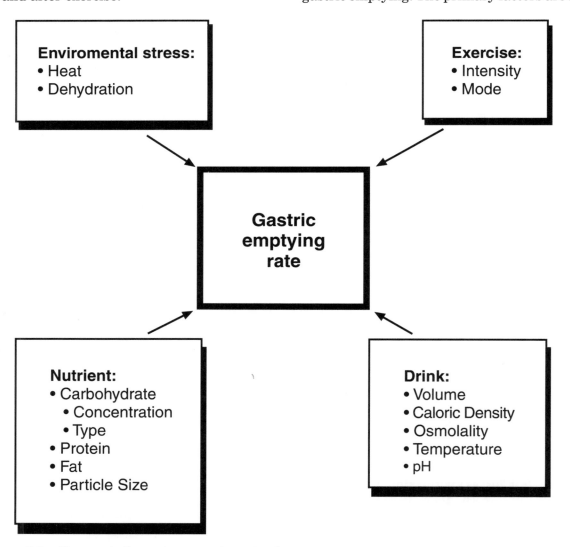

Figure 8.2 Factors influencing gastric emptying rate.
Reprinted from Gisolfi and Ryan 1996.

volume, osmolality, carbohydrate type and concentration, and exercise intensity (Costill 1990; Gisolfi and Ryan 1996). Individual variability in gastric emptying is also important, as Gisolfi and Duchman (1992) discovered. They found that one subject emptied 80% of a 500-ml solution of water in 15 min, while another emptied only 20% of the solution in 15 min. However, both emptied similar amounts of the solution by 30 min. This type of individuality in gastric emptying emphasizes two points:

1. Methods for assessing gastric emptying need to measure gastric emptying rates repeatedly over a designated period.

2. Fluid recommendations for athletes need to be individualized based on gastrointestinal complaints, past experience with fluid intake during exercise, sweat rates, and fluid needs.

Gastric Volume

Gastric volume is one of the strongest regulators of gastric emptying. The greater the volume of fluid consumed, the greater the rate of gastric emptying. This relationship apparently holds true up to a volume of about 600 ml (Costill 1990). Above this point, a further increase in volume may not increase the rate of gastric emptying. Since an average person can empty approximately 40 ml of water per min from the stomach, or 2.4 L/h, consuming too much fluid during exercise is usually not a limiting factor for most athletes (Gisolfi and Ryan 1996). In fact, most athletes have trouble drinking enough fluids during exercise. Note that consuming a large volume of fluid helps speed gastric emptying compared to sipping small amounts of fluids over the same time period.

Osmolality

Osmolality is negatively correlated with gastric emptying—adding carbohydrates or other nutrients to a solution generally slows emptying from the stomach compared to **isotonic solutions** (those containing electrolytes equivalent in osmolarity to that of body fluid). Since most oral rehydration solutions and sport beverages are low in sodium (35-110 mg/8 oz, or 132-416 mg/L) and in osmolality (<400 mOsm/L), they do not inhibit water absorption (Gisolfi et al. 1995). For example, when Brouns et al. (1995) compared six solutions with equal carbohydrate content but different osmolalities, ranging from 240-390 mOsm/L, they found that all drinks emptied from the stomach at similar rates. The effects of different carbohydrates on osmolality have also been studied since glucose polymers (frequently used in sport drinks) have a lower osmolality than glucose. The formulation of a rehydration beverage must balance a number of factors: it must be low in osmolality to improve gastric emptying and absorption, yet must provide carbohydrates for energy and salts to improve palatability and fluid retention.

Carbohydrate Concentration and Type

The effects of carbohydrate on gastric emptying and fluid absorption in the small intestine have been extensively studied, since sport and rehydration beverages include various types of carbohydrates. Because little fluid is absorbed in the stomach, the fluid must leave the stomach and move to the small intestine where fluid absorption can occur. Any factor that decreases gastric emptying may also decrease absorption since a fluid cannot be absorbed until it leaves the stomach. In general, as the carbohydrate concentration of a fluid increases, gastric emptying decreases. Depending on the research examined, the effect of low concentrations of carbohydrate solutions (2-8%) on gastric emptying is variable. These differences in gastric emptying rates can be explained by the differing research methods used in various studies—for example, the type of test drink, the volume consumed, different types of carbohydrates and/or electrolytes used, time of administration, varying osmolalities, and sample timing. For example, Vist and Maughan (1994) found that even low concentrations of glucose (2% solution) slowed gastric emptying compared to water (but the difference was *not* statistically significant); higher glucose concentrations (>2%) significantly decreased gastric emptying. In a follow-up study, Vist and Maughan (1995) reported that both osmolality and carbohydrate content influenced gastric emptying, but that carbohydrate content had a greater influence than osmolality. It appears that the type of carbohydrate may have less effect than the amount of carbohydrate added to a solution.

Although carbohydrate may slow gastric emptying, it appears to enhance fluid and sodium absorption in the small intestine (Gisolfi and Duchman 1992; Gisolfi et al. 1991; Gisolfi et al. 1995). Glucose is actively transported in the gut by a sodium energy-dependent transport system. As carbohydrate and sodium are absorbed, water follows. Thus, transported carbohydrate, co-transported with sodium, is the primary method for promoting water absorption from a sport drink or oral rehydration solution (Schedl et al. 1994). Although the composition of a beverage can affect gastric emptying, solutions containing 2-6% simple carbohydrate of various types (glucose, sucrose, fructose, maltodextrins, or various combinations of these sugars) are generally emptied quickly from the stomach and absorbed as well as or better than water (Gisolfi and Ryan 1996; Gisolfi et al. 1992). Therefore, carbohydrate-electrolyte beverages of low concentration (≤ 6% carbohydrate) should not compromise fluid replenishment during exercise (Ryan et al. 1998). Moreover, numerous research studies indicate that these substances improve exercise performance by providing additional energy substrate (see chapter 2, which also discusses intestinal absorption of different types of carbohydrates). Finally, Ploutz-Snyder et al. (1999) studied the gastric emptying rates of various carbohydrate-electrolyte replacement beverages with and without carbonation. They found that noncarbonated carbohydrate-electrolyte beverages and water leave the gut sooner than lightly carbonated carbohydrate-electrolyte beverages or carbonated cola.

Exercise Intensity and Type

Although low-to-moderate intensity exercise (~30-70% $\dot{V}O_2$max) for 60-90 min appears to have little effect on gastric emptying and intestinal absorption (Gisolfi et al. 1991; Schedl et al. 1994), high-intensity exercise (>70% $\dot{V}O_2$max) delays gastric emptying (Gisolfi and Ryan 1996). Different *types* of physical activity may also alter the ability and ease with which fluids can be consumed and the way fluids are emptied from the stomach. For example, runners typically have lower fluid intakes compared to cyclists because it is more difficult to drink while running and fluid movement in the stomach can be uncomfortable. This means runners generally consume less fluid, which in turn can affect gastric emptying. On the other hand, running may aid gastric emptying by increasing mechanical movement of fluids in the stomach and thereby increasing intragastric pressure (Puhl and Buskirk 1998). Running intensity may also influence intestinal permeability (Pals et al. 1997) and reduce blood flow to the gut—both of which may explain some of the gastrointestinal distress associated with intense running. Thus, the amounts of fluid consumed, and the effect of a particular sport on gastric emptying and gastrointestinal distress, depend on the nature and intensity of the sport, the type of movement involved, and the amount of fluid consumed.

Dehydration, Hypohydration, and Hyponatremia

Dehydration is a decrease in total body water, which occurs anytime that fluid intake does not keep up with fluid loss. For example, during exercise, **involuntary dehydration** occurs: since most active people tend to drink only enough to assuage their thirst, they do not consume enough water or other fluids to offset the water losses that occur due to sweating. The amount of water or fluid they consume does not return them to a state of **euhydration** (normal hydration). Most people end an exercise session in a state of dehydration that must be corrected by eating and drinking during the post-exercise period. Thirst is not an adequate guide to fluid requirements.

The effect of dehydration on exercise performance and physiological functions within the body has been well documented. Table 8.3 summarizes these effects. Dehydration increases hemoconcentration, blood viscosity and osmolality, core body temperature, and heart rate, while decreasing stroke volume (Montain and Coyle 1992).

Dehydration hastens the onset of fatigue and makes any given exercise intensity appear harder than if the individual were well hydrated

Table 8.3 **Physiological Responses to Dehydration**

Increase in . . .
Gastrointestinal distress
Plasma osmolality
Blood viscosity
Heart rate
Core temperature at which sweating begins
Core temperature at which blood flow increases in skin
Core temperature at a given exercise intensity
Muscle glycogen use

Decrease in . . .
Plasma volume
Splanchnic and renal blood flow
Central blood volume
Central venous pressure
Stroke volume
Cardiac output
Sweat rate at a given core temperature
Maximal sweat rate
Skin blood flow at a given core temperature
Performance
Endurance capacity (exercise to exhaustion)

Reprinted from Murray 1995.

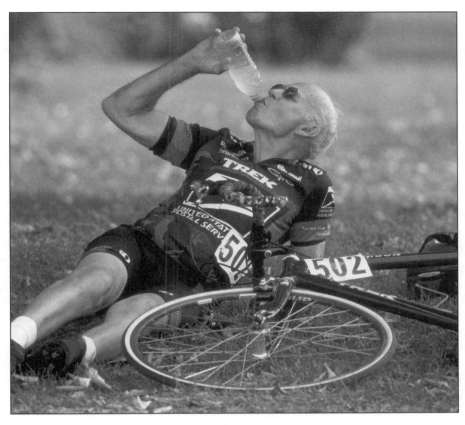

Dehydration is one of the most common nutritional problems that athletes face. Drinking adequate fluids is imperative for good exercise performance.

(Maughan 1992). In addition, glycogen is used more rapidly when a person exercises while dehydrated. *The most serious effect of progressive dehydration, however, is that reduced blood flow to the skin limits the body's ability to sweat.* This in turn reduces the body's ability to cool itself, which increases core body temperature and the risk of heat illness and collapse—and, in rare situations, life-threatening heatstroke (Sutton 1990). "Heat-Related Disorders" (page 226) outlines various types of heat-related disorders, as well as factors that increase risk for heat illness. Dehydration—where 3% or more of body weight is lost—can cause significant reductions in cardiac output since the reduction in stroke volume can be greater than the increase in heart rate (American College of Sports Medicine [ACSM] 1996). Figure 8.3 gives an overview of the effects of continued dehydration on thirst, on the ability to perform work, and on physiological functions.

As one becomes progressively dehydrated, from which body water pools does the water come? According to an early study by Costill et al. (1976), who dehydrated subjects using a combination of cycling exercise and heat exposure, low levels of dehydration remove water primarily from the extracellular space. As body water losses increase, a proportionally greater percentage of water comes from the intracellular spaces. When Costill's subjects lost 9% of their body weight due to dehydration, ~50% of the lost water came from intracellular water. This means that body cells, especially muscle cells that are 70% water, were being depleted of the water necessary to maintain metabolic functions—perhaps one reason why dehydration hinders exercise performance. Researchers have also examined the effect of exercise, without prior dehydration, on change in body water compartments (Maw et al. 1998). When subjects cycled for 50 min at moderate intensity (50% $\dot{V}O_2$max) in a cool environment (60°F, or 14.4°C), fluid losses came primarily from the extracellular fluid. When they repeated the protocol in a hot environment (97°F, or 36.2°C), 23% of the fluid losses came from the intracellular environment. Thus, progressive dehydration in well-hydrated people doing moderate exercise primarily depletes extracellular fluid; when the stress of heat is added, some fluid is drawn from the intracellular space.

Heat-Related Disorders

Heat Syncope

The dizziness experienced with this condition is due to the pooling of blood in the vasodilated periphery in unacclimatized people who stand for long periods. Dehydration is not a prerequisite for this disorder, however—it generally occurs when individuals stand for long periods of time in the heat, stop suddenly after a race, or stand suddenly from a lying position (Sutton 1990).

Heat Cramps

These skeletal muscle spasms occur several hours after a strenuous exercise event where sweat losses and fluid intakes were high, urine volume was low, and sodium intake was inadequate to replace losses. Cramps usually occur in the legs, arms, or abdominal wall long after a person has cooled down from the exercise. Although the specific mechanism for heat cramps is not known, it is associated with sodium depletion (Sutton 1990). Sunstroke, heat cramps, and heat exhaustion are possible with prolonged exposure or physical activity in temperatures between 90-105°F (~32-41°C) (National Weather Service 1998).

Heat Exhaustion and Heatstroke

Plasma volume decreases during exercise, reducing blood flow from the muscles to the skin—which in turn compromises the body's ability to dissipate the heat generated during exercise and to adequately cool itself. The result is that the body's heat production exceeds its ability to dissipate heat—and core body temperature rises to ≥104°F (≥40°C). Dehydration exacerbates these physiological changes and contributes to heat-related problems. Think of these two illnesses as a continuum, where heat exhaustion can lead to heatstroke (heat exhaustion is less severe than heatstroke, which can lead to loss of consciousness and even death). Early symptoms of heat injury are excessive sweating, headache, nausea, dizziness, a gradual impairment of consciousness, and difficulty concentrating. *Along with an increased core body temperature (≥104°F or 40°C) and hot, dry skin, altered mental status is the universally accepted sign that distinguishes exertional heatstroke from heat exhaustion* (Shapiro and Seidman 1990). Environmental conditions that predispose exercisers to heat exhaustion or heatstroke are hot, humid, windless conditions or unseasonably hot conditions to which the people are not acclimatized. Sunstroke, heat cramps, or heat exhaustion are likely, and heatstroke possible, with prolonged exposure or physical activity in temperatures ranging from 105-130°F (41-54°C). If the temperature rises to ≥130°F (54°C), heatstroke/sunstroke is highly likely with continued exposure (National Weather Service 1998). People are more susceptible to heatstroke if they are unfit, overweight, dehydrated, unacclimatized to the heat, or ill. Finally, children and the elderly are more susceptible to heat-related injury because they have less sensitive homeostatic mechanisms for fluid balance (Sutton 1990).

Studies of exertional heat illness in military recruits show that risk was greatest when temperatures rose to >65°F (18°C), strenuous exercise was done (e.g., running), or if recruits had heat stress exposure on previous days (Kark et al. 1996). For new recruits, a body mass index (BMI) >22 and a 1.5-mi run time >12 min also increased the risk of heat illness (Gardner et al. 1996).

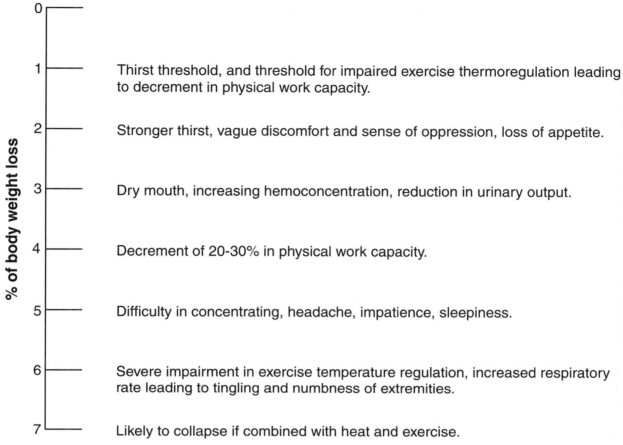

Figure 8.3 Adverse effects of dehydration on work capacity.
Reprinted from Greenleaf 1992.

Environmental conditions have a dramatic effect on fluid losses. As temperature and humidity rise, exercising becomes harder and risks of heat-related problems rise. Table 8.4 outlines the effects of air temperature, relative humidity, and solar radiation on potential environmental heat hazards. As the wet bulb globe temperature rises, the risks of exercising in the heat also rise. **Wet bulb** is an index of relative humidity (the method for calculating wet bulb globe temperature follows). **Dry bulb** is an index of ambient temperature (the actual air temperature measured on a thermometer). If the dry bulb and wet bulb temperatures are the same, the air has a humidity of 100% and evaporation is impossible. The **black bulb** is an index of heat radiation from the environment (e.g., from the sun). The combination of these three temperatures into a single factor is known as the **wet bulb globe temperature (WBGT).**

WBGT = 0.7(wet bulb temperature) + 0.2(black bulb temperature) + 0.1(dry bulb temperature)

The greatest contributor to the WBGT is humidity (wet bulb), while the ambient temperature (dry bulb) contributes the least. Thus, it is easier and safer to exercise in a hot environment with a low humidity than in a hot environment with a high humidity. For example, it is easier to exercise in Arizona when the temperature is 90°F with 10% humidity (heat index <90°F), than it is to exercise in Alabama when the temperature is 90°F with 90% humidity (heat index = 122°F). As the humidity rises, it is harder for the body to cool itself through evaporation of sweat from the skin. Those of us who have no access to wet and black bulb temperatures can use the Heat Index Chart in figure 8.4 to calculate a rough index of the WBGT by using just the air temperature and relative humidity. The one part of the WBGT that this chart does not include is the effect of

Table 8.4 Exercise Recommendations for Various Wet Bulb Globe Temperatures (WBGTs)

Wet bulb globe temperature	Exercise recommendation	Comments
Less than 80°F (~ <27°C)	All can exercise	Activities may be performed by most individuals without a risk of heat problems.
80 to 85°F (~27 to 29°C)	Exercise with caution	Take frequent water breaks. Look for signs of heat illness (dizziness, rapid heart rate, nausea, chilling, headache, and decreased coordination). Do not attempt distances greater than 10 km when WBGT >82°F (28°C).
85 to 88°F (~29 to 31°C)	Limited exercise	Unconditioned and unacclimatized individuals should suspend activity; those still exercising should take frequent water breaks.
Greater than 88°F (~ >31°C)	Suspend exercise	Suspend all activities or move indoors to a cooler environment.

WBGT = 0.7(wet bulb temperature) + 0.2(black bulb temperature) + 0.1(dry bulb temperature); dry bulb temperature measures the ambient room temperature; wet bulb temperature measures the temperature when the bulb is moist (relative humidity); black bulb temperature measures radiated heat (this bulb absorbs the radiated heat).

Adapted from Pivarnik and Palmer 1994.

radiated heat. For this reason, it is important to remember that exercising in the direct sunlight increases the temperature. The United States National Weather Service (1998) developed this chart to alert Americans to the dangers of developing heat-related illnesses when temperatures rise. As the air temperature and the humidity rise, the heat index values increase. For example, when the air temperature is 86°F (~30°C) and the relative humidity is 40%, it feels like 85°F (~29°C). If it is 86°F (~30°C) and the relative humidity is 95%, it feels like 108°F (~42°C). As indicated by the Heat Index Chart, exercising outside on such a day can pose a real health danger. *Since the heat index values were devised for shady, light wind conditions, exposure to full sunshine can increase heat index values by up to 15°F (~6°C).* Strong winds, especially combined with very hot dry air, can also increase heat index values. Always consider the environmental conditions when exercising outside in the heat, and take appropriate precautions to avoid heat-related illnesses.

The term **hypohydration** is frequently used to refer to the **voluntary dehydration** that many athletes self-impose before a competitive exercise event. This is usually done in order to make weight for a particular sport (e.g., wrestling, rowing, boxing, or horse racing) or to improve muscle definition and physical appearance (e.g., bodybuilders before competition). Hypohy-

dration can negatively affect exercise performance and health even more than the involuntary dehydration discussed previously since, in this case, the individual *begins* the competition depleted of body water and then experiences further dehydration during the competition. The result can be muscle fatigue, loss of concentration, and poor exercise performance. For example, a wrestler may lose 6-11 lb (3-5 kg) of his body weight 3 d prior to weigh-in, and another 2.2 lb (1 kg) or more during the match. While most wrestlers try to rehydrate after weigh-in but before their match begins, total rehydration is not always possible. Their ability to rehydrate depends on the level of hypohydration earlier imposed and the amount of time between weigh-in and competition. Some wrestlers experience severe dehydration by the end of their match, especially if they're competing indoors under conditions that increase sweat rate and water loss.

Using dehydration to lose weight can have serious consequences. "Dehydration-Related Deaths in Three Collegiate Wrestlers in 1997" (page 230) demonstrates the potential lethality of severe dehydration.

Hyponatremia refers to abnormally low plasma sodium concentrations (<130 mmol/L). This condition usually occurs when excess water accumulates, relative to sodium, in the extracellular water compartments of the body. General symptoms of hyponatremia are fatigue

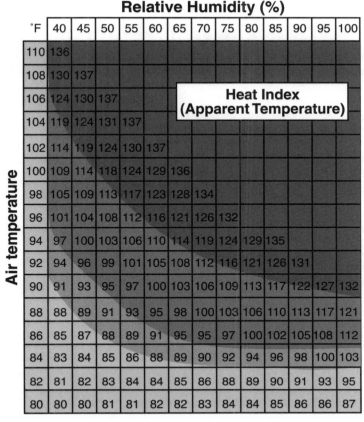

Relative Humidity (%)

°F	40	45	50	55	60	65	70	75	80	85	90	95	100
110	136												
108	130	137											
106	124	130	137										
104	119	124	131	137									
102	114	119	124	130	137								
100	109	114	118	124	129	136							
98	105	109	113	117	123	128	134						
96	101	104	108	112	116	121	126	132					
94	97	100	103	106	110	114	119	124	129	135			
92	94	96	99	101	105	108	112	116	121	126	131		
90	91	93	95	97	100	103	106	109	113	117	122	127	132
88	88	89	91	93	95	98	100	103	106	110	113	117	121
86	85	87	88	89	91	95	95	97	100	102	105	108	112
84	83	84	85	86	88	89	90	92	94	96	98	100	103
82	81	82	83	84	84	85	86	88	89	90	91	93	95
80	80	80	81	81	82	82	83	84	84	85	86	86	87

Air temperature

Heat Index (Apparent Temperature)

With prolonged exposure and/or physical activity

Extreme Danger

Heatstroke or sunstroke highly likely

Danger

Sunstroke, muscle cramps, and/or heat exhaustion likely

Extreme Caution

Sunstroke, muscle cramps, and/or heat exhaustion possible

Caution

Fatigue possible

Figure 8.4 This Heat Index Chart provides general guidelines for assessing the potential severity of heat stress. Individual reactions to heat will vary. It should be remembered that heat illness can occur at lower temperatures than indicated on the chart. In addition, studies indicate that susceptibility to heat illness tends to increase with age.

How to use the Heat Index Chart:

1. Across the top locate the relative humidity (%).
2. Down the left side of the chart locate the air temperature (°F).
3. Follow across and down to find the *apparent temperature*. Apparent temperature is the combined index of heat and humidity. It is an index of the body's sensation of heat caused by the temperature and humidity. In other words, it is what the temperature "feels like" to the body.
4. Note: Exposure to full sunshine can increase heat index values by up to 15°F.

Reprinted from National Weather Service 1998.

and nausea (Armstrong et al. 1993); in severe cases, it can result in grand mal seizures, respiratory arrest, acute respiratory distress syndrome, and coma (Noakes et al. 1990). While there are many clinical causes of hyponatremia, during exercise it usually seems to result from prolonged endurance exercise in a warm environment in which the individual does not replace adequate sodium but drinks excessive amounts of low-sodium fluids. These individuals' fluid-electrolyte control mechanisms either are defective or are overwhelmed by the environmental conditions and the intense exercise (Armstrong et al. 1993). For example, in 1996

a woman developed hyponatremia during an all-day hike in the heat of the Grand Canyon in Arizona, consuming only bottled water and low-sodium foods (Richards 1996). Noakes et al. (1990) reported that in the 1986 and 1987 Comrades Marathon in South Africa, 9% of collapsed runners had hyponatremia. Although there are a number of research papers reporting hyponatremia in individual athletes (Armstrong et al. 1993), the overall incidence of hyponatremia in athletes and active individuals is very low. Nevertheless, athletes still need to be aware of the importance of replacing electrolytes lost in sweat.

■ HIGHLIGHT ■

Dehydration-Related Deaths in Three Collegiate Wrestlers in 1997

During late autumn of 1997, three previously healthy collegiate wrestlers living in different states died while engaging in programs of rapid weight loss to qualify for competition. In the hours before the official weigh-in, all three wrestlers engaged in weight-loss regimens that promoted dehydration. They also restricted fluid and food intake and tried to maximize sweat losses by wearing vapor-impermeable suits under cotton warm-ups and by exercising vigorously in hot environments. Remick et al. (1998) compiled the complete details of these three cases for the Centers for Disease Control and Prevention.

Case 1

In North Carolina, a 19-year-old wrestler attempted to lose 15 lb (6.8 kg) in a 12-h period so he could compete in the 195-lb (88.6-kg) weight class of a wrestling tournament. His preseason weight was 233 lb (106 kg), and over the next 10 weeks he lost 23 lb (10.5 kg). Using the weight-loss regimen described above, this wrestler lost 9 lb (4 kg) in 8 h. After a 2-h rest, he exercised for another hour, at which time he felt poorly and stopped exercising. Within an hour he went into cardiac arrest and died.

Case 2

In Wisconsin, a 22-year-old wrestler attempted to lose 4 lb (1.8 kg) in a 4-h period so he could compete in the 153-lb (69.5-kg) weight class of a tournament. His preseason weight was 178 lb (81 kg); over the next 10 weeks he lost 21 lb (9.5 kg), of which 8 lb (3.6 kg) were lost 3 d prior to his death. On the day of his death, he initiated the weight-loss regimen described above and lost 3.6 lb (1.6 kg) in 3 h. During this time he complained of shortness of breath but continued to exercise. After resting for 30 min, he resumed exercising again but stopped 30 min later because he was not feeling well. He then became unresponsive, went into cardiac arrest, and could not be resuscitated.

Case 3

In Michigan, a 21-year-old wrestler attempted to lose 6 lb (2.7 kg) in a 3-h period in order to compete in the 153-lb (69.5-kg) weight class of a wrestling tournament. His preseason weight was 180 lb (82 kg); over the next 13 weeks he lost 21 lb (9.5 kg), of which 11 lb (5 kg) were lost 2 d prior to his death. On the day of his death, he initiated the weight-loss regimen described above, lost 2.3 lb (1 kg) in 1.5 h, and weighed 156.7 lb (71.2 kg). He then participated in wrestling practice; after practice, he continued the same weight-loss regimen. Within the next 75 min, he lost another 2 lb (0.9 kg). He then took a 15-min rest and continued to exercise for another hour, at which time he stopped to weigh himself. A few minutes later, his legs became unsteady. He became incommunicative, went into cardiac arrest, and died.

Fluid and Electrolyte Recommendations for Exercise

Exercise increases the loss of water and electrolytes from the body. Even small amounts of dehydration (1% loss of body weight) can increase cardiovascular stress and limit the body's ability to cool itself (ACSM 1996). These physiological changes increase the probability that exercise performance will be compromised. This section outlines fluid recommendations for before, during, and after exercise. The recommendations assume that the active person, regardless of skill level, is beginning the exercise event well fed and hydrated. Anyone who has dehydrated prior to exercise in order to make weight, or has been ill or dieting prior to the event, should change the recommendations herein to account for his or her current state of hydration and nutrition. Since people typi-

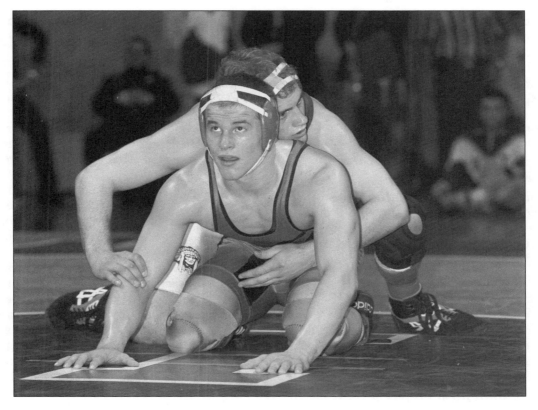

Weight-category sports often encourage athletes to lose weight through dehydration before exercise starts. This practice can negatively affect exercise performance and health.

cally are weak and dehydrated following illness and dieting, they should do all they can to nourish and hydrate themselves before exercising.

Fluid Needs Before Exercise

The American College of Sports Medicine (ACSM) has recently published a position stand on exercise and fluid replacement (1996). They recommend that athletes and active individuals consume 14-20 oz (400-600 ml) of fluid 2 h before exercising. This level of fluid intake should ensure adequate hydration and allow time for the excretion of excess fluid as urine before an exercise event. It should also help to correct any fluid imbalance that may have been present before exercise and help delay or avoid the detrimental effects of dehydration during exercise. In hot weather, an additional ~8-16 oz (250-500 ml) may be needed (Murray 1998). One way to check an individual's level of hydration is to monitor urine color, odor, and volume. *If the urine has a strong odor or dark color, or urine volume is low, then the athlete may be dehydrated, and additional fluid (~16 oz or 500 ml) should be consumed.* According to recent research monitoring athletes over a 42-h period, urine color is the best field indicator of hydration and was as effective or better than urine volume in predicting fluid balance in athletes (Armstrong et al. 1998). People should continue to drink until their urine is either "very pale yellow" or "pale yellow" in color. Body mass of athletes with this urine color should be within 1% of the well-hydrated baseline body mass (Armstrong et al. 1998). However, Kovacs et al. (1999) found that urine color was not a good indicator of hydration up to 6 h post-exercise. The length of time required post-exercise for urine color to indicate good hydration status may vary depending on the level of dehydration that occurs during exercise, the amount of fluid consumed post-exercise, and environmental conditions. Illness and various food and sport supplements—especially vitamin supplements—can produce dark urine with a strong odor; in these cases, urine color cannot be used as a guide to hydration level. When urine color can no longer be used, urine volume may be the only field indicator of hydration level available. If this is the case, an athlete needs to drink adequate fluids to produce 1-2 L of urine per day.

lways want to know what to drink, drink, and when to drink before type and amount of fluid you rec- ld depend on a number of factors, which are listed below (along with questions that help determine more specific needs):

- *The time of fluid ingestion:* How much time before the exercise event begins?

- *Environmental conditions:* Is the weather hot, cold, or humid?

- *Individual level of acclimation to the weather:* Is the athlete well adapted to the environment in which the exercise is occurring? Has he or she been exercising and training in this environment for longer than 2 weeks?

- *Type and intensity of activity to be engaged in:* Is the event of long duration and of high intensity?

- *Current nutritional status:* Is the athlete coming to the exercise event well fed and hydrated?

- *Individual fluid preferences:* What fluids does the athlete prefer to drink? In the past, what fluids have caused gastrointestinal distress during exercise?

If athletes are well hydrated and fed, well acclimated to the weather conditions, and in good health, and if the upcoming exercise is moderate in intensity and duration, then they can consume water, a sport drink, or fruit juice before the event. However, if they are dehydrated, need additional energy, or will be participating in strenuous activity, or if the environmental conditions are extreme, then they should consume an oral rehydration beverage or sport drink. These beverages provide both fluid and energy for the upcoming challenge. The sodium and flavoring in these drinks increases palatability, which may improve fluid intake. The closer a person is to an exercise event, the more water or a sport drink becomes the fluid of choice. More concentrated carbohydrate beverages (≥10% carbohydrate) like soda pop, fruit juices, or fruit drinks may not empty adequately from the stomach before exercise begins. Of course, you should always consider an individual's needs and preferences— concerning both amounts and types of fluids— when you recommend fluids. Some people are subject to severe gastrointestinal distress during strenuous exercise and may need to avoid items that aggravate this condition. These athletes usually tolerate sport drinks rather well.

Fluid Needs During Exercise

The goal of drinking fluids during exercise is to maintain plasma volume and electrolytes, prevent abnormal elevation in heart rate and core body temperature, and provide fuel to the working muscles. This in turn may prevent or delay fatigue and the fluid imbalances that occur during exercise. As mentioned earlier, the most serious effect of exercise-induced dehydration is the abnormal rise in core body temperature (i.e., >104°F or 40°C), due to the inability to dissipate heat.

The effectiveness of an oral rehydration solution depends on factors such as exercise duration and intensity, the volume and composition of the fluid, environmental conditions, feeding frequency, and the nutritional status of the individual before exercise. No single rehydration solution can meet the needs of all active individuals in all exercise situations. However, general recommendations can be made regarding fluid intake during exercise. The guidelines in the ACSM position stand are given below under "Endurance Exercise." You can modify these recommendations to meet individual needs and differing environmental conditions.

Endurance Exercise

During endurance exercise, fluid intake should match or exceed sweat loss—yet athletes who are allowed to drink ad libitum (as much as they desire) during exercise tend to replace only two-thirds of the water lost in sweat. This typically results in dehydration levels of 2-5% (based on decreases in total body weight). For example, while runners may drink only ~6.5 oz (200 ml) during a 2-h race in a cool environment, water losses can range from 1-2 L/h. This loss of fluid can decrease exercise performance and increase heart rate, core body temperature, and muscle glycogen use. Hargreaves and colleagues (1996) studied five trained men during 2 h of cycling at 67% $\dot{V}O_2$max on two different cycling tests—one with water provided, one with no fluids. Compared to the trial with no fluid intake, exercise with water intake significantly decreased heart rate, rectal temperature, muscle temperature, and muscle glycogen utilization. Net muscle glycogen utilization also decreased by 16% when water was ingested, which may help explain why fluid intake during exercise can improve exercise performance.

The ACSM position stand (1996) on exercise and fluid replacement recommends that during exercise lasting longer than 1 h, fluids containing both carbohydrate and electrolytes (primarily sodium chloride) be consumed at 600-1050 ml/h (20-36 oz). The sport drink or fluid replacement solution should contain 4-8% carbohydrate and 0.5-0.7 g of sodium per liter. The carbohydrate provides energy during exercise, while the sodium improves palatability and replaces lost electrolytes. These fluids should also be cool and flavor-enhanced to increase consumption. Ideally, fluid intake should begin early in an exercise event and occur frequently (~ every 15-20 min; 150-350 ml or 5-12 oz); however, not every sport allows for frequent fluid intakes. The beneficial effect of carbohydrate-containing sport drinks on exercise performance has been well established and is discussed in detail in chapter 2. Athletes should become familiar with their own sweat losses during exercise under various environmental conditions by measuring weight before and again after exercise. They should then strive to consume enough fluid during exercise to prevent or minimize these weight losses. Although some people may have difficulty consuming this volume of fluid, they should at least be aware of their ideal goal for fluid intake.

Intermittent Exercise and Team Sports

Sports involving intermittent exercise are usually team sports in which high-intensity exercise is interspersed with rest or with lower-intensity exercise. Examples include volleyball, soccer, basketball, American football, and ice hockey but can also include sports such as ice skating, gymnastics, swimming, and tennis. The duration and intensity of these sports vary dramatically but can last anywhere from 60 min to 2 h. These sports can produce sweat rates as high as those in endurance sports and usually involve high-intensity exercise that relies heavily on muscle glycogen. Moreover, many of these sports are played indoors, where higher temperatures can contribute to increased sweat losses. Unlike endurance sports, in which the athlete usually dictates fluid intake, intermittent exercise sports usually restrict fluid consumption to breaks in play or between events.

Fluid intake during intermittent sports has not been studied as extensively as fluid intake during endurance sports. Research on the effect of fluid intake during intermittent or high-intensity exercise (>80% $\dot{V}O_2$max) has found that beverages containing electrolytes and carbohydrate can improve exercise performance and prevent dehydration. Laboratory research has attempted to mimic the team sport environment by interspersing high-intensity work with lower-intensity exercise over an extended period. Davis and colleagues (1997) had subjects repeatedly cycle for 1 min at 120-130% $\dot{V}O_2$max, separated by 3 min of rest, until fatigued. They repeated this protocol on two different occasions: one with a carbohydrate-electrolyte replacement beverage and one with a water placebo. In the carbohydrate trial, subjects received an 18% carbohydrate solution before exercise began and a 6% carbohydrate solution during exercise. In the carbohydrate trial, time to fatigue was 27 min longer than with the water placebo. In addition, during the carbohydrate trial, subjects were able to complete 21 1-min high-exercise bouts compared to only 14 bouts with the water placebo. Nicholas et al. (1995) did a similar study using shuttle running. Subjects completed 75 min of exercise, which included five 15-min periods of intermittent running (sprinting interspersed with periods of jogging and walking). This was then followed by a run to fatigue. Consumption of a beverage containing electrolytes and 6.9% carbohydrate during the shuttle running increased time to fatigue by 33% compared to a noncarbohydrate placebo.

Researchers have also examined the effect of fluid intake on exercise performance, and the physiological factors associated with dehydration, in high-intensity exercise (usually ≥80% $\dot{V}O_2$max) lasting ≤1 h. Ball et al. (1995) found that, in a 50-min simulated cycle time trial, a 7% carbohydrate solution increased subjects' peak power and mean power output compared to a water placebo. These data were supported by a study done by Jeukendrup et al. (1997), who fed a 7.6% carbohydrate-electrolyte beverage or a water placebo to athletes during cycle time trials lasting approximately 1 h. Subjects cycled faster and did more work when they drank a carbohydrate solution than when they drank a water placebo. The above studies tested athletes after an overnight fast; the results in well-fed athletes might be different.

In summary, it appears that consuming fluids—especially carbohydrate-electrolyte beverages—increases exercise performance in high-intensity exercise or team sports where intermittent play is done over an extended period. The effect on performance may be especially profound if high-intensity exercise is done in a hot environment that increases sweat loss (Morris et al. 1988), since even a 1.8% decrease in body weight can impair exercise at high intensities (Walsh et al. 1994). Consumption of a sport beverage may be especially beneficial for the athlete who is dehydrated, fasted, or has poor glycogen stores before a high-intensity event. A number of recent review articles have discussed the role of fluids in team sports and intermittent exercise (Burke 1997; Burke and Hawley 1997; Kirkendall 1998; Maughan and Leiper 1994; Shi and Gisolfi 1998).

Fluid Needs After Exercise

What is required to bring an individual back to a state of euhydration after exercise is over? The goal of post-exercise rehydration is to replace the water and electrolytes lost during exercise—which vary dramatically from person to person and depend on exercise intensity, frequency, duration, and environmental conditions. In general, athletes can replace water and electrolytes by consuming adequate water and food during the recovery period. If no food is consumed, either by choice or circumstances, then any fluid consumed should contain electrolytes, especially sodium (~50 mmol/L), and carbohydrate (Maughan and Shirreffs 1997). The sodium improves fluid retention in the body, while the carbohydrate enhances intestinal uptake of sodium and water and helps replace muscle and liver glycogen. *The volume of fluid consumed should be greater than the volume of sweat lost* since losses of fluid in the urine and in respiration also need to be covered (Shirreffs et al. 1996). Shirreffs et al. (1996) found that athletes needed to consume 150% of the body mass losses that occurred during exercise to be at fluid balance 6 h after exercise ended. These athletes were dehydrated by 2.06% of body mass by exercising in a hot, humid environment at approximately 60% $\dot{V}O_2$max for 35-40 min (figure 8.5).

A number of studies have examined the effect of various electrolyte replacement beverages, water, and other fluids on restoration of fluid balance after exercise. Gonzalez-Alonso et al. (1992) found that a dilute carbohydrate-electrolyte solution (6% carbohydrate, 20 mmol/L sodium, 3 mmol/L potassium) was more effective in promoting post-exercise rehydration than plain water or Diet Coke. The

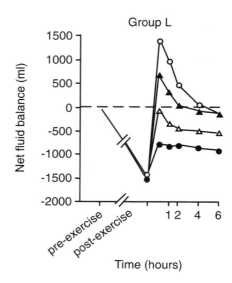

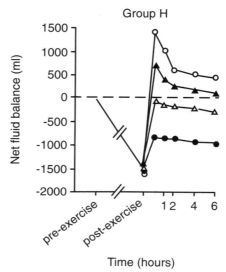

- ● Trial A - 50% replacement
- △ Trial B - 100% replacement
- ▲ Trial C - 150% replacement
- ○ Trial D - 200% replacement

Figure 8.5 Net fluid balance calculated from the volumes of sweat loss, fluid ingestion, and urine output in 12 male volunteers, dehydrated by 2.06% of body mass by intermittent cycle exercise, consuming four different drink volumes equivalent to 50% (trial A), 100% (trial B), 150% (trial C), and 200% (trial D) of body mass lost. Subjects consumed these four different drink volumes on four separate weeks; in each trial, six subjects received drink L (23 mmol/L of sodium) and six received drink H (61 mmol/L of sodium). The top panel shows the results for group L and the lower panel shows the results of group H.

Reprinted from Shirreffs et al. 1996.

carbohydrate-electrolyte beverage produced the smallest urine volume, indicating that it promoted the greatest retention of fluid. Brouns and colleagues (1998) confirmed these results. They examined the effect of three different fluid replacement beverages—a carbohydrate-electrolyte drink (Isostar), a low-sodium mineral water, or a caffeinated soft drink (Coca Cola)—on fluid replacement in the first 2 h following cycling in the heat. The cola and the water trials produced the greatest urinary losses of sodium, potassium, chloride, magnesium, and calcium during the 2-h recovery period, while the carbohydrate-electrolyte drink resulted in sodium, magnesium, and calcium retention, and no change in potassium and chloride retention. The researchers concluded that ingesting either water or caffeinated cola after exercise resulted in a negative electrolyte balance; that caffeine-containing beverages abetted urinary magnesium and calcium losses; and that a carbohydrate-electrolyte drink containing moderate amounts of sodium, magnesium, and calcium helped maintain electrolyte balance.

Athletes who have time to eat and drink after exercise can effectively restore fluid balance without consuming carbohydrate-electrolyte sport drinks (Maughan et al. 1996). The meal should provide adequate electrolytes and water or other fluids. In general, alcohol is not recommended as a fluid replacement beverage after exercise, primarily due to its diuretic effect. One recent research project found that moderate amounts of alcohol (beer containing ≤ 2% alcohol; volume equal to 150% of estimated sweat losses) did not negatively impact rehydration after exercise, but these data are not particularly relevant to most people since, in the United States, beer typically contains about 5% alcohol, with the lowest levels being around 3.2%. The data also showed that drinks containing 4% alcohol delayed the recovery process (Shirreffs and Maughan 1997). *If* athletes can find any beer containing ≤2% alcohol to drink after a long run, it apparently will not adversely affect their fluid balance.

These are the best current recommendations for post-exercise rehydration:

• Sodium chloride should be consumed either in food or in a carbohydrate-electrolyte beverage after exercise is over (Maughan and Leiper 1995). Fluids should be palatable and the appropriate temperature for the occasion.

Cool, flavored fluids tend to increase fluid intake.

• The amount of fluid consumed should equal 100-150% of the fluid lost in sweat—that is, for every pound (0.45 kg) of body weight lost due to sweating, about 15-23 oz (0.45-0.68 L) of fluid need to be consumed.

• If no food is consumed post-exercise, then a carbohydrate-electrolyte beverage should be used to rehydrate. Food consumed with adequate amounts of water can adequately restore fluid balance after exercise. Both sodium and fluid volume are important in restoring fluid balance after exercise (Shirreffs et al. 1996).

• *Small* amounts of alcohol can be used in moderation by the athlete post-exercise without adversely affecting rehydration efforts; however, excessive amounts can inhibit rehydration and are not recommended. No athlete is encouraged to consume alcohol after exercise.

Although the above recommendations seem very straightforward, it is not always easy for athletes to adequately refuel and rehydrate after exercise. Burke (1996) has outlined some of the factors that interfere:

• *Fatigue:* The athlete is too tired to eat and drink. Fatigue can interfere with the ability and interest to obtain and consume food or fluids.

• *Loss of appetite:* This occurs especially if stress and fatigue levels are high.

• *Limited access:* Suitable foods/beverages often are unavailable at an exercise venue. If the athlete will not eat the food or drink the beverages available, post-exercise recovery will be significantly impaired. It is always helpful for athletes, coaches, or parents to bring acceptable foods and fluids to the sporting event.

• *Other post-exercise commitments:* Coaches' meetings, drug tests, equipment maintenance, mandatory study periods, cool-down activities, medical treatments such as physical therapy—these activities can prevent athletes from obtaining adequate food and drink post-exercise.

• *Postcompetition social activities:* These often take precedence over the consumption of water and food (e.g., excessive alcohol intake without adequate food and other fluids).

Fluid Needs in Hot and Cold Environments

Exercise stresses the body's ability to regulate body heat and fluid balance. Exercise in the heat increases the risk of dehydration, as core body temperature and sweat rates rise. Training and heat acclimatization can increase sweat rates by 10-20% (Gisolfi 1993), or 200-300 ml/h more than the 1-2 L/h of sweat typically lost during high-intensity exercise. Exercising in the heat also increases the use of body glycogen as a fuel source, hastens the onset of fatigue and rate of perceived exertion, and impairs mental performance (Murray 1995). Of course, all these changes can result in decreased physical performance—or, in some cases, heat illness or heatstroke (see "Heat-Related Disorders," page 226). Ideally, athletes need 10-14 d of training in hot humid environments to adequately acclimate (Armstrong and Maresh 1991). Here are several recommendations to help athletes maintain fluid balance in the heat and acclimate to hot environments:

- Increase fluid intake to match or exceed sweat rates. Athletes should monitor urine color or weigh before and after exercise—and replace fluids lost during exercise. A daily morning weigh-in can also be helpful during the days of acclimation to determine if fluid balance is being maintained. If body weight is reduced by 2-3%, extra fluids are needed. If body weight is reduced by 4-6%, a reduction in exercise training and additional fluid intake may be required (Armstrong and Maresh 1991). Remember that small levels of dehydration (as little as a 2% loss of body weight) can significantly decrease the desire and ability to perform physical activity.

- Increase sodium intake if total daily sodium from food and beverages is less than 3 g/d (Armstrong and Maresh 1991). One way to increase sodium and fluid intakes is to use a carbohydrate-electrolyte sport drink before, during, and after exercise in the heat. These beverages provide low amounts of sodium, increase total fluid intake, and provide additional energy in the form of carbohydrate. Another way to increase sodium intake is to eat adequate amounts of food, including foods high in sodium (pickles, salty snacks, processed foods such as canned soups, stews, chili).

- Be aware of the signs and symptoms of heat stress and illness—prevention is the best treatment.

Less has been written on the body's response to cold weather exercise; however, exercising in cold environments stresses the body's thermoregulation mechanisms. If exercise in the cold is combined with high altitudes, the metabolic stresses on the body are extremely high, escalating the demand for adequate fuel and fluid intake. Murray (1995) has described how exercising in cold environments can compromise fluid balance. Cold can increase urinary fluid losses at the same time fluid intake is reduced. In the cold there may be less of a desire to drink and the need to drink less obvious; fluids may be less available; or fluid intake may be purposefully reduced to avoid having to go to the bathroom. This is especially true for athletes who may have to disrobe from many layers of clothing in order to urinate or travel some distance to find a restroom. Finally, exercising in the cold can increase fluid losses through respiration since the partial pressure of water vapor in cold air is less than that of warm air. This change in water vapor sets up a pressure gradient for water loss so that, when cold air is exhaled, it is immediately saturated with water vapor from the body. This can result in significant water loss from the body through respiration (~0.2-1.5 L/d). Exercising in cold temperatures also can produce high sweat losses, especially if heavy insulated clothing is worn.

Fluid and Electrolyte Needs for Children and Adolescents

Probably over 50% of children and adolescents participate in some type of competitive athletics, either at school or in the community (Squire 1990). Health professionals are constantly encouraging schools and communities to keep their children active to prevent obesity and promote good health. However, children and adults respond differently to exercise and have different fluid requirements. Dr. Oded Bar-Or and colleagues at McMaster University in Ontario have extensively studied the responses of children to exercise, especially in the heat (Bar-Or and Unnithan 1994; Wilk and Bar-Or 1996; Wilk et al. 1998). They have found that children are less efficient thermoregulators than adults, especially when they exercise in warm environments. Compared to adults, children acclimatize more slowly, have a higher **set point** (i.e., change in rectal temperature at which sweating starts) and a lower sweat rate, produce more metabolic heat per kilogram of body weight during exercise, and have greater physiological impairment from dehydration. Playing in the heat stresses a child's thermoregulatory mechanisms much more than those of an adult playing with the child. If you as an adult feel hot, your child is probably *very* hot! And just like adults, when children exercise they often do not drink adequate amounts of fluid to maintain fluid balance, leading to involuntary dehydration. For these reasons, active children need to learn the importance of adequate fluid intake before, during, and after exercise. "Keeping Children Well Hydrated During Exercise" (below) provides some important guidelines for anyone who works with children.

Sport Drinks/Fluid Replacement Beverages

There is no general agreement among researchers on the optimal formulation of a sport drink; neither is there an "ideal" beverage that will satisfy all conditions (Gisolfi and Duchman 1992). We don't even know exactly how much any particular individual needs to drink for a particular exercise event (Maughan 1992). Ideally, the optimal sport drink for any one person would depend on the duration and intensity of the exercise, the environmental conditions, and the characteristics of the individual (Maughan 1992). Table 8.5 lists the carbohydrate, electrolyte, and osmolality contents of current sport drinks. Although we do not have an "optimal" sport drink or oral rehydration solution, any drink listed in table 8.5 that contains both electrolytes and carbohydrate (at concentrations ≤8%) can enhance fluid balance.

The primary reasons for using a beverage containing electrolyte and carbohydrate are to maximize fluid intake, replace electrolyte losses, and provide carbohydrate for energy and for rapid replacement of muscle and liver glycogen both during and after exercise (Marriott 1994). These beverages can be helpful in a number of situations, depending on the individual, the event, and the environment. Listed below are a number of exercise situations in which you may want to recommend use of a fluid replacement beverage or sport drink (Marriott 1994):

- To provide adequate fluid intake *before* exercise in which dehydration may occur; this is especially important if the athlete has poor fluid balance before beginning exercise.
- To provide adequate fluid, electrolytes, and carbohydrate *during* exercise or physical work under various environmental

■ HIGHLIGHT ■

Keeping Children Well Hydrated During Exercise

Children can maintain euhydration during prolonged and intermittent exercise if they drink 4 oz of fluid (120 ml) every 15-20 min (Bar-Or and Unnithan 1994). Children should be encouraged to drink fluids (~4-8 oz, or roughly 120-240 ml) before exercise; and after exercise, they should drink ~16 oz of fluid (roughly 0.5 L) for every pound (0.5 kg) lost. They should be reminded that *thirst is not a good indicator of fluid needs*. Like adults, children can learn to monitor their urine color as an indicator of fluid balance.

Fluids should be flavored, palatable, and cool. Research shows that children aged 9-13 years prefer flavored beverages (especially grape flavor) over water (Meyer et al. 1994). Flavored beverages containing sodium and carbohydrate promote adequate fluid intake and help maintain fluid balance during exercise in the heat better than unflavored or flavored water (Rivera-Brown et al. 1999; Wilk and Bar-Or 1996; Wilk et al. 1998). However, water is a good beverage, especially if other fluids are not available or if the exercise intensity is low and of short duration.

Be aware of the early signs of dehydration in active children. Look for dry lips and tongue, dark yellow urine, fatigue and apathy, muscle cramps, infrequent urination, and sunken eyes.

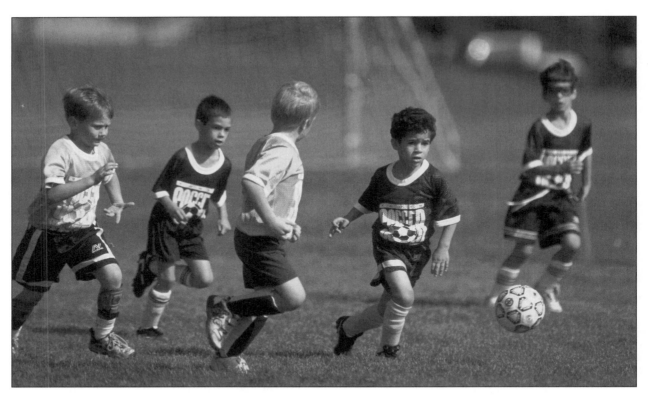

Children overheat and become dehydrated more quickly than adults. They should be encouraged to drink adequate fluids before, during, and after exercise.

Table 8.5 Carbohydrate and Electrolyte Contents of Sport Drinks, Soft Drinks, Juices, and Water

Beverage	Carbohydrate (g/L)	Carbohydrate %	Sodium (mg/L)	Potassium (mg/L)	Osmolality (mOsm/kg)
Demineralized water	0	0	0	0	5-8
Diet Pepsi[a]	0	0	99	23	41
AllSport (Pepsico)[c]	56	5.6	155	155	280-330[b]
Gatorade[c]	60	6	400	120	320-360
Isostar[c]	76	7.6	724	211	~305
PowerAde (Coca-Cola)[c]	80	8.0	118	135	280-350[b]
Sprite	110	11.0	97	0	560-590
Coca Cola[a]	113	11.3	23	10	550-650
Orange juice (fresh)	109	10.0	11	2096	~670
Cranberry juice cocktail	154	15.4	21	193	~700
Beer (Miller Genuine Draft)	37	3.7	20	—	~840
Beer (Miller Genuine Draft Light)	10	1.0	17	—	—

Most solutions also contain chloride, biocarbonate, citrate, and phosphate. Beverages are ranked by carbohydrate concentration (%).
[a]Also contains caffeine: Coke has 130 mg/L of caffeine; Diet Pepsi has 101 mg/L.
[b]Values were estimated.
[c]Sport drinks that contain less than 10% carbohydrate, and electrolytes in appropriate amounts for good fluid absorption.

Adapted from Greenleaf 1994; Brouns et al. 1998; data from product manufacturers and Food Processor Version 7.11, ESHA Research, Salem, OR.

conditions—especially if high temperature or humidity will increase sweat rates; and especially if the athlete has low electrolyte intakes before exercise or high electrolyte losses due to illness, diarrhea, or vomiting or is not heat-acclimated before exercise.

- To provide rapid rehydration following exercise or between exercise bouts when it is difficult to consume food.

- To maintain blood glucose levels during exercise. This is especially important if an individual has poor glycogen stores before exercise.

- To provide energy, in the form of carbohydrate, to people who are not well fed before exercise due to the unavailability of food or due to illness, vomiting, or diarrhea.

Chapter in Review

There is no question that maintaining fluid balance during exercise is important for exercise performance and good health. The amount, type, and timing of fluid intake both before and during exercise depend on a number of factors related to a person's level of fitness and general health and to the exercise environment. After exercise is over it is also important to make sure that adequate energy, fluids, and electrolytes are available in the food and drink consumed to replenish the body for the next exercise event. Inadequate fluid intake before, during, and after exercise is one of the most common nutritional problems facing athletes, especially those who work and train in extreme environments. Teaching athletes the importance of fluid balance, how to monitor their own level of dehydration, and how to adequately replace fluids are some of the most important skills you can impart to them.

Before you recommend an oral rehydration solution or sport drink to an athlete, judge its formulation in terms of how it will influence gastric emptying and intestinal absorption of fluids, as well as how it fits the athlete's requirements for fluid and energy before, during, and after exercise. Finally, consider the intensity and duration of the athlete's exercise before making fluid recommendations. In general, a fluid replacement drink should provide low concentrations of carbohydrate for energy and of sodium for palatability—and it should taste good.

Today's marketplace is filled with fluid replacement beverages, sport drinks, fruit juices and drinks, soda pop, and bottled water. Picking the right drink for the right situation can be confusing. All of these beverages provide fluid, while some provide energy and electrolytes. What you choose will depend on the athletes' individual preferences, their nutrient needs, the type of exercise in which they are participating, and the exercise environment. If athletes cannot or will not consume food after exercise, sport drinks are an excellent source of energy and fluids.

KEY CONCEPTS

 1. Understand the function and regulation of water and electrolyte balance within the body, and the adverse health effects of dehydration, hypohydration, and hyponatremia.

Body water makes up a significant proportion of body weight (~60%); it functions as a transport medium, a structural part of body tissues, a lubricant, and a component of chemical reactions. Body water is found both inside (intracellular) and outside (extracellular) the cells. Electrolytes help maintain this distribution of water within and outside the cells. Balance of water and electrolytes within the body is maintained by endocrine and neurological control mechanisms. Especially during exercise, optimal fluid balance is required to maintain plasma volume and electrolyte balance—and fluid balance depends on the rate and content of fluid intake and on the rates of gastric emptying and of intestinal absorption. Dehydration, which occurs when there is a decrease in total body water, hastens the onset of fatigue and degrades exercise performance. Hypohydration occurs when athletes voluntarily dehydrate before an exercise competition to make weight or improve aesthetic appearance. Hypohydration can also negatively affect exercise performance and health. During exercise, hyponatremia (low plasma sodium concentrations) occurs when excess water is consumed and sodium intake is low or losses are high. General symptoms of mild hyponatremia are fatigue and nausea.

 ## 2. Identify the fluid and electrolyte recommendations for exercise.

Two hours before exercise, athletes should consume ~16 oz (500 ml) of fluid; this amount should increase if the weather is hot or the individual is poorly hydrated. During exercise, athletes should consume ~21-43 oz/h (600-1200 ml/h) of fluid, or enough to replace fluid losses. The goal of the post-exercise rehydration period is to replace the water and electrolytes lost during exercise. This can be achieved by consuming both food and beverages during the post-exercise period. The amount of fluid consumed should be 100-150% of the fluid lost during exercise. Athletes should continue to drink fluids until the urine is pale yellow. Consuming a sport beverage during the post-exercise period helps replace fluid and electrolyte losses and provides carbohydrate for energy and glycogen replacement.

 ## 3. Understand the role of sport drinks in preventing and maintaining fluid balance before, during, and after exercise.

The primary reasons for using an electrolyte-carbohydrate beverage before, during, and after exercise are to maximize fluid balance and replace electrolyte losses; to provide carbohydrate for energy and maintenance of blood glucose during exercise; and to rapidly replace muscle and liver glycogen after exercise.

KEY TERMS

black bulb
dehydration
dry bulb
euhydration
extracellular water
heat cramps
heat exhaustion and heatstroke
heat syncope
hypohydration
hyponatremia
interstitial fluid
intracellular water

intravascular water
involuntary dehydration
isotonic solutions
osmolality
osmolarity
osmotic pressure
set point
transcellular water
voluntary dehydration
wet bulb
wet bulb global temperature (WBGT)

References

American College of Sports Medicine (ACSM). Authors: Convertino VA, Armstrong LE, Coyle EF, Mack GW, Swaka MN, Senay LC, Sherman WM. ACSM Position Stand: Exercise and fluid replacement. Med Sci Sports Exerc 1996;28:i-vii.

Armstrong LA, Curtis WC, Hubbard W, Francesconi RP, Moore R, Askew EW. Symptomatic hyponatremia during prolonged exercise in heat. Med Sci Sports Exerc 1993;25:543-9.

Armstrong LA, Maresh CM. The induction and decay of heat acclimatization in trained athletes. Sports Med 1991;12:302-12.

Armstrong LA, Soto JAH, Hacker FT, Casa DJ, Kavouras SA, Maresh CM. Urinary indices during dehydration, exercise, and rehydration. Int J Sport Nutr 1998;8:345-55.

Ball TC, Headley SA, Vanderburgh PM, Smith JC. Periodic carbohydrate replacement during 50 min of high-intensity cycling improves subsequent sprint performance. Int J Sport Nutr 1995;5:151-8.

Bar-Or O, Unnithan VB. Nutritional requirements of young soccer players. J Sport Sci 1994;12:S39-S42.

Brouns F, Kovacs EMR, Senden JMG. The effect of different rehydration drinks on post-exercise electrolyte excretion in trained athletes. Int J Sports Med 1998;19:56-60.

Brouns F, Senden J, Beckers EJ, Saris WH. Osmolarity does not effect the gastric emptying rate of oral rehydration solutions. J Parenter Enteral Nutr 1995;19:403-6.

Burke LM. Nutrition for post-exercise recovery. Aust J Sci Med Sport 1996;29:3-10.

Burke LM. Fluid balance during team sports. J Sport Sci 1997;15:287-95.

Burke LM, Hawley JA. Fluid balance in team sports. Guidelines for optimal practices. Sports Med 1997;24:38-54.

Costill DL. Gastric emptying of fluids during exercise. In: Gisolfi CV, Lamb DR, eds. Perspectives in Exercise and Science and Sport Medicine: Fluid Homeostasis During Exercise. Indianapolis, IN: Benchmark Press, 1990:97-121.

Costill DL, Cote R, Fink W. Muscle water and electrolytes following varied levels of dehydration in man. J Appl Physiol 1976;40:6-11.

Davis JM, Jackson DA, Broadwell MS, Query JL, Lambert CL. Carbohydrate drinks delay fatigue during intermittent, high-intensity cycling in active men and women. Int J Sport Nutr 1997;7:261-73.

Food Processor (software program), Version 7.11. ESHA Research, Salem, OR.

Gardner JW, Kark JA, Karnei K, et al. Risk factors predicting exertional heat illness in male Marine Corps recruits. Med Sci Sports Exerc 1996;28:939-44.

Gisolfi CV. Water requirements during exercise in the heat. In: Marriott BM, ed. Nutritional Needs in Hot Environments. Washington, DC: National Academy Press, 1993:87-96.

Gisolfi CV, Duchman SM. Guidelines for optimal replacement beverages for different athletic events. Med Sci Sports Exerc 1992;24:679-87.

Gisolfi CV, Ryan AJ. Gastrointestinal physiology during exercise. In: Buskirk ER, Puhl SM, eds. Body Fluid Balance: Exercise and Sport. Boca Raton, FL: CRC Press, 1996:19-51.

Gisolfi CV, Spranger KJ, Summers RW, Schedl HP, Bleiler TL. Effects of cycling exercise on intestinal absorption in humans. J Appl Physiol 1991;71:2518-27.

Gisolfi CV, Summers RW, Schedl HP, Bleiler TL. Intestinal water absorption from select carbohydrate solutions in humans. J Appl Physiol 1992;73:2142-50.

Gisolfi CV, Summers RW, Schedl HP, Bleiler TL. Effect of sodium concentration in a carbohydrate-electrolyte solution in intestinal absorption. Med Sci Sports Exerc 1995;27:1414-20.

Gonzalez-Alonso J, Heaps CL, Coyle EF. Rehydration after exercise with common beverages and water. Int J Sport Med 1992;13:399-406.

Greenleaf JE. Problem: thirst, drinking behavior and involuntary dehydration. Med Sci Sports Exerc 1992;24:645-56.

Greenleaf JE. Environmental issues that influence intake of replacement beverages. In: Marriott BM, ed. Fluid Replacement and Heat Stress. Committee on Military Nutrition Research, Food and Nutrition Board, Institute of Medicine. Washington, DC: National Academy Press, 1994:195-214.

Hargreaves M, Dillo P, Angus D, Febbraio MA. Effect of fluid ingestion on muscle metabolism during prolonged exercise. J Appl Physiol 1996;80:363-6.

Horswill CA. Effective fluid replacement. Int J Sport Nutr 1998;8:175-95.

Jeukendrup A, Brouns F, Wagenmakers AJM, Saris WHM. Carbohydrate-electrolyte feedings improve 1 h time trial cycling performance. Int J Sports Med 1997;18:125-9.

Kark JA, Burr PQ, Wenger CB, Gastaldo E, Gardner JW. Exertional heat illness in Marine Corps recruit training. Aviat Space Environ Med 1996;67:354-60.

Kirkendall DT. Fluid and electrolyte replacement in soccer. Clin Sports Med 1998;17:729-38.

Kleinman LI, Lorenz JM. Physiology and pathophysiology of body water and electrolytes. In: Kaplan LA, Pesce AI, eds. Clinical Chemistry: Theory, Analysis and Correlation. St. Louis: C.V. Mosby Company, 1996:439-63.

Kovacs EMR, Senden JMG, Brouns F. Urine color, osmolality and specific electrical conductance are not accurate measures of hydration status during post-exercise rehydration. J Sports Med Phys Fitness 1999;39:47-53.

Marriott BM, ed. Fluid Replacement and Heat Stress. Committee on Military Nutrition Research, Food and Nutrition Board, Institute of Medicine. Washington, DC: National Academy Press, 1994.

Maughan RJ. Fluid balance and exercise. Int J Sport Med 1992;13:S132-S135.

Maughan RJ, Leiper JB. Fluid replacement requirements in soccer. J Sports Sci 1994;12:S29-S34.

Maughan RJ, Leiper JB. Sodium intake and post-exercise rehydration in man. Eur J Appl Physiol 1995;71:311-9.

Maughan RJ, Leiper JB, Shirreffs SM. Restoration of fluid balance after exercise-induced dehydration effects of food and fluid intake. Eur J Appl Physiol 1996;73:317-25.

Maughan RJ, Shirreffs SM. Recovery from prolonged exercise: restoration of water and electrolyte balance. J Sport Sci 1997;15:297-303.

Maw GJ, MacKenzie IL, Taylor NAS. Human body-fluid distribution during exercise in hot, temperate and cool environments. Acta Physiol Scand 1998;163:287-304.

Meyer F, Bar-Or O, Salsberg A, Passe D. Hypohydration during exercise in children: effect of thirst, drink preference and rehydration. Int J Sport Nutr 1994;4:22-35.

Montain SJ, Coyle EF. Influence of graded dehydration on hyperthermia and cardiovascular drift during exercise. J Appl Physiol 1992; 73:1340-50.

Morris JG, Nevill ME, Lakomy HKA, Nicholas C, Williams C. Effect of a hot environment on performance of prolonged, intermittent, high-intensity shuttle running. J Sport Sci 1998;16:677-86.

Murray R. Fluid needs in hot and cold environments. Int J Sport Nutr 1995;5:S62-S73.

Murray R. Fluid needs of athletes. In: Berning JR, Steen SN, eds. Nutrition for Sport and Exercise. Gaithersburg, MD: Aspen Publishers, 1998:143-53.

National Weather Service, National Oceanic and Atmospheric Administration, Dept. of Commerce, Heat Index Chart. December 1998. [URL: **http://www.nws.noaa.gov**]

Nicholas CW, Williams C, Phillips G, Nowitz A. Influence of ingesting a carbohydrate-electrolyte solution on endurance capacity during intermittent, high intensity shuttle running. J Sport Sci 1995;13:282-90.

Noakes TD, Norman RJ, Buck RH, Godlonton J, Stevenson K, Pittaway D. The incidence of hyponatremia during prolonged ultraendurance exercise. Med Sci Sports Exerc 1990;22:165-70.

Pals KL, Chang R, Ryan AJ, Gisolfi CV. Effect of running intensity on intestinal permeability. J Appl Physiol 1997;82:571-6.

Pivarnik JM, Palmer RA. Water and electrolyte balance during rest and exercise. In: Wolinsky I, ed. Nutrition in Exercise and Sport. Boca Raton, FL: CRC Press, 1994: 245-62.

Ploutz-Snyder L, Foley J, Ploutz-Snyder R, Kanaley J, Sagendorf K, Meyer R. Gastric gas and fluid emptying assessed by magnetic resonance imaging. Eur J Appl Physiol 1999;79:212-20.

Puhl SM, Buskirk ER. Nutrient beverages for physical performance. In: Wolinsky I, ed. Nutrition in Exercise and Sport. Boca Raton, FL: CRC Press, 1998:277-314.

Remick D, Chancellor K, Pederson J, Zambraski EJ, Sawka MN, Wenger CD. Hyperthermia and dehydration-related deaths associated with intentional rapid weight loss in three collegiate wrestlers—North Carolina, Wisconsin, and Michigan, November-December 1997. CDC Morbidity and Mortality Weekly Report 1998;47(6):105-8.

Richards L. Disturbing trend: hiker ill from too much water. Arizona Republic, 1996 (April 27).

Rivera-Brown AM, Gutierrez T, Gutierrez JC, Frontera WR, Bar-Or O. Drink composition, voluntary drinking, and fluid balance in exercising, trained, heat-acclimatized boys. J Appl Physiol 1999;86(1):78-84.

Ryan AJ, Lambert G, Shi X, Chang RT, Summers RW, Gisolfi CV. Effect of hypohydration on gastric emptying and intestinal absorption during exercise. J Appl Physiol 1998;84:1581-8.

Sawka MN, Pandolf KB. Effects of body water loss in physiological function and exercise performance. In: Lamb DR, Gisolfi CV, eds. Perspectives in Exercise and Science and Sport Medicine: Fluid Homeostasis During Exercise. Indianapolis, IN: Benchmark Press, 1990:1-38.

Schedl HP, Maughan RJ, Gisolfi CV. Intestinal absorption during rest and exercise: implications for formulating an oral rehydration solution (ORS). Med Sci Sports Exerc 1994; 26:267-80.

Senay LC. Water and electrolytes during physical activity. In: Wolinsky I, ed. Nutrition in Exercise and Sport. Boca Raton, FL: CRC Press, 1998:257-76.

Shapiro Y, Seidman DS. Field and clinical observations of exertional heat stroke patients. Med Sci Sports Exerc 1990;22:6-14.

Shi X, Gisolfi CV. Fluid and carbohydrate replacement during intermittent exercise. Sports Med 1998;25:157-72.

Shirreffs SM, Maughan RJ. Restoration of fluid balance after exercise-induced dehydration: effects of alcohol consumption. J Appl Physiol 1997;83:1152-8.

Shirreffs SM, Taylor AJ, Leiper JB, Maughan RJ. Post-exercise rehydration in man: effects of volume consumed and drink sodium content. Med Sci Sports Exerc 1996;28: 1260-71.

Squire DL. Heat illness: fluid and electrolyte issues for pediatric and adolescent athletes. Pediatr Clin North Am 1990;37:1085-109.

Sutton JR. Clinical implications of fluid imbalance. In: Lamb DR, Gisolfi CV, eds. Perspectives in Exercise and Science and Sport Medicine: Fluid Homeostasis During Exercise. Indianapolis, IN: Benchmark Press, 1990:425-53.

Vist GE, Maughan RJ. Gastric emptying of ingested solutions in man: effect of beverage glucose concentration. Med Sci Sports Exerc 1994;26:1269-73.

Vist GE, Maughan RJ. The effect of osmolality and carbohydrate content on the rate of gastric emptying of liquids in man. J Physiol 1995;486:523-31.

Wade CE. Hormonal control of body fluid volume. In: Buskirk ER, Puhl EM, eds. Body Fluid Balance: Exercise and Sport. Boca Raton, FL: CRC Press, 1996:53-73.

Walsh RM, Noakes TD, Hawley JA, Dennis SC. Impaired high-intensity cycling perfor-

mance time at low levels of dehydration. Int J Sports Med 1994;15:392-8.

Wilk B, Bar-Or O. Effect of drink flavor and NaCl on voluntary drinking and hydration in boys exercising in heat. J Appl Physiol 1996;80:1112-7.

Wilk B, Kriemler S, Heidemaire K, Bar-Or O. Consistency in preventing voluntary dehydration in boys who drink a flavored carbohydrate-NaCl beverage during exercise in the heat. Int J Sport Nutr 1998;8:1-9.

Zambraski EJ. The kidney and body fluid balance during exercise. In: Buskirk ER, Puhl EM, eds. Body Fluid Balance: Exercise and Sport. Boca Raton, FL: CRC Press, 1996:75-95.

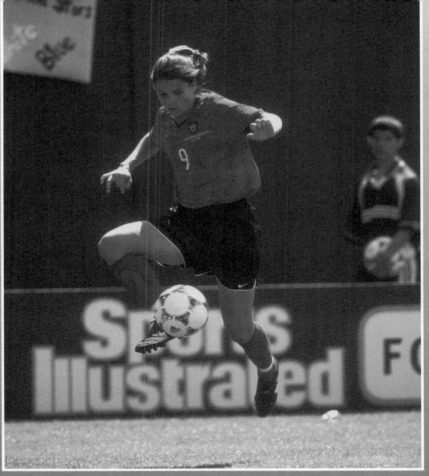

© Frank DiBrango

CHAPTER 9

B-Complex Vitamins Important in Energy Metabolism

After reading this chapter you will be able to

- understand the exercise-related functions and dietary requirements of the B-complex vitamins;
- discuss the rationale for increased need for B-complex vitamins in active individuals;
- identify the dietary and biochemical assessment methods for the B-complex vitamins;
- discuss how exercise may alter B-complex vitamin requirements in active people; and
- explain the relationship between B-complex vitamins and exercise performance.

Do you take vitamin or mineral supplements? If you answer yes, *why* are you supplementing? How did you know which supplement to buy? People give many different reasons for supplementing with vitamins and minerals. If you were to ask friends or clients why they supplement, here are some of the responses you might hear:

- They supplement as an insurance policy because they do not eat right.
- They think the food supply lacks sufficient vitamins and minerals.
- They think supplements will give them extra energy.
- They supplement to prevent disease or to treat a particular health problem.
- They think active people need more vitamins than sedentary individuals.
- They think people under high stress need more vitamins and minerals.

At least 25% of Americans appear to use dietary supplements daily, and as many as 35-40% use them occasionally. For people engaged in physical activity, the estimates are as high as 50% (Sobal and Marquart 1994). In some sports, like bodybuilding, 60-100% of the participants use supplements. This high use of supplements has created a $4 billion industry that constantly bombards the public with advertisements. In addition, newspapers and TV news programs frequently report studies about nutrients that can prevent cancer, improve health, or prevent fatigue. It is not surprising that American consumers are confused about whether they should use vitamin or mineral supplements. As a health professional, you will be constantly asked about supplements, especially if you are working with active individuals. How do you sort through this information overload? How can you make the best recommendations to people who ask you about supplements? How do you respond to the athlete who wants to know whether exercise increases the need for vitamins, or whether supplementation will improve exercise performance? (See "Guidelines for Recommending Vitamin Supplements," page 267.)

This chapter addresses these questions, specifically examining whether exercise increases the need for the **B-complex vitamins** (thiamine, riboflavin, vitamin B_6, niacin, pantothenic acid, and biotin) required in energy metabolism. Because these vitamins are especially impor-

tant in the production of energy, they are grouped together in one chapter (vitamin B_{12} and folate are also B-complex vitamins but, due to their critical role in blood formation, are covered in chapter 12).

First, we review the exercise-related functions and dietary requirements of each vitamin. Then we briefly cover whether active people have increased needs. Next we review the methods for assessing vitamin status—including the dietary sources of each nutrient, the typical intakes reported in active individuals, and the biochemical assessment parameters typically measured. Then we address the impact of vitamin deficiency or marginal vitamin status on exercise performance and work. Finally, we examine whether vitamin supplementation in healthy individuals enhances exercise performance.

Because most B-complex vitamins are cofactors for metabolic reactions that produce energy, it is natural to hypothesize that exercise increases the need for these nutrients. In fact, the 1989 Recommended Dietary Allowances (RDAs) for most of these nutrients were based on intakes of energy (thiamine, riboflavin, and niacin catalyze steps in energy metabolism) and protein (vitamin B_6 is involved in protein synthesis and glycogen metabolism). As people become more physically active, it is reasonable to think that they will consume more energy and protein and, in the process, consume more of these vitamins. Yet this is not always true. If people make poor dietary choices, they may not increase their consumption of these micronutrients as much as they increase their energy and protein intakes. Moreover, if they increase physical activity but restrict energy intake (as happens often with people who are dieting), the need for the vitamins may increase while their dietary intake actually declines.

Exercise-Related Functions and Dietary Requirements

To discuss why exercise might increase the need for these vitamins, we must first understand their role in energy metabolism. Figure 9.1 shows how thiamine, riboflavin, vitamin B_6, niacin, pantothenic acid, and biotin each is a cofactor in one or more of the metabolic pathways that produce energy during exercise. Table 9.1 lists each vitamin, its active form in the body, the various metabolic pathways for which

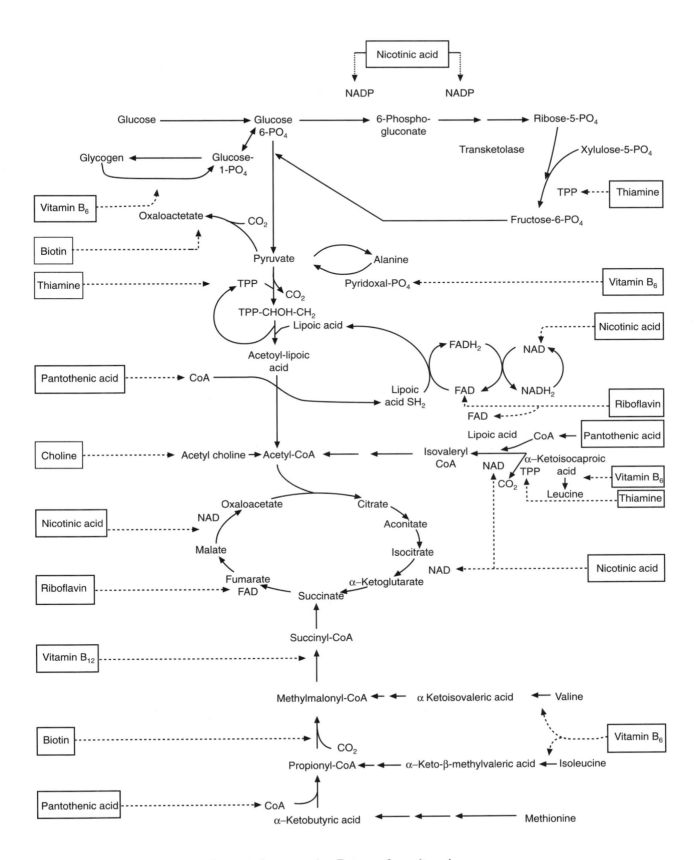

Figure 9.1 Metabolic pathways that require B-complex vitamins.

Table 9.1 Exercise-Related Metabolic Functions and Examples of Enzymes for These Functions That Require B-Complex Vitamins As Cofactors

Vitamin	Active form of vitamin	Functions of vitamin related to exercise	Metabolic pathways that require the vitamin	Major enzymes that require the vitamin as a cofactor
Thiamine (B$_1$)	Thiamine pyrophosphate (TPP)	Energy production from protein, fat, and carbohydrate	Carbohydrate, BCAAs, and fat metabolism	Pyruvate dehydrogenase; α-keto-glutarate decarboxylase; branched-chain α-keto decarboxylase
Riboflavin (B$_2$)	Flavin mononucleotide (FMN); Flavin-adenine dinucleotide (FAD)	Energy production from protein, fat, and carbohydrate; conversion of vitamin B$_6$ and folate to their active forms	Carbohydrate, protein, and fat metabolism (TCA cycle, electron transport)	Acyl-CoA dehydrogenase; succinate dehydrogenase; glycerol dehydrogenase; pyruvate dehydrogenase
Vitamin B$_6$	Pyridoxine, pyridoxal, pyridoxamine; pyridoxal-5′-phosphate (PLP) is active cofactor	Transamination of amino acids, release of glucose from glycogen, glucose-alanine cycle, gluconeogenesis	Protein and carbohydrate metabolism	Glycogen phosphorylase; transaminases
Niacin (B$_3$) nicotinic acid	Nicotinamide adenine dinucleotide (NAD); nicotinamide adenine dinucleotide phosphate (NADP)	Energy production from protein, fat, and carbohydrate	TCA cycle, glycolysis, pentose phosphate pathway	Lactate dehydrogenase; glucose-6-phosphate dehydrogenase; 3-phosphoglyceraldehyde dehydrogenase; glutamine dehydrogenase
Pantothenic acid	Coenzyme A (CoA); acyl carrier protein (ACP)	Energy metabolism from fat and carbohydrate	β-oxidation of fats, TCA cycle, glycolysis	CoA and ACP function as carriers of acyl groups
Biotin		Energy production from protein, carbohydrate metabolism, and fat synthesis	Gluconeogenesis, fatty acid synthesis, and amino acid degradation	Pyruvate carboxylase; acetyl-CoA carboxylase; propionyl-CoA carboxylase; 3-methylcrotonyl-CoA carboxylase

See the following references for additional information on the exercise-related functions of these vitamins: Clarkson 1998; Peifer 1997; Sampson 1997; Thomas 1997.

it is required, and some of the specific enzymes that require the vitamin as a cofactor. The following section briefly discusses the specific exercise-related function of each of the B-complex vitamins involved in energy metabolism.

Thiamine

Thiamine is important for the metabolism of both carbohydrate and the **branched-chain amino acids (BCAAs)**. The active form of thiamine in the body is **thiamine pyrophosphate (TPP)**. Thiamine is a coenzyme for the pyruvate dehydrogenase complex that catalyzes the conversion of pyruvate to acetyl-CoA (see figure 9.1), which can then enter the **tricarboxylic acid (TCA)** cycle for metabolism. Thiamine is also a coenzyme for α-ketoglutarate decarboxylase, an enzyme responsible for the formation of succinyl-CoA in the TCA cycle. Thus, thiamine helps in the oxidation of both carbohydrate and fat through this cycle. Finally, thiamine is required for branched-chain α-keto decarboxylase, an enzyme responsible for the catabolism of the BCAAs. Physical activity stresses these energy-producing metabolic pathways. Because thiamine requirements are linked to energy metabolism (especially CHO metabolism), the 1989 RDA for thiamine was expressed in terms of energy intake (mg/1000 kcal), with 0.5 mg of thiamine required per 1000 kcal consumed per day. This value was then extrapolated to the estimated minimum energy requirements for men and women. Thus, the 1989 RDA was 1.5 mg/d for adult men and 1.1 mg/d for adult women, with a minimum of 1.0 mg/d required for all adults. An additional 0.4 and 0.5 mg/d are recommended during pregnancy and lactation, respectively (Food and Nutrition Board 1989; Tanphaichitr 1994).

In 1998, the RDA for thiamine was decreased for men but not for women (Food and Nutrition Board 1998). The new thiamine RDA for adult men and women (19-50 years) is 1.2 mg/d for men (see table 9.2). One reason for the decrease for men is that the new RDA for thiamine was no longer based on energy intake (see "How Does the Dietary Reference Intake [DRI] Differ From the Recommended Dietary Allowance [RDA]?" on page 257). However, this does not diminish the importance of thiamine for carbohydrate metabolism. It merely means that active people, especially those consuming high levels of energy or carbohydrate, may need more thiamine than the current RDA.

Riboflavin

Riboflavin is necessary for the synthesis of two important coenzymes in the body—**flavin mononucleotide (FMN)** and **flavin adenine dinucleotide (FAD)**. These coenzymes are especially important in the metabolism of glucose, fatty acids, glycerol, and amino acids for energy. Because exercise stresses the biochemical pathways that metabolize these substrates, it has been hypothesized that riboflavin requirements are higher in people who exercise. Riboflavin is also involved in the conversion of pyridoxine (vitamin B_6) and folate to their coenzyme forms (Leklem 1988). Like thiamine, the 1989 RDA for riboflavin was expressed in terms of energy intake, with 0.6 mg of riboflavin recommended for every 1000 kcal consumed—or 1.7 mg/d for adult men and 1.3 mg/d for adult women, with a minimum recommended intake of 1.2 mg/d. Because pregnancy and lactation increase energy demands, an additional 0.3 mg/d was recommended during pregnancy and an additional 0.4-0.5 mg/d during lactation (McCormick 1994; Food and Nutrition Board 1989).

In 1998, the RDA for riboflavin was revised downward for both adult men and women (19-70 years), to 1.3 mg/d for men and 1.1 mg/d for women (see table 9.2) (Food and Nutrition Board 1998). One of the reasons for the lower RDA is that the new RDA for riboflavin was no longer based on energy intake (see "How Does the Dietary Reference Intake [DRI] Differ From the Recommended Dietary Allowance [RDA]?" on page 257). This change was due to limited research on how riboflavin requirements change over a large range of energy intakes and body sizes. It is well known that riboflavin plays an important role in energy metabolism; the new RDAs for riboflavin were adjusted to reflect differences in average energy requirements and in body size and to reflect the energy requirements of pregnancy and lactation. The change does not diminish the importance of riboflavin for energy metabolism in active individuals who may need more riboflavin than the current RDA.

Vitamin B₆

Vitamin B_6 plays a major role in metabolic pathways required during exercise. It is required in the metabolism of proteins and amino acids and in the release of glucose from stored glycogen. **Pyridoxal-5'-phosphate (PLP),** the most metabolically active form of vitamin B_6, can be measured in the blood. PLP is a cofactor for transversases, transaminases, decarboxylases, and other enzymes used in the metabolic transformations of amino acids. During exercise, the gluconeogenic process involves the breakdown of amino acids for energy in the muscle and the conversion of lactic acid to glucose in the liver. The breakdown of muscle glycogen for energy during exercise is another function of vitamin B_6 that is directly related to energy production. Vitamin B_6 must be present to release glucose-1-phosphate from muscle glycogen (Leklem 1985; Leklem 1994; Manore 1994). Once you know the functions of vitamin B_6, it is easy to understand why adequate vitamin B_6 is so important for exercise. Because vitamin B_6 is directly involved in amino acid metabolism, the 1989 RDA for vitamin B_6 was expressed in terms of protein intake. This means that the more protein you consume, the more vitamin B_6 you need (mg/d). The 1989 RDA for vitamin B_6 was based on a dietary vitamin B_6 intake of 0.016 mg per g of protein. This ratio was determined to be adequate to ensure good vitamin B_6 status. The 1989 RDA for vitamin B_6 was established by using twice the RDA for protein (126 g/d for men and 100 g/d for women). The recommendation for adults 25 years of age or older was calculated to be 2.0 mg/d for men and 1.6 mg/d for women. As with thiamine and riboflavin, vitamin B_6 requirements increase slightly with pregnancy and lactation (Food and Nutrition Board 1989, 1998; Leklem 1994).

In 1998, the RDA for vitamin B_6 was revised downward, to 1.3 mg/d for both men and women (ages 19-50 years) (Food and Nutrition Board 1998). One reason for the decrease was that the new RDA was no longer based on protein intake (see "How Does the Dietary Reference Intake [DRI] Differ From the Recommended Dietary Allowance [RDA]?" on page 257), and the biochemical cut-off points for status were changed. This change was due to discrepancies in the research data on the relationship between protein and vitamin B_6 intake. However, this does not diminish the importance of vitamin B_6 for protein or carbohydrate metabolism. *It just means that active individuals, especially active women, may need to consume significantly more vitamin B_6 than the new RDA calls for.* In fact, recent research suggests that the vitamin B_6 requirements for women are greater than 0.016 mg/g of protein (Hansen et al. 1997). In this study, sedentary women consuming 85 g/d of protein (1.16 g/kg body weight) required a minimum of 1.3 mg/d of vitamin B_6 to maintain adequate vitamin B_6 status. A second study done by Huang et al. (1998) found that sedentary young women consuming 96 g/d of protein (1.55 g/kg body weight) required 1.94 mg vitamin B_6 per day—or approximately 0.019 mg/g of protein. It should be noted that these research studies were published after the new 1998 vitamin B_6 RDA was set.

Niacin

Niacin, also known as nicotinic acid and nicotinamide, serves as the precursor for two coenzymes—**nicotinamide adenine dinucleotide (NAD)** and **NAD phosphate (NADP)**. These two coenzymes are found in all cells and are required for production of energy through glycolysis, the TCA cycle, electron transport, and the pentose pathway (figure 9.1). They are also involved in the β-oxidation of fats and the synthesis of proteins.

The body's requirement for niacin can be met in two ways. It can be consumed in the diet from food or made in the body from the essential amino acid tryptophan (hence the RDA for niacin is reported in **niacin equivalents (NEs)** instead of just milligrams of niacin per day); it takes about 60 mg of tryptophan to make 1 mg of niacin or 1 NE (see "Calculating Total NE Intake," page 251). To calculate total NE in the diet, you need to know the amounts of both preformed niacin and tryptophan consumed.

Because niacin is so involved in energy production, the 1989 RDA for niacin was expressed as niacin equivalents per 1000 kcal (6.6 NE/1000 kcal). For adults 19-50 years of age, the 1989 RDA for niacin was 19 NE/d (i.e., the equivalent of 19 mg niacin/d) for men and 15 NE/d for women (Food and Nutrition Board 1989). In 1998, the RDA for niacin was changed to 16 NE/d for men of all ages and 14 NE/d for women of all ages (Food and Nutrition Board 1998). Although the 1998 RDA for niacin is not based on energy intake, niacin is still important for the oxidation of fuels for energy.

Pantothenic Acid

All tissues can convert pantothenic acid to its biologically functional forms—**coenzyme A (CoA)** and **acyl carrier protein (ACP)**. CoA and ACP function as carriers of acyl groups. Acetyl-CoA is formed from attachment of acetate to CoA. Acetyl-CoA is involved in many

■ HIGHLIGHT ■

Calculating Total NE Intake

Many computerized nutrient analysis programs now calculate the total NE (niacin equivalents) of the diet being analyzed. If you are using an analysis program that does not do this, you can still figure out the total intake of niacin in your diet by using the calculation given below. The simple fact to keep in mind is that 1 NE = *either* 60 mg tryptophan *or* 1 mg niacin.

Total NE = niacin intake + (tryptophan intake/60)

where both intakes are measured in mg/d.

Here is a sample calculation for total NE in a diet containing 1696 kcal/d:

Niacin intake = 18.9 mg/d

Tryptophan intake = 630 mg/d

Therefore total NE = 18.9 + (630/60) = 29.4 NE/d

This person is consuming *the equivalent of* 29.4 mg niacin/d (17.3 mg/1000 kcal); one-third of the niacin intake comes from tryptophan. Foods like milk that are low in preformed niacin but high in tryptophan can still significantly add to total niacin intake.

---

energy-producing metabolic pathways, such as glycolysis, β-oxidation, and the TCA cycle. Pantothenic acid is also involved in gluconeogenesis and in the synthesis of steroid hormones, acetylcholine, fatty acids, and membrane phospholipids. Finally, pantothenic acid is involved in protein degradation and amino acid synthesis. Since pantothenic acid is widely distributed in foods, human deficiencies are rare. There is no RDA set for pantothenic acid; however, there is an estimated adequate intake (AI) recommendation of 5 mg/d (Food and Nutrition Board 1998).

Biotin

Biotin serves as an essential cofactor for several key carboxylase enzymes required for metabolism of glucose, fat, and protein. For example, in gluconeogenesis, pyruvate carboxylase requires biotin; in fatty acid synthesis, acetyl-CoA carboxylase is the biotin-dependent enzyme. Biotin is also required for the degradation of some amino acids (isoleucine, valine, methionine, and leucine) and odd-carbon fatty acids. The conversion of biotin to its active coenzyme requires both magnesium and adenosine triphosphate (ATP). Like pantothenic acid, biotin is widely distributed in foods; deficiencies are rare since only small amounts are needed daily. There is no RDA

for biotin, but an estimated AI of 30 μg/d is recommended (Food and Nutrition Board 1998).

Rationale for Increased Need for Active Individuals

Because exercise stresses metabolic pathways that use these B-complex vitamins, it has been suggested that the requirements for these vitamins are increased in athletes and active individuals. Theoretically, exercise could increase the need for these nutrients in the following ways:

- Alter absorption of the nutrient due to decreased transit time.
- Increase the turnover, metabolism, or loss of the nutrient in urine or sweat.
- Increase the need due to the biochemical adaptations associated with training.
- Increase mitochondrial enzymes that require the nutrients as cofactors.
- Increase the need for the nutrient for tissue maintenance and repair.
- Increase the need due to biochemical adaptations associated with changes in the composition of the diet (higher carbohydrate and/or protein intakes).

251

■ HIGHLIGHT ■

B-Complex Vitamins: Pharmacological Effects and Toxic Levels

High intakes of some of the water-soluble B-complex vitamins can have pharmacological effects unrelated to the role they play as essential micronutrients. High intakes of these vitamins can be toxic in some cases.

Thiamine

There is no evidence of thiamine toxicity from oral supplementation. Because there appears to be little risk for thiamine toxicity, the new 1998 Dietary Reference Intakes (DRIs) set no Tolerable Upper Intake Level (UL) for thiamine (Food and Nutrition Board 1998). However, parenteral doses at 100 times the RDA may cause headache, convulsions, weakness, paralysis, cardiac arrhythmia, and allergic reactions (Combs 1992; Food and Nutrition Board 1998; Tanphaichitr 1994).

Riboflavin

There is no evidence of riboflavin toxicity from food or supplements since the human gut can absorb only about 20-27 mg in a single dose (Food and Nutrition Board 1998; McCormick 1994). Thus, there is no UL set for riboflavin.

Vitamin B_6

Chronic high doses of vitamin B_6 (>250 mg/d for many months) in the treatment of some diseases have resulted in a few cases of neurotoxicity (Leklem 1994). Toxicity symptoms include depression, fatigue, irritability, headaches, numbness, damage to nerves leading to loss of reflexes and sensations, and difficulty walking. Because of this risk of neurotoxicity, the 1998 DRIs include a UL of 100 mg/d for vitamin B_6 (Food and Nutrition Board 1998).

Niacin

For years, physicians have prescribed niacin in doses of 1.5-3.0 g/d to treat high blood lipids. Side effects can include flushing of the skin, hyperuricemia, abnormal liver function, and low blood glucose levels (Swendseid and Jacob 1994). The high doses of niacin used to lower blood lipids also negatively affect substrate use during exercise, which lowers exercise performance. Niacin supplementation decreases the ability to burn fat during exercise, thus increasing the amount of carbohydrate required for energy (Health et al. 1993; Lewis 1997; Murray et al. 1995). Because of the flushing that occurs with high doses of niacin, the 1998 DRIs include a UL of 35 mg/d (Food and Nutrition Board 1998).

Pantothenic Acid and Biotin

Since both appear to be relatively safe even at high intakes, no UL has been set for these two vitamins. For pantothenic acid there is no evidence of toxicity in humans even with relatively high intakes (e.g., 10 g/d).

There is some biochemical evidence of poor vitamin status for these nutrients in active people (see table 9.3), but the research has been limited and equivocal. Poor nutritional status may occur in some active people because of long-term marginal dietary intakes associated with either poor dietary choices or reduced energy intake. Inconsistencies in these studies may also be related to differences in experimental designs, which can differ according to

- degree of dietary control,
- type and intensity of exercise used,
- type and number of status indices measured,
- level of regular physical activity in which subjects engage,
- type of subjects included, and
- whether or not a control group was included.

Exercise increases both energy and protein needs, which may in turn increase the total daily need for thiamine, riboflavin, vitamin B_6, and niacin in active people. Dietary intakes of these vitamins even by athletes should be adequate unless the individuals make poor dietary choices or restrict their energy intake.

Unfortunately, as people increase their training regimens, they do not always correspondingly increase their consumption of energy, protein, or vitamins/minerals.

Assessment of Vitamin Status

To determine a person's vitamin status, one needs to measure a number of parameters. Ideally, these measurements should include biochemical assessments (both direct and indirect) along with dietary intake data (see table 9.2). The following section discusses the most common assessment parameters—including biochemical, dietary intake, and food source data—

Table 9.2 **Assessment Indices for Evaluating Vitamin B_6, Riboflavin, Thiamine, and Niacin Status**

Indices	Suggested value for poor status
Vitamin B_6	
Plasma pyridoxal phosphate (PLP)	<30 nmol/L[1] or <20 nmol/L[3]
Plasma total vitamin B_6	<40 nmol/L[1]
Urinary 4-pyridoxic acid (4-PA)	<3.0 µmol/d[1,3]
Urinary total vitamin B_6	<0.5 µmol/d[1]
Erythrocyte alanine transaminase activity coefficient (EALTAC)	>1.25[1,3]
Erythrocyte aspartate transaminase activity coefficient (EASTAC)	>1.80[1] or >1.60[3]
1989 Recommended Dietary Allowance (RDA)[2]	
Adult men (≥15 years)	2.0 mg/d
Adult women (≥15 years)	1.6 mg/d
1998 RDA[3]	
Adult men (19-50 years)	1.3 mg/d
Adult women (19-50 years)	1.3 mg/d
Riboflavin	
Plasma riboflavin	<0.24 umol/L or <240 nmol/L
Erythrocyte riboflavin	<270 nmol/L [1,3]
Erythrocyte glutathione reductase activity coefficient (EGRAC)	>1.25 or >1.4[3]
Urinary riboflavin per gram of creatinine (Cr): low status	<30 µg/g Cr[1] or 19-27 µg/g Cr[3]
Urinary riboflavin per gram of creatinine (Cr): deficient status	<19 µg/g Cr[3]
Urinary riboflavin	
per 24 h	<40 µg/d
per 6 h	<10 µg/6 h[4]
1989 RDA (based on a consumption of 0.6 mg of riboflavin/1000 kcal)[2]	
Adult men (15-50 years)	1.7 mg/d
Adult women (11-50 years)	1.3 mg/d
1998 RDA[3]	
Adult men (19-70 years)	1.3 mg/d
Adult women (19-70 years)	1.1 mg/d

(continued)

Table 9.2 *(continued)*

Indices	Suggested value for poor status
Thiamine	
Plasma thiamine	<98 nmol/L or <10 ng/ml[1]
Erythrocyte thiamine: marginal deficiency	70-90 nmol/L[3]
Erythrocyte thiamine: deficiency	<70 nmol/L[3]
Thiamine pyrophosphate (TPP) % stimulation: marginal deficiency	15-24%[3]
Thiamine pyrophosphate (TPP) % stimulation: deficiency	≥25%[3]
Erythrocyte transketolase activity coefficient (ETKAC): marginal deficiency	1.20-1.25[3]
Erythrocyte transketolase activity coefficient (ETKAC): deficiency	>1.25[3]
Urinary thiamine per gram of creatinine (Cr): marginal deficiency	40-100 µg/g Cr[3]
Urinary thiamine per gram of creatinine (Cr): deficiency	<5 µg/g Cr[3]
Urinary thiamine	
per 24 h: marginal deficiency	27-66 µg/d[3]
per 24 h: deficiency	<27 µg/d[3]
per 6 h	<10 µg/6 h[4]
1989 RDA (based on a consumption of 0.5 mg/1000 kcal)[2]	
Adult men (15-50 years)	1.5 mg/d
Adult women (11-50 years)	1.1 mg/d
1998 RDA[3]	
Adult men (19-50 years)	1.2 mg/d
Adult women (19-50 years)	1.1 mg/d
Niacin	
Urinary N'-methylnicotinamide (NMN): low status	5.8-17.5 µmol/d[3]
Urinary N'-methylnicotinamide (NMN): deficient status	<5.8 µmol/d[3]
NMN/N'-methyl-2-pyridone-5-carboxylamide (2-pyridone) ratio[4]	
Acceptable niacin status	1.0-4.0
Niacin deficiency or low status	<1.0
1989 RDA (based on 6.6 niacin equivalents (NE)/1000 kcal)[2]	
Adult men (15-50 years)	19 mg NE/d
Adult women (15-50 years)	15 mg NE/d
1998 RDA[3]	
Adult men (all ages)	16 mg NE/d
Adult women (all ages)	14 mg NE/d

[1]Values are from Fischbach 1996.

[2]Values are the 1989 RDAs for the vitamins (Food and Nutrition Board 1989). For vitamin B_6, the RDA is based on a vitamin B_6:protein ratio of 0.032 mg/d protein for adult males consuming 126 g protein/d, and females consuming 100 g protein/d.

[3]Values are the 1998 RDAs for the vitamins and the new cut-off values for low or deficient status for urine and blood parameters (FNB 1998).

[4]Values are from Gibson 1990.

for thiamine, riboflavin, vitamin B_6, and niacin. Because dietary intake data are poor for pantothenic acid and biotin, these two nutrients have not often been measured in active people. There are no research data indicating poor status for these two nutrients in healthy active individuals, probably because of their widespread distribution in food.

For premenopausal females, phase of the menstrual cycle can alter energy and nutrient intakes. Because some blood and urinary assessment parameters for vitamins are influenced by recent nutrient intakes, studies examining nutrient status should consider the phase of the menstrual cycle. Martini and colleagues (1994) found significant increases in energy, protein, carbohydrate, fat, vitamin D, riboflavin, potassium, phosphorus, and magnesium intakes in the midluteal phases versus the midfollicular phases in women studied over four to six ovulatory menstrual cycles.

Biochemical Assessment of Vitamin Status

Biochemical tests can reflect the body's stores of a nutrient as well as the amount of the vitamin lost from the body in urine, feces, or sweat. (When possible, researchers and clinicians like to include *functional measurements* of vitamin status—i.e., measurements of the *availability* of the vitamin to function as a coenzyme within the body.) Biochemical measurements can be direct (measurement of blood, urine, or fecal concentration of the vitamin or its metabolite) or indirect (measurement of an enzyme that requires the vitamin as a cofactor or measurement of that enzyme's functional activity). The typical dietary intake of the vitamin should also be determined. One should measure as many assessment parameters as possible, including both indirect and direct measurements, plus dietary data. Table 9.2 specifically outlines all the various

Table 9.3   **Incidence of Low or Marginal Vitamin B$_6$, Riboflavin, Thiamine, and Niacin Status in Studies of Nonsupplemented Active People**

Study	Assessment indices[1]	No. subjects	Type of subjects	Low status (%)	Dietary vitamin (mg/d)[2]
Vitamin B$_6$					
Fogelholm et al. 1993	EASTAC (>2.00) EAST basal	42	Active subjects[3]	43	—
Guilland et al. 1989	EASTAC (>1.99) Plasma PLP	55	Male athletes	35 17	1.5 ± 0.1
Telford et al. 1992	EASTAC	86		59	—
Rokitzki, Sagredos, Reub, Cufi, and Keul 1994	EASTAC (>1.50) Urinary 4-PA (<2.73 μmol/g Cr) Whole blood B$_6$	57	Athletes[3]	5 18	1.36-5.40[4]
Weight et al. 1988	Plasma PLP	30	Female athletes	0[5]	1.7 ± 0.6
Riboflavin					
Fogelholm et al. 1993	EGRAC (>1.30) EGR basal	42	Active subjects[2]	57	—
Guilland et al. 1989	EGRAC (>1.20)	55	Male athletes	4	2.1 ± 0.2
Keith and Alt 1991	EGRAC (>1.20) Urinary riboflavin	13	Female athletes	0[5]	1.9 ± 0.9
Rokitzki, Sagredos, Keck et al. 1994	EGRAC (>1.50) Whole blood riboflavin Urinary riboflavin	62	Athletes[3]	0[5]	1.4-2.5[4]
Weight et al. 1988	EGRAC (>1.15)	30	Male runners	0[5]	1.8 ± 1.8
Thiamine					
Fogelholm et al. 1993	ETKAC (>1.20)	42	Active subjects[2]	12	—
Guilland et al. 1989	ETKAC (>1.20)	55	Male athletes	17	1.5 ± 0.1
Weight et al. 1988	TPP Stim. (>25%) ETK basal	30	Male runners	0[5]	1.5 ± 0.5
Niacin					
Weight et al. 1988	Plasma niacin	30	Male runners	0[5]	20.4 ± 5.6

[1] See table 9.2 for description of assessment parameters and normal values. In addition, different cut-off values for poor status vary depending on the biochemical assessment parameter used and the laboratory. Telford et al. (1992) do not provide the EASTAC cut-off value used to determine poor status.

[2] Mean ± SD or range of intakes.

[3] Included both males and females.

[4] Researchers used 7-d weighed food records.

[5] Zero means none of the individuals had poor status. Values reported are a range of intakes for various male and female athletes.

assessment parameters that might be used in assessing status for the vitamins discussed in this chapter, along with cut-off points for poor status.

Thiamine

The most widely used biochemical assessment parameter for thiamine is the measurement of **erythrocyte transketolase activity coefficient (ETKAC). Erythrocyte transketolase** is a thiamine-dependent enzyme; without adequate thiamine, activity of the enzyme declines. ETKAC is determined by first measuring the basal activity of the enzyme (without the added coenzyme) and then by measuring the enzyme activity (with added coenzyme). The activity coefficient, or percentage of stimulation, is determined by dividing the stimulated enzyme activity by the basal enzyme activity. A *high* activity coefficient indicates *poor* or marginal nutritional status. The criteria used for interpreting ETKAC depend on the laboratory and the biochemical method used. An activity coefficient of 1.0-1.15 is generally considered normal, 1.16-1.20 is considered marginal thiamine deficiency, and >1.20 is considered severely deficient (Gibson 1990). Thiamine can also be measured in urine, whole blood, or plasma. Thiamine in the urine does not adequately reflect body stores but is a better index of dietary intake (Gibson 1990).

Riboflavin

Riboflavin status is determined by measuring a number of blood and urine parameters. The most common measurements are urinary excretion of riboflavin, erythrocyte riboflavin levels, and the determination of **erythrocyte glutathione reductase activity coefficient (EGRAC).** EGRAC is increasingly used as an index of subclinical riboflavin deficiency. As with thiamine, the activity coefficient is calculated by dividing the enzyme activity (with added cofactor FAD) by the basal enzyme activity (without added cofactor FAD). Thus, a *high* EGRAC indicates *impaired* riboflavin status and has been confirmed using human depletion studies (Soares et al. 1993). The evaluation criteria for EGRAC vary depending on the laboratory. The cut-off value frequently used for adequate status is <1.2, while low status is 1.2-1.4 and deficient status is >1.4 (McCormick 1994). Low levels of riboflavin excretion also indicate deficiency (table 9.2) (McCormick 1994). Although some researchers question whether the standard reference values for sedentary individuals are appropriate for active people (Rokitzki, Sagredos, Keck et al. 1994), this hypothesis has not yet been tested.

Vitamin B₆

Like riboflavin, vitamin B_6 status is determined by measuring a number of blood and urine parameters. The most relevant direct measures of vitamin B_6 status are plasma PLP, total plasma vitamin B_6, and **urinary 4-pyridoxic acid (4-PA).** Indirect measures include evaluation of either **erythrocyte alanine transaminase activity coefficient (EALTAC) or erythrocyte aspartate transaminase activity coefficient (EASTAC)**, with activation by PLP (both enzymes require PLP as a cofactor) (see table 9.2). As with thiamine and riboflavin, *high* activity coefficients indicate *poor* status. At least two biochemical measures should be used to assess vitamin B_6 status, and dietary intakes of vitamin B_6 and protein should be measured (Leklem 1990).

Niacin

Currently, there are no functional assessment measurements for niacin status. Blood concentrations of niacin and niacin metabolites are quite low and appear to be better indicators of recent dietary intakes than long-term status (Gibson 1990; Swendseid and Jacob 1994). The best index available for assessing niacin status measures the two major end products of niacin metabolism found in the urine: **N'-methylnicotinamide (NMN)** and **N'-methyl-2-pyridone-5-carboxylamide (2-pyridone).** Both compounds are derived from either dietary niacin or the nicotinic acid ribonucleotide made from tryptophan within the body. It is estimated that healthy adults excrete about 20-30% of niacin as NMN and 40-60% as 2-pyridone (Gibson 1990). Both urinary metabolites decrease with niacin deficiency. Urine 2-pyridone can decrease to nearly zero before clinical signs of deficiency appear, while urinary excretion of NMN decreases after clinical signs appear. A low urinary concentration of NMN (<0.8 mg/d) is the standard criterion used to indicate poor niacin status and is much easier to measure clinically than 2-pyridone (Fischbach 1996; Swendseid and Jacob 1994). Sometimes the urinary ratio of 2-pyridone:NMN is used to assess niacin status. A ratio <1.0 indicates low niacin status, while an acceptable ratio is between 1.0-4.0 (Gibson 1990).

How Does the Dietary Reference Intake (DRI) Differ From the Recommended Dietary Allowance (RDA)?

In 1989, the Food and Nutrition Board of the National Research Council published the last complete set of RDAs for all nutrients, defining RDAs as "the levels of intake of essential nutrients that, on the basis of scientific knowledge, are judged by the Food and Nutrition Board to be adequate to meet the known nutrient needs of practically all healthy persons (p. 1, Food and Nutrition Board 1989). In the past, the RDAs were regularly updated to reflect new scientific knowledge. We are now in a transition period in which the RDAs are being replaced with a set of **Dietary Reference Intakes (DRIs)**. *This change was made to reflect the growing body of scientific evidence that nutrient requirements may change in chronic disease.* The DRI committee for each group of nutrients establishes reference intakes, periodically updating the recommendations according to newer scientific data. Currently, we have new guidelines for calcium and related nutrients (vitamin D, phosphorous, magnesium, and fluoride) and the B-complex nutrients (thiamine, riboflavin, niacin, vitamin B_6, folate, vitamin B_{12}, pantothenic acid, biotin, and choline). Since the DRIs were established in 1998 for the B-complex vitamins, we give both the more recent DRIs and the 1989 RDAs for the B-complex vitamins throughout this chapter. The next few paragraphs explain the new guidelines.

Recommended Dietary Allowance

The RDA is the intake that meets the nutrient need of *almost all of the healthy individuals in a specific age and gender group.* It should be used in guiding people to achieve adequate nutrient intake aimed at decreasing the risk of chronic disease. It is based on estimates of average requirements, plus an increase to account for the variation within a particular group. Available scientific evidence allowed the DRI committee to calculate RDAs for phosphorus, magnesium, thiamine, riboflavin, niacin, vitamin B_6, folate, and vitamin B_{12}.

Adequate Intake

When sufficient scientific evidence is not available to estimate an average requirement, adequate intakes (AIs) have been set. Individuals should use the AI as a goal for intake where no RDAs exist. The AI is derived though experimental or observational data that show a mean intake, *which appears to sustain a desired indicator of health* (e.g., calcium retention in bone) *for most members of a population group.* For example, AIs have been set for infants through 1 year of age using the average observed nutrient intake of populations of breast-fed infants as the standard. The committee set AIs for calcium, vitamin D, fluoride, pantothenic acid, biotin, and choline.

Estimated Average Requirement (EAR)

The EAR is the intake that *meets the estimated nutrient need of half the individuals in a specific group.* This figure is used as the basis for developing the RDA and is used by nutrition policy makers in evaluating the adequacy of nutrient intakes of a group and for planning how much the group should consume.

Tolerable Upper Intake Level (UL)

The UL is the *maximum intake by an individual that is unlikely to pose risks of adverse health effects in almost all healthy individuals in a specified group.* It is not a recommended level of intake—there is no established benefit for individuals to consume nutrients at levels above the RDA or AI. For most nutrients, this figure refers to total intakes from food, fortified food, and nutrient supplements.

Dietary Intakes of Active Individuals

Few researchers have investigated thiamine, riboflavin, vitamin B_6, or niacin intakes by athletes. As you are read about these studies, remember that B-complex vitamin data from older research (before about 1989) are usually incomplete because good nutrient databases were not available. In addition, few researchers have looked at intakes of biotin or pantothenic acid in active people. In general, studies examining dietary intakes of active males report adequate intakes of thiamine, riboflavin, vitamin B_6, and niacin (Lewis 1997; Manore in press). These adequate intakes can be attributed to the relatively high energy intakes in active males. Only Guilland et al. (1989) reported low mean intakes of vitamin B_6 in young male athletes (20 years old); 67% of their subjects consumed less than 100% of the 1989 RDA (2 mg/d) and had a vitamin B_6:protein ratio of 0.013. No studies reported low mean thiamine, riboflavin, or niacin intakes in active males. Only two studies (DeBolt et al. 1988; Faber and Benade 1991) reported that 5-18% of their subjects were consuming less than the 1989 RDA for thiamine and riboflavin. There are no reports of low intakes of thiamine, riboflavin, or niacin expressed as mg/1000 kcal/d. It appears that the high energy consumption of active men keeps dietary intakes of all these vitamins high, usually 1.5-2.0 times the RDA.

As expected, dietary intakes of these vitamins are generally lower in active females than males; yet most studies report adequate intakes for thiamine, riboflavin, and niacin (Manore in press). Only Kaiserauer et al. (1989) reported thiamine, riboflavin, and niacin to be low in their amenorrheic runners, while Beals and Manore (1998) reported low niacin intakes (less than two-thirds of the 1989 RDA) in only 10% of their female athletes (n = 49). Dietary intake data for vitamin B_6 in active females is more variable, yet most studies report mean intakes greater than two-thirds of the 1989 RDA. Lower dietary intakes of vitamin B_6 usually accompany energy intakes <1900 kcal/d (Kaiserauer et al. 1989; Rucinski 1989). *It appears that unless a person is restricting energy intake or consuming a diet high in refined foods, nutrient intakes of thiamine, riboflavin, vitamin B_6, and niacin appear to be adequate.*

Dietary Sources

The water-soluble B-complex vitamins occur in a variety of animal and plant products and in a number of different biochemical forms. Their bioavailability depends on factors such as the dietary form of the vitamin, other substances in the diet, drugs a person is taking, age, and the person's general health. Several of the B-complex vitamins are sensitive to environmental conditions, which can alter the amount of the vitamin in foods. For example, light easily destroys riboflavin—which is why milk, a food high in riboflavin, is packaged in opaque containers. *Other B-complex vitamins, such as biotin, vitamin B_6, thiamine, and pantothenic acid, can easily be destroyed by heating, cooking, and milling processes; or they can be lost in cooking water. Any cooking process that exposes food to heat (canning, heat curing, cooking) or milling, or that discards cooking fluids, may reduce the amounts of these vitamins.* The amount of a vitamin absorbed by the gut and made available to the body may be very different from the amount of the vitamin measured in the raw food.

In general, B-complex vitamins are found in the germ and bran portions of whole grains, meat products, and fortified or enriched cereals and grains (see "Enriched and Fortified Foods," page 259). More specifically, thiamine is abundant in lean pork, yeast, legumes, and enriched cereals and breads. Riboflavin is found in eggs, lean meats, milk, milk products, broccoli, and enriched breads and cereals. Vitamin B_6 is plentiful in meats (especially chicken and tuna) and in plant foods such as beans, cereals, and brown rice. In the typical American diet, approximately 40% of dietary vitamin B_6 comes from animal products and 60% from plants. The highest amounts of niacin occur in meats and in the bran portion of grains. In the typical American diet, meats, fish, and poultry contribute about half the niacin equivalents consumed. Other good sources of niacin are whole grains, legumes and seeds (peanuts), enriched and fortified breads and cereals, peaches, potatoes, and mushrooms. Vegetables are rich sources of niacin (per kilocalorie). Since they can provide substantial amounts of niacin *if* consumed in abundance, vegetarians can obtain adequate amounts of niacin if they chose their foods carefully.

Pantothenic acid and biotin are widespread in foods. Dietary sources particularly high in pantothenic acid are meats (especially liver and heart), baker's yeast, wheat and rice bran, mushrooms, nuts (cashews and peanuts), soybeans, broccoli, and avocados. Grains are good

■ HIGHLIGHT ■

Enriched and Fortified Foods

Enriched Foods

When grain is milled, the germ and bran are removed. Since many of the vitamins and minerals are in this portion of the grain, the refined product is less nutritious. White flour and white rice have fewer vitamins and minerals than whole wheat flour or brown rice. In the 1940s, the Food and Drug Administration (FDA) mandated that some of the nutrients lost during the milling and refining of flour be replaced by enrichment. In the milling process, these nutrients (thiamine, riboflavin, niacin, and iron) are added back to the refined product at levels specifically established by the FDA. In Canada, all refined flour is also enriched with these nutrients. If you read package labels, you will notice that enriched flour is added to many products such as bread, pasta, doughnuts, muffins, and cookies. Besides flour, many milled grain products, such as rice and corn, are also enriched.

Fortified Foods

Fortification is the addition of a vitamin or mineral to a food product during processing. The FDA of the United States does not mandate this process except for folic acid in flour, breads, and grains. Canada's regulations, different from those in the United States, were under review as of 1999. In the United States, manufacturers can add any amount of any vitamin or mineral to their products. They can add micronutrients that may not naturally occur in the original product, or they can add additional levels to what is already present. For example, many cereals are fortified with 100% of the RDA for selected vitamins and minerals. Orange juice is now fortified with calcium and additional vitamin C. Even some candies are now being fortified with vitamin C! The manufacturer determines which foods will be fortified and the amount of fortification.

Sport and diet foods have been especially targeted for fortification with vitamins, minerals, or both. The level of fortification depends on the products, but many manufacturers add 25-100% of the RDA or DRI of various nutrients to sport bars and meal-replacement products. Most fat-free cookies, breakfast bars, muffins, and granola bars are fortified to some extent.

---

sources of the vitamin, but it is located in the outer layers, which are frequently removed with milling. Like pantothenic acid, biotin is widely distributed in foods but in low concentrations. Foods that contribute most to our dietary intake of biotin are brewer's yeast, milk, cheese, liver, egg yolks, nuts (peanuts and walnuts), lentils, soybeans, and some vegetables (cauliflower, spinach, peas) and grains (oats, wheat bran, sorghum). Small amounts of biotin are also produced in the intestinal tract of humans. A substance in raw eggs—avidin—interferes with biotin absorption and decreases biotin status. But since avidin is unstable in heat, cooked eggs cause no threat to biotin status.

B-complex vitamins are frequently added to commercially prepared foods at 25-100% of the RDA per serving. This means that consuming

fortified cereals, breakfast bars, sport bars and drinks, or energy shakes and/or meal-replacement products (e.g., Ensure, Boost, GatorPro) will dramatically increase total dietary intakes. Individuals who "watch their weight" or engage in physical activity frequently use these types of products. In addition, many multivitamin or vitamin/mineral supplements contain 100% or more of the RDA for these nutrients. Since many Americans use dietary supplements, the total intake of these vitamins in the diet may be increasing regardless of dietary choices.

Vitamin Deficiency in Active Individuals

Because B-complex vitamins are important to energy production during exercise, it is assumed that individuals with poor status (poor dietary intakes and poor biochemical assessment values) will have a reduced ability to perform physical activity (see "Vitamin Deficiencies and Their Symptoms," below). A number of studies have supported this hypothesis. Van der Beek et al. (1994) depleted 24 healthy men of thiamine, riboflavin, and vitamin B_6 over an 11-week metabolic feeding period, then examined the effects of the multiple deficiencies on physical performance. Depletion of these three vitamins had the following effects on exercise performance:

- 12% decrease in maximal work capacity ($\dot{V}O_2$max)

■ HIGHLIGHT ■

Vitamin Deficiencies and Their Symptoms

Thiamine

Beriberi is associated with low dietary intake of thiamine. The disease affects the cardiovascular, gastrointestinal, and nervous systems. Clinical signs and symptoms include mental confusion, altered carbohydrate metabolism, increased levels of tissue and plasma pyruvate, anorexia, muscular weakness, peripheral paralysis, edema, muscle wasting, tachycardia, and enlarged heart (Food and Nutrition Board 1989). In the United States, people at greatest risk for thiamine deficiency are alcoholics, renal patients, the chronically ill, and anyone who consumes a diet high in processed foods (which are typically low in thiamine). Enrichment of white flour has eliminated much of the risk for beriberi in the United States.

Riboflavin

No single disease is associated with low dietary intakes of riboflavin. Low intakes are associated with lesions around the mouth, general dermatitis, and normocytic anemia (Food and Nutrition Board 1989). Riboflavin is essential for the conversion of vitamin B_6 and niacin to their active forms.

Vitamin B_6

Like riboflavin, vitamin B_6 has no unique clinical deficiency disease associated with low intakes. Deficiency symptoms, which are usually connected with other B-complex vitamin deficiencies, are convulsions, neurological symptoms, dermatitis, and anemia (Food and Nutrition Board 1989). If high protein intakes accompany low vitamin B_6 intakes, the deficiency will appear sooner.

Niacin

Pellagra is associated with niacin deficiency. Early symptoms include weakness, lassitude, anorexia, digestive disturbances, and mental symptoms of anxiety, depression, irritability, and forgetfulness (Gibson 1990). Later stages of the disease are characterized by dermatitis, diarrhea, inflammation of the mucous membranes, dementia, and in some cases death (Food and Nutrition Board 1989) (the disease is frequently called the "disease of the four Ds"). The symptoms are due to a lack of energy for muscle control and neural functions. Although prevalent in the southern United States in the early 1900s, pellagra is now rare due to the enrichment of white flour and government programs that provide food to the poor. People still at risk for the disease are malnourished alcoholics, some elderly individuals, and those using isoniazid or 3-mercaptopurine for the treatment of tuberculosis or leukemia, respectively (Gibson 1990). The disease is usually associated with poor intakes of all the B-complex vitamins and poor protein intakes.

Pantothenic Acid and Biotin

There are no deficiency diseases associated with low intakes of pantothenic acid or biotin.

- 7% decrease in **onset of blood lactate accumulation (OBLA)**

- 12% decrease in oxygen consumption at OBLA

- 9% decrease in peak power

- 7% decrease in mean power

This study supports earlier research that identified individuals with subclinical vitamin deficiencies and assessed their ability to do work before and after vitamin supplementation. After measuring vitamin B_6 and riboflavin status in boys (n = 124, ages 12-14 years), Suboticanec and colleagues (1990) found that 24% had poor vitamin B_6 status (EASTAC >2.00) and 19% had poor riboflavin status (EGRAC >1.20). A subgroup (n = 37) of the original sample pool was then given 2 mg of vitamin B_6 (pyridoxine) 6 d/week for 2 mo. A second subgroup (n = 38) was given 2 mg of riboflavin 6 d/week for 2 mo. At the beginning and end of each treatment period, physical work capacity was measured on a bicycle ergometer. The researchers reported a significant negative correlation ($p = 0.036$) between $\dot{V}O_2$max and EASTAC (a measure of vitamin B_6 status) (figure 9.2)—as vitamin B_6 status improved (EASTAC got smaller), work

capacity also improved ($\dot{V}O_2$max got larger). Although the results for riboflavin appeared similar to those for vitamin B_6, the negative correlation did not reach statistical significance. These data suggest that subclinical deficiencies of vitamin B_6 (and possibly riboflavin) negatively affect aerobic capacity in young boys. When the vitamin deficiency is corrected through either diet or vitamin supplementation, work capacity improves. In summary, these studies suggest that deficiencies of thiamine, riboflavin, or vitamin B_6 may decrease the ability to do work, especially maximal work.

Exercise and Vitamin Requirements

How do you determine if exercise increases the need for vitamins? The most common types of research studies that have examined this question are the following:

- Metabolic diet studies of sedentary and active individuals (for more details, see "What Is a Metabolic Diet Study? How Do These Studies Assess Vitamin Requirements?" on page 264).

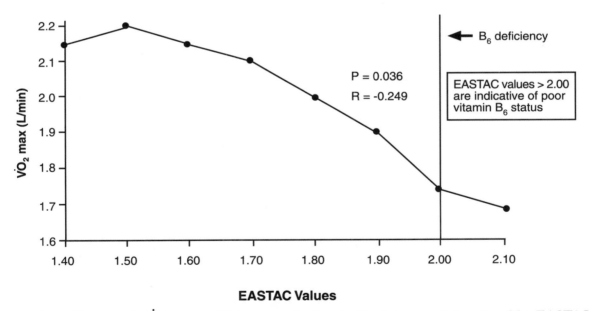

EASTAC Values

Figure 9.2 Changes in $\dot{V}O_2$max with improved vitamin B_6 status, as determined by EASTAC, in young boys 12-15 years of age. This graph shows the relationship between vitamin B_6 status, using erythrocyte aspartic transaminate activity coefficient (EASTAC), and $\dot{V}O_2$max before and after supplementation of 2 mg vitamin B_6 for 6 d/week for 2 mo. $\dot{V}O_2$max improved significantly with supplementation as status improved until EASTAC values reached 1.4-1.5. EASTAC values > 2.00 indicate poor vitamin B_6 status.

Adapted from Suboticanec et al. 1990.

- Cross-sectional studies comparing nutrient intakes and status of active versus sedentary individuals.
- Intervention studies examining nutrient intakes and statuses of sedentary people who begin an exercise program. These studies try to determine if vitamin status decreases as these people become more physically fit.
- Intervention studies examining nutrient intakes and statuses of sedentary people who start a diet (reduced energy intake) and exercise program for weight loss. These studies try to determine if status decreases as these individuals lose weight and become more physically fit.

Metabolic Diet Studies

Metabolic studies are the most controlled way to answer the question posed above. With this approach, a researcher feeds a known amount of the vitamin to both sedentary and active individuals and determines if subsequent nutrient statuses are different. If vitamin status decreases in active people compared to controls, or if more of the vitamin is required to maintain status, it would appear that active individuals need more of the vitamin. In this section, we evaluate metabolic studies that have examined riboflavin and vitamin B_6 statuses of both sedentary and active people under controlled conditions. To date there have been no metabolic studies of thiamine, niacin, pantothenic acid, or biotin status in active and sedentary people.

Based on a series of metabolic studies in active women, it appears that exercise, dieting, and diet plus exercise increase the need for riboflavin above the 1989 RDA (0.6 mg/1000 kcal or 1.3 mg/d). The current RDA is set at 1.1 mg/d (Food and Nutrition Board 1998), which is lower than the 1989 RDA. Belko et al. (1983) at Cornell University were first to examine riboflavin requirements of active people. Measuring riboflavin status (EGRAC and urinary riboflavin excretion) in young women fed various levels of riboflavin over a 12-week period, they found that weight-stable women who exercised (running) for 20-50 min 6 d/week needed at least 1.1 mg riboflavin/1000 kcal (~2.4 mg/d) to maintain good riboflavin status. Even when the women were not exercising and receiving the 1989 RDA (0.6 mg/1000 kcal) they demonstrated poor riboflavin status. Mean EGRAC values remained normal (<1.25) when the

women exercised only at the higher intake levels of riboflavin (about 2.3 times the 1989 RDA) (figure 9.3). This study was followed by two others (Belko et al. 1984; Belko et al. 1985) in which young overweight women were placed on a metabolic diet providing 1200-1250 kcal/d and various levels of riboflavin intake (0.8-1.6 mg/1000 kcal) (figure 9.4). Dieting for weight loss increased the amount of riboflavin required to maintain good status in these women; when dieting was combined with exercise, even more riboflavin was required. The researchers concluded that 1.6 mg of riboflavin/1000 kcal is required to maintain good riboflavin status in women who both diet and exercise (3 h/week at 75-85% of maximal heart rate). Finally, Winters et al. (1992) examined the effect of moderate exercise (2.5 h/week at 75-85% of maximal heart rate) on riboflavin status of active women 50-67 years old. All subjects consumed a metabolic diet that provided adequate energy for weight maintenance (1800-2000 kcal/d) at two levels of riboflavin (0.6 and 0.9 mg/1000 kcal) for 5 weeks. Exercise increased the amount of riboflavin required to maintain good status (0.9 mg of riboflavin/1000 kcal or ~1.8 mg/d). *It appears that both exercise and dieting for weight loss increase riboflavin requirements above the RDA. Combining exercise (2.5-5 h/week) with dieting (~1250 kcal/d) increases the riboflavin required for good status even more (1.6 mg/1000 kcal, or 2 mg/d).* These studies all examined the riboflavin requirements of women engaged in *moderate* exercise (2.5-5 h/week). No metabolic data are available for people who participate in more strenuous exercise.

A number of metabolic studies have examined vitamin B_6 requirements of active and sedentary people—leading to the conclusion that approximately 1.5-2.3 mg/d of vitamin B_6 are required to maintain PLP concentrations above the cut-off value of 30 nmol/L (Leklem 1990). The 1989 RDA for vitamin B_6 was 1.6 mg/d for women and 2.0 mg/d for men, while the 1998 RDA is 1.3 mg/d for both men and women (Food and Nutrition Board 1998). For example, a metabolic study by Dreon and Butterfield (1986) examined vitamin B_6 status in active and sedentary men consuming 4.2 mg/d of vitamin B_6. The active men were running either 5 or 10 mi/day (8-16 km/d). Although vitamin B_6 status did not change as running mileage increased, the men were consuming three times the current RDA for vitamin B_6. Manore et al. (1987) examined vitamin B_6 status in three groups of women

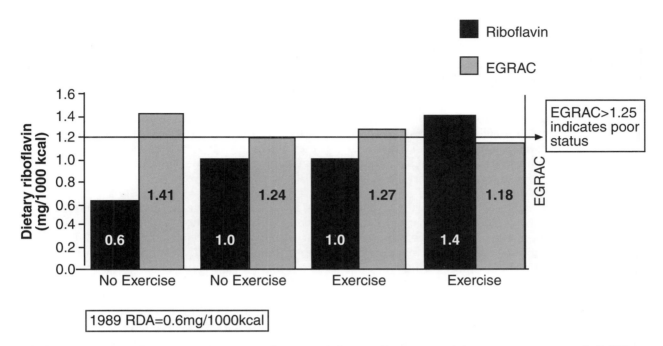

Figure 9.3 Riboflavin requirements for exercising and nonexercising young women fed different levels of riboflavin. Each nonexercising period was 2 weeks, and each exercise period was 3 weeks. Shaded bars indicate dietary riboflavin intake; nonshaded bars indicate the erythrocyte glutathione reductase activity coefficient (EGRAC). EGRAC values > 1.25 indicate poor riboflavin status.

Adapted from Belko et al. 1983.

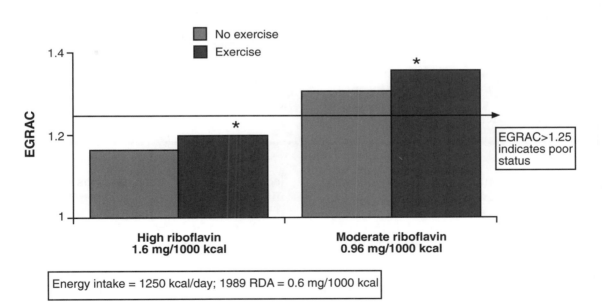

Figure 9.4 Riboflavin requirements for exercising and nonexercising young women consuming a 1250 kcal/d metabolic weight-loss diet with either high (1.6 mg/1000 kcal) or moderate (0.96 mg/1000 kcal) riboflavin intake. EGRAC was used to determine riboflavin status (EGRAC > 1.25 indicates poor riboflavin status). The 1989 RDA for riboflavin was 0.6 mg/1000 kcal/d. Exercise significantly increased EGRAC compared to nonexercise ($p < 0.05$). More riboflavin was needed to maintain good riboflavin status during exercise.

Adapted from Belko et al. 1985.

■ HIGHLIGHT ■

What Is a Metabolic Diet Study? How Do These Studies Assess Vitamin Requirements?

The purpose of a metabolic diet study is to determine how vitamin assessment parameters change under controlled conditions when the dietary intake of a nutrient is closely controlled. In these studies, all foods eaten by study participants are prepared in a metabolic research kitchen. These studies may last for weeks or months. All food is weighed to within 0.1 g and carefully recorded. Subjects are usually required to either live at the research facility (all physical activity is monitored) or come to the research facility for all their meals. In addition, body weight is measured daily to prevent any increase or decrease in weight. If weight does change, energy intake is altered so that the subject returns to the baseline weight. This must be done without altering the intake of the vitamin being studied. During this time, vitamin biochemical assessment parameters are also measured (such as blood, urine, and fecal material). This may require that the subject collect all 24-h urine and fecal samples throughout the study. An example: you might design the following study to determine if active and sedentary women have different vitamin requirements.

Feed active women (all of equal fitness levels and exercising the same number of hours/week) and sedentary females three different diets that provide three different levels of vitamin B_6: vitamin B_6 below the RDA (1.0 mg/d) for 3 weeks; vitamin B_6 at the level of the RDA (1.3 mg/d) for 3 weeks; vitamin B_6 above the RDA (1.6 mg/d) for 3 weeks. Ideally, you would like to randomly assign these diets, with a 6-week "washout" period between diets. (The RDA for vitamin B_6 should provide adequate amounts of the vitamin for normal healthy women.) Feeding a metabolic diet means that subjects are fed *all* the food they eat during the study period and are monitored to *make sure they eat all the food.* The amount of vitamin B_6 in the food is determined by biochemical assessment. You would collect blood and 24-h urine samples throughout the study period and make sure all subjects maintain baseline body weights. You would determine nutritional status for each of the diets to test which of the diets provide adequate vitamin B_6 to keep assessment parameters within normal range. You would also compare vitamin status between groups for each of the diets. If the active women have poor status on 1.3 mg/d of vitamin B_6, while the sedentary subjects have adequate status on this level, you would conclude that the RDA is not adequate for the active individuals.

(active young, sedentary young, sedentary old) who were fed two levels of vitamin B_6 over a 7-week period. Throughout the study, the active women continued to exercise (2-4 h/week). At baseline, the young active subjects and the sedentary older subjects had lower plasma PLP concentrations (indicating poor vitamin status) compared to the young sedentary subjects. For all groups, mean plasma PLP concentrations improved when they were fed a metabolic diet providing either 2.3 or 10.0 mg/d of vitamin B_6. The only differences observed between the active and sedentary groups were that the active females lost more vitamin B_6 as 4-PA.

Manore et al. (1987) also measured changes in plasma PLP concentrations during a 20-min exercise period at 80% $\dot{V}O_2$max. For all sub-

jects, plasma PLP concentrations increased significantly during exercise (figure 9.5) and then returned to baseline within 60 min. A number of other studies have confirmed this phenomenon (Crozier et al. 1994; Hofmann et al. 1991; Leklem and Schultz 1983). While the metabolic reason for this increase in PLP concentrations during exercise is not known, animal studies reveal a shift in the vitamin from the liver to the muscle. The increase in plasma PLP concentrations during exercise increases the probability that PLP will be metabolized in the liver to 4-PA and lost in the urine (Crozier et al. 1994). Thus, exercise can increase the turnover and loss of vitamin B_6. Researchers have documented higher urinary 4-PA losses in active individuals compared to sedentary controls, and

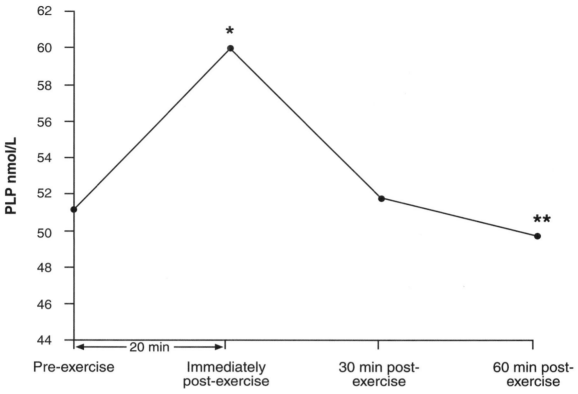

Figure 9.5 Changes in plasma pyridoxal phosphate (PLP) concentrations during 20 min of exercise (80% $\dot{V}O_2$max) in active and sedentary females consuming a metabolic diet containing 2.3 mg/d vitamin B_6. Plasma PLP increased with exercise and then decreased to baseline 60 min post-exercise. PLP levels immediately post-exercise were significantly higher than those at all other times, and PLP levels 60 min post-exercise were significantly lower than the levels of PLP immediately post-exercise ($p < 0.05$).

Adapted from Manore et al. 1987.

after strenuous exercise (Crozier et al. 1994; Manore 1994). Rokitzki, Sagredos, Reub, Buchner, and Keul (1994) recently calculated, based on urinary 4-PA excretion concentrations, that marathon runners lose approximately 1 mg of vitamin B_6 during a 26.2-mi race. Yet no one has documented a decrease in plasma PLP concentrations due to exercise-induced 4-PA losses. In general, any loss of vitamin B_6 due to exercise is small and could easily be replaced by eating one to two servings of a high vitamin B_6 food. However, as table 9.4 illustrates, some individuals (especially the elderly) have poor plasma PLP concentrations on their self-selected free-living diets, and numerous studies have documented lower vitamin B_6 status in the elderly (Lowik et al. 1989; Manore et al. 1989; Ribaya-Mercado et al. 1991) and in individuals with various chronic diseases such as arthritis (Roubenoff et al. 1995) and diabetes (Manore et al. 1991; Manore in press). No one

has determined if active individuals with chronic diseases, such as diabetes or arthritis, have higher requirements for vitamin B_6.

The effect of combining exercise and dieting for weight loss has also been examined to a limited extent for vitamin B_6. Fogelholm, Koskinen et al. (1993) found a significant decrease in vitamin B_6 status in male elite wrestlers after 3 weeks of dieting (1700 kcal/d) but no changes in thiamine and riboflavin status. However, the authors provided no dietary intake data for vitamin B_6; thus, the poor status may have been due to poor dietary intakes during the dieting period combined with high physical activity. Van Dale et al. (1990) examined the effect of a 14-week diet (900 kcal/d) or of diet plus exercise in 12 obese men (mean age = 40 years). Plasma PLP concentrations significantly decreased in the diet-plus-exercise group (54.5 to 40.0 nmol/L) compared to the diet-only group (49.8 to 48.7 nmol/L). Riboflavin and thiamine

Table 9.4 **Mean Fasting Concentrations of Plasma Pyridoxal-5'-Phosphate (PLP) in Active and Sedentary Women on Their Free-Living Diets and on Metabolic Diets Providing Either 2.3-2.4 or 10 mg/d of Vitamin B$_6$**

Groups	PLP[1] (nmol/L)
Active young (n = 5)	
Free-living diet	42 ± 14
2.3-2.4 mg B$_6$/d	48 ± 9
10 mg B$_6$/d	175 ± 24
Sedentary young (n = 5)	
Free-living diet	35 ± 15
2.3-2.4 mg B$_6$/d	61 ± 24
10 mg B$_6$/d	203 ± 56
Sedentary old (n = 5)	
Free-living diet	30 ± 12
2.3-2.4 mg B$_6$/d	44 ± 18
10 mg B$_6$/d	181 ± 41

[1]All values are mean ± SD. A plasma PLP concentration <30 nmol/L is considered low.

Adapted from Manore et al. 1987.

status decreased in both groups, but the only statistically significant changes were for riboflavin status in the diet-plus-exercise group. However, the dietary intakes of vitamin B$_6$ and thiamine were below the 1989 RDA for the last 9 weeks of the study, while riboflavin intake was at the 1989 RDA.

Vitamin Status of Active Individuals

If exercise increases the need for the B-complex vitamins involved in energy metabolism, then active individuals should have poor status while consuming the RDA for these vitamins. This section examines the research available on the vitamin status (thiamine, riboflavin, vitamin B$_6$, niacin) of nonsupplementing active individuals consuming free-living diets.

Table 9.3 outlines recent studies examining the nutritional status of active individuals who consume free-living diets with no supplemental intakes of thiamine, riboflavin, vitamin B$_6$, or niacin. The number of assessment parameters measured for each study varies, but most studies that report poor status use more than one biochemical measurement and dietary intake of the vitamin. For vitamin B$_6$, the number of active people with poor status ranged from 0-60% in five studies. To date, Telford et al. (1992) have reported the most athletes with poor vitamin B$_6$ status. They studied 86 male and female athletes before and after an 8-mo training period during which half consumed a multivitamin/mineral supplement and a matched group took a placebo. They found that 60% of the athletes had poor vitamin B$_6$ status before any supplementation occurred. There are fewer reported incidences of poor status for the other B-complex vitamins in active people consuming a free-living diet. There are no well-controlled studies of pantothenic acid or biotin status in active people. One report from Finland (Fogelholm, Ruokonen et al. 1993) examined vitamin B$_6$, riboflavin, and thiamine status in 42 physically active college students (18-32 years) before and after 5 weeks of vitamin B-complex supplementation. At the beginning of the study, 43% had poor vitamin B$_6$ status, 57% had poor riboflavin status, and 12% had poor thiamine status. Supplementation significantly improved status measurements for all three vitamins. These data suggest that some active individuals have poor vitamin status while consuming a free-living diet. Research also indicates that exercise can decrease vitamin status in individuals who already have poor or marginal vitamin status (Soares et al. 1993).

Vitamins and Exercise Performance

A number of researchers have examined whether vitamin and/or mineral supplements improve exercise performance. These types of studies are difficult to do because so many factors besides diet can affect performance. In addition, there are many ways to measure performance. The major flaw in most studies is that they did not control for nutritional status before adding supplements to athletes' diets; when the study began, some athletes may already have had good nutritional status, while others had poor status. If initial nutritional status is not controlled, there is no way to un-

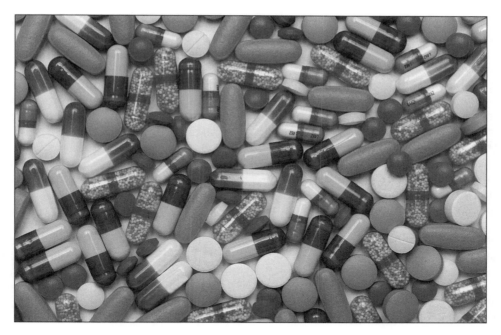

Many athletes supplement with vitamins and minerals without critically evaluating the supplements they buy or their own nutritional needs.

ambiguously determine the effect of the supplement on performance.

The following is an example of an early project that tested whether supplementation improved exercise performance. Barnett and Conlee (1984) examined the effect of a commercial dietary supplement on endurance performance in 20 male runners. For 4 weeks, subjects were given either a placebo or a supplement containing vitamins, minerals, amino acids, and a fatty acid complex. The study was "double blind"—neither the subjects nor the researchers knew who was on which treatment. Before and after the 4-week treatment period, subjects performed a 60-min submaximal treadmill run (65-70% $\dot{V}O_2$max) and a max $\dot{V}O_2$

■ HIGHLIGHT ■

Guidelines for Recommending Vitamin Supplements

The following questions will help you determine whether you should recommend vitamin supplements for an active person:

- Is current dietary intake of the vitamin adequate?
- Is there any indication for increased need?
- Is the amount recommended below the toxic level?
- Are any nutrient-nutrient or drug-nutrient interactions indicated?
- Why does the athlete want to supplement?
- Is the athlete willing to make dietary changes that would improve vitamin intakes?
- What is the cost of the supplement? What is the cost of getting the nutrient from food?
- Can the nutrient be easily obtained in food by making simple dietary changes that are acceptable to the athlete?

test. There were no differences between groups in blood concentrations of glucose, free fatty acids, and lactate during exercise, or in the amount of glycogen used during exercise. The supplement had no effect on maximum oxygen consumption. The authors concluded that the supplement had no beneficial effect on exercise performance. The major problems with this study are that (1) the researchers did not determine the subjects' nutritional status before the study began, (2) neither diet nor exercise training was controlled during the study, and (3) the supplement contained 33 different nutrients. It is not surprising that the supplement had no effect on performance: there were too many uncontrolled variables.

To date there are no data to support improved exercise performance in individuals who supplement with vitamins or minerals *as long as nutrient status was good before supplementation began.* For example, if you already have good vitamin B_6 status, supplementing with more vitamin B_6 will not improve your exercise performance. However, if your vitamin B_6 status is poor, then improvement in vitamin B_6 status, through either diet or supplements, may improve exercise performance above that seen in the "subclinical" state. Once vitamin status has normalized, additional supplementation will not continue to improve performance.

Chapter in Review

We started this chapter by asking two questions about vitamin supplementation and exercise. This section summarizes the research available to answer these questions.

Does exercise increase the need for B-complex vitamins in active healthy individuals? Research on the micronutrient needs of active people has been limited, with most of the work done in athletes. It appears that ribo-

flavin requirements increase with exercise, dieting, and dieting plus exercise in both young and older women doing moderate activity. No data are available on men or for individuals exercising more strenuously. Exercise alters vitamin B_6 metabolism by increasing plasma concentrations of PLP during exercise, which in turn may increase the loss of vitamin B_6 through urinary 4-PA excretion. But the amount of vitamin B_6 needed to cover losses or increased need is small (<1 mg/d in individuals running a 26.2-mi marathon) and can be easily met through good food choices. In addition, exercise appears to cause a redistribution of vitamin B_6 from the liver to the muscles. The exact reason for this redistribution is not known. The data on changes in thiamine status with exercise are limited, but some cross-sectional studies suggest a small percentage of active individuals can have poor status. There are few or no data on the effect of exercise on niacin, pantothenic acid, or biotin status.

Little research has been done on the effect of combining both diet and exercise for weight loss on micronutrient status of thiamine, riboflavin, vitamin B_6, or niacin. If people are restricting energy intake for weight loss, or are making poor dietary choices, dietary intakes of these nutrients will probably be low. Finally, no data are available on the effect of exercise or dieting plus exercise on B-complex vitamin status of people with chronic health problems, such as diabetes or hypertension.

Does supplementation with B-complex vitamins improve exercise performance? In active individuals who already have good nutritional status, there are no data to support improved exercise performance with vitamin or mineral supplementation. However, if a person has marginal nutritional status, supplementation may improve performance by improving nutritional status and the availability of cofactors in the energy metabolism pathways.

KEY CONCEPTS

 1. Understand the exercise-related functions and dietary requirements of the B-complex vitamins.

The B-complex vitamins (thiamine, riboflavin, vitamin B_6, niacin, pantothenic acid, and biotin) are cofactors for various enzymes in the metabolic pathways that produce energy from protein, carbohydrate, and/or fat during exercise. In 1998, new joint DRIs between the United States and Canada were established for the B-complex vitamins, which included new

RDAs for thiamine (1.2 mg/d for men; 1.1 mg/d for women), riboflavin (1.3 mg/d for men; 1.1 mg/d for women), vitamin B_6 (1.3 mg/d for men and women), and niacin (16 NE/d for men; 14 NE/d for women). Pantothenic acid and biotin do not have RDAs, but AIs have been established: 5 mg/d for pantothenic acid and 30 μg/d for biotin.

2. Discuss the rationale for increased need for B-complex vitamins in active individuals.

Theoretically, exercise may increase or alter the need for B-complex vitamins in several ways. Exercise stresses many of the metabolic pathways that require these micronutrients. Exercise training may result in muscle biochemical adaptations that increase micronutrient need. Exercise may also increase the turnover of these micronutrients, increasing their loss from the body. Finally, higher intakes of micronutrients may be required to cover increased needs for the repair and maintenance of lean tissue mass in athletes.

3. Identify the dietary and biochemical assessment methods for the B-complex vitamins.

Determination of vitamin status for an individual requires measurement of a number of parameters, including biochemical markers of status and levels of dietary intake. The biochemical markers should reflect the body's stores of the vitamin and the amount of the vitamin lost from the body in urine, feces, or sweat. If available, functional measurements of vitamin status should be included. The most widely used biochemical assessment parameter for thiamine is ETKAC. The most common biochemical measures of riboflavin status are urinary excretion of riboflavin, erythrocyte riboflavin concentrations, and the determination of EGRAC. For vitamin B_6, the most common assessment measures are plasma PLP, total vitamin B_6, and urinary 4-PA. Measurement of EASTAC and EALTAC are indirect measures of vitamin B_6 status. Good biochemical assessment measures for niacin, biotin, and pantothenic acid are not available.

4. Discuss how exercise may alter B-complex vitamin requirements in active people.

Exercise may slightly increase the need for some of the B-complex vitamins (thiamine, riboflavin, vitamin B_6) by one to two times the current RDA, but this increased need can generally be met by the higher energy intakes required of athletes to maintain body weight. Combining dieting for weight loss and exercise may further increase the need for these vitamins. Vitamin supplementation is recommended for active people who consume low-energy diets or diets high in processed foods, or who restrict dietary intake of fruits, vegetables, or whole grains.

5. Explain the relationship between B-complex vitamins and exercise performance.

Vitamin status is one of many factors that can influence an individual's exercise performance. No data are available to support improved exercise performance in people who supplement with B-complex vitamins *if* vitamin status was good before supplementation. Exercise performance may be improved with supplementation if B-complex vitamin status was poor prior to supplementation.

KEY TERMS

acyl carrier protein (ACP)
adequate intake (AI)
B-complex vitamins

beriberi
branched-chain amino acid (BCAA)
coenzyme A (CoA)

(continued)

dietary reference intake (DRI)
erythrocyte alanine transaminase activity coefficient (EALTAC)
erythrocyte aspartate transaminase activity coefficient (EASTAC)
erythrocyte glutathione reductase activity coefficient (EGRAC)
erythrocyte transketolase
erythrocyte transketolase activity coefficient (ETKAC)
estimated average requirement (EAR)
flavin adenine dinucleotide (FAD)
flavin mononucleotide (FMN)
NAD phosphate (NADP)

niacin equivalent (NE)
nicotinamide adenine dinucleotide (NAD
N'-methyl-2-pyridone-5-carboxylamide (2-pyridone)
N'-methylnicotinamide (NMN)
onset of blood lactate accumulation (OBLA)
pellagra
pyridoxal-5'-phosphate (PLP)
recommended dietary allowance (RDA)
thiamine pyrophosphate (TPP)
tolerable upper intake level (UL)
tricarboxylic acid (TCA)
urinary 4-pyridoxic acid (4-PA)

References

Barnett DW, Conlee RK. The effects of a commercial dietary supplement on human performance. Am J Clin Nutr 1984;40:586-90.

Beals KA, Manore MM. Nutritional status of female athletes with subclinical eating disorders. J Am Diet Assoc 1998;98:419-25.

Belko AZ, Meredith MP, Kalkwarf HJ, et al. Effects of exercise on riboflavin requirements: biological validation in weight reducing women. Am J Clin Nutr 1985;41:270-7.

Belko AZ, Obarzanek E, Kalwarf HJ, et al. Effects of exercise on riboflavin requirements of young women. Am J Clin Nutr 1983;37:509-17.

Belko AZ, Obarzanek E, Roach B, et al. Effects of aerobic exercise and weight loss on riboflavin requirements of moderately obese, marginally deficient young women. Am J Clin Nutr 1984;40:553-61.

Clarkson PM. Exercise and the B vitamins. In: Wolinsky I, Hickson JF, eds. Nutrition in Exercise and Sport. Boca Raton, FL: CRC Press, 1998:179-95.

Combs GF. The Vitamins: Fundamental Aspects in Nutrition and Health. New York: Academic Press, 1992.

Crozier PG, Cordain L, Sampson DA. Exercise-induced changes in plasma vitamin B-6 concentrations do not vary with exercise intensity. Am J Clin Nutr 1994;60:552-8.

DeBolt JE, Singh A, Day BA, Deuster PA. Nutritional survey of the U.S. Navy SEAL trainees. Am J Clin Nutr 1988;48:1316-23.

Dreon DM, Butterfield GE. Vitamin B-6 utilization in active and inactive young men. Am J Clin Nutr 1986;43:816-24.

Faber M, Benade AJ. Mineral and vitamin intake in field athletes (discus-, hammer-, javelin-throwers and shot-putters). Int J Sports Med 1991;12:324-7.

Fischbach F. A Manual of Laboratory and Diagnostic Tests. Philadelphia: Lippincott-Raven Publishing, 1996.

Food and Nutrition Board, National Research Council. Recommended dietary allowances 10th ed. Washington, DC: National Academy Press, 1989.

Food and Nutrition Board, Institute of Medicine. Dietary reference intakes: thiamine, riboflavin, niacin, vitamin B-6, folate, vitamin B-12, pantothenic acid, biotin, and choline. Washington, DC: National Academy Press, 1998.

Fogelholm GM, Koskinen R, Laakso J, Rankinen T, Ruokonen I. Gradual and rapid weight loss: effects on nutrition and performance in male athletes. Med Sci Sports Exerc 1993;25:371-7.

Fogelholm M, Ruokonen I, Laakso JT, Vuorimaa T, Himberg JJ. Lack of association between indices of vitamin B-1, B-2 and B-6 status and exercise-induced blood lactate in young adults. Int J Sport Nutr 1993;3:165-76.

Gibson RS. Principles of Nutritional Assessment. New York: Oxford University Press, 1990.

Guilland JC, Penaranda T, Gallet C, Boggio V, Fuchs F, Klepping J. Vitamin status of young athletes including the effects of supplementation. Med Sci Sports Med 1989;21:441-9.

Hansen CM, Leklem JE, Miller LT. Changes in vitamin B-6 status indictors of women fed a constant protein diet with varying levels of vitamin B-6. Am J Clin Nutr 1997;66:1379-87.

Health EM, Wilcox AR, Quinn CM. Effects of nicotinic acid on respiratory exchange ratio and substrate levels during exercise. Med Sci Sports Exerc 1993;25:1018-23.

Hofmann A, Reynolds RD, Smoak BL, Villanueva VG, Deuster PA. Plasma pyridoxal and pyridoxal 5'-phosphate concentrations in response to ingestion of water or glucose polymer during a 2-h run. Am J Clin Nutr 1991;53:84-9.

Huang Y, Chen W, Evans MA, Mitchell ME, Shultz TD. Vitamin B-6 requirement and status assessment of young women fed a high-protein diet with various levels of vitamin B-6. Am J Clin Nutr 1998;67:208-20.

Kaiserauer S, Snyder AC, Sleeper M, Zierath J. Nutritional, physiological, and menstrual status of distance runners. Med Sci Sports Exerc 1989;21:120-5.

Keith RE, Alt LA. Riboflavin status of female athletes consuming normal diets. Nutr Res 1991;11:727-34.

Leklem JE. Physical activity and vitamin B-6 metabolism in men and women: Interrelationship with fuel needs. In: Reynolds RD, Leklem JE, eds. Vitamin B-6: Its Role in Health and Disease. New York: AR Liss, 1985:221-41.

Leklem JE. Vitamin B-6: of reservoirs, receptors and requirements. Nutri Today 1988; Sept/Oct:4-10.

Leklem JE. Vitamin B-6: a status report. J Nutr 1990;120;1503-7.

Leklem JE. Vitamin B-6. In: Shils ME, Olson JA, Shike M, eds. Modern Nutrition in Health and Disease. Philadelphia: Lea and Febiger, 1994:383-94.

Leklem JE, Shultz TD. Increased plasma pyridoxal 5'-phosphate and vitamin B-6 in male adolescents after a 4500-meter run. Am J Clin Nutr 1983;38:541-8.

Lewis RD. Riboflavin and niacin. In: Wolinsky I, Diskell JA, eds. Sports Nutrition: Vitamins and Trace Minerals. Boca Raton, FL: CRC Press, 1997:57-73.

Lowik MRH, van den Berg H, Westenbrink S, et al. Dose-response relationships regarding vitamin B-6 in elderly people: a nationwide nutritional survey (Dutch Nutritional Surveillance System). Am J Clin Nutr 1989;50:391-9.

Manore MM. The effect of physical activity on thiamine, riboflavin, and vitamin B-6 requirements. Am J Clin Nutr (in press).

Manore MM. Vitamin B-6 and exercise. Int J Sport Nutr 1994;4:89-103.

Manore MM, Leklem JE, Walter MC. Vitamin B-6 metabolism as affected by exercise in trained and untrained women fed diets differing in carbohydrate and vitamin B-6 content. Am J Clin Nutr 1987;46:995-1004.

Manore MM, Vaughan LA, Carroll SS, Leklem JE. Plasma pyridoxal 5-phosphate concentration and dietary vitamin B-6 intake in free-living, low-income elderly people. Am J Clin Nutr 1989;50:339-45.

Manore MM, Vaughan LA, Leklem JE, Felicetta JV. Changes in plasma pyridoxal phosphate (PLP) in diabetic, hypertensive and hypertensive-diabetic men fed a constant vitamin B-6 diet. FASEB Journal 1991;5:A586 (abstract).

Martini MC, Lampe JW, Slavin JL, Kurzer MS. Effect of the menstrual cycle on energy and nutrient intake. Am J Clin Nutr 1994;60:895-9.

McCormick DB. Riboflavin. In: Shiles ME, Olson JA, Shike M, eds. Modern Nutrition in Health and Disease. Philadelphia: Lea and Febiger, 1994:366-75.

Murray R, Bartoli WP, Eddy DE, Horn MK. Physiology and performance responses to nicotinic-acid ingestion during exercise. Med Sci Sports Exerc 1995;27:1057-62.

Peifer JJ. Thiamin. In: Wolinsky I, Driskell JA, eds. Sports Nutrition. Vitamins and trace minerals. Boca Raton, FL: CRC Press, 1997:47-55.

Ribaya-Mercado JD, Russell RM, Sahyoun N, Morrow FD, Gershoff SN. Vitamin B-6 requirements of elderly men and women. J Nutr 1991;121:1062-74.

Rokitzki L, Sagredos A, Keck E, Sauer B, Keul J. Assessment of vitamin B2 status in performance athletes of various types of sports. J Nutr Sci Vitaminol 1994;40:11-22.

Rokitzki L, Sagredos AN, Reub F, Buchner M, Keul J. Acute changes in vitamin B-6 status in endurance athletes before and after a marathon. Int J Sport Nutr 1994;4:154-65.

Rokitzki L, Sagredos AN, Reub F, Cufi D, Keul J. Assessment of vitamin B-6 status of strength and speedpower athletes. J Am Coll Nutr 1994;13:87-94.

Roubenoff R, Roubenoff RA, Selhub J, et al. Abnormal vitamin B-6 status in rheumatoid cachexia. Arthritis Rheum 1995;38:105-9.

Rucinski A. Relationship of body image and dietary intake of competitive ice skaters. J Am Diet Assoc 1989;89:98-100.

Sampson DA. Vitamin B-6. In: Wolinsky I, Driskell JA. eds. Sports Nutrition. Vitamins and Trace Minerals. Boca Raton, FL: CRC Press, 1997:75-84.

Sobal J, Marquart LF. Vitamin/mineral supplement use among athletes: a review of the literature. Int J Sport Nutr 1994;4:320-34.

Soares MJ, Satyanarayana K, Bamji MS, Jacob CM, Ramana YV, Rao SS. The effect of exercise on the riboflavin status of adult men. Br J Nutr 1993;69:541-51.

Suboticanec K, Stavljenic A, Schalch W, Buzina R. Effects of pyridoxine and riboflavin supplementation on physical fitness in young adolescents. Int J Vitam Nutr Res 1990;60:81-8.

Swendseid ME, Jacob RA. Niacin. In: Shils ME, Olson JA, Shike M, eds. Modern Nutrition in Health and Disease. Philadelphia: Lea & Febiger, 1994:377-82.

Tanphaichitr V. Thiamin. In: Shils ME, Olson JA, Shike M, eds. Modern Nutrition in Health and Disease. Philadelphia: Lea & Febiger, 1994:359-65.

Telford RD, Catchpole EA, Deakin V, McLeay AC, Plank AW. The effect of 7 to 8 months of vitamin/mineral supplementation on the vitamin and mineral status of athletes. Int J Sport Nutr 1992;2:123-34.

Thomas EA. Pantothenic acid and biotin. In: Wolinsky I, Driskell JA, eds. Sports Nutrition. Vitamins and trace minerals. Boca Raton, FL: CRC Press, 1997:97-100.

van Dale D, Schrijver J, Saris WHM. Changes in vitamin status in plasma during dieting and exercise. Int J Vitam Nutr Res 1990; 60:67-74.

van der Beek EJ, van Dokkum W, Wedel M, Schrijver J, van den Berg H. Thiamine, riboflavin and vitamin B-6: impact of restricted intake on physical performance in man. J Am Coll Nutr 1994;13:629-40.

Weight LM, Noakes TD, Labadarios D, Graves J, Jacobs P, Berman PA. Vitamin and mineral status of trained athletes including the effects of supplementation. Am J Clin Nutr 1988;47:186-91.

Winters LRT, Yoon JS, Kalkwarf HJ, et al. Riboflavin requirements and exercise adaptation in older women. Am J Clin Nutr 1992;56:526-32.

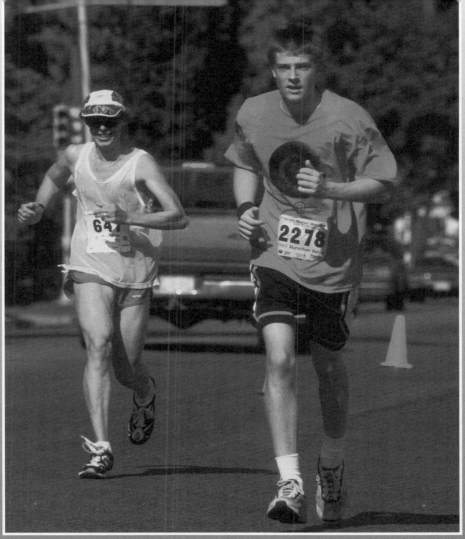
© Paul T. McMahon

CHAPTER 10

Antioxidant Nutrients

After reading this chapter you should be able to

- define free radicals;
- list the enzymes involved in antioxidant activities, and describe the reactions in which they participate;
- discuss the nutrients involved in antioxidant activities;
- describe the methods used to assess oxidative damage;
- describe the proposed rationale for increased antioxidant need among active people;
- discuss how antioxidants play a role in chronic diseases; and
- discuss the relationship between antioxidants and athletic performance.

273

The health benefits of antioxidant nutrients are widely published in both scientific and popular literature. Antioxidants have been purported to protect active people from oxidative tissue damage, reduce risks of cancer and heart disease, and even to slow or reverse the aging process. Is there scientific evidence to support these claims? Should people, particularly active people, increase their consumption of foods high in antioxidants, take antioxidant supplements, or both?

This chapter attempts to answer these questions. We define antioxidants and describe in detail the specific nutrients involved in the antioxidant process. And we closely examine the claim that consuming antioxidants enhances athletic performance.

Actions of Antioxidants

Antioxidants are nutrients that act to prevent oxidative damage resulting from **free radical** formation (see "Definition of Free Radicals," below). Antioxidants can

- scavenge free radicals;
- remove the catalysts that accelerate oxidative reactions, thus minimizing the formation of free radicals;
- repair the damage resulting from oxidation; and
- bind free metal ions to prevent them from reacting with reactive species.

In order to have a clearer understanding of how antioxidants work, you must understand how free radicals are formed. Mitochondrial oxidation usually occurs by four single electron-transfer reactions, starting from NADH and ending with a final product of water (Alberts et al. 1989) (figure 10.1). The electron transfer occurs within the **electron transport chain (ETC, or respiratory chain)**, which is located in the inner mitochondrial membrane. As fig-

■ HIGHLIGHT ■

Definition of Free Radicals

A free radical is a molecule with an unpaired electron in its outer orbit, or valence shell. Free radicals are naturally produced during normal respiration and can be generated in response to exposure to toxic substances (e.g., ozone, alcohol, UV rays, etc.). Free radicals are highly reactive and can create a chain reaction that produces even more free radicals! This chain reaction occurs when a free radical reacts with a stable compound in order to pair its unpaired electron with an electron from the stable compound (table 10.1). If free radicals are produced in excess and not neutralized by the antioxidant systems present in the human body, then cellular damage can occur.

A number of free radicals and reactive oxygen species have been identified. Some of these include

- superoxide radical ($O_2 \cdot^-$),
- hydroxyl radical ($OH \cdot$),
- hydrogen peroxide (H_2O_2)—not a free radical, but can be involved in reactions that cause the production of free radicals,
- singlet oxygen ($^1O_2$), and
- hydroperoxyl free radical ($ROOH \cdot$).

Table 10.1 reviews the processes that form these reactive species, which can damage lipids in membranes (**lipid peroxidation**), resulting in cell damage and possibly cell death. Free radicals are also purported to cause damage to cell proteins, particularly those associated with genetic material. Free radicals also may destroy endothelial cells that line blood vessels, damage the lungs, and accelerate the aging process (Cutler 1984; Halliwell and Gutteridge 1984; Halliwell and Gutteridge 1985; Tate and Repine 1984).

Antioxidant defense systems, including enzymes and nutrients that possess antioxidant properties, help prevent oxidative damage.

Table 10.1 **Reactions That Form Free Radicals and Other Reactive Oxygen Species**

(1) Superoxide radical is formed when an electron is added to an oxygen molecule:

$$O_2 + e^- = O_2^{.-}$$

(2) Hydroxyl radical is formed when hydrogen peroxide reacts with $O_2^{.-}$ in the presence of free metal ions (e.g., Fe^{3+} or Cu^{2+}), or when water reacts with $O_2^{.-}$:

$$O_2^{.-} + H_2O_2 \overset{Fe, Cu}{=} O_2 + OH^. + OH^-$$
$$H_2O + 1/2\ O_2^{.-} = 2OH^.$$

(3) Hydrogen peroxide is formed by joining two hydroxyl radicals or by superoxide radicals generated in aqueous solutions:

$$OH^. + OH^. = H_2O_2$$
$$2O_2^{.-} + 2H^+ = H_2O_2 + O_2$$

(4) Singlet oxygen is formed when one of the six electrons in the outer shell of an oxygen molecule moves into a higher energy orbit using energy released from a nearby chemical reaction or from exposure to radiation.

(5) Hydroperoxyl free radical is formed through a series of reactions involving a lipid, protein, or nucleotide:

(a) the hydroxyl radical attacks an organic compound (RH), forming a carbon-centered radical ($R^.$):

$$RH + OH^. = R^. + H_2O$$

(b) a peroxyl radical is formed from $R^.$ reacting with oxygen:

$$R^{.-} + O_2 = ROO^.$$

(c) a hydroperoxyl radical is formed when the peroxyl radical reacts with a surrounding molecule (either a protein or lipid):

$$ROO^{.-} + RH = R^. + ROOH$$

Adapted from Karlsson 1997.

ure 10.1 shows, the ETC comprises a series of electron carriers, including cytochrome c, **ubiquinone** (i.e., **coenzyme Q$_{10}$**), and the following three enzyme complexes:

- **NADH dehydrogenase complex:** Accepts electrons from NADH and passes them to ubiquinone, which then transfers its electrons to the b-c$_1$ enzyme complex.

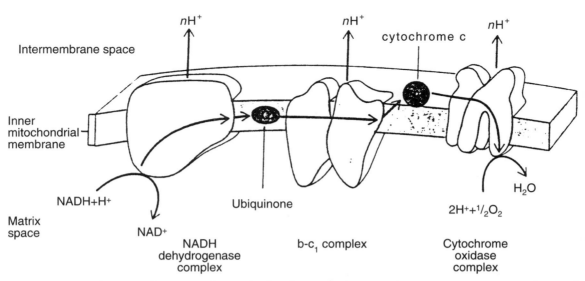

Figure 10.1 The flow of electrons through the three major respiratory enzyme complexes during the transfer of two electrons from NADH to oxygen. Ubiquinone and cytochrome c serve as carriers between the complexes.

Reprinted from Alberts et al. 1989.

- The **b-c₁ enzyme complex:** Accepts electrons from ubiquinone and passes them to cytochrome c, which carries its electrons to the cytochrome oxidase complex.
- *Cytochrome oxidase complex:* Accepts electrons from cytochrome c and passes them on to oxygen to form water.

Electrons (e⁻) can be accepted in the electron transport process in two ways: through tetravalent reduction of oxygen to water and through alternative univalent pathways. No oxygen intermediates are formed during the tetravalent process. During normal cellular respiration, most of the O_2 is reduced to form water via the tetravalent reaction; however, electrons can escape from various locations along the electron transport chain. Oxygen can accept these escaped electrons in an alternate univalent reaction that results in formation of the **superoxide radical**, which can be further reduced to potentially harmful species—**hydrogen peroxide** and **hydroxyl radical** (figure 10.2). It has been estimated that 4-5% of the oxygen consumed in mitochondrial oxidation may form oxygen species with unpaired electrons (Jenkins and Goldfarb 1993). These highly reactive oxygen species can produce more free radicals, including other reactive oxygen species.

Enzymes Involved in Antioxidant Activities

Numerous defense systems protect the body against excessive oxidative damage. The defenses include enzymatic systems—such as superoxide dismutase (SOD), catalase (CAT), glutathione peroxidase (GPX), glutathione reductase (GR), and peroxidase—located in the extracellular, membranous, and intracellular components of cells. Figure 10.3 provides a visual representation of the antioxidant defense system in relation to the cell. The defenses are widespread and strategically placed within the cell—for instance, SOD is located in both the cytoplasm and the mitochondrion,

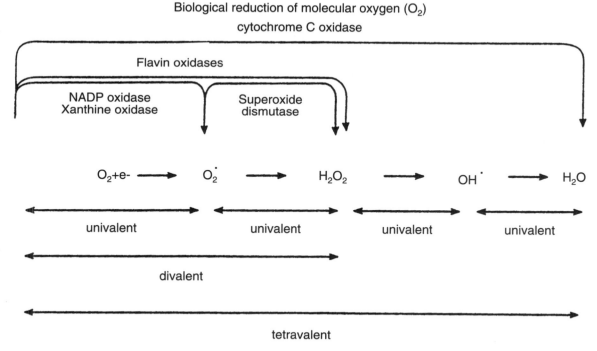

Figure 10.2 Molecular oxygen can participate in univalent, divalent, and tetravalent reactions in mitochondrial metabolism. Respiration and water formation is the normal and tetravalent reaction. Water can also be formed by four consecutive univalent reactions, which produces oxygen-centered radicals as well as hydrogen peroxide (H_2O_2). Hydrogen peroxide provokes radical (OH·) formation from water.

Adapted from Karlsson 1997.

where it can convert the superoxide radical to hydrogen and oxygen in both lipid and aqueous media.

The antioxidant defense enzymes require minerals as cofactors, including

- copper (Cu), which is part of the structure of cytosolic SOD;
- iron (Fe), which is part of the structure of CAT;
- manganese (Mn), which is part of the structure of mitochondrial SOD; and
- zinc (Zn), which is part of the structure of cytosolic SOD.

Deficiencies of these minerals can result in reduced activities of the corresponding antioxidant enzymes. *Note also that unbound forms of certain minerals, such as iron and copper, can enhance oxidative damage.*

Enzymatic Defense Systems

- ***Superoxide dismutase (SOD):*** Accelerates the conversion of superoxide radical to hydrogen peroxide.
- ***Catalase (CAT):*** Removes hydrogen peroxide.
- ***Glutathione:*** A substrate (not an enzyme) involved in the removal of hydrogen

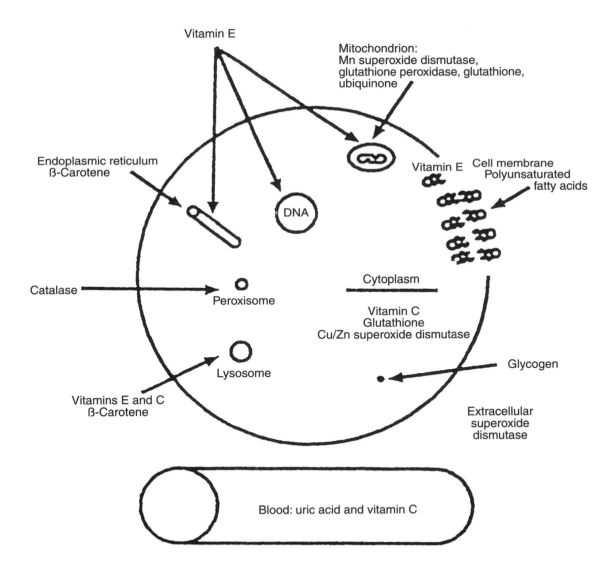

Figure 10.3 Antioxidant defense.
Reprinted from Jenkins 1993.

peroxide and the reduction of lipid hydroperoxides. The oxidized form of glutathione is abbreviated GSSG; the reduced form is abbreviated GSH.

- *Glutathione peroxidase (GPX):* Removes hydrogen peroxide and reduces lipid hydroperoxides.
- *Glutathione reductase (GR):* Converts oxidized glutathione (GSSG) back to reduced glutathione (GSH).
- *Peroxidase (no abbreviation):* Rids the body of excess hydrogen peroxide.

Superoxide dismutase provides one line of defense in the mitochondria and cytosol. This enzyme acts to accelerate the conversion of the superoxide radical to hydrogen peroxide and oxygen, as illustrated in equation 1:

(SOD)

Equation 1 $2O_2{\cdot}^- + 2H^+ \rightarrow H_2O_2 + O_2$

Catalase, located in peroxisomes and possibly in myocardial mitochondria, removes hydrogen peroxide by converting it to water and oxygen:

(CAT)

Equation 2 $2H_2O_2 \rightarrow 2H_2O + O_2$

Glutathione peroxidase and glutathione reductase are substrate-enzyme complexes located in the mitochondria and cytosol. GPX removes hydrogen peroxide by using it to oxidize reduced glutathione (GSH). GPX also reduces lipid hydroperoxides to hydroxy acids, as in equations 3 and 4:

(GPX)

Equation 3 $2GSH + H_2O_2 \rightarrow GSSG + 2H_2O$

(GPX)

Equation 4 $ROOH + 2GSH \rightarrow ROH + H_2O + GSSG$

where R is any organic backbone of a hydroperoxide.

Equation 3 is probably the major reaction that processes the hydrogen peroxide formed in the SOD reaction of equation 1 (Gutteridge and Halliwell 1994). Glutathione reductase converts oxidized glutathione (GSSG) back to reduced glutathione (GSH), as illustrated in equation 5:

(GR)

Equation 5 $GSSG + NADPH \rightarrow GSH + NADP$

Peroxidases are enzymes that use hydrogen peroxide to oxidize a given substrate (S), thus ridding the body of excess hydrogen peroxide. This action is illustrated in equation 6:

(peroxidase)

Equation 6 $SH_2 + H_2O_2 \rightarrow S + 2H_2O$

where S is any reduced substrate.

The reactions in equations 1 through 6 represent only a few of the functions these enzyme systems perform. Many of these enzyme systems are also involved in the repair of damage caused by free radicals and in regenerating other protective antioxidant nutrients. For instance, GPX metabolizes damaged lipids from membranes, which can then be replaced by healthy fatty acids, and GSH assists in recycling both vitamins E and C (Gutteridge and Halliwell 1994).

Nutrients Involved in Antioxidant Activities

In addition to enzyme systems, many micronutrients are also involved in the antioxidant process. While vitamins E, C, and beta-carotene are well-known antioxidants, other nutrients (including many minerals) also help remove free radicals (table 10.2).

Vitamin E

Vitamin E is an essential fat-soluble vitamin that includes eight compounds classified as tocopherols and tocotrienols, with each compound having a different biological activity (Meydani et al. 1997). **Alpha-tocopherol** is considered the most biologically active vitamin E compound, with its primary function identified as an antioxidant.

Vitamin E performs many antioxidant functions in the body. Some of the primary functions of vitamin E are listed below (Gutteridge and Halliwell 1990; Kanter 1995; Karlsson 1997):

- Halts lipid peroxidation
- Quenches singlet oxygen
- Stabilizes the superoxide radical
- Stabilizes the hydroxyl radical
- Spares selenium and protects beta-carotene from destruction

Table 10.2 **Nutrients Involved in Antioxidant Activities**

Nutrient	Primary antioxidant functions
Vitamin E (alpha-tocopherol)	Halts lipid peroxidation
Vitamin C (ascorbic acid)	Quenches singlet oxygen, regenerates the reduced form of vitamin E
Beta-carotene	Quenches singlet oxygen
Selenium	Part of the glutathione peroxidase enzyme system
Ubiquinone (reduced coenzyme Q_{10})	Scavenges peroxyl radicals
Copper	Part of the Cu-Zn SOD enzyme complex (in cytosol)
Zinc	Part of the Cu-Zn SOD enzyme complex (in cytosol)
Iron	Part of the catalase enzyme system
Manganese	Part of the Mn-SOD enzyme complex (in mitochondria)

- May stabilize membrane structure

The primary role of vitamin E is to protect the polyunsaturated fatty acids (PUFAs) in biological membranes against oxidative damage. Vitamin E interrupts the chain reaction of lipid peroxidation, helping to maintain membrane stability and fluidity and protecting cellular structures against oxidative damage.

Methods of Assessment

Currently there are no biochemical indices that accurately reflect dietary vitamin E intakes or body stores of vitamin E. Tocopherol values can be measured in serum, erythrocytes, platelets, and tissues such as liver or adipose (Gibson 1990). Although serum tocopherol concentration is often used as an index of vitamin E status, concentrations can vary significantly and are closely associated with serum lipid levels. Serum tocopherol values vary with age, physiological state, and method of analysis; a wide range of values is reported for apparently healthy individuals.

Measurement of tocopherol in erythrocytes is technically difficult, and there appears to be little justification for using it to indicate vitamin E status. Tocopherol concentrations in platelets and tissues appear promising as accurate indicators of vitamin E status, but more research needs to be done to confirm their usefulness; however, assessing tissue tocopherol levels is invasive and not appropriate for use in large populations.

Two indirect assessments of vitamin E status are the **erythrocyte hemolysis test** and **breath pentane measurements** (Gibson 1990). Hemolysis rates are inversely related to serum tocopherol levels; one weakness of this test is that changes in the status of other nutrients, such as folic acid, can also increase erythrocyte hemolysis. The breath pentane test measures exhalation of the aliphatic hydrocarbons ethane and pentane as indirect indicators of linolenic and linoleic acid oxidation—which is positively correlated with vitamin E deficiency. The use of aliphatic hydrocarbons as indicators of oxidative damage is discussed in more detail later in this chapter.

Dietary Sources, Recommended Intakes, and Supplementation Products

Primary food sources for vitamin E include certain vegetable oils, green leafy vegetables, nuts, wheat germ, and whole grains. The results of NHANES II found that fats and oils, vegetables and fruits, meat, poultry, fish, and fortified breakfast cereals were the major contributors to vitamin E intake among U.S. adults (Murphy et al. 1990). While animal pro-ducts are generally poor sources of vitamin E, they are consumed more frequently by adults and thus contribute more to vitamin E intakes in the U.S. diet. Although nuts are a good source of vitamin E, their consumption is low in the U.S. diet.

Vitamin E deficiencies are rare in humans and occur primarily in infants with fat-malabsorption syndromes. The RDAs for vitamin E—10 mg and 8 mg for men and women, respectively (Food and Nutrition Board 1989) (see "Units of Expression for Vitamin E," page 280)—appear adequate to maintain normal function and protect PUFAs from lipid peroxidation (Meydani et al. 1997). But vitamin E requirements rise with higher intakes of PUFAs. Since many athletes and active people consume a diet that is moderately high in fat (25-35% of total kilocalories from fat), and since they utilize more oxygen than sedentary people, vitamin E requirements for active people may be higher than the RDA. While it is possible to consume adequate vitamin E from dietary sources, Murphy et al. (1990) found that median intakes of the U.S. population were only 73% and 68% of the RDA for men and women, respectively—69% of men and 80% of women in this survey consumed less than the RDA for vitamin E. Vitamin E supplements are available to the general public. Unlike supplementation with other fat-soluble vitamins, vitamin E supplements appear to be safe. Few side effects have been reported for doses as high as 3 g/d, which is 300 and 375 times the RDA for men and women, respectively (Meydani et al. 1997).

Vitamin C

Vitamin C, also known as ascorbic acid or **ascorbate**, is an essential water-soluble vitamin. While plants and most mammals are capable of synthesizing their own vitamin C, humans (and other primates) lack **gulonolactone oxidase,** the enzyme that catalyzes the final step in vitamin C synthesis (Chatterjee et al. 1975). Scurvy is the primary vitamin C deficiency disease in humans. Vitamin C plays many important roles in the body, including that of an antioxidant.

Vitamin C functions as an antioxidant primarily in the extracellular fluid (Bendich et al. 1986). The suggested antioxidant actions of vitamin C include the following:

- Stabilizes the hydroxyl radical
- Quenches singlet oxygen
- Reduces the oxidized form of vitamin E
- Reduces nitrosamines to harmless species
- May help protect the lungs from ozone and cigarette smoke (see "Vitamin C and Cigarette Smoking," page 281)

Vitamin C may also help prevent the metal ion-induced oxidation of low-density lipoproteins (LDL) (Jialal et al. 1990)—an important role, since LDL oxidation significantly increases the risk of atherosclerosis. The associations between antioxidants and cardiovascular disease are discussed in more detail later in this chapter.

Under certain circumstances vitamin C can also act as a **prooxidant**—a substance that *increases* the production of free radicals and enhances oxidative damage. When administered at very low concentrations in vitro, vitamin C increased iron-induced lipid peroxidation in rat myocardial cells (Link et al. 1987). Herbert (1993a) asserted that vitamin C is a powerful prooxidant in the presence of high body iron stores (perhaps 6-10% of Americans are genetically predisposed to enhanced iron absorption and high body iron stores). Increased serum concentrations of vitamin C augment the release of catalytic iron from ferritin; the released iron then accelerates oxidative damage. Thus, *combining vitamin C supplements with iron supplements may be a poor, and possibly hazardous, choice for people with high iron stores or at risk for hemochromatosis.* "The Relationship Between Vitamin C and Iron" (page 282) reviews the potentially dangerous prooxidant relationship between iron and vitamin C.

Methods of Assessment

The most commonly used measure of vitamin C status is **serum ascorbic acid concentrations** (Gibson 1990). Only fasting blood samples are used since recent dietary intake of vitamin C influences serum levels (serum levels increase proportionally for small doses up to 150 mg). As with many other vitamins, serum ascorbic acid concentrations are not accurate indicators

■ HIGHLIGHT ■

Units of Expression for Vitamin E

Vitamin E is expressed using three primary units of measurement: international units (IU), milligrams (mg), and α-tocopherol equivalents (α-TE). *The activity of 1 mg of the acetate form of synthetic α-tocopherol is defined as equal to 1 IU of vitamin E.* When referring specifically to the diet, vitamin E activity is expressed as α-TE (Food and Nutrition Board 1989). The relationship between these units is simple: 1 mg is equal to 1 IU, and 1 α-TE is equal to 1 mg. The units used in this chapter follow those reported in the cited research papers.

■ HIGHLIGHT ■

Vitamin C and Cigarette Smoking

Serum vitamin C concentrations are depressed in smokers and those exposed to secondhand smoke. Cigarette smoke contains numerous oxidants, and vitamin C is depleted in both active smokers and in those exposed to secondhand smoke (Tribble et al. 1993). The RDA for vitamin C is 60 mg/d, with a higher recommendation of 100 mg/d suggested for smokers.

Vitamin C helps protect against the harmful effects of cigarette smoking through three mechanisms:

1. Improving endothelium-dependent vasodilation (Heitzer et al. 1996)
2. Reducing adhesiveness of monocytes to endothelium cells (Weber et al. 1996)
3. Decreasing oxidative damage (Reilly et al. 1996)

All three of these actions can help reduce the risk of cardiovascular disease in smokers. Smokers have a diminished vasodilator response to chemical and mechanical stressors, which affects blood flow and blood pressure. Reducing the adhesiveness of monocytes to endothelial cells may prevent the inflammatory response in the vessel wall resulting from cigarette smoke, which in turn could reduce the initiation and development of atherosclerosis. As oxidation of serum lipids is strongly associated with increased risk of cardiovascular disease, any mechanism by which oxidative damage can be reduced will be beneficial. Note: the health benefits of vitamin C described here were accomplished with 2 g per day of vitamin C over 5-10 d—much higher than the 100 mg/d recommended for smokers.

Although vitamin C can reduce some of the risks associated with cigarette smoking, the risk factors associated with regular cigarette smoking far outweigh vitamin C's ability to fight oxidation-related damage. It is encouraging, however, to know there are protective steps smokers can take while "breaking the habit."

of vitamin C status in persons consuming chronically high levels of the vitamin. Serum levels do not increase proportionally with higher doses, as a result of significantly increased renal clearance with high intakes (Harris et al. 1973). Blood levels of vitamin C eventually peak and fail to increase even when greater amounts of vitamin C are consumed. However, serum vitamin C is an adequate indicator of chronically low vitamin C intakes. Several non-nutritional factors can lower serum vitamin C concentrations, including cigarette smoking, oral contraceptive use, acute stress, surgery, and chronic inflammatory diseases.

A more reliable indicator of tissue stores of vitamin C is **leukocyte ascorbic acid concentration** since this measure is less affected by short-term fluctuations in dietary intake of vitamin C. The assay is technically difficult, however, and requires relatively large samples of blood (Gibson 1990). While **urinary excretion** of vitamin C reflects recent dietary intake, it is not a sensitive indicator of vitamin C status. Measurement of **capillary fragility** has also been used as a functional test of vitamin C status: a blood pressure cuff is applied to the upper arm, and the pressure at which hemorrhages appear on the skin is noted. This test is inconsistent, and other diseases can cause capillary fragility; thus, it is not a sensitive and reliable test of vitamin C status. *The most reliable method of assessing vitamin C status is* ***isotope dilution*** (Baker et al. 1971). An oral dose of ^{14}C- or ^{13}C-labeled ascorbic acid is administered, and the specific activity of blood or urine ascorbate is measured over 24-48 h. This method has been used to establish total body pool vitamin C levels.

Dietary Sources, Recommended Intakes, and Supplementation Products

Fruits and vegetables are the best sources of vitamin C. In particular, broccoli, oranges, strawberries, grapefruit juice, red bell peppers, and kiwi fruit are excellent sources. Raw fruits and vegetables usually have a higher density

The Relationship Between Vitamin C and Iron

Vitamin C promotes the absorption of iron from the digestive tract by capturing iron and keeping it in the ferrous form (Fe^{2+}), which is the form that is more readily absorbed. In addition, vitamin C can mobilize iron from body stores in situations where people have high iron body stores, which can result in **iron-induced cardiac failure**. The death of three athletes from iron-induced cardiac failure may have resulted from taking megadoses of vitamin C (Herbert 1993b; also see chapter 12).

What is the mechanism by which iron and other metals form free radicals? When iron and other metals are in the free or unbound form, they are capable of forming free radicals through the "iron-catalyzed Haber-Weiss reaction" (McCord and Day 1978). The net reaction is

$$O_2\cdot + H_2O_2 \rightarrow O_2 + OH\cdot + OH^-$$

Iron catalyzes this reaction as follows:

$$Fe^{3+} + O_2\cdot \rightarrow Fe^{2+} + O_2$$

$$Fe^{2+} + H_2O_2 \rightarrow Fe^{3+} + OH\cdot + OH^-$$

It is important to understand that, depending on the body's chemistry, vitamin C and other "antioxidants" can also act as prooxidants. It is critical that people have their iron status assessed before taking supplemental iron and doses of vitamin C greater than 1-2 g/d. Herbert (1993b) stated that 12% of Americans have excess iron levels, and taking large doses of vitamin C can be harmful by increasing oxidative damage and causing other complications resulting from excessive circulating free iron.

of vitamin C because vitamin C is destroyed by heat. *Thus, reducing cooking time of vegetables will assist in preserving the vitamin C content.* It is also important to store produce in airtight, closed containers, as vitamin C is easily oxidized. Severe vitamin C deficiencies are rare in the United States due to the availability of food sources high in this nutrient. There is no evidence that active people consume inadequate amounts of vitamin C; in fact, individuals who consume fruits and vegetables on a regular basis have no difficulty consuming more than the RDA (60 mg/d) for vitamin C. It has been suggested, however, that the RDA is not adequate for most individuals due to the loss of vitamin C in foods from heat and light exposure. The increased use of vitamin C to fight the damage from smog, cigarette smoke, and other environmental pollutants may also contribute to higher vitamin C needs (Kanter 1995). Increasing oxygen consumption and free radical production by exercising may further burden the antioxidant systems, increasing an active person's need for vitamin C above the current RDA. However, active people who regu-

larly consume fruits and vegetables are most likely getting adequate vitamin C from dietary sources.

Vitamin C supplements are easily available and relatively inexpensive. As vitamin C is water-soluble, it can be consumed in doses much higher than the RDA with minimal side effects. However, people taking more than 2-3 g/d may suffer from a variety of side effects including nausea, diarrhea, abdominal cramps, and erythrocyte hemolysis. An additional risk with **megadoses** of vitamin C is iron overload toxicity (see "The Relationship Between Vitamin C and Iron," above). There is no evidence that consuming heavy doses (greater than 1 g/d) of vitamin C prevents colds, although vitamin C has been shown to reduce blood histamine (Johnston et al. 1992). Since histamine can suppress the immune response, this is one possible mechanism by which vitamin C may affect immune system responses.

Other Functions Related to Exercise

Vitamin C has a variety of functions in the body besides its antioxidant properties:

- Is essential for collagen synthesis; collagen is the dominant protein of connective tissues and is the matrix on which teeth and bones are formed.
- Plays a yet unidentified role in the stress response—possibly associated with vitamin C's role in production of norepinephrine and thyroxin and its role as an antioxidant during increased immune system activity.
- Assists with amino acid metabolism.
- Increases absorption of dietary iron (ferric iron) or non-heme iron.
- Improves symptoms of upper-respiratory infections in sedentary people and ultramarathon runners (Bucca et al. 1992; Peters et al. 1993).

These functions are important to maintain the health of sedentary and active people. Supporters of supplementation insist that adequate intakes of vitamin C can be accomplished only by taking dietary supplements. However, a person can consume more than four times the RDA by eating a combination of 1 medium orange, 1 cup of chopped, cooked broccoli (from fresh), and 1/2 cup of raw red bell pepper (or 1 cup of raw green bell pepper). The combined vitamin C from all these foods is approximately 265 mg, an intake level that is very achievable in the daily diet. Regularly consuming a diet containing only a few fruits and vegetables will result in lower than recommended vitamin C intakes and low serum concentrations of vitamin C.

Beta-Carotene and Vitamin A

Beta-carotene is one of many compounds classified as **carotenoids**. Carotenoids are part of the red, orange, and yellow pigments found in many fruits and vegetables. They are fat-soluble, transported in the blood by lipoproteins, and stored in the fatty tissues of the body. Beta-carotene, the most researched carotenoid, is a precursor to vitamin A. This means that vitamin A can be produced in the body from β-carotene. Like vitamin A, β-carotene has antioxidant properties. There are actually over 600 carotenoids in nature, including **lycopene** (found in tomatoes) and **lutein** (found in green leafy vegetables), which may have antioxidant properties more potent than β-carotene.

Beta-carotene performs its functions in the lipid portion of cell membranes and in LDL particles. In addition to quenching singlet oxy-gen, β-carotene quenches hydroperoxyl radicals and protects against lipid peroxidation. Beta-carotene is a relatively weak antioxidant in comparison to vitamin E. As previously mentioned, there are numerous other carotenoids that may be stronger antioxidants than β-carotene. More studies on these carotenoids need to be conducted to fully understand their role in antioxidant metabolism.

Vitamin A protects LDL-cholesterol (LDL-C) against oxidation and may reduce oxidative damage in infants who are vitamin A deficient (Livrea et al. 1995; Schwarz et al. 1997). Vitamin A is a much weaker antioxidant than β-carotene, and vitamin A supplementation in individuals without deficiency is highly toxic. In contrast, β-carotene can be taken in supplemental doses with very low risk of toxicity. One side effect of large doses of β-carotene is yellowing of the skin. This condition is called hypercarotenemia, or carotenosis, and appears to be reversible and harmless. Although β-carotene is converted to vitamin A in the body, high doses of β-carotene do not result in toxic levels of vitamin A. Thus, most of our discussion focuses on β-carotene's actions as an antioxidant.

Methods of Assessment

New methods have been developed to measure carotenoid concentrations in the blood. High-performance liquid chromatography is the predominant method used to assess carotenoid concentrations. The six most common carotenoids identified in human blood are listed below (Epler et al. 1992; Epler et al. 1993):

- Beta-carotene
- Alpha-carotene
- Lutein
- Zeaxanthin
- Cryptoxanthin
- Lycopene

Newer methods have led to even greater specificity and selectivity for less common carotenoids (Sharpless et al. 1996).

Analyses of serum β-carotene concentrations have shown that most people have levels ranging from 0.2 to 0.6 μmol/L, with smokers having lower concentrations than nonsmokers. Women in general, and men and women who consume recommended amounts of fruits and vegetables, have higher serum levels of β-carotene (Burri 1997). Plasma carotenoid concentrations fluctuate throughout the menstrual cycle, with concentrations lowest at menses and significantly higher thereafter (Forman et al. 1996). Beta-carotene concentrations appear to peak in the late follicular phase. These results emphasize the importance of tracking menstrual cycle status when measuring carotenoid concentrations in premenopausal women.

Dietary Sources, Recommended Intakes, and Supplementation Products

The best sources of β-carotene are dark green leafy vegetables such as spinach; deep orange fruits such as cantaloupe and apricots; and vegetables such as winter squash, carrots, sweet potatoes, and broccoli. While average intakes in the United States and Europe are 2-4 mg/d, median intakes are much lower than this range (Burri 1997). Nebeling et al. (1997) reported that the average intake of lutein (from dark green leafy vegetables) decreased from 1987 to 1992, particularly in Caucasian women. Accompanying this decreased lutein intake was an increase in the intake of foods rich in lycopene and β-carotene. People who eat recommended amounts of fruits and vegetables (five servings/d) have a much higher intake of β-carotene, with values averaging 10 mg/d or more. At present, there is no RDA for β-carotene, but some researchers have recommended that an intake of 6-10 mg/d is sufficient to increase serum levels of β-carotene to concentrations associated with reduced risks of diseases. These levels are achievable through the diet; table 10.3 lists foods rich in β-carotene.

Beta-carotene supplements are commonly sold in combination with other antioxidant nutrients. Although intakes of 6-10 mg/d are associated with reduced risk for cancer and heart disease in epidemiological studies, clinical trials designed to study β-carotene's effects on disease status have supplemented with larger doses of 15-30 mg/d. These doses were shown to be harmful to heavy smokers and alcohol drinkers (Albanes et al. 1995; Alpha-Tocopherol, Beta-Carotene Cancer Prevention Study Group [ABCPSG] 1994; Omenn et al. 1996). Skin yellowing, a common side effect of high β-carotene intakes, occurred in 20-25% of the participants in these trials. At this time, there are no definitive data suggesting that people benefit from β-carotene supplementation. It appears that consuming *a combination of five servings of fruits and/or vegetables per day* will maintain healthy levels of β-carotene in the blood.

Selenium

Selenium is a trace mineral whose primary action is associated with the antioxidant enzyme glutathione peroxidase (GPX). GPX is termed the "selenium-dependent enzyme." Remember that GPX removes hydrogen peroxide, reduces lipid hydroperoxides, and prevents damage to RNA and DNA, thus acting as an important protector against oxidative damage (Ji 1995). As GPX cannot carry out its function without adequate selenium, this mineral plays a critical role in antioxidant metabolism.

Methods of Assessment

Plasma or serum selenium levels generally reflect short-term selenium status and are a measure of acute dietary changes in selenium. The best index of long-term selenium status is whole blood selenium concentrations since low blood levels reflect chronic deficiencies of selenium

Table 10.3 **Food Sources of Beta-Carotene**

Foods	Serving size	Beta-carotene (mg/serving)
Kale, boiled and drained	1 cup (130 g)	16.4
Sweet potato, baked in skin	1 medium (114 g)	14.9
Carrots, chopped, raw	1 medium (72g)	7.6
Winter squash, baked	1 cup (205 g)	3.1
Cantaloupe, cubes	1 cup (160 g)	2.6
Spinach, raw	1 cup (30 g)	2.0
Broccoli, chopped, raw	1 cup (88 g)	0.4

Adapted from DIETSYS, version 3.7, National Cancer Institute, Bethesda, MD, 1996.

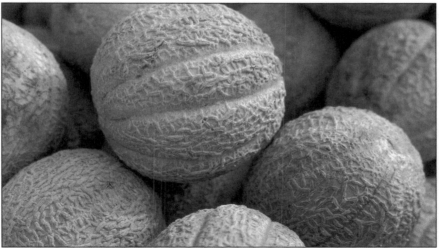

Dark green, yellow, and orange fruits and vegetables, such as cantaloupe, are high in β-carotene.

(Gibson 1990). Erythrocyte levels of selenium can also be used to indicate long-term status. Urinary selenium levels over a 24-h period are generally used to indicate selenium toxicity and industrial exposure (Glover 1967; Hojo 1981).

GPX activity can be used as a functional index of selenium status in people with habitually low dietary intakes. Whanger et al. (1988) compared blood selenium concentrations and GPX activity in individuals from New Zealand, Oregon, and South Dakota—locations representing people with low, moderate, and high selenium exposure, respectively. Blood selenium concentrations and GPX activity were found to be significantly lower in subjects from New Zealand as compared to the other two locations. While GPX activity of the subjects from New Zealand was lower than for the other locations, no differences were found between subjects from Oregon or South Dakota—suggesting that GPX activity is an appropriate indicator of selenium status only in people with below-normal levels of selenium.

Dietary Sources, Recommended Intakes, and Supplementation Products

The results of the study by Whanger et al. (1988) illustrated that selenium intakes can vary considerably by geographic location. Areas known to have soil depleted of selenium include parts of China, New Zealand, and parts of Finland. Low selenium intakes have been linked with various diseases in these areas, including Keshan disease, certain cancers, and cardiovascular disease (Whitney and Rolfes 1996). Selenium content of U.S. soils varies con-

siderably. Selenium deficiencies are rare in the United States for two primary reasons: (1) Most people consume foods from various parts of the country; and (2) most Americans eat meat that comes from multiple geographic areas, and meat is an excellent source of selenium. The most important food sources of selenium are seafoods, meat (including muscle, liver, and kidney), and some grain products (depending on where they were grown).

Olson (1986) reported that the margin between selenium toxicity and deficiency is much narrower than for other trace minerals. Toxicity can easily result from supplementation. The RDA for selenium is 70 μg/d for men and 55 μg/d for women. Doses of at least 1 mg or more per day are considered toxic, and a maximum safe dose of 5 μg/d per kg body weight is recommended for adults (Olson 1986). Multivitamin/mineral supplements typically contain 50-200 μg of selenium per dose.

Other Nutrients With Antioxidant Properties

In addition to the nutrients already discussed, several others appear to play a role in antioxidant metabolism. Some of them are not antioxidants, but are important cofactors in reactions that protect the body against oxidative damage. These nutrients include the minerals discussed on page 279 (table 10.2).

Karlsson (1997) has identified several such nutrients as "unofficial" vitamins. One that has received considerable attention as an antioxidant is ubiquinone, or coenzyme Q_{10} (although

Table 10.4 Compounds in Food That Have Been Attributed Antioxidant and Disease-Fighting Properties

Compound	Food source	Function
Allylic sulfides	Garlic and onion	Glutathione precursor
Carotenoids	Carrots, parsley, vegetables	Antioxidant, vitamin A precursor
Bioflavonoids	Tea, red wine, vegetables, fruits	Antioxidants (catechins, tannins)
Indoles	Cabbage, brussels sprouts	Block steroid hormone synthesis
Thiocyanates	Horseradish, radish	Detoxification
Limonoids	Citrus fruits	Detoxification
Lycopenes	Tomatoes	Antioxidants
Monoterpenes	Vegetables	Antioxidants

Reprinted from Karlsson 1997.

not established as a vitamin, it is sometimes referred to as vitamin Q) (see "Coenzyme Q_{10} As an Antioxidant and Ergogenic Aid," below). Table 10.4 lists other potential antioxidant compounds, their food sources, and suggested functions. These substances are currently under study. Some of these compounds are called **bioflavonoids**—substances found in tea, red wine, and certain fruits and vegetables that may have antioxidant properties. The compounds listed in table 10.4 are generally referred to as **phytochemicals**—a term that in general simply means a chemical from a plant but which is often used more specifically to refer to compounds that may protect against diseases such as heart disease and cancer.

Assessment of Oxidative Damage

It is difficult to assess oxidative damage within body tissues and cells. Free radicals are highly reactive and short-lived; only recently have techniques been developed that could *directly* measure free radical production or activity. Most assays measure secondary by-products—

■ HIGHLIGHT ■

Coenzyme Q_{10} As an Antioxidant and Ergogenic Aid

Coenzyme Q_{10}, or ubiquinone, is a naturally occurring lipid-soluble compound that is part of the electron transport chain, or ETC (refer to figure 10.1). It transfers electrons from NADH to the b-c$_1$ enzyme complex in the ETC. Coenzyme Q_{10} has been identified as the rate-limiting electron shuttle in the ETC. It is touted as an ergogenic aid, with claims that increasing coenzyme Q_{10} levels with supplementation will increase electron flux through the ETC—which will result in enhanced production of ATP and work output. Studies of coenzyme Q_{10} as an ergogenic aid are equivocal, with some showing benefits of supplementation (Amadio et al. 1991; Fiorella et al. 1991; Guerra et al. 1987; Zeppilli et al. 1991) and others finding no effect (Braun et al. 1991; Snider et al. 1992).

Coenzyme Q_{10} is also claimed to scavenge free radicals and reduce lipid peroxidation (Folkers, Vadhanavikit and Mortensen 1985; Folkers, Wolaniuk et al. 1985; Greenberg and Frishman 1988; Karlsson 1987; Langsjoen and Folkers 1990). *It is important to emphasize that these claims are derived from studies of people recovering from a heart attack and from in vitro studies of oxidative damage related to myocardial ischemia / reperfusion, cardiomyopathies, and muscular dystrophy.* In vivo studies with healthy adults have not been performed to confirm coenzyme Q_{10}'s role as an antioxidant.

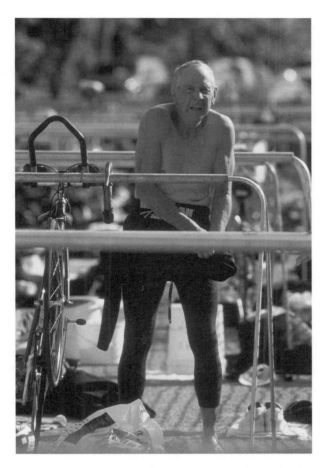

Aging may increase the need for antioxidants.

in the blood, urine, or breath—that result from oxidative damage at the cellular level.

Measuring Free Radical Production

Direct techniques to assess free radical production in humans have only recently become available. Both **electron spin resonance** and **paramagnetic resonance spectrometry** detect superoxide radicals and can be used in vivo or in vitro. As the superoxide radicals spin, they emit a signal. These procedures measure the peak of the resonance signal as an indicator of superoxide radical production (Alessio 1993) and show great promise for enhancing our understanding of oxidative damage during exercise. The invasive nature, high cost, and sophisticated equipment needed, however, limit the widespread use of these techniques at the present time.

Markers of Lipid Peroxidation

Tests available to assess lipid peroxidation are indirect, measuring the secondary reaction products of lipid peroxidation. These tests are not foolproof, and Kneepkens et al. (1994) claimed that the sensitivity and specificity of most such tests are questionable. Standard procedures for these tests need to be established, as do further studies of their validity.

One test of lipid peroxidation is the assessment of **conjugated dienes**. Once the chain reaction of lipid peroxidation is initiated, dienes are immediately formed. While conjugated dienes have been measured in exercising humans (Duthie et al. 1990), these products are very difficult to determine in human blood and urine (Gutteridge and Halliwell 1990). The accuracy of the appearance of conjugated dienes as a marker of lipid peroxidation is also questionable as these dienes can be derived from sources other than the peroxidation of lipids (Kneepkens et al. 1994).

Lipid hydroperoxides are the major initial products of lipid peroxidation (see table 10.1). Decomposition products of hydroperoxides can be measured in the blood as an indicator of lipid peroxidation. The most common decomposition product that is assessed is **malonaldehyde (MDA)**, which is measured by its reaction with thiobarbituric acid (Kneepkens et al. 1994). The products generated are referred to as **thiobarbituric acid reactive substances (TBARSs)**. This assay technique is relatively simple to perform, which most likely contributes to its widespread use. The reliability and validity of the procedure are questionable, however, and it should be used in conjunction with other markers (Kneepkens et al. 1994).

Another commonly used marker of lipid peroxidation is **aliphatic hydrocarbons,** which are measured in a person's breath. While numerous aliphatic hydrocarbons are produced in the human body, the best markers of lipid peroxidation are **ethane** and **pentane**. Since other aliphatic hydrocarbons are produced in the colon, and the concentration of hydrocarbons in ambient air is similar to that of breath, the mere presence of random hydrocarbons in the breath does not necessarily indicate lipid peroxidation. Ethane and pentane are considered specific markers of lipid peroxidation, however, since ethane is the main product of the peroxidation of linolenic acid and other omega-3 fatty acids, while pentane is the main product of the peroxidation of linoleic and arachidonic acids (omega-6 fatty acids). Therefore, ethane and pentane appear to be adequate markers for peroxidation of the majority of the polyunsaturated fatty acids in the human body (Kneepkens et al. 1994).

Other Markers of Oxidative Stress

Changes in antioxidant enzymes can be used to assess the functional activity of the antioxidant system. Changes in the reduced form of glutathione (GSH) can be measured to indicate the activity of the glutathione peroxidase (GPX) system. A decrease in GSH and an increase in GSSG (the oxidized form of glutathione) indicate an increase in the activity of the glutathione antioxidant defense system. The activity of specific antioxidant enzymes can also be measured. These enzymes include GPX, SOD, CAT, and GR (see page 277-278 for definitions). Increases in these enzyme activities indicate an increase in the antioxidant activity of the body, suggesting that free radical production and oxidative damage have occurred.

Rationale for Increased Antioxidant Need Among Active Individuals

Ken is a triathlete who has come to you for nutritional advice because soreness and fatigue have been interfering with his training sessions. He has also been plagued with numerous upper-respiratory infections over the previous six months, coinciding with an increase in training volume and intensity. While he has sought medical treatment for the symptoms of the infections, the causes of the soreness, fatigue, and infections remain unidentified. Ken's fellow competitors suggested that he take antioxidant supplements to ward off the possible weakening of his cellular defense systems due to heavy training and to improve his ability to train and compete. Ken's questions to you include:

- Will antioxidant supplements improve his health and performance?
- If yes, what are the best antioxidant supplements he can take?
- How much should he take if he decides to supplement?

This scenario highlights two very important questions: (1) Do athletes and highly active people have a higher requirement for antioxi-

dants? (2) If so, why is their need increased? The suggestion that athletes have an increased need for antioxidants stems from three primary assumptions:

- Athletes generate excessive free radicals through heavy physical training as they consume more oxygen than sedentary individuals.
- The antioxidant systems in place are not sufficient to cope with the increased free radical production that accompanies heavy training.
- Athletes in urban areas may need even more antioxidants than those in rural areas since high levels of air pollution can increase free radical production.

Support for Increased Need

Research data suggest that acute exercise increases free radical production. Exercise also increases oxygen consumption ($\dot{V}O_2$), which increases the activity of cellular respiration. Increasing the rate of oxygen consumption and electron flux leads to increased free radical production and the leaking of reactive oxygen species out of the electron transport chain (Alessio 1993; Davies et al. 1982; Jenkins 1988). Other factors that may lead to increased free radical production during exercise include an increase in catecholamines (including epinephrine) that can produce free radicals and an increase in lactic acid, which can convert the superoxide radical into the highly damaging hydroxyl radical (Demopoulos et al. 1986). Tissue damage from intense exercise can also lead to lipid peroxidation of membranes and free radical production via the inflammation response (Clarkson 1995).

Two ways to assess the effects of exercise on free radical production are (1) measuring free radical production directly or measuring the secondary by-products of free radical production and (2) measuring changes in antioxidant enzyme systems. A number of excellent articles describe the effects of acute exercise and exercise training on free radicals and antioxidant enzyme systems in more detail (Alessio 1993; Clarkson 1995; Ji 1995; Kanter 1994).

Effects of Acute Exercise on Antioxidant Systems

Much of the research conducted in the areas of exercise, free radical production, and antioxidant metabolism has used animal models. While use of animal models in this area of research does not appear to be highly controversial, studies including humans as subjects are the ideal way to examine antioxidant activities during exercise in humans. The results discussed here will focus primarily on studies of humans during exercise.

As previously reviewed, a variety of methods can be used to quantify free radical production. Each method has its limitations, and no one best marker is available. The majority of studies in humans have used indirect markers of lipid peroxidation to indicate free radical production and consequent damage (e.g., MDA, TBARSs, expired hydrocarbons). In addition, the use of various forms and intensities of exercise, use of different markers of free radical production, and the assessment of various tissues have led to inconsistent results. These inconsistencies make it difficult to confirm with confidence the relationships among exercise, free radical damage, and lipid peroxidation. They also make it difficult to prescribe specific antioxidant nutrient recommendations to active people. Despite these limitations, there is evidence supporting an increase in free radical production and lipid peroxidation during exercise.

Two studies using the direct measures of electron spin resonance and electroparamagnetic resonance found an increase in free radical production with exercise in animals (Davies et al. 1982; Jackson et al. 1985). Measurement of lipid peroxidation using expired pentane and TBARSs confirms that free radical production and subsequent lipid peroxidation may increase with acute exercise in humans. Early work by Dillard et al. (1978) showed that expired pentane increased with exercise intensity; obvious increases occurred at 75% $\dot{V}O_2$max. Pincemail et al. (1990), studying one subject, found a significant increase in pentane expiration following maximal exercise. Leaf et al. (1997) also found significant increases in expired ethane and pentane at approximately 72% $\dot{V}O_2$max; the levels remained elevated to maximal exercise. Exposure to high altitude increases expired pentane production, and exercise at high altitude combined with poor energy intakes may exacerbate this condition (Simon-Schnass 1992). Many other researchers have reported increases in TBARSs (or MDA) as a result of exercise in humans (Kanter et al. 1988; Lovlin et al. 1987; Maughan et al. 1989).

Changes in antioxidant enzyme concentrations also occur as a result of acute exercise.

Erythrocyte and blood levels of GSH appear to decrease with acute exercise, accompanied by an increase in GSSG in some instances (Duthie et al. 1990; Goldfarb 1993). Increases in erythrocyte GR activity after moderate exercise have also been reported. These changes indicate an increase in the activity of the glutathione antioxidant enzyme system (refer to equations 3, 4, and 5 on page 278) and suggest that exercise increases the production of hydrogen peroxide and lipid hydroperoxides.

Yet there is contradictory evidence. Dernbach et al. (1993) found no increase in TBARS with intense training in rowers, while Sahlin et al. (1992) found no increase in MDA levels with either isometric or dynamic exercise. In the study by Leaf et al. previously mentioned (1997), researchers found no significant increase in MDA levels despite significant changes in expired hydrocarbons. Numerous factors may influence the degree of lipid peroxidation that occurs with exercise, partly explaining the inconsistencies in these studies:

- *Exercise intensity:* Intense, acute, maximal bouts may increase lipid peroxidation more than moderate exercise.

- *Type of exercise:* Eccentric contractions may increase free radical production and subsequent damage as compared to concentric muscle contractions (Dekkers et al. 1996).

- *Training status of subjects:* Untrained persons performing intense exercise may experience more lipid peroxidation than trained athletes.

- *Different methods used:* Methods are imperfect, and it is inappropriate to compare data from different assessment techniques; furthermore, the anatomical source of sampled tissue will affect results.

- *Nutritional status of subjects:* This strongly affects their responses to exercise.

- *Antioxidant status of the subjects:* There are many *interrelated* antioxidant systems, and it is virtually impossible to control the levels of each before beginning an exercise test.

Effects of Chronic Exercise Training on Antioxidant Systems

As increases in mitochondrial enzymes and oxidative capacity occur with endurance training, the potential for oxidative damage is greater in the trained athlete. There is evidence that antioxidant enzyme activity increases with training; controversy exists, however, as to whether the increases in antioxidant activity are sufficient to protect the system from the increased oxidative damage that may accompany exercise training. Antioxidant nutrient pools within the body may also change with training. In animals, muscle levels of vitamin E have been shown to decrease with endurance training; these levels may also depend on initial vitamin E status. Training may conserve vitamin E in a deficient animal as compared to an untrained animal with vitamin E deficiency.

Cross-sectional data show a significant positive correlation between $\dot{V}O_2$max and activities of antioxidant enzymes; and trained athletes appear to have higher SOD, GPX, and CAT activities than untrained individuals (Jenkins 1993; Mena et al. 1991). Results of training studies show a reduction in MDA levels (i.e., lipid peroxidation) (Yagi 1992) and increased activities of CAT and GR (Evelo et al. 1992; Ohno et al. 1988). These changes indicate that the trained system adapts to increased oxygen consumption with complementary changes in the protective antioxidant enzymes. However, more studies need to be conducted to assess if the adaptations with training are sufficient to protect against oxidative damage.

Antioxidant Deficiencies and Exercise

Most studies of nutritional deficiencies and their effects on exercise performance have been conducted with animals. Studying nutrient deficiencies in humans is limited by ethical considerations. It is important to note that antioxidant nutrient deficiencies are rare in sedentary animals or humans consuming a nutritionally adequate diet (Ji 1995). Since exercise reduces stored levels of vitamin E (Bowles et al. 1991; Kumar et al. 1992; Packer 1986), it has been speculated (but not demonstrated) that highly active individuals may be predisposed to antioxidant nutrient deficiency if adequate dietary intakes are not achieved (Packer 1986).

What effects do antioxidant deficiencies have on oxidative damage and exercise performance? Selenium deficiency resulted in increased lipid peroxidation in the liver and muscle of rats (Ji et al. 1988) but appears to have no effect on acute exercise performance or endurance capacity (Ji et al. 1988; Lang et al. 1987). Vitamin E deficiency increases exercise-induced oxidative damage (Davies et al. 1982; Gohil et al. 1986; Goldfarb 1993; Quintanilha et al. 1982) and also decreases endurance performance in animals (Davies et al. 1982). Very few data exist regarding the effects of vitamin C deficiency on exercise-induced oxidative damage, but Packer (1984, 1986) found myocardial oxidative capacity and endurance time to be reduced in animals deficient in vitamin C.

Deficiencies of vitamins E, C, and β-carotene are rare. Studies that have measured the vitamin A, C, or E status of athletes using blood samples have found no evidence of deficiencies (Cohen et al. 1985; Fogelholm et al. 1992; Guilland et al. 1989; Weight et al. 1988). While many athletes exceed the RDA for these nutrients, those with poor energy or dietary intakes and weight concerns, and those who eat little or no fruits or vegetables, may not consume adequate antioxidant nutrients and may require supplementation. However, studies assessing the nutritional status and antioxidant nutrient intake patterns in these higher-risk athletes need to be performed before recommendations for supplementation can be made.

At the present time, there does not appear to be enough evidence to support the suggestion that active individuals are deficient in antioxidant nutrients. We need more research to assess the antioxidant nutrient status of the general population using objective measures. It is not known whether exercise training improves antioxidant protection to an extent sufficient to protect against increases in oxidative damage that may accompany regular, vigorous physical training. Until these questions can be answered, it is unwise to make sweeping recommendations regarding antioxidant needs of active people.

Potential Risks Associated With Antioxidant Supplementation

While it appears that supplementing antioxidant deficiencies is beneficial in restoring cellular functions, supplementation can be associated with a variety of health risks. Herbert (1994) reviewed the "antioxidant supplement myth" and suggested that the following risks are associated with antioxidant supplementation:

- ***Vitamin E supplementation:*** Exacerbation of autoimmune and immune diseases such as asthma, allergies, diabetes, and rheumatoid arthritis.

- *Vitamin C supplementation (in combination with high iron intake):* Promotion of kidney stones and increased risk of iron-induced cardiac failure or of hemochromatosis (see "The Relationship Between Vitamin C and Iron," page 282).
- *Beta-carotene supplementation:* Increased rates of lung cancer and mortality due to cardiovascular disease.

Herbert (1994) emphasizes that these risks are associated with supplemental intakes, not an increased intake of antioxidants from food. He attributes the problems with supplement pills to "unbalanced chemistry," in that pills are not equally balanced between the oxidized and reduced states of the specific nutrient. It is important for the reader to understand that the issues raised by Herbert represent one individual's interpretation of the research literature. Other reputable scientists and health professionals hold opposing views. Since evidence does exist to suggest that supplementation with antioxidant nutrients may be harmful in certain circumstances, consumers should exercise caution when considering supplementation.

Antioxidants and Chronic Diseases

Antioxidant nutrients are purported to reduce the risk of many chronic diseases such as cardiovascular disease and diabetes. Contrary to popular opinion, there is no conclusive evidence that consuming antioxidant nutrients in amounts greater than recommended will prevent or cure certain chronic diseases. The purpose of this section is to familiarize the reader with known associations among specific antioxidant nutrients and chronic diseases and to review the mechanisms by which antioxidant nutrients may act to reduce risks for these diseases.

Cardiovascular Disease

The highly publicized results of epidemiological studies (Gaziano et al. 1990; Stampfer et al. 1992) showing significant relationships between intake of antioxidant nutrients and reduced incidence of cardiovascular events have led the general public to assume that there is a cause-and-effect relationship between antioxi-

dants and cardiovascular disease. It is important to stress that *associations* among variables in these studies do not prove cause and effect. At the present time, there are no published results from large experimental studies supporting a definitive role of antioxidant nutrients in the prevention of heart disease. (For a discussion of different types of epidemiological studies, refer to "Different Types of Epidemiological Studies," page 292). Indirect evidence and correlational findings, however, highlight the roles antioxidant nutrients may play in the progression of heart disease. The following risk factors for heart disease have been associated with low intakes of antioxidant nutrients:

- Oxidation of LDL-cholesterol
- Reduced serum levels of HDL-cholesterol
- Hypertension
- Insulin insensitivity and type II diabetes
- Reperfusion injury associated with an ischemic event
- Impaired vasomotor tone as it relates to arterial stiffness and coronary artery spasm
- Increased platelet adhesiveness

One factor that has been theorized to contribute significantly to atherosclerosis is the oxidation of LDL-cholesterol. Atherosclerosis first appears as fatty streaks along the arterial wall; these fatty streaks are initiated from damage incurred to the endothelium. Oxidized LDL-cholesterol attaches to the damaged areas of the endothelium and contributes to perpetual damage to the vascular wall over many years. This damage results in the formation of plaque and the development of atherosclerosis (Gutteridge and Halliwell 1994). Vitamin E has been shown to decrease the oxidation of LDL-cholesterol in humans (Dieber-Rotheneder et al. 1991; Jialal and Grundy 1992), while vitamin C and β-carotene were found to inhibit LDL-cholesterol oxidation in vitro (or in cellular preparations).

Some epidemiological studies have shown an association between increased vitamin C intakes and elevated HDL-cholesterol levels (Dallal et al. 1989; Jacques et al. 1987). In addition, the administration of 1-2 g/d of vitamin C has significantly increased HDL-cholesterol levels in some, but not all, studies (Buzzard et al. 1982; Heine and Norden 1979; Horsey et al. 1981). A strong correlation between low serum

■ HIGHLIGHT ■

Different Types of Epidemiological Studies

Can all epidemiological studies be defined as experimental in nature? What determines whether an epidemiological study is an experimental research study? An experiment is a scientific project in which the investigator attempts to control all factors that affect the outcome of interest (Rothman 1986). In addition, conditions of interest are manipulated in an experiment. Rothman (1986) provides an excellent review of types of epidemiological studies that can be classified as experimental or nonexperimental. Experimental studies include randomized clinical trials (RCTs) and community intervention trials. Nonexperimental epidemiological studies include case-control and many cohort studies. Projects that are descriptive or observational in nature are considered nonexperimental studies.

Due to many ethical constraints, use of certain experimental designs is limited in much of epidemiological research. According to Rothman (1986), these constraints include

- the inability to limit the research subjects' exposure to potential preventives of disease, and
- the inappropriateness of depriving subjects of the preferable form of treatment or of any preventive that is not included in the study.

Because of researchers' inability to control many confounding variables, it is critical that they report the results of nonexperimental epidemiological research in a way that emphasizes the limitations of the study. It is also important for readers to understand that an *association* between antioxidant nutrients and disease risks does not prove cause and effect. While nonexperimental epidemiological studies provide the scientific community with invaluable information, the results of these studies need to be distributed with a clear explanation of the implications to health and disease status. For example, an epidemiological study that looks at a large population *in retrospect* and finds a correlation between one lifestyle variable and a disease is a nonexperimental study that can provide important information on which to base future experimental studies, but that does not prove cause and effect. Merely observing a strong correlation between smoking and heart disease, for instance, does not *prove* that smoking is a causative factor. But, inspired by such nonexperimental data, one could design an experimental epidemiological study: identify a large group of smokers and follow them for 10 years, helping all who wish to kick the habit; then compare heart disease data between those who kept smoking and those who quit. If the latter group had significantly less heart disease, those data would be more persuasive in claiming a causal relationship.

vitamin C levels and high blood pressure has also been reported (McCarron et al. 1984; Salonen et al. 1988; Yoshioka et al. 1984), but no large-scale, long-duration clinical trials have been conducted. Thus, it is unknown at this time if there is a cause-and-effect relationship between vitamin C levels and blood pressure.

Diabetes is a well-known risk factor for cardiovascular disease, and associations between elevated serum glucose and oxidative stress have been reported in humans with diabetes (Williamson et al. 1993). It is theorized that the altered glucose metabolism that accompanies

diabetes may be related to peroxidation. Administration of 900 mg/d of vitamin E for 4 mo resulted in improvements in glucose clearance and disposal in individuals with non-insulin dependent diabetes mellitus (Paolisso et al. 1993). Similar benefits of vitamin E supplementation were observed in elderly nondiabetic subjects (Paolisso et al. 1994).

Antioxidants may also play a role in reducing the damage from **reperfusion injury**, which results from an ischemic event such as a myocardial infarction or stroke. Once ischemia occurs, reoxygenation of the tissue is critical to slow the death of the cells. Restoring oxygen to cells results in oxidative stress and subsequent excessive production of free radicals, and the consequent damage has been termed reoxygenation, or reperfusion injury. Vitamin E supplementation has been shown to reduce oxidative damage resulting from the reperfusion associated with coronary artery bypass surgery (Cavarocchi et al. 1986; Ferriera et al. 1991). Other mechanisms through which antioxidants may reduce risk of cardiovascular disease include altering platelet adhesiveness and vasomotor tone. Supplementation with vitamins C and E may decrease the "stickiness," or aggregability, of platelets (Bordia and Verma 1985; Salonen et al. 1991; Steiner and Anastasi 1976; Steiner and Mower 1982), and vitamin C supplementation was found to improve endothelium-dependent arterial dilation in individuals with established coronary heart disease (Levine et al. 1996). Thus, antioxidant nutrients may play a role in altering the development of cardiovascular disease; however, there is no evidence to support that antioxidant supplements can prevent or cure cardiovascular disease.

Cancer

The process of transforming normal cells into cancerous cells occurs through multiple stages. While the exact functions of antioxidant nutrients in cancer prevention or reversal are unknown, these nutrients may play a role in preventing initiation by detoxifying carcinogens or blocking their actions; they may also affect the various stages of cancer development. Most intervention studies have been conducted to study the effects of antioxidant supplements on precancerous lesions, which is controversial. It is imperative that when precancerous lesions are used as midpoint markers in intervention studies, the lesions must be strongly linked with the eventual development of cancer. Burri (1997) emphasized that studies showing a reduction in midpoint markers of cancer and heart disease are not equal to results showing a reduction in the incidence of these diseases. Well-designed studies would ideally include midpoint markers of disease progression and documentation of disease incidence.

Epidemiological studies have shown that β-carotene and vitamins A, C, and E have significant associations with certain cancers. Low dietary intakes and serum levels of vitamin C and

β-carotene are related to increased incidence of cervical dysplasia (a precancerous lesion of cervical cancer) (Harris et al. 1986; Wassertheil-Smoller et al. 1981; Wylie-Rosett et al. 1984). Vitamin A and β-carotene can lead to remission of precancerous lesions of oral cancer (Stich et al. 1988). Vitamins C and E may also reduce the risk of stomach cancer through their role in blocking the formation of nitrosamines and other carcinogenic agents in the stomach (Mirvish 1986). Erhardt et al. (1997) found that humans fed a diet high in dietary fat and meat and low in dietary fiber had a significant decrease in plasma levels of β-carotene and vitamin C. This diet also resulted in a significant production of hydroxyl radicals in the feces and a higher concentration of iron in the feces. In contrast, the same subjects fed a vegetarian diet low in dietary fat and high in fiber had higher serum concentrations of β-carotene and vitamin C and a lower serum MDA concentration, indicating less lipid peroxidation on this diet.

Results from four large-scale intervention studies do not support benefits of antioxidant supplements in reducing risks of cancer or heart disease (Albanes et al. 1995; ABCPSG 1994; Blot et al. 1995; Blot et al. 1993; Hennekens et al. 1996; Omenn et al. 1996). The only study showing positive results was the Linxian study (Blot et al. 1995; Blot et al. 1993), in which rates of stomach and esophageal cancers were reduced, as was overall mortality, in middle-aged Chinese men and women. The Physicians' Health Study (Hennekens et al. 1996) showed no effect of β-carotene supplementation on cancer, heart disease, or overall mortality. In contrast, the Alpha-Tocopherol and Beta-Carotene (ATBC) study (Albanes et al. 1995; ABCPSG 1994) and the beta-Carotene and Retinol Efficacy Trial (CARET) (Omenn et al. 1996) found negative results of mixed antioxidant supplements. The ATBC study found an increase in lung cancer rates and overall mortality, with no effect on heart disease, while the CARET study was ended early due to a trend toward increased mortality and cancer rates associated with supplementation. Heavy smokers and drinkers seemed to be particularly vulnerable to the negative effects of supplementation in these studies. From the results of these studies, it appears that more research needs to be conducted on the effects of antioxidants (from food and supplemental sources) on cancer before conclusive recommendations regarding intakes of these nutrients can be made.

Cataracts

Cataract is defined as "a dysfunction of the lens due to partial or complete opacification" (Taylor 1993). Cataracts are formed when proteins in the lens of the eye are damaged. As the lens proteins have an extremely long life, they are exposed to many damaging factors. These damaged proteins accumulate, aggregate, and precipitate, which causes **opacification** of the lens (Taylor 1993). Some have suggested that free radical damage resulting from repeated exposure to oxygen and ultraviolet light may contribute to development of cataracts (Harding and van Heyningen 1987).

As a person ages, the levels of antioxidants and activity of antioxidant enzymes decline. The activity of proteases (enzymes that remove damaged proteins) also decreases with age. Thus, the combination of increased oxidative damage and a reduced capacity to protect against this dam-

age leads to opacification of the lens. Studies have shown individuals with cataracts to have lower serum concentrations of vitamins E, C, and β-carotene (Jacques and Chylack 1991; Jacques et al. 1988). Moreover, individuals taking vitamin C and E supplements (400 IU vitamin E and 300-600 mg vitamin C) had a significantly lower risk of cataracts than those not taking supplements (Robertson et al. 1989). Thus, antioxidant nutrients—particularly vitamins C and E—may reduce the risk of cataracts in older people by providing the lens of the eye with additional protection from oxidative damage. For further discussion of antioxidants and the aging process, see "Antioxidants and Aging," below.

Antioxidants and Performance

The popularity of supplementation and prevalent use of performance-enhancing products

HIGHLIGHT

Antioxidants and Aging

Can antioxidants slow the aging process? Can duration and quality of life be enhanced by the use of antioxidant supplements? These are very important questions since the elderly are the fastest growing age group in the United States. The free radical theory of aging suggests that free radicals are the primary cause of aging; if this assumption holds true, then reducing oxidative damage should reduce the progression of the aging process. Aging is associated with decreased activities of antioxidant enzymes in most body tissues (Ji 1995). Interestingly, the activities of antioxidant enzymes such as SOD, CAT, and GPX reportedly are enhanced in aging skeletal muscle. Despite this magnified activity in skeletal muscle, lipid peroxidation is higher in aging muscle than in young muscle (Ji et al. 1990). It has been speculated that antioxidant enzymes become less efficient in protecting the body with age.

Despite findings of decreased ability to fight free radical damage with age, no studies have reported prolonged life as a result of antioxidant supplementation. However, there is strong support for increasing the RDAs for many nutrients among the elderly due to the reduced food intake and impairment of nutrient absorption and metabolism with increasing age. In addition to the diseases discussed in this chapter, osteoporosis and impaired immune function are related to nutritional factors. Memory performance and cognitive function are also related to antioxidant and B-vitamin intakes (La Rue et al. 1997; Perrig et al. 1997). It is possible that many elderly individuals would benefit from vitamin and mineral supplementation to improve nutritional status.

Because elderly people differ physiologically according to age, sex, health status, and physical activity status, Blumberg (1991) suggested separate RDAs for age brackets such as 51-60, 61-70, 71-80, and 81-90 years. He proposed that the recommendations for micronutrients need to be higher among the elderly if the goal of the RDAs is to maximize health. Since antioxidants and other nutrients have been associated with reduced risks for chronic diseases, it may be that supplementation, while not increasing the *duration* of life, will enhance the *quality* of life. Studies focusing on the interactions among antioxidants, life span, and morbidity need to be conducted in order to determine the impact of antioxidant nutrients on the aging process.

emphasize the competitive athlete's strong desire to win at any cost. As discussed throughout this chapter, specific antioxidant nutrients may reduce free radical production and subsequent tissue damage while exercise training may enhance the protective capabilities of the antioxidant system. While this information is interesting, the most important question for many athletes is, "Does the use of antioxidant supplements enhance performance?"

Antioxidant Supplementation and Performance

It is theorized that consuming antioxidant supplements will augment the antioxidant defenses even beyond the increases caused by regular training. It may also be that "weekend warriors," or occasional exercisers, may benefit from antioxidant supplements. In fact, it has been suggested that the occasional exerciser will benefit even more from supplementation than the trained athlete because the former has a less developed antioxidant defense system than the latter (Clarkson 1995).

Most studies investigating the effects of antioxidant supplementation on performance have focused on vitamins E and C. Although many studies have shown that supplementation with vitamin E reduces markers of lipid peroxidation with exercise (Dillard et al. 1978; Kanter et al. 1993; Kumar et al. 1992; Packer 1984; Sumida et al. 1989; Tappel 1973), others have shown no effect (Helgheim et al. 1979; Kanter and Eddy 1992; Warren et al. 1992; Witt et al. 1992). No studies of vitamin C supplementation in humans have included measurements of oxidative damage, and most have assessed its impact in combination with other antioxidant nutrients.

One study of swimmers found that 14 d of selenium supplementation resulted in a smaller increase in MDA and an enhancement in the glutathione system (Dragen et al. 1990).

Although antioxidant supplementation seemed to reduce oxidative damage in some studies, the impact on performance does not appear to be significant. Numerous studies of vitamin E supplementation in swimmers have shown no effect on performance (Lawrence et al. 1975; Sharman et al. 1976; Sharman et al. 1971; Shephard et al. 1974; Talbot and Jamieson 1977) with similar results reported for cycling exercise to exhaustion (Sumida et al. 1989) and $\dot{V}O_2$max levels of hockey players (Watt et al.

1974). While some studies of vitamin C supplementation show improvements in performance, they contain major design flaws that make interpretation of their results unreliable. Well-controlled studies of vitamin C supplementation show no improvements in performance (Gey et al. 1970; Keith and Merrill 1983; Keren and Epstein 1980), and vitamin C restriction over 3 weeks in healthy men did not affect $\dot{V}O_2$max or the accumulation of blood lactate (van der Beek et al. 1990). Selenium supplementation was found to have no effect on endurance exercise training (Tessier et al. 1995). Coenzyme Q_{10} supplementation has also failed to improve performance or training capacity (Braun et al. 1991; Weston et al. 1997). Likewise, there is no evidence to support any relationship between vitamin A and exercise, and the effects of β-carotene supplementation have not been studied in regard to exercise performance.

Two areas where antioxidant supplementation may affect exercise performance are with altitude exposure and in conditions of extremely high ambient temperatures. Simon-Schnass and Pabst (1988) found that vitamin E supplementation reduced lipid peroxidation and improved performance in hypoxic environments. Kotze et al. (1977) and Strydom et al. (1976) found that vitamin C supplementation in South African miners enhanced acclimatization to high ambient temperatures and reduced rectal temperature and total sweat output. It is possible that antioxidant supplementation is beneficial under extreme environmental conditions. Note also that nutritional status of people working in these extreme conditions may also be compromised due to poor appetite and limited food availability, emphasizing the link between adequate nutritional status and exercise performance.

Recommendations for Antioxidant Intake

Is there sufficient evidence to warrant making recommendations for antioxidant nutrients? Since available evidence to argue for supplementation appears inadequate at this time, recommendations appear premature. Yet some researchers strongly suggest that research data justify recommendations for antioxidant nutrients (Ji 1995). Lachance (1996) advocated increasing the RDAs of vitamins C, E, and β-carotene, suggesting that new recommendations be based on ideal diets recommended in government documents to prevent various diseases (Lachance 1992). Table 10.5 lists the present RDAs and the suggested optimal intakes of vitamins C, E, and β-carotene. While Lachance's recommendation for vitamin C is similar to that already discussed earlier in this chapter, his suggestion for vitamin E is much lower.

Table 10.5 is not provided as a definitive recommendation for antioxidant supplementation but rather as an illustration of how opinions differ regarding the adequacy of present RDAs. New RDAs will be published for these nutrients in 2000. There are several concerns regarding the safety of antioxidant supplementation, including

- toxicity risks of certain nutrients,
- impact of long-term supplementation on health,
- bioavailability of supplement pills, and
- potential interactions among nutrients.

Although vitamin A is known to be highly toxic, higher doses of vitamins E, C, and β-carotene appear to be tolerable. Intakes of 200-600 mg/d, 1-2 g/d, and 30-90 mg/d for vitamin E, vitamin C, and β-carotene, respectively, have been reported with no side effects. Unfortunately, most studies of supplementation are short-term (4-8 weeks), and the impact of long-term supplementation in humans is not known. The effects of supplementation are dependent upon the supplement's bioavailability, which can change depending upon the nutritional status of the individual. Many environmental factors can affect a person's need for antioxidant nutrients, including environmental pollution, certain medications, smoking, disease status, and exposure to herbicides.

Finally, interactions among antioxidant nutrients are unknown. Does consuming these nutrients in combination have a synergistic effect? Does supplementation with these nutrients reduce absorption or activity of other nutrients? These questions need to be answered before definitive recommendations can be made. However, it is prudent for all people, including highly trained athletes and recreationally active individuals, to consume a diet that contains a wide variety of foods. Meeting the American Cancer Society's recommendation of eating a *combination of five fruits and/or vegetables per day* will result in many people's meeting and exceeding the RDA for antioxidant nutrients. Multivitamin and mineral supplements can also be used to safely supplement diets.

Chapter in Review

We started this chapter with questions regarding the role of antioxidants in health and performance. From the information discussed in this chapter, the following conclusions can be made:

- Antioxidant nutrients are important to minimize damage resulting from free radical formation.
- Deficiencies of antioxidant nutrients can result in increased oxidative damage and may increase the risk for various diseases. Furthermore, poor antioxidant status probably impairs physical performance.
- There is no evidence that antioxidant supplementation improves performance in well-fed, healthy adults who have good overall nutritional status and good antioxidant status.

Table 10.5 **Current RDAs and Proposed Recommended Intakes of Select Antioxidant Nutrients**

Nutrient	RDA[1]	Recommended intake[2]
Vitamin C	60 mg/d (nonsmokers)	220 mg/d
Vitamin E	8 mg/d (women) 10 mg/d (men)	23 mg/d
Beta-carotene	Not applicable[3]	5.7 mg/d

[1]Food and Nutrition Board 1989.
[2]Lachance 1992.
[3]No recommended dietary allowance has been defined for beta-carotene.

- Epidemiological studies indicate that healthy individuals may benefit from antioxidant supplementation; however, more experimental clinical trials need to be performed to establish a cause-and-effect relationship between antioxidant nutrients and reduced disease risk.

While consuming two to three times the RDA for most antioxidant nutrients appears to cause little harm, people should discuss supplementation of these products with a qualified medical professional as some individuals may respond adversely to supplementation.

KEY CONCEPTS

1. Define free radicals.

A free radical is a molecule with an unpaired electron in its outer orbit. Free radicals are highly reactive and can damage cells when produced in excess.

2. List the enzymes involved in antioxidant activities, and describe the reactions in which they participate.

The enzymatic antioxidant defense systems include (1) superoxide dismutase, which accelerates the conversion of the superoxide radical to hydrogen peroxide; (2) catalase, which removes hydrogen peroxide; (3) glutathione, which assists in the removal of hydrogen peroxide and reduction of lipid hydroperoxides; (4) glutathione peroxidase, which removes hydrogen peroxide and reduces lipid hydroperoxides; (5) glutathione reductase, which converts oxidized glutathione back to reduced glutathione; and (6) peroxidase, which rids the body of excess hydrogen peroxide.

3. Discuss the nutrients involved in antioxidant activities.

Vitamin E halts lipid peroxidation and protects polyunsaturated fatty acids. Vitamin C quenches singlet oxygen and regenerates the reduced form of vitamin E. Beta-carotene quenches singlet oxygen. Selenium is part of the glutathione peroxidase enzyme system. Other nutrients that act as antioxidants include coenzyme Q_{10}, copper, zinc, iron, and manganese.

4. Describe the methods used to assess oxidative damage.

Electron spin resonance and paramagnetic resonance spectrometry are used to assess superoxide radical production. Markers of lipid peroxidation include conjugated dienes, lipid hydroperoxides, malonaldehyde (or TBARSs), and the aliphatic hydrocarbons ethane and pentane. Changes in antioxidant enzymes can also indicate the functional activity of the antioxidant system.

5. Describe the proposed rationale for increased antioxidant need among active people.

It is suggested that active people's higher oxygen consumption leads to excessive free radical production—and that such people need more antioxidants because their existing antioxidant systems are not sufficient to cope with the elevated levels of free radicals. Active people may also have higher exposure to environmental pollutants, which again can increase the need for antioxidants.

6. Discuss how antioxidants play a role in chronic diseases.

Heart disease risk factors—such as hypertension, oxidation of LDL-cholesterol, type II diabetes, and reperfusion injury with an ischemic event—have been associated with low intakes of antioxidant nutrients. Low intakes of vitamin C and E have been associated with certain cancers, but recent studies have not indicated that supplementation prevents or reduces the risk for these cancers. Vitamins C and E may reduce the risk of cataracts in older individuals by providing the lens of the eye with additional protection from oxidative damage.

7. Discuss the relationship between antioxidants and athletic performance.

Although antioxidant supplementation is popular among many athletes and active people, there are no data to suggest that supplementing with antioxidants improves athletic performance in healthy individuals with good nutritional status. A nutritionally balanced diet is critical to optimal performance, and eating a combination of five fruits and vegetables per day will result in most people's meeting or exceeding the RDA for antioxidants.

KEY TERMS

aliphatic hydrocarbons
alpha-tocopherol
antioxidants
ascorbate
beta-carotene
bioflavonoids
breath pentane measurements
capillary fragility
carotenoids
catalase (CAT)
cataract
conjugated dienes
electron spin resonance
electron transport chain (ETC, or respiratory chain)
erythrocyte hemolysis test
ethane
free radical
glutathione
glutathione peroxidase (GPX)
glutathione reductase (GR)
gulonolactone oxidase
hydrogen peroxide
hydroperoxyl free radical
hydroxyl radical

iron-induced cardiac failure
isotope dilution
leukocyte ascorbic acid concentration
lipid hydroperoxides
lipid peroxidation
lutein
lycopene
malonaldehyde (MDA)
megadose
opacification
paramagnetic resonance spectrometry
pentane
peroxidase
phytochemicals
prooxidant
reperfusion injury
singlet oxygen
serum ascorbic acid concentrations
superoxide dismutase (SOD)
superoxide radical
thiobarbituric acid reactive substance (TBARS)
ubiquinone (coenzyme Q_{10})
urinary excretion

References

Albanes D, Heinonen OP, Huttunen JK, et al. Effects of alpha-tocopherol and beta-carotene supplements on cancer incidence in the Alpha-Tocopherol Beta-Carotene Cancer Prevention Study. Am J Clin Nutr 1995;62(suppl.):1427S-30S.

Alberts B, Bray D, Lewis J, Raff M, Roberts K, Watson JD. Molecular Biology of the Cell. 2nd ed. New York: Garland Publishing, 1989.

Alessio HM. Exercise-induced oxidative stress. Med Sci Sports Exerc 1993;25(2):218-24.

Alpha-Tocopherol, Beta-Carotene Cancer Prevention Study Group. The effect of vitamin E and beta-carotene on the incidence of lung cancer and other cancers in male smokers. N Engl J Med 1994;330:1029-35.

Amadio E, Palermo R, Peloni G, Littarru G. Effect of CoQ_{10} administration on VO_2max and diastolic function in athletes. In: Folkers K, Littarru G, eds. Biomedical and Clinical Aspects of Coenzyme Q. Amsterdam: Elsevier, 1991:525-33.

Baker EM, Hodges RE, Hood J, Sauberlich HE, March SC, Canham JE. Metabolism of [14]C- and ^{3}H-labeled L-ascorbic acid in human scurvy. Am J Clin Nutr 1971;24:444-54.

Bendich A, Machlin LJ, Scandurra O, Burton GW, Wayner DDM. The antioxidant role of vitamin C. Adv Free Radical Biol Med 1986;2:419-44.

Blot WJ, Li J, Taylor PR, Guo W, Dawsey SM, Li B. The Linxian trials: mortality rates by vitamin-mineral intervention group. Am J Clin Nutr 1995;62(suppl.):1424S-6S.

Blot WJ, Li JY, Taylor PR, et al. Nutrition intervention trials in Linxian, China: supplementation with specific vitamin/mineral combinations, cancer incidence, and disease-specific mortality in the general population. J Natl Cancer Inst 1993;85:1483-92.

Blumberg JB. Considerations of the recommended dietary allowances for older adults. Clin Appl Nutr 1991;1(4):9-18.

Bordia AK, Verma SK. Effects of vitamin C on platelet adhesiveness and platelet aggregation in coronary artery disease patients. Clin Cardiol 1985;8:552-4.

Bowles DK, Torgan CE, Kehrer JP, Ivy JI, Starnes JW. Effects of acute, submaximal exercise on skeletal muscle vitamin E. Free Rad Res Commun 1991;14:139-43.

Braun B, Clarkson P, Freedson P, Kohl R. Effects of coenzyme Q_{10} supplementation on exercise performance, VO_2max, and lipid peroxidation in trained cyclists. Int J Sport Nutr 1991;1:353-65.

Bucca C, Rolla G, Farina JC. Effect of vitamin C on transient increase of bronchial responsiveness in conditions affecting the airways. Ann NY Acad Sci 1992;669:175-86.

Burri BJ. Beta-carotene and human health: a review of current research. Nutr Res 1997;17(3):547-80.

Buzzard IM, McRoberts MR, Driscoll DL, Bowering J. Effects of dietary eggs and ascorbic acid on plasma lipid and lipoprotein cholesterol levels in healthy young men. Am J Clin Nutr 1982;36:94-105.

Cavarocchi NC, England MD, O'Brien JF, et al. Superoxide generation during cardiopulmonary bypass: is there a role for vitamin E? J Surg Res 1986;40:519-27.

Chatterjee IB, Majumder AK, Nandi BK, Subramanian N. Synthesis and some major functions of vitamin C in animals. Ann NY Acad Sci 1975;258:24-47.

Clarkson PM. Antioxidants and physical performance. Crit Rev Food Sci Nutr 1995;35 (1&2):131-41.

Cohen JL, Potosnak L, Frank O, Baker H. A nutritional and hematological assessment of elite ballet dancers. Phys Sportsmed 1985;13:43-54.

Cutler RG. Antioxidants, aging, and longevity.

In: Pryor WA, ed. Free Radicals in Biology. London: Academic Press, 1984:371-428.

Dallal GE, Choi E, Jacques PF, Schaefer EJ, Jacob RA. Ascorbic acid, HDL cholesterol and apolipoprotein A-I in an elderly Chinese population in Boston. J Am Coll Nutr 1989;8:69-74.

Davies KJA, Quintanilha AT, Brooks GA, Packer L. Free radicals and tissue damage produced by exercise. Biochem Biophys Res Commun 1982;107:1198-205.

Dekkers C, van Doornen LJP, Kemper HCG. The role of antioxidant vitamins and enzymes in the prevention of exercise-induced muscle damage. Sports Med 1996;21(3):213-38.

Demopoulos HB, Santomier JP, Seligman ML, Pietronigro DD. Free radical pathology: rationale and toxicology of antioxidants and other supplements in sports medicine and exercise science. In: Katch FI, ed. Sport, Health, and Nutrition. Champaign, IL: Human Kinetics, 1986:139-89.

Dernbach AR, Sherman WM, Simonsen JC, Flowers KM, Lamb DR. No evidence of oxidant stress during high-intensity rowing training. J Appl Physiol 1993;74(5):2140-5.

Dieber-Rotheneder M, Puhl H, Waeg G, Striegl G, Esterbauer H. Effect of oral supplementation with D-alpha tocopherol on the vitamin E content of human LDL resistance to oxidation. J Lipid Res 1991;1325-32.

DIETSYS (software progrm), version 3.7. 1996. National Cancer Institute, Bethesda, MD.

Dillard CJ, Litov RE, Savin WM, Dumelin EE, Tappel AL. Effects of exercise, vitamin E, and ozone on pulmonary function and lipid peroxidation. J Appl Physiol Respir Enviorn Exerc Physiol 1978;45(6):927-32.

Dragen I, Dinu V, Mohora M, Cristea E, Plesteanu E, Stroescu V. Studies regarding the antioxidant effect of selenium on top swimmers. Rev Roum Physiol 1990;27:15-25.

Duthie GG, Robertson JD, Maughan RJ, Morrice PC. Blood antioxidant status and erythrocyte lipid peroxidation following distance running. Arch Biochem Biophys 1990;282:78-83.

Epler KS, Sander L, Zeigler RG, Wise SA, Craft NE. Evaluation of reversed-phase liquid chromatographic columns for the recovery and selectivity of selected carotenoids. J Chromatogr 1992;595:89-101.

Epler KS, Ziegler RG, Craft NE. Liquid chromatographic method for the determination of carotenoids, retinoids and tocopherols in human serum and in food. J Chromatogr 1993;619:37-48.

Erhardt JG, Lim SS, Bode JC, Bode C. A diet rich in fat and poor in dietary fiber increases the in vitro formation of reactive oxygen species in human feces. J Nutr 1997;127:706-9.

Evelo CTA, Palmen NGM, Artur Y, Janssen GME. Changes in blood glutathione concentrations, and in erythrocyte glutathione reductase and glutathione S-transferase activity after running training and after participation in contests. Eur J Appl Physiol 1992;64:354-8.

Ferriera RF, Milei J, Liesuy S, Flecha BG, et al. Antioxidant action of vitamins A and E in patients submitted to coronary artery bypass surgery. Vascular Surgery 1991;25:191-5.

Fiorella P, Bargossi M, Grossi G, et al. Metabolic effects of coenzyme Q_{10} treatment in high level athletes. In: Folkers K, Littarru G, Yamagami T, eds. Biomedical and Clinical Aspects of Coenzyme Q. Amsterdam: Elsevier, 1991:513-20.

Fogelholm GM, Himberg J, Alopaeus K, Gref C, Laakso JT, Lehto JJ, Mussalo-Rauhamaa H. Dietary and biochemical indices of nutritional status in male athletes and control. J Am Coll Nutr 1992;11:181-91.

Folkers K, Vadhanavikit S, Mortensen SA. Biochemical rationale and myocardial tissue data on the effective therapy of cardiomyopathy with Coenzyme Q_{10}. Proc Natl Acad Sci USA 1985;82:901-4.

Folkers K, Wolaniuk J, Simonsen R, Morishita M, Vadhanavikit S. Biochemical rationale and the cardiac response of patients with muscle disease to therapy with Coenzyme Q_{10}. Proc Natl Acad Sci USA 1985;82:4513-6.

Food and Nutrition Board. Institute of Medicine. Recommended Dietary Allowances. 10th ed. Washington, DC: National Academy Press, 1989.

Forman MR, Beecher GR, Muesing R, et al. The fluctuation of plasma carotenoid concentrations by phase of the menstrual cycle: a controlled diet study. Am J Clin Nutr 1996;64:559-65.

Gaziano M, Manson JAE, Ridker PW, Buring JE Hennekens CH. Beta carotene therapy for chronic stable angina. Circulation 1990; 82 (suppl III):201 (abstract).

Gey GO, Cooper KH, Bottenberg RA. Effect of ascorbic acid on endurance performance and athletic injury. J Am Med Assoc 1970;211:105-11.

Gibson RS. Principles of Nutritional Assessment. New York: Oxford University Press, 1990.

Glover JR. Selenium in human urine: a tentative maximum allowable concentration for industrial and rural populations. Ann Occupational Hygiene 1967;10:3-14.

Gohil K, Packer L, deLumen B, Brooks GA, Terblanche SE. Vitamin E deficiency and vitamin C supplementation: exercise and mitochondrial oxidation. J Appl Physiol 1986;60:1986-91.

Goldfarb AH. Antioxidants: role of supplementation to prevent exercise-induced oxidative stress. Med Sci Sports Exerc 1993;25:232-6.

Greenberg SM, Frishman WH. Coenzyme Q_{10}: a new drug for myocardial ischemia? Medic Clin NA 1988;72(1):243-58.

Guerra G, Ballardini E, Lippa S, Oradei A, Littarru G. Effect of the administration of ubidecarenone over the maximum consumption of oxygen and on the physical performance in a group of young cyclists. Med Sport 1987;40:359-64.

Guilland JT, Penaranda C, Gallet V, Boggio F, Fuchs, Klepping J. Vitamin status of young athletes including the effects of supplementation. Med Sci Sports Exerc 1989;21:441-9.

Gutteridge JMC, Halliwell B. The measurement and mechanism of lipid peroxidation in biological systems. Trends Biochem Sci 1990;15:129-35.

Gutteridge JMC, Halliwell B. Antioxidants in Nutrition, Health, and Disease. Oxford: Oxford University Press, 1994.

Halliwell B, Gutteridge JMC. Oxygen toxicity, oxygen radicals, transition metals and disease. Biochem J 1984;219:1-14.

Halliwell B, Gutteridge JMC. Free Radicals in Biology and Medicine. Oxford: Clarendon Press, 1985:139-89.

Harding JJ, van Heyningen R. Epidemiology and risk factors for cataract. Eye 1987; 1:537-41.

Harris A, Robinson AB, Pauling L. Blood plasma L-ascorbic acid concentration for oral l-ascorbic acid dosage up to 12 grams per day. Int Res Commun Sys 1973;1:24.

Harris RWC, Forman D, Doll R, Vessey MP, Wald NJ. Cancer of the cervix uteri and vitamin A. Br J Cancer 1986;83:653-9.

Heine H, Norden C. Vitamin C therapy in hyperlipoproteinemia. Int J Vit Nutr Res 1979;19(suppl.):45-54.

Heitzer T, Just H, Münzel T. Antioxidant vitamin C improves endothelial dysfunction in chronic smokers. Circulation 1996;94:6-9.

Helgheim I, Hetland O, Nilsson S, Ingjer F, Stromme SB. The effects of vitamin E on serum enzyme levels following heavy exercise. Eur J Appl Physiol 1979;40:283-9.

Hennekens CH, Buring JE, Manson JE, et al. Lack of effect of long-term supplementation with beta-carotene on the incidence of malignant neoplasms and cardiovascular disease. N Engl J Med 1996;334:1145-9.

Herbert V. Dangers of iron and vitamin C supplements. J Am Diet Assoc 1993a;93:526-7.

Herbert V. Does mega-C do more good than harm, or more harm than good? Nutr Today 1993b;28(1):28-32.

Herbert V. The antioxidant supplement myth. Am J Clin Nutr 1994;60:157-8.

Hojo Y. Evaluation of the expression of urinary selenium level as ng. Se/mg creatinine and the use of single-void urine as a sample for urinary selenium determinations. Bull Environ Contamination Toxicol 1981;27:213-20.

Horsey J, Livesley B, Dickerson JWT. Ischaemic heart disease and aged patients: effects of ascorbic acid on lipoproteins. J Hum Nutr 1981;35:53-8.

Jackson MJ, Edwards RHT, Symons MCR. Electron spin resonance studies of intact mammalian skeletal muscle. Biochem Biophys Acta 1985;847:185-90.

Jacques PF, Chylack LT, Jr. Epidemiologic evidence of a role for the antioxidant vitamins and carotenoids in cataract prevention. Am J Clin Nutr 1991;53(suppl.):352S-5S.

Jacques PF, Chylack LT, Jr., McGandy RB, Hartz SC. Nutritional status in persons with and without senile cataract: blood vitamin and mineral levels. Am J Clin Nutr 1988;48:152-8.

Jacques PF, Hartz SC, McGandy RB, Jacob RA, Russell RM. Ascorbic acid, HDL, and total plasma cholesterol in the elderly. J Am Coll Nutr 1987;6:169-74.

Jenkins RR. Free radical chemistry: relationship to exercise. Sports Med 1988;5:156-70.

Jenkins RR. Exercise, oxidative stress, and antioxidants: a review. Int J Sport Nutr 1993;3:356-75.

Jenkins RR, Goldfarb A. Introduction: oxidant stress, aging, and exercise. Med Sci Sports Exerc 1993;25(2):210-2.

Ji LL. Exercise and oxidative stress: role of the cellular antioxidant systems. Ex Sport Sci Rev 1995;23:135-66.

Ji LL, Dillon D, Wu E. Alteration of antioxidant enzymes with aging in rat skeletal muscle and liver. Am J Physiol 1990;258:R918-R923.

Ji LL, Stratmen FW, Lardy HA. Antioxidant enzyme systems in rat liver and skeletal muscle. Arch Biochem Biophys 1988;263:150-60.

Jialal I, Grundy SM. The effect of dietary supplementation with alpha-tocopherol on the oxidative modification of low density lipoprotein. J Lipid Res 1992;6:899-906.

Jialal I, Vega GL, Grundy SM. Physiologic levels of ascorbate inhibit the oxidative modification of low density lipoprotein. Atherosclerosis 1990;82:185-91.

Johnston CS, Martin LJ, Cai X. Antihistamine effect of supplemental ascorbic acid and neutrophil chemotaxis. J Am Coll Nutr 1992;11:172-6.

Kanter MM. Free radicals, exercise, and antioxidant supplementation. Int J Sport Nutr 1994;4:205-20.

Kanter M. Free radicals and exercise: effects of nutritional antioxidant supplementation. Ex Sport Sci Rev 1995;23:375-97.

Kanter MM, Eddy DE. Effect of antioxidant supplementation on serum markers of lipid peroxidation and skeletal muscle damage following eccentric exercise. Med Sci Sports Exerc 1992;24:S17 (abstract).

Kanter MM, Lesmes GR, Kaminsky LA, Laham-Saeger J, Nequin ND. Serum creatine kinase and lactate dehydrogenase changes following an eighty kilometer race: relationship to lipid peroxidation. Eur J Appl Physiol 1988;57:60-3.

Kanter MM, Nolte LA, Holloszy JO. Effects of an antioxidant vitamin mixture on lipid peroxidation at rest and postexercise. J Appl Physiol 1993;74:965-9.

Karlsson J. Heart and skeletal muscle ubiquinone or CoQ$_{10}$ as a protective agent against radical formation in man. Adv Myochem 1987;1:305-18.

Karlsson J. Antioxidants and Exercise. Champaign, IL: Human Kinetics, 1997.

Keith RE, Merrill E. The effects of vitamin C on maximal grip strength and muscular endurance. J Sports Med 1983;23:253-6.

Keren G, Epstein Y. The effect of high dosage vitamin C intake on aerobic and anaerobic capacity. J Sports Med 1980;20:145-8.

Kneepkens CMF, LePage G, Roy CC. The potential of the hydrocarbon breath test as a measure of lipid peroxidation. Free Rad Biol Med 1994;17(2):127-60.

Kotze HF, van der Walt WH, Rogers GG, Strydom NB. Effects of plasma ascorbic acid levels on heat acclimatization in man. J Appl Physiol 1977;42:711-6.

Kumar CT, Reddy VK, Prasad M, Thyagaraju K, Redanna P. Dietary supplementation of vitamin E protects heart tissue from exercise-induced oxidant stress. Mol Cell Biochem 1992;111:109-15.

Lachance PA. Diet-health relationship. In: Finely JW, Robinson SF, and Armstrong DJ, eds. Food Safety Assessment. ACS Symposium Series N. 484. Washington, DC: American Chemical Society, 1992:278-96.

Lachance PA. Future vitamin and antioxidant

RDAs for health promotion. Prev Med 1996;25:46-7.

Lang JK, Gohil K, Packer L, Burk RF. Selenium deficiency, endurance exercise capacity, and antioxidant status in rats. J Appl Physiol 1987;63:2532-5.

Langsjoen PH, Folkers K. Long-term efficacy and safety of coenzyme Q_{10} therapy for idiopathic dilated cardiomyopathy. Am J Cardiol 1990;65:521-3.

La Rue A, Koehler KM, Wayne SJ, Chiulli SJ, Haaland KY, Garry PJ. Nutritional status and cognitive functioning in a normally aging sample: a 6-y reassessment. Am J Clin Nutr 1997;65:20-9.

Lawrence JD, Bower RC, Riehl WP, Smith JL. Effects of alpha-tocopherol acetate on the swimming endurance of trained swimmers. Am J Cli Nutr 1975;28:205-8.

Leaf DA, Kleinman MT, Hamilton M, Barstow TJ. The effect of exercise intensity on lipid peroxidation. Med Sci Sports Exerc 1997;29(8):1036-9.

Levine GN, Frei B, Koulouris SN, Gerhard MD, Keaney JF, Vita JA. Ascorbic acid reverses endothelial vasomotor dysfunction in patients with coronary artery disease. Circulation 1996;93:1107-13.

Link G, Pinson A, Kahane I, Hersko C. Iron loading modifies the fatty acid composition of cultured rat myocardial cells and liposomal vesicles: effect of ascorbate and alpha-tocopherol on myocardial lipid peroxidation. J Lab Clin Med 1987;114:243-9.

Livrea MA, Tesoriere L, Bongiorno A, Pintaudi AM, Ciaccio M, Riccio A. Contribution of vitamin A to the oxidation resistance of human low density lipoproteins. Free Rad Biol Med 1995;18(3):401-9.

Lovlin R, Cotte W, Pyke I, Kavanagh M, Belcastro AN. Are indices of free radical damage related to exercise intensity? Eur J Appl Physiol 1987;56:313-6.

Maughan RJ, Donnelly AE, Gleeson M, Whiting PH, Walker KA, Clough PJ. Delayed-onset muscle damage and lipid peroxidation in man after a downhill run. Muscle Nerve 1989;12:332-6.

McCarron DA, Morris DC, Henry HJ, Stanton JL. Blood pressure and nutrient intake in the United States. Science 1984;224:1392-8.

McCord JM, Day ED, Jr. Superoxide dependent production of hydroxyl radical catalyzed by iron-EDTA complex. FEBS Lett 1978;86:139-42.

Mena P, Maynar M, Gutierrez JM, Maynar J, Timon J, Campillo JE. Erythrocyte free radical scavenger enzymes in bicycle professional racers. Adaptation to training. Int J Sports Med 1991;12:563-6.

Meydani M, Fielding RA, Fotouhi N. Vitamin E. In: Wolinsky I, Driskell JA, eds. Sports Nutrition: Vitamins and Trace Elements. Boca Raton: CRC Press, 1997:119-35.

Mirvish SS. Effects of vitamins C and E on N-nitroso compound formation, carcinogenesis and cancer. Cancer 1986;58:1842-50.

Murphy SP, Subar AF, Block G. Vitamin E intakes and sources in the United States. Am J Clin Nutr 1990;52:361-7.

Nebeling LC, Forman MR, Graubard BI, Snyder RA. Changes in carotenoid intake in the United States: the 1987 and 1992 National Health Interview Surveys. J Am Diet Assoc 1997;97:991-6.

Ohno YH, Yahata T, Sato Y, Yamamura K, Taniguchi N. Physical training and fasting erythrocyte activities of free radical scavenging enzyme systems in sedentary men. Eur J Appl Physiol 1988;57:173-6.

Olson OE. Selenium toxicity with emphasis on man. J Am Coll Toxicol 1986;5:45-70.

Omenn GS, Goodman GE, Thornquist MD, et al. Effects of a combination of beta-carotene and vitamin A on lung cancer and cardiovascular disease. N Engl J Med 1996;334:1150-5.

Packer L. Vitamin E, physical exercise and tissue damage in animals. Med Biol Helsinki 1984;62:105-9.

Packer L. Oxygen radicals and antioxidants in endurance training. In: Benzi G, Packer L, Siliprandi N, eds. Biochemical Aspects of Physical Exercise. New York: Elsevier, 1986:73-92.

Paolisso G, D'Amore A, Giugliano D, Ceriello A, Varricchio M, D'Onofrio F. Pharmacologic doses of vitamin E improve insulin action in healthy subjects and non-insulin-dependent diabetic patients. Am J Clin Nutr 1993;57:650-6.

Paolisso G, Di Maro G, Galzerano D, Cacciapuoti F, Varricchio G, Varricchio M, D'Onofrio F. Pharmacological doses of vitamin E and insulin action in elderly subjects. Am J Clin Nutr 1994;59:1291-6.

Perrig WJ, Perrig P, Stähelin HB. The relation between antioxidants and memory performance in the old and very old. J Am Geriatr Soc 1997;45:718-24.

Peters EM, Goetzsche JM, Grobbelaar B, Noakes TD. Vitamin C supplementation reduces the incidence of postrace symptoms of upper-respiratory-tract infection in ultramarathon runners. Am J Clin Nutr 1993;57:170-4.

Pincemail J, Camus G, Roesgen A, et al. Exercise induces pentane production and neutrophil activation in humans: effect of propranolol. Eur J Appl Physiol 1990;61:319-22.

Quintanilha AT, Packer L, Davies JMS, Racanelli T, Davies KJA. Membrane effects of vitamin E deficiency: bioenergetics and surface charge density studies of skeletal muscle and liver mitochondria. Ann NY Acad Sci 1982;399:32-47.

Reilly M, Delanty N, Lawson JA, FitzGerald GA. Modulation of oxidant stress in vivo in chronic cigarette smokers. Circulation 1996;94:19-25.

Robertson JM, Donner AP, Trevithick JR. Vitamin E intakes and risk of cataract in humans. Ann NY Acad Sci 1989;570:372-82.

Rothman KJ. Modern Epidemiology. Boston: Little, Brown 1986:51-76.

Sahlin K, Cizinsky S, Warholm M, Hoberg J. Repetitive static muscle contractions in humans—a trigger of metabolic and oxidative stress? Eur J Appl Physiol 1992;64:228-36.

Salonen JT, Salonen R, Ihanainen M, et al. Blood pressure, dietary fats, and antioxidants. Am J Clin Nutr 1988;48:1226-32.

Salonen JT, Salonen R, Seppaenen K, et al. Effects of antioxidant supplementation on platelet function: a randomized pair-matched, placebo-controlled, double-blind trial in men with low antioxidant status. Am J Clin Nutr 1991;53:1222-9.

Schwarz KB, Cox JM, Sharma S, et al. Possible antioxidant effect of vitamin A supplementation in premature infants. J Pediatr Gastroenterol Nutr 1997;25(4):408-14.

Sharman IM, Down MG, Norgan NG. The effects of vitamin E on physiological function and athletic performance of trained swimmers. J Sports Med 1976;16:215-25.

Sharman IM, Down MG, Sen RN. The effects of vitamin E and training on physiological function and athletic performance in adolescent swimmers. Br J Nutr 1971;26:265-76.

Sharpless KE, Thomas JB, Sander LC, Wise SA. Liquid-chromatographic determination of carotenoids in human serum using an engineered C-30 and a C-18 stationary phase. J Chromatogr 1996;678:187-95.

Shephard RJ, Campbell R, Pimm P, Stuart D, Wright GR. Vitamin E, exercise, and the recovery from physical activity. Eur J Appl Physiol 1974;33:119-26.

Simon-Schnass IM. Nutrition at high altitude. J Nutr 1992;122:778-81.

Simon-Schnass I, Pabst H. Influence of vitamin E on physical performance. Int J Vit Nutr Res 1988;58:49-54.

Snider I, Bazzarre T, Murdoch S, Goldfarb A. Effects of coenzyme athletic performance system as an ergogenic aid on endurance performance to exhaustion. Int J Sport Nutr 1992;2:272-86.

Stampfer MJ, Manson JAE, Colditz GA, Speizer FE, Willett WC, Hennekens CH. A prospective study of vitamin E supplementation and risk of coronary disease in women. Circulation 1992;86(suppl. 4):I-463.

Steiner M, Anastasi J. Vitamin E: an inhibitor of the platelet release reaction. J Clin Invest 1976;57:732-7.

Steiner M, Mower R. Mechanism of action of vitamin E on platelet function. Ann NY Acad Sci 1982;393:289-99.

Stich HF, Rosin MP, Hornby AP, Mathew B, Sankaranarayanan R, Nair MK. Remission of oral leukoplakias and micronuclei in tobacco/betel quid chewers treated with beta carotene and with beta carotene plus vitamin A. Int J Cancer 1988;42:195-9.

Strydom NB, Kotze HF, van der Walt WH, Rogers GG. Effect of ascorbic acid on rate of heat acclimatization. J Appl Physiol 1976;41:202-5.

Sumida S, Tanaka K, Kitao H, Nakadomo F. Exercise-induced lipid peroxidation and leakage of enzymes before and after vitamin E supplementation. Int J Biochem 1989;21:835-8.

Talbot D, Jamieson J. An examination of the effect of vitamin E on the performance of highly trained swimmers. Can J Appl Sport Sci 1977;2:67-9.

Tappel A. Lipid peroxidation damage to cell components. Fed Proc 1973;32:1870-5.

Tate RM, Repine JE. Phagocytes, oxygen radicals, and lung injury. In: Pryor WA, ed. Free Radicals in Biology. London: Academic Press, 1984:199-209.

Taylor A. Cataract: relationships between nutrition and oxidation. J Am Coll Nutr 1993;12(2):138-46.

Tribble DL, Giuliano LJ, Fortmann SP. Reduced plasma ascorbic acid concentrations in non-smokers regularly exposed to environmental tobacco smoke. Am J Clin Nutr 1993;58:886-90.

van der Beek EJ, van Dokkum W, Schrijver J, Wesstra A, Kestemaker C, Hermus RJJ. Controlled vitamin C restriction and physical performance in volunteers. J Am Coll Nutr 1990;9:332-9.

Warren JA, Jenkins RR, Packer L, Witt EH, Armstrong RB. Elevated muscle vitamin E does not attenuate eccentric exercise-induced muscle injury. J Appl Physiol 1992;72:2168-75.

Wassertheil-Smoller S, Romney SL, Wylie-Rosett J, et al. Dietary vitamin C and uterine cervical dysplasia. Am J Epidemiol 1981;114:714-24.

Watt T, Romet TT, McFarlane I, McGuey D, Allen C, Goode RC. Vitamin E and oxygen consumption. Lancet 1974;2:354 (abstract).

Weber C, Erl W, Weber K, Weber PC. Increased adhesiveness of isolated monocytes to endothelium is prevented by vitamin C intake in smokers. Circulation 1996;93:1488-92.

Weight LM, Noakes TD, Labadarios D, Graves J, Jacobs P, Berman PA. Vitamin and mineral status of trained athletes including the effects of supplementation. Am J Clin Nutr 1988;47:186-91.

Weston SB, Zhou S, Weatherby RP, Robson SJ. Does exogenous coenzyme Q_{10} affect aerobic capacity in endurance athletes? Int J Sport Nutr 1997;7:197-206.

Whanger PD, Beilstein MA, Thomson CD, Robinson MF, Howe M. Blood selenium and glutathione peroxidase activity of populations in New Zealand, Oregon, and South Dakota. FASEB J 1988;2:2996-3002.

Whitney EN, Rolfes SR. Understanding Nutrition. 7th ed. Minneapolis: West Publishing, 1996.

Williamson JR, Chang K, Frangos M, et al. Hyperglycemic pseudohypoxia and diabetic complications. Diabetes 1993;42(6):801-13.

Witt EH, Reznick AZ, Viguie CA, Starke-Reed P, Packer L. Exercise, oxidative damage and effects of antioxidant manipulation. J Nutr 1992;122:766-73.

Wylie-Rosett JA, Romney SL, Slagle S, et al. Influence of vitamin A on cervical dysplasia and carcinoma in situ. Nutr Cancer 1984;6:49-57.

Yagi K. Lipid peroxides and exercise. Med Sport Sci 1992;37:40-4.

Yoshioka M, Matsushita T, Chumen Y. Inverse association of serum ascorbic acid level and blood pressure on rate of hypertension in male adults aged 30-39 years. Int J Vit Nutr Res 1984;54:343-7.

Zeppilli P, Merlino B, DeLuca A, et al. Influence of coenzyme Q_{10} on physical work capacity in athletes, sedentary people, and patients with mitochondrial disease. In: Folkers K, Littarru G, Yamagami T, eds. Biomedical and Clinical Aspects of Coenzyme Q. Amsterdam: Elsevier, 1991:541-545.

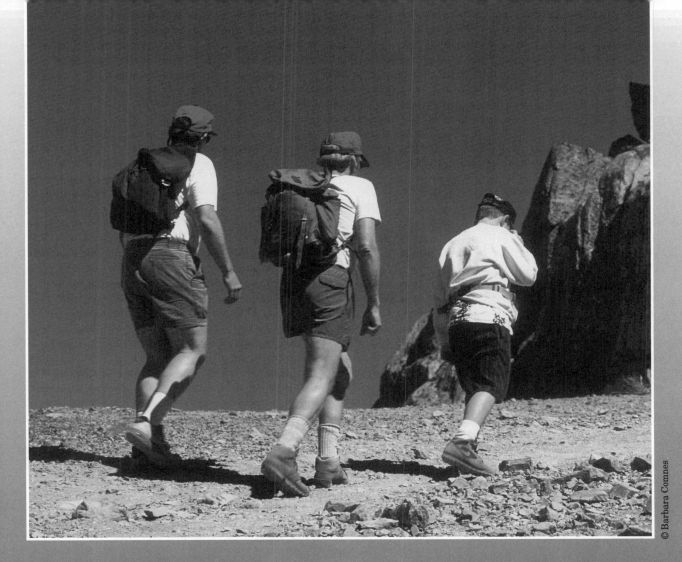

CHAPTER 11

Minerals and Exercise

After reading this chapter you will be able to

- identify the exercise-related functions, dietary requirements, and food sources of minerals;
- explain the rationale for increased need of certain minerals in active people;
- understand the assessment methods for zinc, magnesium, and chromium; and
- discuss the zinc, magnesium, and chromium status of active people.

Do you take a mineral supplement? If so, which supplement(s) do you use? What prompted you to begin supplementing? Active people have been bombarded with advertisements about supplements, especially mineral supplements like calcium (Ca) and iron (Fe). But what about minerals such as zinc (Zn), magnesium (Mg), copper (Cu), and chromium (Cr)? Do you need to supplement with these as well? Because minerals are different from vitamins in a number of ways, the decision to supplement with minerals requires different decision-making criteria.

This chapter addresses these questions and specifically looks at the requirements for iron, zinc, magnesium, copper, and chromium in active people. Because these minerals are especially important for the metabolism of macronutrients and the production of energy, they are grouped together in one chapter. Chapter 12 discusses the blood-building minerals (such as iron and copper) in detail; here we will discuss only their role in energy metabolism. Chapter 13 covers the minerals that help build bone, especially magnesium and calcium. In this chapter, we discuss magnesium only as it relates to energy metabolism and exercise-related functions unrelated to bones. Chapter 10 covers selenium in its role as an antioxidant.

In this chapter, we first review the exercise- and energy-related functions—and the dietary requirements and sources—of each mineral. Then we briefly cover the rationale for increased need in active people. Next we discuss how minerals differ from vitamins in their bioavailability, homeostatic mechanisms, and use by the body. We review the methods for assessing mineral status, including the biochemical assessment parameters measured. Then we review the mineral intakes of active people and address the impact of mineral deficiency or marginal mineral status on exercise performance. Finally, we examine whether exercise increases the mineral requirements of active people and whether mineral supplementation in healthy individuals enhances exercise performance.

Exercise-Related Functions, Dietary Requirements, and Food Sources

In order to discuss why exercise might increase a person's need for minerals, we must first explain the role of minerals in energy metabolism, their exercise-related functions, and their role in the maintenance of good health. Table 11.1 lists each mineral discussed in this chapter, the various metabolic pathways that require the mineral, and some of the specific enzymes that need it as a cofactor. Zinc, magnesium, iron, and copper are especially important for the metabolic pathways involved in energy metabolism and for the maintenance, building, and repair of muscle tissues. Chromium is important for glucose metabolism and optimal insulin action. The following section briefly discusses the specific exercise- and energy-related function of each of these minerals. Since chapter 12 reviews iron and copper in detail, only their role in energy metabolism is discussed here.

Iron

One of the primary functions of iron is the transport of oxygen in red blood cells, but it is also important for energy metabolism during exercise. Approximately 74% of the body's iron is in hemoglobin and myoglobin, while only 1% is found in oxidative enzymes (Lukaski 1995)—yet this 1% is vital to energy metabolism and is as important in energy production during exercise as is the delivery of oxygen via hemoglobin (table 11.1). Chapter 12 describes the dietary requirements for iron and its food sources.

Copper

Although copper is important for proper iron metabolism (see chapter 12) and hemoglobin production, like iron it is also important for energy metabolism. Copper is an important cofactor for the enzymes of the electron transport pathway (and therefore for production of energy). Copper is also required for **superoxide dismutase (SOD)**, an antioxidant enzyme that helps protect cells against oxidative damage. Finally, copper is important for the synthesis and maintenance of collagen. Chapter 12 describes the dietary requirements of copper and its food sources.

Zinc

Zinc is a cofactor for over 300 enzymes in the human body (Prasad 1995). Tables 11.1 and 11.2 list some of these enzymes and their related functions. Zinc is important in the structure and function of biomembranes and helps to stabilize the structures of **ribonucleic acid**

Table 11.1 **Exercise and Energy-Related Metabolic Functions of Minerals (Zinc, Magnesium, Iron, Copper, and Chromium)**

Mineral	Common form of the mineral in food and body	Functions related to exercise	Major enzymes or pathways that require the mineral as a cofactor
Zinc (Zn)	Zn^{2+}	Zn-containing enzymes function in carbohydrate, lipid, protein, and nucleic acid metabolism.	Lactate dehydrogenase, carbonic anhydrase, malate dehydrogenase, carboxypeptidase, alkaline phosphatase, alcohol dehydrogenase, glutamate dehydrogenase, superoxide dismutase
Magnesium (Mg)	Mg^{2+}	Mg-containing enzymes are involved in the glycolytic pathway, β-oxidation of fat, protein synthesis, metabolism, ATP hydrolysis, electrolyte balance, muscle contractions, and second-messenger systems.	Hexokinase, phosphofructokinase, pyruvatekinase, pyruvate dehydrogenase complex, acyl-CoA synthase
Iron (Fe)	Ferric iron (Fe^{3+}—oxidized iron), ferrous iron (Fe^{2+}—reduced iron)	Required for numerous enzymes involved in energy production during exercise. Required for the synthesis of hemoglobin and myoglobin.	Pyruvate oxidase, mitochondrial cytochromes, cytochrome P-450, ribonucleotide reductase, tyrosine and proline hydrolase, monoamine oxidase, catalase, glucose 6-phosphatase, 6-phosphogluconate dehydrogenase
Copper (Cu)	Found in three oxidation states: Cu^{0}, Cu^{1+}, Cu^{2+}, with Cu^{2+} being most common in nature	Cu is an important component of hemoglobin and myoglobin and is required for the proper utilizations of iron. Important for electron transport enzymes, enzymes involved in collagen synthesis, and synthesis of norepinephrine. Cu is also required to protect cells against oxidative damage.	Cytochrome-c oxidase, superoxide dismutase, protein-lysine 6-oxidase, dopamine-β-monooxygenase
Chromium (Cr)	Cr^{3+}, as part of glucose tolerance factor (GTF)	Potentiates the effect of insulin.	No chromium-dependent enzymes identified at this time

See the following references for more information on the exercise-related functions of these minerals: Haymes 1998; Haymes and Clarkson 1998; Reeves 1997; Weaver and Rajaram 1992.

(RNA), deoxyribonucleic acid (DNA), and ribosomes. Zinc is also important for growth and repair of tissue, maintenance of the immune response, and energy metabolism during exercise (King and Keen 1994). For example, zinc is required for protein metabolism, glucose utilization, insulin secretion, and lipid metabolism (Lukaski 1997). Because of these roles, zinc seriously affects energy substrate utilization during exercise and the building and repair of protein tissues after exercise. Zinc also plays an important role in hormone metabolism and is required for the production, storage, and secretion of growth hormone, thyroid hormones, gonadotropins, sex hormones, prolactin, and corticosteroids (Lukaski 1997). Finally, zinc is important for wound healing and skin integrity, skeletal and brain development, proper taste perception, reproduction, and gastrointes-

tinal function. Zinc occurs in all body tissues, 95% being within the cells. The amount of zinc in muscle varies, but the highest concentrations are found in slow-twitch, oxidative skeletal muscle fibers. Zinc is also found in high concentrations within bone tissue. Bone zinc levels appear to be the most responsive to changes in dietary intake and may reflect a gradual decline in total body zinc when zinc intake is poor (Lukaski 1997).

The body needs to absorb ~5 mg zinc/d to maintain the total body zinc pool of ~1.5-2.5 g. Since zinc absorption is estimated to be about 33% under controlled conditions (Cousins 1996), dietary zinc recommendations need to be higher than the actual amount absorbed. The current Recommended Dietary Allowance (RDA) for zinc is 15 mg/d for adult men and 12 mg/d for adult women aged ≥19 years (Food and

Table 11.2 **Zinc-Dependent Enzymes and Their Functions**

Specific enzyme	Function	Tissue
Carboxypeptidase	Digestion of dietary protein	Pancreas
Carbonic anhydrase	Acid/base balance	Numerous tissues
Alkaline dehydrogenase	Phosphate hydrolysis	Numerous tissues
Alcohol dehydrogenase	Metabolism of alcohol	Liver, kidney
Superoxide dismutase	Antioxidant	Liver
Lactate dehydrogenase	Conversion of lactate to pyruvate	Liver, muscle cells
Malate dehydrogenase	Metabolism of macronutrient	TCA cycle of the cells
Glutamate dehydrogenase	Transamination of amino acids	Numerous tissues/cells

Nutrition Board 1989). The RDA for zinc is similar to the zinc content of the typical mixed diet of North American adults (10-15 mg/d), which appears to provide adequate zinc to maintain zinc balance. An additional 3 mg/d are recommended during pregnancy, and an additional 7 mg/d during the first 6 mo of lactation (Food and Nutrition Board 1989).

Animal products, especially meat, provide 70% of the dietary zinc intake in the United States (King and Keen 1994). Within this food group, shellfish (especially oysters), beef, and other red meats have the highest zinc content by weight. See table 11.3 for the zinc content of commonly consumed foods. As you can see from this table, oysters have the highest zinc content at 28.2 mg in 3 oz (85 g) compared to 4.4 mg in 3 oz of ground beef. Red meats are higher in zinc than white meats like turkey, chicken, and some fish such as tuna or haddock. Cereal grains are the primary plant sources of zinc, and provide approximately 13% of the zinc intake in the United States (Lukaski 1997). Most of the zinc in cereal grains is in the bran and germ portions of the kernel. If these are removed with milling, then a significant portion of the zinc is lost. For example, whole wheat bread provides 0.5 mg of zinc per slice, while white bread provides less than half that amount (0.2 mg/slice). Note, however, that the zinc in cereal grains is less bioavailable due to the fiber and phytic acid content of cereals, which can inhibit zinc absorption. Although some breakfast cereals are fortified with zinc and can provide 25-100% of the RDA in one serving, the bioavailability of this zinc may be low due to the cooking process used in making these products. This cooking process, called extrusion cooking, inhibits the degradation of phytic acid in the gut and causes less efficient absorption of zinc (King and Keen 1999). Other dietary factors that may alter the

bioavailability of zinc in the diet are high supplemental intakes of iron, calcium, or tin; the tannic acid in tea and coffee; and caffeine. Fats, oils, soft drinks, alcohol, and most candies are low in zinc. Likewise, drinking water is also typically low in zinc. Recently, zinc-containing cold lozenges (~13 mg zinc/lozenge, dose = 6 lozenges/d) have been marketed as a way of reducing the severity of colds. Using the lozenges as recommended would result in ~80 mg of zinc/d. Chronic zinc intakes as low as 50 mg/d can induce secondary copper deficiency from competition between copper and zinc for absorption (Keen and King 1999). Caution should be used when supplementing with zinc, especially chronically high intakes.

Magnesium

As with zinc, magnesium is found throughout the body and plays a role in hundreds of enzymes and cellular functions (table 11.1). The most important exercise-related functions of magnesium are energy metabolism, protein synthesis, and neuromuscular transmission and activity. Magnesium is required for the glycolytic pathway, the synthesis and oxidation of fatty acids and proteins, adenosine triphosphate (ATP) hydrolysis, and for the formation of cyclic adenosine monophosphate (cAMP), a second-messenger system within cells (Lukaski 1995; Shils 1994). Several key enzymes in the glycolytic pathway require magnesium (hexokinase, phosphofructokinase, and pyruvate kinase); in the tricarbolic acid (TCA) cycle, pyruvate dehydrogenase requires magnesium. The first step in β-oxidation of fatty acids also requires magnesium for the acyl-CoA synthase complex (Shils 1994, 1996, 1999). It is clear that magnesium plays a vital role in substrate metabolism and in the production of energy for

Table 11.3 Zinc and Magnesium Content of Commonly Consumed Foods

Foods	Serving size	Zinc (mg/serving)	Magnesium (mg/serving)
Meats and fish			
Pacific oysters, steamed, medium	3 oz (85 g)	28.2	37.4
Ground beef (19% fat), fried	3 oz (85 g)	4.4	17.1
Beef chuck roast, choice, cooked	3 oz (85 g)	5.7	16.2
Beef steak, sirloin, choice/lean, cooked	3 oz (85 g)	5.6	27.2
Pork, cured bacon, cooked	3 oz (85 g)	2.8	20.4
Pork, cured ham, roasted	3 oz (85 g)	2.0	16.2
Pork, fresh rump roast, lean, cooked	3 oz (85 g)	2.6	24.5
Pork chop loin, blade, cooked	3 oz (85 g)	2.9	12.8
Pork chop, center cut, lean, fried	3 oz (85 g)	1.3	17.2
Chicken, boneless, roasted	3 oz (85 g)	1.8	21.3
Chicken, boneless breast, cooked	3 oz (85 g)	0.9	23.0
Chicken, boneless, thigh, cooked	3 oz (85 g)	2.2	20.4
Turkey, boneless, skinless, cooked	3 oz (85 g)	2.6	22.1
Turkey, dark meat, cooked	3 oz (85 g)	3.8	20.4
Turkey, white meat, cooked	3 oz (85 g)	1.8	23.9
Tuna, canned in water	3 oz (85 g)	0.8	24.7
Lobster, steamed	3 oz (85 g)	2.5	29.8
Shrimp, steamed	3 oz (85 g)	1.3	28.9
Salmon, sockeye, broiled	3 oz (85 g)	0.4	26.4
Dairy			
Milk, 2%	1 cup (244 g)	1.0	33.4
Yogurt, low-fat	1 cup (244 g)	2.2	42.9
Cottage cheese, 2% fat	1 cup (225 g)	1.0	13.6
Cheese, cheddar	1 oz (28g)	0.9	7.9
Cheese, Monterey Jack	1 oz (28 g)	0.8	7.7
Cereals, grains, and nuts			
Oatmeal, cooked	1 cup (234 g)	1.2	56.2
Shredded Wheat cereal	1 cup (43 g)	1.4	37.4
Cornflakes cereal	1 cup (25 g)	0.1	3.3
Total wheat cereal, General Mills	1 cup (40 g)	20.0	42.8
All-Bran cereal	1/3 cup (26 g)	5.5	71.7
Cheerios cereal, General Mills	1 cup (23 g)	2.8	24.7
Total Corn Flakes, General Mills	1 cup (40 g)	20.0	10.4
Almonds, dry roasted	1/4 cup (35 g)	1.7	104.9
Peanuts, dry roasted	1/4 cup (37 g)	1.2	64.2
Peanut butter, smooth	1 tbsp (16 g)	0.5	25.4
Walnuts, English	1/4 cup (30 g)	0.8	50.7
Sunflower seeds	1/4 cup (36 g)	1.8	127.4
Brewer's yeast	1 tbsp (8 g)	0.6	18.5

(continued)

Table 11.3 *(continued)*

Foods	Serving size	Zinc (mg/serving)	Magnesium (mg/serving)
Bread and pasta			
Whole wheat bread	1 slice (28 g)	0.5	24.1
White bread	1 slice (28 g)	0.2	6.9
English muffin	1 each (57 g)	0.4	12.0
Whole wheat bagel, small	1 each (55 g)	1.3	59.4
Pasta, cooked	1 cup (115 g)	0.6	20.1
Fruit			
Banana, medium	1 each (118 g)	0.2	34.2
Apple, medium	1 each (138 g)	0.1	6.9
Blueberries, fresh	1 cup (145 g)	0.1	7.3
Orange, large	1 each (184 g)	0.1	18.4
Vegetables			
Broccoli, cooked	1 cup (156 g)	0.6	37.4
Carrots, cooked	1 cup (156 g)	0.5	20.3
Green peas, cooked	1 cup (160 g)	1.9	62.4
Potato, baked	1 each (156 g)	0.5	39.0
Potato, mashed with whole milk	1 cup (210 g)	0.6	37.9
Tomato, whole	1 each (128 g)	0.1	13.5
Beans and legumes			
White beans, cooked	1/2 cup (90 g)	1.0	60.9
Pinto beans, cooked	1/2 cup (85 g)	0.9	47.0
Pork and beans in tomato sauce	1/2 cup (127 g)	7.4	44.3
Hummus	1/2 cup (123 g)	1.4	35.7

Data from Food Processor, Version 7.02, ESHA Research, Salem, OR, 1997.

physical activity. Magnesium also is required for membrane stability, energy-dependent membrane transport, muscle contractions, protein synthesis, immune response, and cardiovascular and hormonal functions (Food and Nutrition Board 1989; Shils 1994, 1996, 1999).

The RDA for magnesium is 400 mg/d for men ages 19-30 years and 420 mg/d for men ages 31-70 years. For women, the RDA for magnesium is 310 mg/d for ages 19-30 years and 320 mg/d for ages 31-70 years (Food and Nutrition Board 1997). The slight increase in the RDA for magnesium with age is attributed to more instances of negative balance in older subjects. It is recommended that pregnant women consume 360-400 mg/d of magnesium and that nursing mothers consume 320-360 mg/d (Food and Nutrition Board 1997). The specific amount of magnesium recommended during pregnancy or lactation depends on age, with younger women (14-18 years) requiring higher amounts of magnesium when they are pregnant or lactating.

Magnesium is widespread in foods but is highest in whole grain cereals, seeds, and legumes. See table 11.3 for magnesium content of various foods and food groups. Since >80% of the magnesium in cereal grains is in the germ and bran, processed cereal products lose much of their magnesium content. A slice of whole wheat bread contains 24 mg of magnesium, while white bread contains only 7 mg/slice. Thus, diets high in processed and convenience foods may be low in magnesium. Dairy and meat products provide moderate amounts of magnesium in adults but can contribute 30-35% of the daily magnesium intake in children and young adults due to their higher consumption of these products (Food and Nutrition Board 1989).

Chromium

Unlike the other minerals discussed so far, the role of chromium in exercise is less well defined. According to current research, chromium's primary biological role is to potentiate the effect of insulin, thereby enhancing the uptake and utilization of protein, fat, and carbohydrate (Nielsen 1994). Chromium is a constituent of a complex called the **glucose tolerance factor (GTF),** which also contains nicotinic acid and various amino acids (Nielsen 1994; Stoecker 1996). Although the exact physiological function of GTF is not known, it has been suggested that it facilitates the binding of insulin to its cellular receptor, increases the insulin receptor number, and improves insulin internalization and sensitivity (Anderson 1997; Clarkson 1997; Stoecker 1996). This in turn would raise glucose levels and increase amino acid and fatty acid uptake after a meal, when insulin is high. The amino acids would be used for tissue building and repair, and the fat and carbohydrate for either energy or storage. The role chromium plays in glucose utilization has been confirmed in chromium-deficient individuals who have impaired glucose tolerance but who show improvement when chromium is added back to the diet. Anderson et al. (1991) placed 11 women and 6 men on a low-chromium diet (<20 μg/d of chromium) or a low-chromium diet plus a chromium supplement (200 μg/d). The subjects used each diet for 4 weeks. The amount of chromium provided in the diet was equivalent to the lowest quartile of normal chromium intake in the United States. Glucose tolerance significantly improved for all subjects initially categorized as hyperglycemic (blood glucose values between 100 and 200 mg/dL were observed 90 min after an oral glucose tolerance test) when they received the chromium supplement. There was no improvement in glucose tolerance when they were on the low-chromium diet alone without supplemental chromium. These data demonstrate that low chromium intakes may lead to detrimental effects on glucose tolerance, insulin, and glucagon in subjects with mildly impaired glucose tolerance.

Chromium is also important for growth, improved blood lipid profiles, synthesis of DNA and RNA, and proper immune function (Stoecker 1996). Some metabolic stressors—such as exercise, pregnancy, lactation, and infection—appear to increase chromium losses in the urine. This increased loss of chromium in the urine would suggest that individuals with these stresses might have greater chromium needs. This in turn might suggest an increased requirement in this population.

There is no RDA for chromium since (1) there are no reliable measures of chromium status, (2) there are no identified enzymes that require chromium, and (3) information regarding the chromium content of food is not available. Without an accurate nutrient database for chromium, it is impossible to assess the chromium content of large populations; thus, data on chromium intake in the United States are limited. With the few data available, the Food and Nutrition Board set an **estimated safe and adequate daily dietary intake (ESADDI)** for chromium at 50-200 μg/d (Food and Nutrition Board 1989). The normal consumption of chromium in the United States is estimated to be 50-60% of the minimum ESADDI of 50 μg/d. Data supporting low chromium intakes in the United States come from smaller studies examining the chromium intake of individuals. Using paired plate analysis, Anderson and Kozlovsky (1985) estimated 7-d mean dietary intakes to be 25 μg/d for women and 33 μg/d for men. It is estimated that the typical chromium intake of self-selected American diets is approximately 15 μg/1000 kcal (Anderson et al. 1992). According to these estimates, an individual consuming a 2000 kcal/d diet would obtain only 30 μg/d of chromium. Additional information supporting low chromium intakes in the United States comes from chromium supplement studies, which indicate that approximately 50% of the subjects show improvement in glucose tolerance with chromium supplementation (Anderson 1997). *These data suggest that the current chromium intake in the United States is not optimal.*

The chromium content of food varies widely and depends on a number of factors, including where the food is grown and what processing techniques are used. The best sources of chromium in our diets are whole grains, some ready-to-eat cereals, mushrooms, brewer's yeast, spices, dark chocolate, and processed meats

(Lefavi et al. 1992). Processing adds chromium to the food through the leaching of chromium from stainless steel (11-30% chromium) containers (Stoecker 1996). Some beers contain high amounts of chromium for the same reason. Unprocessed meats, poultry, fish, and dairy products are low in chromium, while fruits and vegetables are more variable in their chromium content. In general, diets high in simple sugars will provide low levels of chromium since these foods have little chromium. Table 11.4 gives the chromium content of selected foods.

Intestinal absorption of chromium is low (approximately 0.5-3%), and absorption increases or decreases within this range depending on the dietary chromium intake. A number of dietary factors appear to alter the availability of dietary chromium. For example, starch and ascorbic acid (vitamin C) increase absorption, while oxalates and phytates may either increase or decrease absorption depending on their concentration in the diet (Stoecker 1996). High simple sugar intakes increase the loss of chromium in urine and decrease chromium absorption, while high iron intakes may alter chromium transport in the blood. Both chromium and iron are transported on transferrin. If transferrin is saturated with iron, then the ability to transport chromium is reduced and chromium must be transported on an alternative protein like albumin (Nielsen 1994). The reverse also appears to be true. High intakes of chromium (>200 μg/d) apparently decrease iron absorption and transport and appear to negatively impact iron status (Lukaski, Bolonchuk et al. 1996). The impact of chromium supplementation on iron status may depend on the level of chromium and iron in the diet, initial iron status, and the length of chromium supplementation. Short-term chromium supplementation (<12 weeks) did not negatively affect iron status in older men engaged in a strength-training program (Campbell et al. 1997).

Rationale for Increased Need for Active Individuals

Because minerals are cofactors for many metabolic reactions that produce energy, it is only natural to hypothesize that exercise increases the need for these nutrients. Minerals are also necessary for other biological functions important for exercise, such as synthesis and repair of muscle tissues, a healthy immune function, and cell reproduction. Finally, by increasing mineral loss in urine or sweat, exercise may alter the body's overall mineral balance and increase the intakes required to maintain good balance.

As people become more physically active, it is logical to assume that they will increase their energy intake—and that their dietary intakes of minerals will likewise increase—so there

Table 11.4   Chromium Content of Selected Foods

Food	Serving size	Chromium (μg/serving)
Cheese, Edam	1 slice (24 g)	0.5
Milk, whole	1 cup (244 g)	2.4
Oysters, raw	3 oz (90 g)	12.6
Cornflakes	1 cup (25 g)	1.8
Bread, whole wheat	1 slice (25 g)	0.8
Brown rice, raw	1/6 cup (66 g)	2.0
Apple, raw, medium	1 each (150 g)	7.5
Mushrooms, white	1/2 cup (35 g)	16.4
Beer	12 oz (360 g)	3.2
Brewer's yeast	1 tbsp (8 g)	3.3
Cocoa	1 tbsp (5 g)	0.7
Wine, white	3.5 oz (102 g)	7.6

Data from Anderson and Guttman 1988.

would be no need for mineral supplements. Unfortunately, this is not always true. If people make poor dietary choices, their mineral intake may not increase in parallel with their higher energy intake. And if people increase physical activity while *restricting* energy intake, as often happens with people who are trying to lose weight, the overall need for minerals may increase while the intake is actually decreasing. Initially it would appear that mineral supplements would solve this problem, yet there are problems with casually adding mineral supplements to the diet. High supplements of one mineral may change the bioavailability and status of another. Because of these mineral-mineral interactions, it is important to examine a person's overall mineral intake before making dietary and supplemental mineral recommendations.

Assessment of Mineral Status

Assessment of mineral status is different from the assessment of vitamin status in a number of ways:

- Bioavailability of dietary minerals is generally less than that of vitamins since a number of dietary factors can inhibit the absorption and the transport of minerals into the system. **Bioavailability** is defined as the proportion of any nutrient in food that is absorbed and utilized.

- For many minerals, total-body homeostasis is controlled, in part, by limiting absorption of the mineral in the gut, thereby increasing the loss of excess mineral in the feces. For most water-soluble vitamins, total-body homeostasis is controlled through urinary excretion of the excess vitamin.

- To protect the body from toxic levels of minerals, absorption decreases as intake increases. The mineral may be absorbed into the intestinal mucosal cell but not transported into the system. In this way, the mineral is lost in the feces when the mucosal cell turns over. Although vitamin absorption also decreases as intake increases, any excess amounts absorbed are excreted in the urine.

- Many minerals are found in trace amounts in the diet. It is difficult to overload with diet alone; toxic levels can be achieved only through supplementation or contamination.

- Some trace minerals, like chromium, occur in quantities so small that they are difficult to measure in food and bodily fluids; it is likewise difficult to accurately predict dietary intake.

- High mineral intakes (many times the RDA) are generally much more toxic than high vitamin intakes.

- Many minerals compete with other minerals for absorption and transport. For example, high zinc intake can inhibit copper absorption when the two minerals are taken simultaneously. This nutrient-nutrient interaction occurs to a lesser extent with vitamins.

- Forms of minerals in food may vary, making minerals more or less bioavailable depending on their dietary source. Although vitamins also come in many different forms, bioavailability is generally less an issue than with minerals.

- Unlike vitamins, many minerals are lost in the sweat. The loss of minerals via sweat may be a contributing factor in total-body mineral balance and may increase mineral requirements.

Biochemical Assessment of Mineral Status

Assessment of an individual's mineral status requires measurement of a number of indices (table 11.5)—usually including, if possible, biochemical measures of body fluids that reflect the body's stores of the nutrient. Determination of the amount of the mineral lost from the body in urine, blood, feces, or sweat must also be done. If available, functional measurements of mineral status should be included (Lukaski 1995; Lukaski and Penland 1996)—that is, measures that determine the *availability* of the mineral to perform a particular physiological function within the body. Is there, for example, enough of the mineral for maximal enzyme activity? Finally, the typical dietary intake of the mineral should be determined. The various forms of the mineral found in the diet should also be assessed if they affect bioavailability. Dietary factors that may increase or decrease bioavailability of the mineral need to be identified, including supplemental vitamins and minerals, drugs, or food supplements. At the present time, assessments of zinc, magnesium, and chromium status are not nearly as well developed as those for iron or for many of the vitamins.

Zinc

Assessment of zinc status is hampered by the lack of a single specific and sensitive biochemical

Table 11.5 Experimental Approaches for Assessment of Human Mineral Nutritional Status

Approach	Variable	Standard
Diet records—7 consecutive days if possible, covering a weeks typical exercise days.	Assessment of daily absolute mineral intake (mg/d) and relative mineral intake (mg/1000 kcal). Assessment of all supplemental mineral intake and all dietary factors that may influence mineral bioavailability.	Average or typical intake greater than 70% of RDA or ESADDI. With the new DRIs, an EAR is calculated. This value is estimated to meet the requirement of 50% of the individuals in a specific life stage or gender group.
Blood biochemical index	Plasma or serum concentrations; mineral-specific enzyme activity in erthrocytes, platelets, or leukocytes; transport proteins for minerals; tissue concentrations.	Within range of values for nutritionally adequate, gender-matched, control subjects.
Excretion/losses	Urinary, fecal, blood, or sweat losses.	Increased absolute (mg/d) or relative (% of daily intake) amounts in some designated time period.
Functional markers	Exposure to a controlled stessor such as exercise, temperature, mineral load, or a mental task.	Perturbation of response to a challenge that affects the performance of an integrated biological system or subsystem

RDA = Recommended Dietary Intake; ESADDI = Estimated Safe and Adequate Daily Dietary Intake; EAR = estimated average requirement; DRI = Dietary reference intake

Adapted from Lukaski 1995; Lukaski and Penland 1996.

or functional test in humans (King 1990; King and Keen 1994, 1999). As table 11.5 outlines, the most common way to determine mineral status is to assess static biochemical parameters, such as plasma or urinary zinc. A second approach is to measure a physiological function, such as the activity a zinc-dependent enzyme like alkaline phosphatase (Lukaski 1997). If enzyme activity is low at baseline but increases with additional zinc, then inadequate zinc was initially available. Other suggested functional measures for zinc are resting metabolic rate, ethanol metabolism, and cognitive performance measures (Lukaski and Penland 1996). Unfortunately, none of these tests has the specificity and reliability necessary to be the standard for zinc assessment. Another suggested method for measuring marginal zinc deficiency is the zinc load test, where a positive response indicates poor zinc status (Gibson 1990). However, this approach is expensive, time-consuming, and impractical for clinical assessment. Since there is no good single assessment parameter for zinc, clinicians often use a combination of biochemical and functional measures to assess status. These assessment parameters should always be accompanied by the measurement of dietary zinc

intakes and any factors that may confound zinc bioavailability.

Plasma and serum are the body fluids most often used for zinc assessment, but these appear to be relatively insensitive to modest changes in dietary zinc intake or to changes in the total-body zinc pool (Lukaski 1997). As zinc deficiency occurs (e.g., low dietary zinc intakes), the body conserves zinc, making serum zinc unreliable as a measure of zinc status. In addition, serum zinc concentrations do not decrease unless dietary zinc intake is so low that the total zinc pool is decreased and homeostasis cannot be maintained. Thus, serum zinc can be thought of as a labile pool of zinc that is part of the total-body zinc pool. The body draws on this pool when intake is low; thus low serum zinc is an indication that the body's labile zinc pool is low and that dietary zinc intake is probably low also. Another problem with using serum or plasma zinc as a measure of zinc status is that a number of other factors, unrelated to poor zinc intake, can alter serum zinc concentrations (see "What Is the Difference Between Serum and Plasma?" on page 315). Exercise, stress, acute infection or inflammation, short-term fasting, or hormonal status can alter the distribution of zinc within the body, thus influencing the amount of zinc in the serum (Gibson 1990; Lukaski 1997). Neither serum nor urinary zinc is a good indicator of marginal zinc deficiency because during times of deficiency each will decrease (serum zinc is considered low at <12 μmol/L) (Gibson 1990; Lukaski 1997).

Since the body maintains homeostatic control of zinc by balancing absorption of dietary zinc with excretion of endogenous secretions in the feces (Cousins 1996; King and Keen 1994, 1999), the intestine is a key tissue in maintaining zinc balance. The body can also lose zinc in the urine and sweat; it has been suggested that active individuals, especially athletes with high sweat rates, have increased zinc losses. Sweat zinc losses appear to depend on the location from which the sweat is collected, on exercise intensity and duration, and on environmental conditions (Lukaski 1995, 1997). Losses of trace minerals in sweat are hard to measure due to their low concentration, the technical problems of measuring total sweat losses, and the high probability of sample contamination from body cells and handling techniques. Given these problems with zinc-sweat measurements, Tipton et al. (1993) measured arm sweat rates in male and female athletes exercising at 50% $\dot{V}O_2$max for 1 h in a neutral and in a hot environment. Sweat zinc concentrations ranged from 0.35-1.5 μg/ml. These figures imply that the zinc lost in 1 L of sweat would range from 0.35-1.5 mg, or 2-13% of total daily recommended zinc intakes. The impact that zinc sweat losses have on total zinc balance depends on total sweat losses, zinc lost through other routes, and total zinc intake.

Magnesium

As with zinc, there is no single, specific, reliable biochemical marker for magnesium status (Shils 1994, 1999). Thus, magnesium status is determined by measuring concentrations of magnesium in body fluids, intact cells, and cell partitions. Dietary magnesium intake should also be determined along with any factor that may alter magnesium bioavailability (e.g., dietary components, drugs, and mineral supplements).

Serum magnesium is the most frequently used index for determining magnesium status, despite its low sensitivity and specificity. One reason for this is that better indices are not available, and serum magnesium does appear to mimic tissue concentrations of magnesium when dietary magnesium is low. This point is illustrated in figure 11.1, where you can see that both serum and urinary magnesium concentrations decrease when magnesium is removed from the diet. However, a number of other factors—such as various diseases and stressors, artificial factors (e.g., dehydration, medications or drugs being used), and diurnal variations—can also alter serum magnesium concentration; thus, it is not an ideal indicator of status. In addition, serum represents only a small portion of the body's total magnesium pool (<1%) (Gibson 1990). Normal serum ranges from 0.8-1.2 mmol/L (Lukaski 1995) and comprises three general components: ionized or unbound magnesium (55% of serum magnesium), complexed magnesium (13%), and bound magnesium (32%) (Gibson 1990; Shils 1994,

■ HIGHLIGHT ■

What Is the Difference Between Serum and Plasma?

Plasma is the noncellular portion of the circulating blood, while serum is the noncellular portion of the blood that is obtained after coagulation of the blood. To obtain plasma, blood is drawn in a tube containing an anticoagulant and then centrifuged (spun). The cells of the blood settle to the bottom of the tube, and the plasma is left on top. To obtain serum, a tube of blood is drawn that does not contain an anticoagulant. The clotting factors in the blood will settle to the bottom of the tube with the cells when the tube is centrifuged; what remains on top is serum. Depending on the biochemical assay being done, you may need serum or plasma. Sometimes either is acceptable. In general, minerals are usually measured in serum to avoid any mineral contamination that might occur due to the additives used as anticoagulants. For example, with zinc and magnesium, usually serum is measured, but plasma is also acceptable as long as the anticoagulant is free of mineral contamination.

1999). Magnesium can be bound to transport proteins such as albumin or globulin, or complexed with other substances in the blood, such as citrate or phosphate. It has been suggested that the level of ionized magnesium may be a more reliable clinical measure of magnesium status (Shils 1994), yet work still needs to be done to validate this as a reliable status marker. Erythrocyte magnesium concentrations are frequently measured and appear to reflect chronic magnesium status since the half-life of the red cell is 120 d and concentrations decrease only after several weeks of poor magnesium intake (Gibson 1990). However, as with serum magnesium, a number of factors unrelated to dietary magnesium can influence erythrocyte magnesium concentrations. More recently, magnesium concentrations of leukocytes and other cell types have been examined, and animal data suggest they reflect muscle tissue magnesium content (Gibson 1990). Unfortunately, current clinical data have not been supportive of this hypothesis (Shils 1994). Urinary magnesium concentrations, in combination with dietary magnesium intake, can be helpful in indicating whether there are increased urinary losses or decreased absorption of magnesium.

Currently, there are no good functional mea-

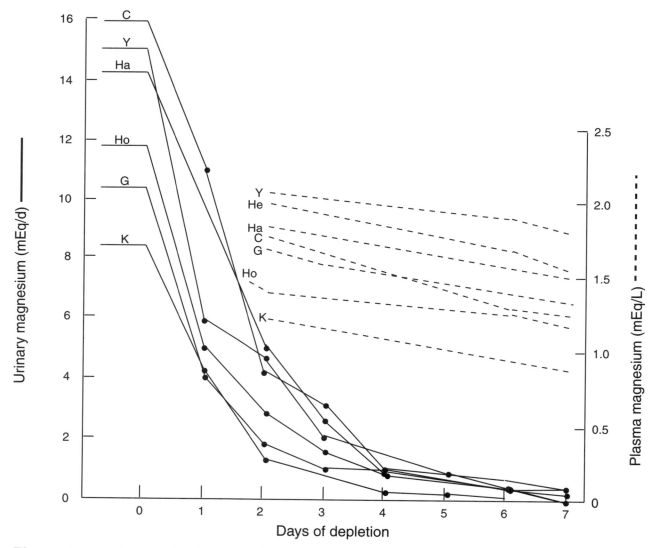

Figure 11.1 Changes in plasma and urinary magnesium concentrations during 1 week of a zero-magnesium diet. The rapid decrease in magnesium excretion is depicted in six subjects. By the 10th day, all plasma values except that of Y were more than 2 standard deviations below the normal mean. Letters indicate individual subjects.

Reprinted from Shils 1994.

sures of magnesium status. Some researchers and clinicians use the magnesium load test as a functional measure of short-term magnesium deficiency (Gibson 1990; Shils 1999). The magnesium load test involves first the infusion of magnesium and then the collection of urinary magnesium for at least 12-24 h. High magnesium retention (20-50% of the magnesium infused) is indicative of magnesium deficiency (Gibson 1990). Unfortunately, this assessment is very expensive, invasive, nonstandardized, and time-consuming, and it is not practical in clinical settings. Since no single reliable assessment measure is available, most clinicians use a combination of static biochemical measures and determination of dietary magnesium intake to assess magnesium status.

The body's magnesium pool can be roughly divided into three areas: approximately 30-35% in the muscles and soft issues, 1% in the extracellular fluid, the rest in the bone (60-65%) (Gibson 1990). The body maintains magnesium homeostasis through both fecal and urinary excretion. With free-living diets containing 234-323 mg/d of magnesium, absorption ranges from 21-27% (Shils 1994). Absorption varies with dietary intake: with low magnesium intakes (7-36 mg/d), absorption increases (65-77%); it decreases (11-14%) with high magnesium intakes (960-1000 mg/d) (Shils 1996). Inhibiting or promoting other dietary components can also influence magnesium absorption. For example, high levels of dietary or supplemental calcium or phosphate may decrease absorption. The kidneys further regulate magnesium homeostasis through urinary magnesium excretion by either increasing or decreasing output, depending on intake, while maintaining blood magnesium concentrations. Like zinc, magnesium is lost in blood and sweat; thus, active individuals with high sweat rates may have increased magnesium losses. Sweat losses of magnesium are estimated to be approximately 7 mg/L, with estimates of 15-18 mg of magnesium lost per day in hot environments (Lukaski 1995). The amount of magnesium lost in the sweat represents approximately 10-15% of total daily magnesium losses (feces, urine, and sweat losses combined), including 4-5% of the daily requirement for men and 5-6% of the requirement for women.

Chromium

At present there are no identified biochemical or clinical methods for assessing chromium sta-tus. Although chromium concentrations can be measured in a number of biological fluids and tissues, none is specific enough to make a good marker of chromium status. In addition, chromium is present in such trace amounts that it is difficult to measure accurately, and contamination can easily occur. Blood or serum chromium concentrations do not appear to reflect tissue concentrations in periods of marginal chromium depletion (Stoecker 1996)—but serum chromium concentrations are low in individuals with chromium deficiency, and high serum concentrations may indicate excessive environmental exposure to chromium. Assessment of hair chromium may reflect endogenous chromium available to the hair, but the samples need to be carefully prepared to prevent chromium contamination from other sources (no bleaches or dyes). In addition, a number of other factors appear to influence hair chromium concentrations, such as age, hair growth rate, pregnancy, and diabetes. Thus, hair chromium does not solely reflect dietary chromium intake. Urinary chromium is frequently used as an index of chromium status because the kidneys appear to regulate chromium homeostasis (Gibson 1990; Stoecker 1996). Unfortunately, changes in urinary chromium better reflect increases in total-body chromium (induced by excessive chromium intakes or exposure) than deficiencies. Urinary chromium can be used to determine if chromium supplements are being used or if an individual has been exposed to high environmental exposure. However, no data are available demonstrating that decreased urinary chromium excretion indicates moderate chromium deficiency (Gibson 1990). A number of confounding factors also affect urinary chromium concentrations, such as diurnal variations, dietary glucose or sucrose intake, salts in the urine, exercise, and trauma (Gibson 1990).

Currently, the best method for diagnosing chromium deficiency is to observe whether chromium supplementation improves glucose tolerance (Gibson 1990). This method requires the administration of two **oral glucose tolerance tests (OGTTs).** The first OGTT determines the baseline response to a glucose load (75 g glucose, or 1 g glucose/kg body weight); the second test is done after supplementing with physiological levels of chromium. After each OGTT, the total area under the curve is determined. If the area under the curve decreases with chromium supplementation, then poor chromium status is indicated. This test is very time-consuming, expensive, requires numerous blood samples, and is not practical for clinical diagnosis.

Dietary Intakes of Active Individuals

The following section briefly reviews the dietary intakes of active individuals for zinc, magnesium, and chromium. Dietary intakes of these minerals are compared to the typical American diet, the 1989 RDAs for zinc and chromium, and the new dietary reference intakes (DRIs) for magnesium. In 1997, a new DRI for magnesium was determined, while the zinc and chromium RDAs were last published in 1989 (Food and Nutrition Board 1989, 1997). Because many studies examining the magnesium intake of active people were done before the new DRIs for magnesium were published, their nutrient intakes are compared to the old 1989 RDA for magnesium. Chapter 12 reviews the dietary intakes of active people for iron and copper.

Zinc

The actual amount of zinc provided by the typical American diet averages about 11-13 mg/d (Moser-Veillon 1990), with an average zinc density of 5 mg/1000 kcal. In general, males select diets that provide approximately 90% of the RDA (15 mg/d), while females self-select diets with approximately 81% of the RDA (12 mg/d). The 1982-1991 Total Diet Studies indicated that for males aged 14-16 years and 25-30 years, zinc intake was at 105% and 108% of the RDA, respectively (Pennington 1996). For females of the same age groups, zinc intake was 83% and 80% of the RDA, respectively. These data further suggest that most adults in the United States consume at least 66% of the RDA for zinc.

Self-reported dietary zinc intakes of active males and male athletes reveal that zinc intake is usually at or above the RDA. Table 11.6 gives the dietary zinc intakes of active men who did not take zinc supplements: no study reported mean intakes in men to be less than two-thirds the RDA, while most reported mean intakes above the RDA. As is true in the general female population, female athletes have zinc intakes below the RDA. Only one study listed in table 11.6 reports mean zinc intakes for active women above the RDA. The lower zinc intakes of active women are usually attributed to their lower intakes of animal products and their lower overall energy intakes. If energy intake is restricted to less than 1900 kcal/d, it

is almost impossible to consume adequate minerals unless a person makes extremely good food choices. This problem is compounded when someone combines low energy intake with low intakes of meat products or with diets high in processed foods. Beals and Manore (1998) demonstrated the effect of reduced energy intake on zinc intake in active women. They found that 88% of their female athletes with a subclinical eating disorder, and 83% of their control athletes, consumed less than the RDA for zinc. However, only 13% of the control athletes, compared with 50% of the eating disordered athletes, consumed less than two-thirds of the RDA for zinc. Thus, energy restriction can significantly affect mineral intake, even for people who are making good food choices.

Magnesium

Magnesium intake of the typical American diet is estimated to be approximately 329 mg/d (94% of the Estimated Average Requirement [EAR]; 78% of the 1997 RDA) for men and 207 mg/d for women (78% of the EAR; 65% of the 1997 RDA). The 1982-1991 Total Diet Studies indicated that for males aged 14-16 years and 25-30 years, magnesium intake was at 75% and 86% of the 1989 RDA, respectively (Pennington 1996). For females of the same age groups, magnesium intake was 65% and 70% of the 1989 RDA, respectively (Pennington 1996). According to the new DRIs for magnesium, these intakes are ~65-85% of the EAR and 53-73% of the RDA, suggesting that most American adults consume at least 66% of the 1997 RDA for magnesium; however, the magnesium intakes of younger females, aged 14-16 years, appear to be low. The magnesium density of the typical American diet is approximately 120 mg of magnesium per 1000 kcal. Based on this nutrient density, the typical man would need to consume 3500 kcal/d, and the typical woman would need to consume 2666 kcal/d, to meet the 1997 RDA for magnesium. These estimates demonstrate the importance of total energy intake on dietary magnesium intake. *People who reduce energy intake without increasing the magnesium density of the diet (milligrams / 1000 kcal) will consume inadequate levels of magnesium.*

The magnesium intake of active people is similar to that reported for the typical adult in the United States. Most studies, published before the new DRIs/RDAs for magnesium were released, report mean magnesium intakes of athletes or active individuals at or above two-thirds of the 1989 RDA, which was 350 mg/d for men and 280 mg/d for women (Clarkson and Haymes 1995; Jensen et al. 1992). Note that the new 1997 RDA for magnesium increased for both men (420 mg/d) and women (320 mg/d), as indicated above. As table 11.6 shows, mean magnesium intakes of male athletes are usually well above the 1989 RDA and the 1997 EAR but are below the 1997 RDA for magnesium. The lowest reported intake levels (Manore et al. 1995) reported mean magnesium intakes at 88% of the 1997 RDA (which is 420 mg/d) and below the EAR (350 mg/d) for males participating in fitness type exercise, and no studies reported mean intakes less than two-thirds of the RDA. The high magnesium intake of male athletes is frequently attributed to their high energy intakes. Table 11.6 shows that mean magnesium intakes of female athletes also appear to be at or near the new EAR but below the RDA for magnesium. As mentioned earlier, if energy intake is restricted, magnesium intakes can be low. For example, Beals and Manore (1998) reported that 54% of their athletes with subclinical eating disorders consumed less than 280 mg/d of magnesium (~88% of the RDA; 106% of the EAR) and 8% consumed less than 184 mg/d (58% of the RDA; ~70% of the EAR). But only 17% of the control athletes consumed less than 280 mg/d of magnesium (~88% of the RDA), and none consumed less than 184 mg/d of magnesium (~70% of the EAR). In this study, the athletes with subclinical eating disorders reported consuming only 1989 kcal/d while the control athletes consumed 2293 kcal/d—closer to the energy requirement needed to meet the RDA for magnesium. Two other studies dramatically demonstrate the effect of low energy intakes on dietary magnesium in female athletes. Baer et al. (1992) reported that eumenorrheic runners consuming 1644 kcal/d took in only 148 mg/d of magnesium (~56% of the EAR), while amenorrheic runners consuming 1912 kcal/d obtained 224 mg/d (84% of the EAR). Kaiserauer et al. (1989) also reported that when female runners consumed less than 1582 kcal/d, 55% of them had magnesium intakes less than the 280 mg/d.

Chromium

Since there are no reliable nutrient databases for chromium, determining chromium intake is difficult, and few researchers have attempted it. As mentioned earlier, Anderson and Kozlovsky (1985) examined the typical chromium intakes of 10 men and 22 women for 7 d using duplicate meal analyses. They found that 90% of the diets contained less than 50 μg/d of chromium. To date, no study has examined dietary chromium intake in active people. However, if we use the chromium data reported for the typical American diet, it is safe to assume that, unless active people are making good dietary choices, chromium intake may be at the low end of the recommended ESADDI (50-200 μg/d).

Nutritional Status of Active People

Attempts to measure zinc and magnesium status in athletes have been hampered by the lack of reliable biochemical indices of status and by the use of varied experimental designs, which make comparing studies difficult (Lukaski 1997). It is therefore difficult to set concise zinc and magnesium recommendations for people engaged in hard exercise training. Although there is little reliable information on assessment of chromium status in active individuals, chromium picolinate supplements have been marketed to athletes to increase muscle mass and to dieters as "fat burners." This type of marketing has made chromium a household word, yet research supporting these claims has not been forthcoming. This section reviews the available research on zinc, magnesium, and chromium status in active individuals.

Zinc

Both acute and chronic exercise appear to significantly affect zinc metabolism. Serum zinc increases immediately after acute strenuous exercise (Anderson et al. 1995; Deuster et al. 1991; Lukaski 1997; Lukaski et al. 1984). Deuster et al. (1991) measured serum zinc concentrations before and after the first women's Olympic marathon trials in May of 1984. Serum zinc concentrations increased 10% above prerace values immediately after exercise but returned to baseline or below baseline concentrations within 30 min to 24 h post-exercise. The magnitude of the increase in serum zinc immediately post-exercise cannot be explained by hemoconcentration alone. It is possible that the increase in serum zinc results from leakage of zinc from damaged muscle tissue into

Table 11.6 **Incidence of Low or Marginal Zinc (Zn) and Magnesium (Mg) Status in Nonsupplemented Active People**

Study	Assessment indices	No. subjects	Type of subjects	Low status (%)	Mean dietary intake (mg/d)	(mg/1000 kcal)	Type of diet record
Zinc							
Beals and Manore 1998[1]	Serum Zn	24	Control female athletes	0%	10.4*	4.9	7-d
		24	SCED female athletes	0%	9.7*	4.5	7-d
Couzy et al. 1990	Serum Zn	6	Male middle-distance runners	0%	—	—	—
Deuster et al. 1989	Plasma and RBC Zn 24-h urinary Zn Oral Zn load	13	Female runners	100%	10.3*	4.4	3-d
Fogelholm, Rehunen et al. 1992	Serum Zn	5	Male elite Nordic skiers	0%	21.9	5.8	28-d
		7	Female elite Nordic skiers	0%	15.8	5.6	28-d
Fogelholm, Himberg et al. 1992	Serum Zn	418	Male athletes	1%	17.5	5.7	FFQ
Fogelholm et al. 1991	Serum Zn RBC Zn	114	Male endurance athletes	0%	17.7	5.9	FFQ
Lukaski et al. 1990	Plasma Zn	13	Male swimmers	0%	15.6	4.6	7-d
		16	Female swimmers	0%	10.4*	4.8	7-d
Lukaski et al. 1996	Plasma Zn	5	Male swimmers	0%	17.6	4.7	3-d
		5	Female swimmers	0%	10.5*	4.9	3-d
Manore et al. 1993	Serum Zn	34	Trained males	0%	13.2*	5.1	9-d
Singh, Moses, and Deuster 1992	Plasma and RBC Zn[2] Urine Zn	11	Active males	0%	10.8*	3.9	4-d
Telford et al. 1992	Serum Zn	44	Athletes[2,3]	2%	—	—	—
Weight et al. 1988	Serum Zn	30	Male runners	0%	13.2*	5.3	5-d

Magnesium

Study	Measure	N	Group	% supplemented			Record
Beals and Manore 1998[1]	Serum Mg	24	Control female athletes	0%	351	153	7-d
		24	SCED female athletes	0%	283*	142	7-d
Fogelholm, Himberg et al. 1992	Serum Mg	418	Male athletes	0%	510	164	FFQ
Fogelholm et al. 1991	Serum Mg RBC Mg	114	Male endurance athletes	0%	548	183	FFQ
Lukaski, Siders et al. 1996	Serum Mg	5	Male swimmers	0%	393*	110	3-d
		5	Female swimmers	0%	269*	125	3-d
Manore et al. 1995	Serum, RBC Mg Urinary Mg	34	Males in 12-week exercise program	0%	330	126	9-d
Singh, Moses, and Deuster 1992	Plasma and RBC Mg[2] Urinary Mg	11	Active males	0%	355*	127	4-d
Telford et al. 1992	Serum Mg	44	Athletes[2,3]	0%	—	—	—
Weight et al. 1988	Serum Mg	30	Male runners	0%	372*	157	5-d

[1]25% of subjects supplemented with some type of vitamin or mineral supplement.

[2]Data from placebo group only (no supplements).

[3]Included both males and females.

FFQ = food frequency questionnaire; SCED = athletes with subclinical eating disorders; RBC = red blood cells.

*Mean value is less than the recommended dietary allowance (RDA). RDA for Zn is 12 mg/d for women and 15 mg/d for men (FNB 1989). RDA for Mg is 320 mg/d for women (19-70 years) and 420 mg/d for men (19-70 years) (FNB 1997).

the extracellular fluid or from a redistribution of zinc from other tissues to the serum (Cordova and Alvarez-Mon 1995; Lukaski 1997; Ohno et al. 1985). The return of serum zinc concentrations to pre-exercise levels or below during the recovery period may be due to increased loss of zinc in the urine, or possibly to the uptake of zinc by other tissues such as the liver or muscles. If exercise causes an increase in urinary zinc losses, then overall zinc balance could be negatively affected. Data reporting increased urinary zinc losses after exercise have been equivocal. For example, Anderson et al. (1984) observed a 50% increase in runners' urinary zinc 1 h after a 10-mi race; other studies have reported no change after exercise (Anderson et al. 1995; Singh, Moses et al. 1992; Buchman et al. 1998). These inconsistencies may result in part from differences in exercise duration and intensity, in the fitness levels of the subjects, and in dietary zinc intakes.

Long-term strenuous exercise can significantly affect zinc metabolism. Athletes, especially endurance athletes, appear to have reduced resting serum zinc concentrations. Dressendorfer and Sockolov (1980) observed that runners (n = 77) had significantly lower serum zinc concentrations than controls (n = 21). Eighteen of the runners (23% of the group) had serum zinc concentrations <11.5 μmol/L. They also reported that *serum zinc concentrations were inversely related to weekly training distance*. These data have been supported by subsequent observations of low resting serum zinc concentrations in athletes (Deuster et al. 1989; Haralambie 1981; Miyamura et al. 1987; Singh et al. 1991). It is possible that these lower serum zinc concentrations are due to one or more of the following factors:

- Endurance athletes have low dietary zinc intakes because their diets are high in carbohydrate and low in meat.

- Endurance athletes have higher zinc losses in sweat.

- Skeletal muscle breakdown in endurance athletes may increase urinary zinc losses.

Although some studies have reported low serum zinc concentrations in athletes, more studies report normal levels in athletes. Table 11.6 lists articles that have reported serum zinc concentrations in active people. Few of these papers reported mean serum zinc concentra-

tions below normal or less than controls (see the column marked "Low status"). Of the studies listed in this table, only Deuster et al. (1989) observed poor zinc status in 13 female runners who averaged 57 mi/week. Their mean dietary zinc intake was 10.3 mg/d (RDA = 12 mg/d), and mean serum zinc concentration was 10.1 μmol/L (<12 μmol/L is considered low). In addition, the runners had significantly higher 24-h urinary zinc concentrations compared to sedentary controls eating similar amounts of zinc. In this study, the lower dietary zinc intakes and the higher urinary zinc losses could have contributed to the lower serum zinc concentrations. Although sweat zinc was not measured, it could also contribute to total zinc losses. Earlier studies have also indicated that intense exercise training depresses serum zinc concentrations, with or without altering urinary zinc losses. Singh et al. (1991) observed a 33% decrease in

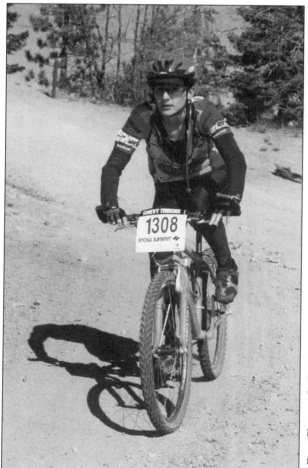

Female athletes may be at risk for low mineral intakes.

serum zinc concentrations in 66 men participating in the United States Navy Seal Hell Week. During this 5-d period, the subjects were allowed only 5 h of sleep while participating in strenuous physical exercise and enduring psychological stress. Energy and zinc intakes were high (5830 kcal/d; 23.6 mg/d of zinc), but urinary zinc losses did not increase during this 5-d period. Miyamura et al. (1987) also monitored 30 United States Army male soldiers during a 34-d intensive training exercise in Hawaii. Subjects consumed approximately 17.3 mg/d of zinc (117% of the RDA). By the end of the training period, serum zinc had decreased 14% and 24-h urinary zinc had increased 171%. *These results suggest that severe exercise training can affect zinc metabolism and could compromise zinc status if continued for an extended period of time, especially if zinc intake is low.*

Another explanation for depressed serum zinc concentrations in some active people may be that the low levels are only transient due to the body's response to changes in exercise intensity or duration. Manore et al. (1993) mea-

sured serum and urinary zinc changes in men participating in either a 12-week aerobic or a 12-week aerobic-anaerobic training program. Serum zinc concentrations significantly decreased by week 6 of the aerobic training program but returned to baseline concentrations by week 12 (figure 11.2). The opposite occurred in the aerobic-anaerobic exercise program, where serum zinc concentrations significantly increased by week 6 but returned to baseline by week 12. These results may help explain the inconsistencies in data regarding changes in plasma or serum zinc levels with different exercise programs (Couzy et al. 1990; Dressendorfer and Sockolov 1980; Lukaski et al. 1990; Singh et al. 1991) and differences between athletes and controls (Fogelholm et al. 1991; Fogelholm, Himberg et al. 1992). When athletes change either the intensity or duration of their exercise, they may undergo a period of adaptation during which zinc homeostasis is altered. If blood samples are taken during this period of adaptation, the values may be abnormal compared to norms or compared to control groups.

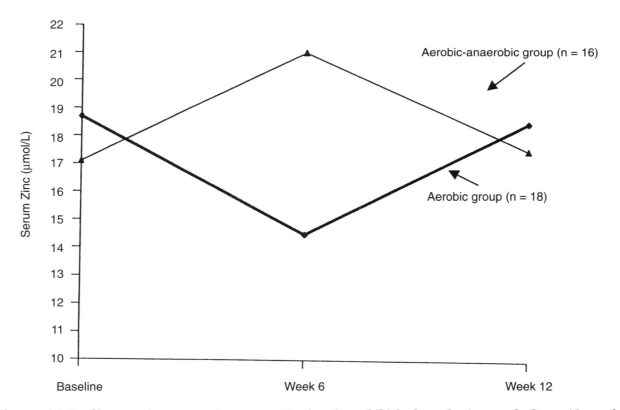

Figure 11.2 Changes in serum zinc concentration (μmol/L) before, during, and after a 12-week aerobic or aerobic-anaerobic training program in previously untrained men.

Reprinted from Manore et al. 1993.

What are the health and performance consequences of low serum zinc? Can low levels affect health and exercise performance? If the muscles have less zinc, then less zinc is available for zinc-dependent enzymes needed for energy production. Zinc is also important to maintain a healthy immune function and decrease the risk of infection. Finally, low serum has been associated with muscular fatigue (Cordova and Alvarez-Mon 1995). Because active people have increased risk of low serum zinc concentrations, they should be careful to assure adequate zinc intakes and to avoid dietary or drug factors that decrease zinc availability. There is no evidence that supplemental zinc improves exercise performance in individuals with good zinc status. If an athlete has poor zinc status, then supplemental zinc may be warranted. Before beginning supplementation, however, an individual should make every effort to improve dietary zinc intake. People who decide to use supplements should use amounts close to the RDA unless there are medical or health reasons to use more. Supplementing with high amounts of zinc (many times the RDA) should be avoided to prevent mineral-mineral interactions.

Magnesium

Acute exercise appears to significantly affect magnesium metabolism. Serum magnesium decreases immediately following acute high-intensity exercise (Deuster et al. 1987) or prolonged endurance exercise (Deuster and Singh 1994; Lijnen et al. 1988; Stendig-Lindberg 1987). Buchman et al. (1998) measured serum magnesium concentrations in 26 male and female runners before and after the 1996 Houston-Tenneco Marathon. They observed a 15% decrease in serum magnesium immediately after exercise as compared to baseline concentrations measured 2 weeks before the marathon. Other researchers have observed decreases in serum magnesium of 2-14% after strenuous exercise (Deuster et al. 1987; Lijnen et al. 1988; Stendig-Lindberg et al. 1987). As with zinc, serum magnesium concentrations appear to return to baseline concentrations within 2-24 h after acute exercise (Deuster et al. 1987; Lijnen et al. 1988). The decrease in serum magnesium concentrations due to acute exercise has been attributed to a transient redistribution of magnesium in the body and/or to losses of magnesium in urine and sweat (Deuster et al. 1987; Lijnen et al. 1988). The

effect of acute exercise on urinary magnesium concentrations varies depending on when the urine samples are collected. Urinary magnesium concentrations appear to decrease during and immediately following strenuous exercise (Buchman et al. 1998) but to increase 21-35% over the next 12-24 h (Deuster et al. 1987; Lijnen et al. 1988). As indicated earlier, exercise also induces magnesium sweat losses, which represent another way active people lose magnesium (Lukaski 1995). Exercise appears to alter magnesium homeostasis. It may cause a temporary redistribution of magnesium within the body; it may also cause a loss of magnesium from the body depending on the exercise intensity and duration. The ability of the body to adjust to these losses and reestablish homeostasis depends on the amount of exercise and the dietary magnesium intake.

Table 11.6 reviews current studies assessing magnesium status in active people. All studies reported mean dietary magnesium intakes at or within 80% of the RDA. No study found mean serum magnesium concentrations to be low. These data indicate that active people appear to maintain good magnesium status as long as magnesium intakes are adequate. If a person is performing hard physical activity and has poor magnesium intake, magnesium status could suffer.

Currently, there is no indication that magnesium supplementation improves serum magnesium concentrations in active people with good magnesium status (Manore et al. 1995; Singh, Moses, and Deuster 1992). No researchers have observed improved exercise performance or time to exhaustion with magnesium supplements (Brilla and Gunter 1995). Brilla and Haley (1992) suggested that magnesium supplementation might improve muscle strength and power; unfortunately, they did not assess magnesium status in this project, making it impossible to determine why muscle strength improved. Was the improvement due to improved magnesium status in people who had poor status initially? Although magnesium supplementation does not appear to benefit active people with good magnesium status, exercise can increase magnesium losses, thereby increasing the risk of poor magnesium status if dietary magnesium intake is not maintained.

Chromium

Since there is no accurate way to assess chromium status, it is not surprising that we know little about the chromium status of active people. A few researchers have examined changes in serum chromium concentrations and urinary chromium losses before and after acute exercise. Exercise appears to increase urinary chromium losses 2-24 h post-exercise (Anderson et al. 1982, 1984, 1988, 1991). If athletes have increased urinary chromium losses, they may be depleting their chromium stores. As indicated earlier, high carbohydrate intakes, especially from simple carbohydrates, also increase urinary chromium losses and decrease chromium absorption (Anderson 1997). Since many athletes (especially endurance athletes) consume high-carbohydrate diets and sport drinks, their levels of exercise added to their high-carbohdyrate diets may be compromising their bodies' chromium balance. Exercise also appears to increase serum chromium concentrations (Anderson et al. 1982, 1984; Gatteschi et al. 1995). This increase may indicate that chromium is being mobilized from body stores in order to improve insulin's effectiveness and enhance glucose uptake during exercise (Clarkson and Haymes 1994). Once chromium is in the blood, it cannot be reabsorbed by the kidneys and therefore is lost in the urine. This mobilization of chromium from tissue stores during exercise may explain the increased urinary chromium losses following acute strenuous exercise. To examine more closely the function of chromium release during exercise, Anderson et al. (1990) fed five different carbohydrate drinks (glucose, uncooked starch, glucose and fructose, uncooked starch and fructose, water and fructose) during exercise. The drink containing only glucose produced the highest insulin response and the greatest urinary chromium losses. These results support the hypothesis that chromium is released during exercise to enhance insulin's action and the uptake of glucose.

Can the increased chromium losses observed with exercise deplete the body of chromium? We do not know. Anderson et al. (1988) observed that trained individuals had lower baseline 24-h chromium losses on nonexercise days than untrained individuals even when carbohydrate and chromium intakes were controlled. These data could be interpreted two ways: (1) Low baseline urinary chromium excretion could mean that trained people have adapted to the chromium losses induced by exercise and are conserving their total-body chromium by reducing urinary losses when they are not exercis-

ing. (2) It could also mean that trained individuals have low chromium stores, and the low baseline chromium excretions on nonexercise days indicate marginal chromium status. At the present time we do not know which of these interpretations is correct. We do know, however, that high-carbohydrate diets can negatively affect chromium balance. Active people need to consume adequate dietary chromium to offset any chromium losses that occur with exercise. If chromium supplements are used, intakes should not exceed the upper limit of the current ESADDI of 200 μg/d. High chromium supplementation appears to negatively impact iron status (Lukaski, Bolonchuk et al. 1996).

Chromium supplements have been marketed to individuals as a "natural" way to increase lean body mass and decrease body fat. The stimulus behind this supplement craze was two reports by Evans (1989) suggesting that chromium supplements improved lean body mass in football players and in weightlifters compared to those receiving a placebo. Unfortunately, these studies did not control diet; they used skinfold measurements to assess changes in lean body mass; and they used small sample sizes. Although these studies were not well controlled, manufacturers have sold millions of chromium supplements using this research to support their claims. Attempts to replicate these studies in active people have failed. A number of researchers have now examined chromium supplements in football players and in people participating in weight control programs and have found no effect on lean body mass (Clancy et al. 1994; Hasten et al. 1992; Hallmark et al. 1996; Lukaski, Bolonchuk et al. 1996; Trent and Thieding-Cancel 1995). One of the best-controlled studies was done by Lukaski, Bolonchuk et al. (1996). In this study, 36 physically active men were involved in a double-blind study (neither researchers nor subjects knew which group the subjects were in) in which they were assigned to one of three groups: placebo (n = 12), chromium chloride supplements (n = 12), and chromium picolinate supplements (n = 12). All subjects participated in a monitored resistance-training program 5 d/week, 60 min/d, for 8 weeks. Diets were monitored at the beginning and end of the training program, and body composition was measured using skinfold measurements and dual-energy X-ray absorptiometry. Finally, blood and urine were collected for measurement of chromium concentrations. The results showed that supplementation had no effect on body composition or on strength gains in these men. Chromium supplementation did increase serum chromium concentrations and urinary chromium excretion regardless of the form of chromium ingested. According to these data, *there appears to be no scientific evidence that chromium supplementation improves lean body mass over a placebo.*

Chapter in Review

We began this chapter with two questions, the first being "Does exercise increase the need for minerals in active healthy people, and do active individuals have poor mineral status?" Current research suggests that exercise does alter the metabolism of zinc, magnesium, and chromium, and may increase mineral losses from the body in sweat and urine; active people have greater losses of minerals from the body than sedentary people. This observation might imply that active individuals have increased requirements for these minerals; yet it appears that, if energy intake is adequate and diets contain a variety of foods, any exercise-induced mineral losses can be met through the diet. Current research indicates that few athletes exhibit poor mineral status while consuming free-living diets. For active people who restrict energy intake, avoid

meat products, or eat a lot of processed foods, mineral intakes may not be adequate. If you have such clients, carefully examine their diets and recommend appropriate *and achievable* dietary changes as well as mineral supplements when necessary. If you recommend supplements, be sure to avoid mineral-mineral interactions. If an athlete wants to use a mineral supplement containing zinc, magnesium, or chromium, make sure they use a multiple mineral supplement that contains these minerals in concentrations close to those recommended by the RDAs. This will help avoid mineral-mineral interactions and the chance of toxic intakes.

Our second question was "Does supplementation with minerals improve exercise performance?" According to current research, there is no evidence that supplementation with iron, zinc, or magnesium improves exercise performance or muscle strength for a person who already has good mineral status. If someone has poor status, supplementation may improve mineral status and therefore his or her exercise performance. Since we know little about the chromium needs of athletes, it is premature to recommend that athletes (especially endurance athletes) supplement with chromium. There is no convincing evidence that chromium supplements improve lean body mass. All studies attempting to duplicate earlier research have failed.

KEY CONCEPTS

 1. Identify the exercise-related functions, dietary requirements, and food sources of minerals.

Zinc, magnesium, iron, and copper are important for the metabolic pathways involved in energy metabolism and for the maintenance, building, and repair of muscle tissue. Chromium is important for glucose metabolism and optimal insulin action. Chapter 12 discusses iron and copper in more detail. New DRIs have been published for magnesium (Food and Nutrition Board 1997) while the 1989 RDAs are still valid for zinc (15 mg/d for men; 12 mg/d for women) and iron (10 mg/d for men; 15 mg/d for premenopausal women). There are no RDAs for chromium or copper; the ESADDI is 50-200 µg/d for chromium and 1.5-3.0 mg/d for copper. Zinc is especially high in animal products, which provide 70% of the dietary zinc in the United States. Magnesium is widespread in foods, especially whole grain cereals, seeds, and legumes. The chromium content of food depends on where the food is grown and the processing techniques used. The best sources of chromium are whole grains, some ready-to-eat cereals, mushrooms, and processed meats.

2. Explain the rationale for increased need of certain minerals in active people.

Minerals are cofactors for many metabolic reactions that produce energy. Minerals are also necessary for the building and repair of muscle tissue, a healthy immune function, and cell reproduction. Exercise may increase the loss of minerals in the sweat and urine, thus altering the body's overall mineral balance and increasing the need for the minerals.

3. Understand the assessment methods for zinc, magnesium, and chromium.

There are no single good measures of zinc or magnesium status and no good functional tests in humans; status is determined by measuring a number of static biochemical parameters (urine, blood, sweat), measuring the activity of a mineral-dependent enzyme, and/or by using a mineral load test. Since there are no identified biochemical or clinical methods for assessing chromium status, the best way to diagnose chromium deficiency is to observe whether chromium supplementation improves glucose tolerance.

4. Discuss the zinc, magnesium, and chromium status of active people.

Self-reported dietary zinc intake data indicate that active men usually have zinc intakes at or above the current RDA, while active women have intakes less than the RDA. Likewise, magnesium intakes in active men are typically near the RDA, while women consume less than the RDA, especially if they restrict energy intake. There are no data reporting the chromium intake of active people. If intakes of these nutrients are low, it usually can be attributed to poor energy intakes or to the elimination of food groups high in these nutrients.

KEY TERMS

bioavailability
deoxyribonucleic acid (DNA)
estimated safe and adequate daily dietary intake (ESADDI)

glucose tolerance factor (GTF)
oral glucose tolerance test (OGTT)
ribonucleic acid (RNA)
superoxide dismutase (SOD)

References

Anderson RA. Nutritional factors influencing the glucose/insulin system: chromium. J Am Coll Nutr 1997;16:404-10.

Anderson RA, Bryden NA, Polansky MM. Dietary chromium intake—freely chosen diets, institutional diets and individual foods. Biol Trace Elem Res 1992;32:117-21.

Anderson RA, Bryden NA, Polansky MM, Deuster PA. Acute exercise effects on urinary losses and serum concentrations of copper and zinc of moderately trained and untrained men consuming a controlled diet. Analyst 1995;120:867-75.

Anderson RA, Bryden NA, Polansky MM, Reiser S. Urinary chromium excretion and insuliogenic properties of carbohydrate. Am J Clin Nutr 1990;51:864-8.

Anderson RA, Bryden NA, Polansky MM, Deuster PA. Exercise effects on chromium excretion of trained and untrained men consuming a constant diet. J Appl Physiol 1988;64:249-52.

Anderson RA, Guttman HN. Trace minerals and exercise. In: Horton ES, Terjung RL, eds. Exercise, Nutrition and Energy Metabolism. New York: MacMillan Publishing Co., 1988:180-95.

Anderson RA, Kozlovsky AS. Chromium intake, absorption and excretion of subjects consuming self-selected diets. Am J Clin Nutr 1985;41:1177-83.

Anderson RA, Polansky MM, Bryden NA. Strenuous running: acute effects on chromium, copper, zinc, and selected clinical variables in urine and serum of male runners. Biol Trace Elem Res 1984;6:327-36.

Anderson RA, Polansky MM, Bryden NA, Canary JJ. Supplemental-chromium effects on glucose, insulin, glucagon, and urinary chromium losses in subjects consuming controlled low-chromium diets. Am J Clin Nutr 1991;54:909-16.

Anderson RA, Polansky MM, Bryden NA, Roginski EE, Patterson KY, Reamer DC. Effect of exercise (running) on serum glucose, insulin, glucagon, and chromium excretion. Diabetes 1982;31:212-6.

Baer JT, Taper LJ. Amenorrheic and eumenorrheic adolescent runners: dietary intake and exercise training status. J Am Diet Assoc 1992;92:89-91.

Beals KA, Manore MM. Nutritional status of female athletes with subclinical eating disorders. J Am Diet Assoc 1998;98:419-25.

Brilla LR, Gunter KB. Effect of magnesium supplementation on exercise time to exhaustion. Med Exerc Nutr Health 1995;4:230-3.

Brilla LR, Haley TF. Effect of magnesium supplementation on strength training in humans. J Am Coll Nutr 1992;11:326-9.

Buchman AL, Keen C, Commisso J, et al. The effects of a marathon run on plasma and urine mineral and metal concentrations. J Am Coll Nutr 1998;17:124-7.

Campbell WW, Beard JL, Joseph LJ, Davey SL, Evans WJ. Chromium picolinate supplementation and resistive training by older men: effects on iron-status and hematologic indexes. Am J Clin Nutr 1997;66:944-9.

Clancy SP, Clarkson PM, DeCheke ME, et al. Effects of chromium picolinate supplementation on body composition, strength and urinary chromium loss in football players. Int J Sport Nutr 1994;4:142-53.

Clarkson PM. Effects of exercise on chromium levels. Is supplementation required? Sports Med 1997;6:341-9.

Clarkson PM, Haymes EM. Trace mineral requirements of athletes. Int J Sport Nutr 1994;4:104-19.

Clarkson PM, Haymes EM. Exercise and mineral status of athletes: calcium, magnesium, phosphorus, and iron. Med Sci Sports Exerc 1995;27:831-43.

Cordova A, Alvarez-Mon M. Behaviour of zinc in physical activity: a special reference to immunity and fatigue. Neurosci Biobehav Rev 1995;19(3):439-45.

Cousins RJ. Zinc. In: Ziegler EE, Filer LJ, eds. Present Knowledge in Nutrition. Washington, DC: ILSI Press, 1996:293-306.

Couzy F, Lafargue P, Guezennec CY. Zinc metabolism in the athlete: influence of training, nutrition and other factors. Int J Sports Med 1990;11:263-6.

Deuster PA, Day BA, Singh A, Douglass L, Moser-Veillon PB. Zinc status of highly trained women runners and untrained women. Am J Clin Nutr 1989;49:1295-301.

Deuster PA, Dolev E, Kyle SB, Anderson RA, Schoomaker EB. Magnesium homeostasis during high-intensity aerobic exercise in men. J Appl Phyiol 1987;62:545-50.

Deuster PA, Kyle SB, Singh A, et al. Exercise-induced changes in blood minerals, associated proteins and hormones in women athletes. J Sports Med Phys Fitness 1991;31:552-60.

Deuster PA, Singh A. Responses of plasma magnesium and other cations to fluid replacement during exercise. J Am Coll Nutr 1994;12:286-93.

Dressendorfer RH, Sockolov R. Hypozinemia in runners. Phy Sportsmed 1980;8(4):97-100.

Evans GW. The effect of chromium picolinate on insulin controlled parameters in humans. Int J Biosocial Med Res 1989;11:163-80.

Fogelholm GM, Himberg JJ, Alopaeus K, et al. Dietary and biochemical indices of nutritional status in male athletes and controls. J Am Coll Nutr 1992;11:181-91.

Fogelholm GM, Laakso J, Lehto J, Ruokonen I. Dietary intake and indictors of magnesium and zinc status in male athletes. Nutr Res 1991;11:1111-8.

Fogelholm M, Rehunen S, Gref C, et al. Dietary intake and thiamin, iron, and zinc status in elite nordic skiers during different training periods. Int J Sport Nutr 1992;2:351-65.

Food and Nutrition Board, Institute of Medicine. Recommended Dietary Allowances, 10th ed. Washington, DC: National Academy Press, 1989.

Food and Nutrition Board, Institute of Medicine. Dietary Reference Intakes: Calcium, phosphorus, magnesium, vitamin D, and fluoride. Washington, DC: National Academy Press, 1997.

Food Processor (software program), Version 7.02. 1997. ESHA Research, Salem, OR.

Gatteschi L, Castellani W, Galvan P, Parise G, Resina A, Rubenni MG. Effects of aerobic exercise on plasma chromium concentrations. In: Kies CV, Driskell JA, eds. Sports Nutrition: Minerals and Electrolytes. Boca Raton, FL: CRC Press, 1995:199-203.

Gibson RS. Principles of Nutritional Assessment. New York: Oxford University Press, 1990.

Hallmark MA, Reynolds TH, DeSouza CA, Dotson CO, Anderson RA, Rogers MA. Effects of chromium and resistive training on muscle strength and body composition. Med Sci Sports Exerc 1996;28:139-44.

Haralambie G. Serum zinc in athletes in training. Int J Sports Med 1981;2:135-8.

Hasten DL, Rome EP, Franks BD, Hegsted M. Effect of chromium picolinate on beginning weight training students. Int J Sport Nutr 1992;2:343-50.

Haymes EM. Trace minerals and exercise. In: Wolinsky I, ed. Nutrition and Exercise and Sport. Boca Raton, FL: CRC Press, 1998:1997-2218.

Haymes EM, Clarkson PM. Minerals and trace minerals. In: Berning JR, Steen SN, eds. Nutrition and Sport and Exercise. Gaithersburg, MD: Aspen Publishers Incorporated, 1998:77-107.

Jensen CD, Zaltas ES, Whittam JH. Dietary intakes of male endurance cyclists during training and racing. J Am Diet Assoc 1992;92:986-8.

Kaiserauer S, Snyder AC, Sleeper M, Zierath J. Nutritional, physiological and menstrual status of distance runners. Med Sci Sports Exerc 1989;21:120-5.

King JC. Assessment of zinc status. J Nutr 1990;120:1474-9.

King JC, Keen CL. Zinc. In: Shils ME, Olson JA, Shike M, eds. Modern Nutrition in Health and Disease. Philadelphia: Lea & Febiger, 1994:214-30.

King JC, Keen CL. Zinc. In: Shils ME, Olson JA, Shike M, Ross AC, eds. Modern Nutrition in Health and Disease. Philadelphia: Lea & Febiger, 1999:223-39.

Lefavi RG, Anderson RA, Keith RE, Wilson GD, McMillan JL, Stone MH. Efficacy of chromium supplementation in athletes: emphasis on anabolism. Int J Sport Nutr 1992;2:111-22.

Lijnen P, Hespel P, Fagard R, Lysens R, Eynde EV, Amery A. Erythrocyte, plasma and urinary magnesium in men before and after a marathon. Eur J Appl Physiol 1988;58:252-6.

Lukaski HC. Micronutrients (magnesium, zinc, and copper): are mineral supplements needed for athletes? Int J Sport Nutr 1995;5:S74-S83.

Lukaski HC. Zinc. In: Wolinsky I, Driskell JA, eds. Sport Nutrition: Vitamins and Trace Elements. Boca Raton, FL: CRC Press, 1997:157-73.

Lukaski HC, Bolonchuk WW, Klevay LM, Milne DB, Sandstead HH. Changes in plasma zinc content after exercise in men fed a low-zinc diet. Am J Physiol 1984;247:E88-E93.

Lukaski HC, Bolonchuk WW, Siders WA, Milne DB. Chromium supplementation and resistance training: effects of body composition, strength, and trace elements status of men. Am J Clin Nutr 1996;63:954-65.

Lukaski HC, Hoverson BS, Gallagher SK, Bolonchuk WW. Physical training and copper, iron and zinc status of swimmers. Am J Clin Nutr 1990;51:1093-9.

Lukaski HC, Penland JG. Functional changes appropriate for determining mineral element requirements. J Nutr 1996;126:2354S-64S.

Lukaski HC, Siders WA, Hoverson BS, Gallagher SK. Iron, copper, magnesium and zinc status as predictors of swimming performance. Int J Sports Med 1996;17:535-40.

Manore MM, Helleksen JM, Merkel J, Skinner JS. Longitudinal change in zinc status in untrained men: effect of two different 12-week exercise training programs and zinc supplementation. J Am Diet Assoc 1993;93:1165-8.

Manore MM, Merkel J, Helleksen JM, Skinner JS, Carroll SC. Longitudinal changes in magnesium status in untrained males: effect of two different 12-week exercise training programs and magnesium supplementation. In: Kies CV, Driskell JA, eds. Sports Nutrition: Minerals and Electrolytes. Boca Raton, FL: CRC Press, 1995:179-87.

Miyamura JB, McNutt SW, Lichton IJ, Wenkam NS. Altered zinc status of soldiers under field conditions. J Am Diet Assoc 1987;87:595-7.

Moser-Veillon PB. Zinc: Consumption patterns and dietary recommendations. J Am Diet Assoc 1990;90:1089-93.

Nielsen FH. Chromium. In: Shils ME, Olson JA, Shike M, eds. Modern Nutrition in Health and Disease. Philadelphia: Lea & Febrger, 1994:264-8.

Ohno H, Yamashita K, Doi R, Yamamura K, Kondo T, Taniguchi N. Exercise-induced changes in blood zinc and related proteins. J Appl Physiol 1985;58:1453-8.

Pennington JAT. Intakes of minerals from diets and foods: is there a need for concern? J Nutr 1996;126:2304S-8S.

Prasad AS. Zinc: an overview. Nutr 1995;11:93-9.

Reeves PG. Copper. In: Wolinsky I, Driskell JA, eds. Sport Nutrition: Vitamins and Trace Elements. Boca Raton, FL: CRC Press 1997:175-87.

Shils ME. Magnesium. In: Shils ME, Olson JA, Shike M, eds. Modern Nutrition in Health and Disease. Philadelphia: Lea & Febiger, 1994:164-84.

Shils ME. Magnesium. In: Shils ME, Olson JA, Shike M, Ross AC, eds. Modern Nutrition in

Health and Disease. Philadelphia: Lea & Febiger, 1999:169-92.

Shils ME. Magnesium. In: Ziegler EE, Filer LJ, eds. Present Knowledge in Nutrition. Washington, DC: ILSI Press, 1996:256-64.

Singh A, Moses FM, Deuster PA. Vitamin and mineral status in physically active men: effects of a high-potency supplement. Am J Clin Nutr 1992;55:1-7.

Singh A, Moses FM, Smoak BL, Deuster PA. Plasma zinc uptake from a supplement during submaximal exercise. Med Sci Sports Exerc 1992;24:442-6.

Singh A, Smoak BL, Patterson KY, LeMay LG, Veillon C, Deuster PA. Biochemical indices of selected trace minerals in men: effect of stress. Am J Clin Nutr 1991;53:126-31.

Stendig-Lindberg G, Shapiro Y, Epstein Y, et al. Changes in serum magnesium concentrations after strenuous exercise. J Am Coll Nutr 1987;6:35-40.

Stoecker BJ. Chromium. In: Ziegler EE, Filer LJ, eds. Present Knowledge in Nutrition. Washington, DC: ILSI Press, 1996:344-52.

Telford RD, Catchpole EA, Deakin V, McLeay AC, Plank AW. The effect of 7 to 8 months of vitamin/mineral supplementation on the vitamin and mineral status of athletes. Int J Sport Nutr 1992;2:123-34.

Tipton K, Green NR, Haymes EM, Waller M. Zinc loss in sweat of athletes exercising in hot and neutral temperatures. Int J Sport Nutr 1993;3:261-71.

Trent JK, Thieding-Cancel D. Effects of chromium picolinate on body composition. J Sports Med Phys Fitness 1995;35:272-80.

Weaver CM, Rajaram S. Exercise and iron status. J Nutr 1992;122:782-7.

Weight LM, Noakes TD, Labadarios D, Graves J, Jacobs P, Berman PA. Vitamin and mineral status of trained athletes including the effects of supplementation. Am J Clin Nutr 1988;47:186-91.

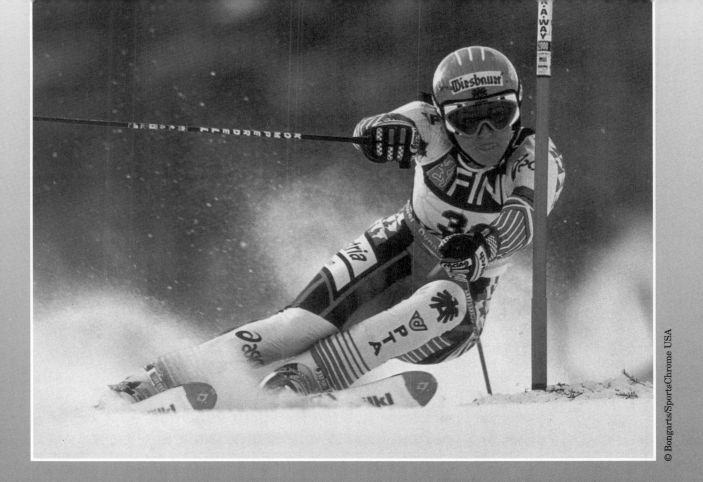

© Bongarts/SportsChrome USA

CHAPTER 12

Micronutrients Important in Blood Formation

After reading this chapter you will be able to

- identify the exercise-related functions, dietary requirements, and food sources of the blood-forming nutrients (iron, copper, folate, and vitamin B_{12});

- explain the rationale for increased need for the blood-building nutrients in active individuals;

- understand the nutrition assessment methods for iron, copper, folate, and vitamin B_{12}; and

- discuss the iron, copper, folate, and vitamin B_{12} status of active individuals.

Without adequate oxygen, the metabolic pathways that produce energy cannot maintain a constant supply of energy to the muscles. The **red blood cells (RBCs)** deliver oxygen to the muscles and transport carbon dioxide back to the lungs. Since the oxygen-carrying capacity of the blood is proportional to the hemoglobin concentration within RBCs, it is important that athletes have an adequate number of RBCs and adequate hemoglobin within each of these cells. If adequate hemoglobin is not available, the athlete's exercise performance can suffer since the ability to deliver oxygen to the tissues during exercise is impaired.

In order for the body to synthesize hemoglobin and produce the red cells that contain hemoglobin, the diet must provide certain micronutrients. Four micronutrients are especially important in hemoglobin synthesis and RBC production—two are minerals (iron and copper), and two are B-complex vitamins (folate and vitamin B_{12}). If the diet is deficient in any of these nutrients, or if the absorption, utilization, or turnover of the nutrients is altered, hemoglobin synthesis and red cell production will be impaired. Because these four nutrients are so interrelated in their roles for the production of hemoglobin and RBCs, we discuss them together in this chapter.

Exercise-Related Functions, Dietary Requirements, and Food Sources

To understand how exercise might increase the need for these nutrients, we must first under-

Table 12.1 Exercise-Related Metabolic Functions That Require Iron, Copper, Folate, or Vitamin B_{12}

Vitamin or mineral	Forms of the vitamin or mineral in food and body	Functions related to exercise	Major enzymes or pathways that require the nutrient as a cofactor
Iron (Fe)	Ferric iron (Fe^{3+}—oxidized iron) Ferrous iron (Fe^{2+}—reduced iron)	Required for hemoglobin and myoglobin production and for numerous enzymes involved in energy production during exercise.	Pyruvate oxidase, mitochondrial cytochromes, cytochrome P-450, ribonucleotide reductase, tyrosine and proline hydrolase, monoamine oxidase, catalase, glucose 6-phosphatase, 6-phosphogluconate dehydrogenase
Copper (Cu)	Found in three oxidation states: Cu^0, Cu^{1+}, Cu^{2+}, with Cu^{2+} being most common in nature.	Required for ceruloplasmin, or ferroxidate I, a plasma protein having ferroxidase activity. Important for electron transport enzymes, enzymes involved in collagen synthesis, and synthesis of norepinephrine.	Cytochrome-c oxidase, superoxide dismutase, protein-lysine-6-oxidase, dopamine-β-monooxygenase
Folate	Folate is typically used to describe food folate, while folic acid is used to identify supplemental folic acid in foods or supplements. Tetrahydrofolate (THF) is the source of active folate coenzymes in the body.	Important for cellular division and cell regeneration—especially the red blood cells, which turn over every 120 d.	Folate coenzymes are required for the synthesis of purines and pyrimidines, including thymidylate, which is incorporated into DNA.
Vitamin B_{12}	Cobalamin	Important for single carbon metabolism required for normal cell division, especially in the methylation of homocysteine to produce methionine. Important for red blood cell production.	Methylmalonyl-CoA mutase, leucine mutase, methionine synthetase

See the following references for additional information on the exercise-related functions of these minerals and vitamins: Benito and Miller 1998; Clarkson 1998; Clarkson and Haynes 1995; McMartin 1997; Selhub and Rosenberg 1996.

stand their role in the formation of hemoglobin and healthy red cells. Table 12.1 outlines how iron, copper, folate, and vitamin B_{12} each plays a role in the formation of red cells or the production of hemoglobin. For the most part, these micronutrients are cofactors for enzymes required for hemoglobin synthesis or cell formation. Folate and vitamin B_{12}, for example, help catalyze reactions related to the production of new cells, including red cells. But there are also nonenzymatic functions—iron is part of the structure of heme in hemoglobin, while copper is required for normal iron transport within the body. Some of these micronutrients are also required for other metabolic pathways or functions associated with exercise (table 12.1). In the following section, we briefly discuss the specific roles each of these nutrients plays in the formation of hemoglobin and red cells and in other functions related to exercise; we also cover dietary requirements and food sources.

Iron

Of all the nutrients related to RBC formation, iron is probably the most familiar to athletes.

This is because iron plays a primary role in the formation of two iron-containing proteins: hemoglobin and myoglobin. **Hemoglobin** is the principal protein constituent of the RBC **(erythrocyte)** and gives blood its red color. A protein synthesized in the bone marrow, hemoglobin comprises four globulin units and four heme units. Hemoglobin is responsible for the red cell's ability to transport oxygen to the muscles and carry carbon dioxide away from the muscles to the lungs. **Heme,** an iron-containing molecule at the center of the hemoglobin unit (figure 12.1), binds oxygen and carbon dioxide reversibly. Hemoglobin contains four of these oxygen-binding heme units (porphyrin rings). **Myoglobin,** a heme protein found in skeletal muscle, increases the rate of oxygen diffusion from the blood to the cells. During iron deficiency, the amount of myoglobin in the muscle is reduced, decreasing the diffusion of oxygen from the RBCs to the mitochondria.

Iron has other metabolic functions related to energy production during exercise (table 12.1). For example, it is a cofactor for enzymes in the electron transport pathway and for enzymes related to carbohydrate and protein metabolism.

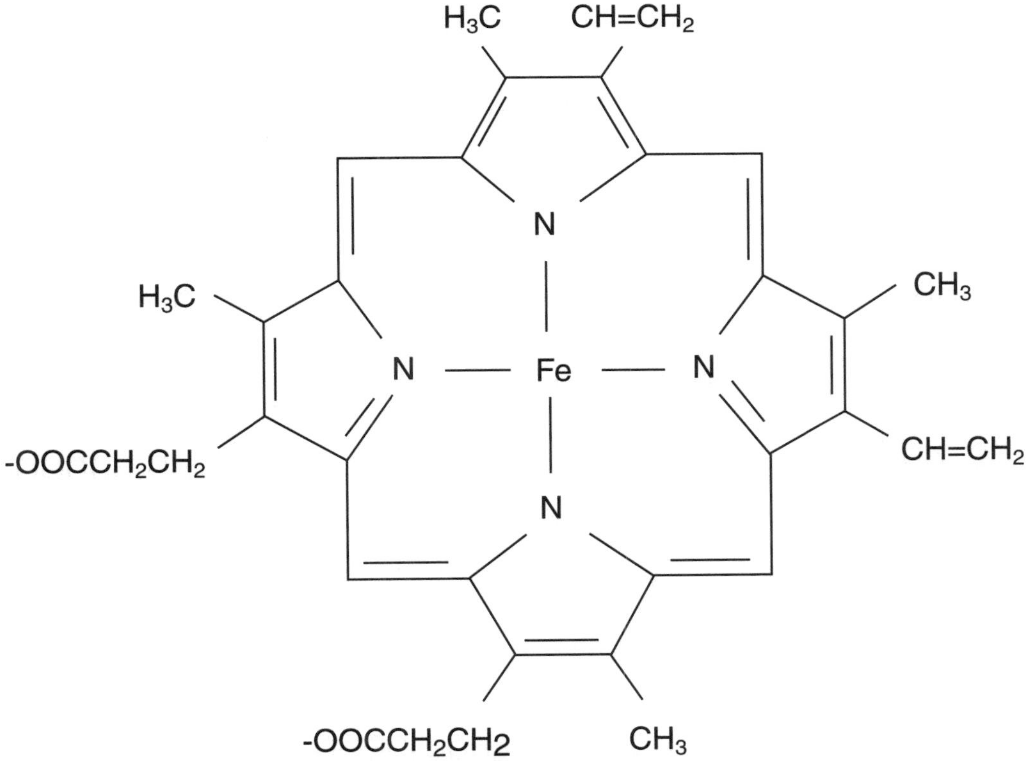

Figure 12.1 Structure of heme, an organometallic complex of protoporphyrin IX and Fe^{2+}.
Reprinted from Schreiber 1989.

Because of the role iron plays in hemoglobin, getting adequate dietary iron is very important, especially for physically active people. Without adequate iron, iron deficiency anemia can develop since there is not enough iron for hemoglobin production (see "Types of Anemia," page 335). This results in a person's feeling tired, weak, and fatigued, and can impair exercise performance. Low or poor dietary iron intake is only one factor that can contribute to the development of anemia in active people. Any condition that increases blood loss, and therefore loss of iron from the body, can also cause anemia (see "Case Studies of Iron Deficiency Anemia," page 346). For example, iron loss due to blood donations, excessive menstrual blood losses, exercise-induced hemoglobinuria or hematuria (increased loss of blood in urine), gastritis (inflammation of the stomach lining, often due to the use of anti-inflammatory drugs), hemorrhoids, or peptic ulcer disease (bleeding of the gastrointestinal tract) can all cause or contribute to anemia. Determining the cause of anemia is not always easy; anemia cannot always be attributed to poor dietary iron intakes.

The current RDA for iron is 15 mg/d for premenopausal women and 10 mg/d for men (Food and Nutrition Board 1989). This dietary recommendation is based on an overall iron absorption rate of 10% and an estimated daily iron turnover of 1.5 mg/d for sedentary women and 1 mg/d for sedentary men. However, the iron turnover rate appears to rise in active individuals. Figure 12.2 outlines the various ways exercise can alter iron losses and turnover in the body. For example, data collected from endurance-trained athletes indicated that iron losses in feces, urine, and sweat were ~1.75 mg/d for men and ~2.3 mg/d for women (Weaver and Rajaram 1992). Females lose more iron than males because of monthly menses; iron losses decrease in cases of amenorrhea. Because of their higher iron turnover, highly active people may have increased risk for iron deficiency, especially if they are

- female athletes,
- long-distance runners, or
- vegetarian athletes.

These groups are at risk for iron deficiency due to decreased iron intake, decreased bioavailability of iron in their diet, or increased iron losses in sweat, blood, urine, or feces.

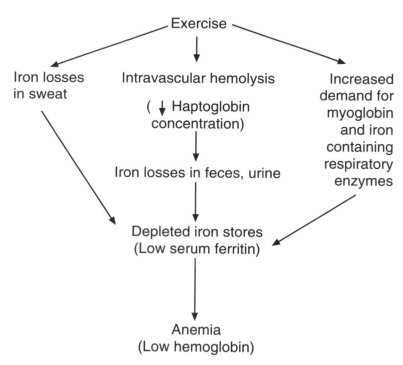

Figure 12.2 Possible mechanisms for exercise-induced iron deficiency.
Reprinted from Weaver and Rajaram 1992.

Dietary iron comes in two forms: heme iron and non-heme iron. Heme iron is the iron bound to hemoglobin or myoglobin in meat, fish, or poultry. This type of iron is much more bioavailable and has a much higher absorption rate (5-35%) than non-heme iron (2-25%). The iron found in animal foods is about 40% heme and 60% non-heme iron. Non-heme iron is the iron found in plant foods, such as breads, grains, legumes, vegetables, and fruit. All the iron found in plant foods is non-heme iron. In general, the typical American diet has an iron density of about 6 mg of iron /1000 kcal consumed. If a diet has a higher iron density, the individual probably consumes iron-fortified foods or eats large amounts of meat, fish, or poultry. Table 12.2 gives some specific examples of dietary sources of heme and non-heme iron and the amount of iron per typical serving.

The bioavailability of iron for absorption from a particular meal depends on several factors that either inhibit or enhance iron absorption; it also depends on current body stores, the amount of iron in the meal, and the chemical nature of the iron (table 12.3). Because so many factors can inhibit iron absorption, dietary iron is much less bioavailable than water-soluble vitamins—which means that improving iron status takes much longer than reversing deficiency in a water-soluble vitamin. Since too

■ HIGHLIGHT ■

Types of Anemia

Anemia is a general term for any condition in which hemoglobin is low. In fact, the word anemia literally means "without blood." Anemia is characterized by too few RBCs or by RBCs that are ill-formed so they cannot properly transport oxygen. Ill-formed RBCs are usually immature (too small) or they contain too little hemoglobin. Either way, the RBCs cannot carry the normal amount of oxygen. There are many different types of anemia caused by a variety of factors, including nutrient deficiencies, bleeding, increased RBC destruction, or defective formation of red cells. Listed below are the major anemias associated with iron, copper, folate, and vitamin B_{12} deficiencies.

Pernicious Anemia

Pernicious anemia is caused by vitamin B_{12} deficiency that arises through lack of intrinsic factor. **Intrinsic factor** is a glycoprotein made in the stomach that aids in the absorption of vitamin B_{12}. Without intrinsic factor, vitamin B_{12} absorption decreases dramatically. Some people naturally produce less intrinsic factor, while others produce less intrinsic factor as they get older. Elderly people have elevated risk for vitamin B_{12} deficiency and for development of macrocytic anemia.

Iron Deficiency Anemia

Iron deficiency anemia is caused by too little iron in the diet, poor iron absorption, or increased loss of iron from the body. In iron deficiency anemia, the body stores are exhausted; the amount of circulating iron has declined; and the person exhibits frank microcytic, hypochromic anemia (small RBCs with inadequate hemoglobin concentration). Diagnosis of iron deficiency anemia is usually based on decreases in the following: blood concentrations of ferritin, transferrin saturation, serum iron levels, hemoglobin, RBC count, mean cell volume (MCV), and hematocrit.

Megaloblastic Anemia

Megaloblastic anemia is associated with a dietary folate deficiency that impairs DNA synthesis. This results in larger than normal red cells (macrocytosis) with increased MCV. Folate deficiency is primarily due to poor dietary folate intake or to drugs that alter intestinal absorption or metabolism of folate.

Table 12.2 Dietary Sources of Heme and Non-Heme Iron

	Iron content (mg)
Animal sources (~40% heme iron, ~60% non-heme iron)	
Beef (all types) (3 oz, cooked)	2.5-3.5
Chicken, white meat (3 oz, cooked)	1
Chicken, dark meat (3 oz, cooked)	1
Chicken, livers (3 oz, cooked)	7
Fish (swordfish) (3 oz, cooked)	1
Pork chops, center cut and boneless (3 oz, cooked)	1
Ham, boneless (3 oz, cooked)	1
Plant sources (100% non-heme iron)	
Breads (whole wheat, bagels, English muffins) (1 slice)	1
Beans (pinto, navy, kidney) (1/2 cup, cooked)	1.5-2.5
Cereals, ready-to-eat, fortified (1 oz)	5-9
Cereals, ready-to-eat, total fortification (1 oz)	10-15
Hummus (1/2 cup)	2
Pasta (all types) (1 cup, cooked)	2
Rice (white) (1 cup, cooked)	2
Raisins (1/4 cup)	1
Spinach (1/2 cup, cooked)	3
Tortilla (10 in. flour)	2.5

much iron can be toxic, the body regulates its total iron stores by regulating iron absorption. If dietary iron intake is high or iron status is good, total iron absorption will decrease to prevent too much iron from being absorbed. *Because some people are at risk for hemochromatosis, iron supplementation should be done with caution* (see "Hemochromatosis: Iron Overload Disease," page 337).

Copper

Copper plays an indirect role in hemoglobin synthesis since it has ferroxidase activity—that is, it helps convert ferrous iron (Fe^{2+}) to ferric iron (Fe^{3+}). In order for iron to be transported in the blood by **transferrin,** an iron transport protein, iron must be in the ferric (Fe^{3+}) form. **Ceruloplasmin,** a plasma protein containing most of the copper in the body, is responsible for this conversion (Milne 1998). Ceruloplasmin also plays a role in the transfer of iron from storage to the blood so that it is available for hemoglobin synthesis. Thus, without adequate copper to synthesize ceruloplasmin, iron cannot be made available for transport within the body, and hemoglobin synthesis does not occur.

Anemia can develop if the diet is low in copper, even if dietary iron is adequate.

In addition to its role in iron metabolism, copper is required for several enzymes important for exercise (table 12.1). It is an essential cofactor for cytochrome-c oxidase, the rate-limiting enzyme in the electron transport chain. In addition, superoxide dismutase, a copper-requiring enzyme, acts as an antioxidant and helps protect the body against free radicals (see chapter 10).

Although there is no current RDA for copper, the estimated safe and adequate dietary intake for adults is 1.5-3.0 mg/d (Food and Nutrition Board 1989). Most of the copper consumed in the American diet is from meat, seafood, vegetables, legumes, peanut butter, nuts, and seeds, with the highest concentrations found in cooked organ meats (~3.8 mg/3 oz serving) and oysters (2.3 mg/3 oz serving) (Reeves 1997). Some ready-to-eat cereals are fortified with copper. As with iron, however, a number of factors can influence copper bioavailability from the diet (Wapnir 1998). For example, vegetables are a major source of copper in the human diet, but they require more extensive digestive enzymatic attack for the

Table 12.3 **Factors That Enhance or Inhibit Iron Absorption**

Enhance iron absorption	Inhibit iron absorption
Heme iron in the diet: • Meat, fish, or poultry in the diet increases absorption of non-heme iron.	Decreased iron demand: • Good iron status
Increased demand for iron in the body: • Pregnancy • Low iron stores • High altitude • High blood loss • High exercise training	Factors in food that complex with iron and decrease availability for absorption: • Phytates and tannins (tea and coffee) • Oxalic acid • Fiber • Soy
Vitamin C in the meal: • Vitamin C promotes absorption of non-heme iron in a meal.	Mineral-mineral interactions. Minerals that compete with iron for transport into intestinal cells: • Zinc • Calcium • Manganese
High gastric acid production, which results in a low stomach pH.	High antacid use, which results in higher stomach pH and greater mineral-mineral interactions.

copper to be released and made available for absorption than the copper found in animal foods. In addition, the milling of grains, the canning of vegetables, and/or the addition of salt or other chemicals for preservation of foods can decrease the copper content of food or its bioavailability. As with iron, fiber and mineral-mineral interactions—especially zinc-copper competitive binding—can decrease copper bioavailability, while vitamin C and pro-tein can increase copper absorption (Reeves 1997; Wapnir 1998).

Typical copper intakes in the United States are reported to be slightly more than 1.0 mg/d—about 1.2-1.3 mg/d for men and 0.9-1.2 mg/d for women (Linder 1996). A recent study that chemically assessed copper intake from the diets of 849 North Americans and Europeans reported that more than 30% of the diets contained less than 1.0 mg/d of copper

■ HIGHLIGHT ■

Hemochromatosis: Iron Overload Disease

Since hemochromatosis is the most prevalent genetic disorder in the United States, iron supplements should be avoided if iron status is good and the diet provides adequate iron. **Hemochromatosis (iron toxicity)** is a genetic disorder that results in an increase in iron absorption. The excess iron accumulates in the body, especially in the liver, heart and pancreas, causing organ damage. If left untreated, hemochromatosis can cause severe health problems such as heart disease, cirrhosis of the liver, or liver cancer. Hemochromatosis was once thought to be a rare disease affecting only white males; however, we now know that it affects one in every 200-300 people. These individuals, who have two copies of the recessive gene (homozygous), absorb about twice as much iron as nonaffected individuals. About one in 8-10 people carries one copy of the gene (heterozygous); these individuals also have increased iron absorption but to a lesser extent, and iron overload is less of an issue (Yip and Dallman 1996). Before taking iron supplements, people should have their iron status checked to make sure they are not at risk for hemochromatosis. Diagnosis of hemochromatosis is usually based on clinically high serum concentrations of ferritin and serum iron and on a high percentage of transferrin saturation (Johnson 1990).

(Klevay et al. 1993). These data suggest that many individuals may have marginal copper intakes.

Folate

Adequate folate intake is very important for athletes because of its roles in RBC production and in tissue repair and maintenance. Specifically, folate functions as a donor or acceptor of one-carbon units in reactions involving nucleotide and amino acid metabolism (Shane 1995) (see table 12.1). Through this role, folate plays a significant part in cell division, especially in tissues with rapid turnover (such as RBCs). Thus, a primary function of folate that directly relates to exercise is the formation of red cells. Folate deficiency leads to **megaloblastic anemia,** which is caused by the failure of the red cell precursors, **megaloblasts,** to replicate into functional red cells (Wagner 1995) (see "Types of Anemia," page 335). The result is abnormally large, **macrocytic red cells** in the blood that cannot effectively transport oxygen or remove carbon dioxide.

Tetrahydrofolate (THF) serves as the source of active folate coenzyme forms required for numerous biological reactions in the body, including red cell formation (Savage and Lindenbaum 1995). Both vitamin B_6 and vitamin B_{12} are required for the conversion of folate to THF (Herbert 1996). A deficiency of folate or of vitamin B_{12} causes a failure of THF synthesis and of folate enzyme production, which leads to impaired DNA synthesis and to development of macrocytic red cells (Savage and Lindenbaum 1995). Because of its role in DNA synthesis, folate is involved in the building and repairing of body tissues, including those damaged due to physical activity. Thus, adequate folate intake ensures that the cells of the body can be replaced and/or repaired when necessary. Finally, low folate intakes have been associated with elevated plasma homocysteine concentrations, which are an important risk factor for the developing premature coronary artery disease and cerebral vascular disease (Scott et al. 1995).

In 1998, the RDA for folate was revised, with the new RDA being 400 μg/d for men and women ≥19 years of age (Food and Nutrition Board 1998). The old 1989 RDA for folate was 200 μg/d for adult men and 180 μg/d for adult women (Food and Nutrition Board 1989). The new RDA was derived using a combination of

blood indexes (Food and Nutrition Board 1998). Although not used as criteria for setting the new folate RDA, high blood homocysteine concentrations and increased risk of neural tube defects are now recognized as associated with low folate intake (Food and Nutrition Board 1998; Green and Jacobsen 1995; Scott et al. 1995). It is now recommended that, to reduce the risk of neural tube defects in newborn babies, women in their childbearing years should obtain an additional 400 μg/d of synthetic folic acid from fortified foods and/or supplements in addition to the folate found in their food (Food and Nutrition Board 1998).

Folate is found in many foods but is especially high in leafy green vegetables (spinach, asparagus, mustard and turnip greens, broccoli), nuts, legumes (peanuts; black-eyed peas; navy, pinto, and kidney beans), and liver. Brewer's yeast is especially high in folate, with one tablespoon containing 300 μg. Thus, one tablespoon of brewer's yeast provides 75% of the 1998 RDA for folate (400 μg/d). The bioavailability of folate in food is approximately 50% (Food and Nutrition Board 1998), but the availability can be further reduced by various cooking procedures. Similar to other water-soluble vitamins, folate can be lost or destroyed by prolonged cooking or canning procedures and acid environments. Today many foods are fortified with synthetic folic acid. For example, most fortified breakfast cereals contain 50-100% of the 1998 RDA for folate. In addition, in 1998 the USDA mandated the fortification of folic acid in enriched breads, flours, corn meals, rice, noodles, macaroni, and other grain products. This synthetic folic acid appears to be highly available for absorption (85% bioavailable). Because our diets contain a mixture of food folate and synthetic folic acid, and because the bioavailability is different between these two types of folate, the amount of folate available for absorption can be determined by calculating **dietary folate equivalents (DFEs).** See "Calculating Dietary Folate Equivalents (DFEs)," page 339.

Vitamin B_{12}

As with folate, the importance of vitamin B_{12} for active people is primarily related to its role in RBC production. Vitamin B_{12}, or **cobalamin,** functions in two primary reactions within the body: (1) Methylcobalamin is required for the methylation of **homocysteine** to re-form the amino acid methionine. Vitamin B_{12} and folate both participate in this reaction since one of the substrates for the reaction is a methylated form of THF (figure 12.3) (Herbert 1996). This is the reason that either folate or vitamin B_{12} deficiency can cause **macrocytic anemia** (see "Types of Anemia," page 335): without vitamin B_{12}, THF cannot be produced; and without THF, normal red cell production does not occur. (2) Cobalamin is required as a cofactor for methylmalonyl-CoA mutase, which converts methylmalonyl-CoA to succinyl-CoA—a reaction required for degradation of some amino acids and fatty acids. Like folate, the primary function of vitamin B_{12} as it relates to exercise is its role in red cell formation. A deficiency of vitamin B_{12} results in **pernicious anemia,** characterized by macrocytic red cells and large megaloblasts (Savage and Lindenbaum 1995) (again, see "Types of Anemia," page 335). Thus, *either a folate or vitamin B_{12} deficiency can limit the synthesis of healthy red cells required for the transport of oxygen during exercise.*

The RDA for vitamin B_{12} was revised in 1998 (Food and Nutrition Board 1998). The 1989 RDA for vitamin B_{12} was 2.0 μg/d (Food and Nutrition Board 1989). The new 1998 RDA is 2.4 μg/d for adults aged 19-50 years. The increase is due, in part, to the new method of deriving the RDA and new information about the bioavailability of dietary vitamin B_{12}. The new RDA is based on a 50% absorption rate for dietary vitamin B_{12}. Because vitamin B_{12} absorption may change with age, it is recommended that adults 50 years or older obtain their daily vitamin B_{12} intake from fortified foods (e.g., fortified breakfast cereals or bars, sport foods) or from supplements (Food and Nutrition Board 1998). Vitamin B_{12} absorption depends on a number of intestinal conditions, including the production of **intrinsic factor,** which can decrease with age. There are few data on the effects of cooking on vitamin B_{12} content; however, it is known that the boiling or cooking of milk reduces vitamin B_{12} content by 50-75% (Food and Nutrition Board 1998).

Vitamin B_{12} is different from the other B-complex vitamins in that it is found only in animal foods, such as milk and dairy products, meat, eggs, fish, and poultry. Vegetarians who avoid all animal products ("vegans") need to obtain vitamin B_{12} through fortified foods or supplements. Foods highest in vitamin B_{12} are shellfish (clams, oysters, mussels, crab, and lobster), fin fish (herring, sardines, trout, mackerel, salmon, and canned tuna), and organ meats (liver, kidney, heart, brains, and tongue). However, these foods are usually limited in the typical American diet. Foods that contribute the most vitamin B_{12} to American diets are dairy (especially milk and yogurt), mixed foods containing meat (sandwiches containing meat and mixed meat dishes), beef, and fortified cereals (Food and Nutrition Board 1998).

Other Nutrients (Vitamin B_6, Protein)

Several other nutrients, such as vitamin B_6 and protein, are required for formation of hemoglobin and RBCs. Vitamin B_6 is important in the formation of the porphyrin ring, which

■ HIGHLIGHT ■

Calculating Dietary Folate Equivalents (DFEs)

Dietary folate has only half the bioavailability of synthetic folic acid. The definition of DFE is as follows: 1 μg of DFE = 1 μg of food folate = 0.5 μg of folic acid taken on an empty stomach or 0.6 μg of folic acid with meals (FNB 1998). To calculate the total intake of DFEs in a person's diet, use the following calculation:

μg of DFE provided = μg of food folate per day + 1.7(μg of synthetic folic acid per day)

Here is an example calculation for total DFEs, for a diet containing 1500 kcal/d:

Assume food folate = 70 μg/d; synthetic folic acid = 224 μg/d

DFEs = 70 μg/d + 1.7(224 μg/d) = 451 μg/d

Of this person's ~451 μg of DFE/d, 84% is from fortified foods (breakfast cereals).

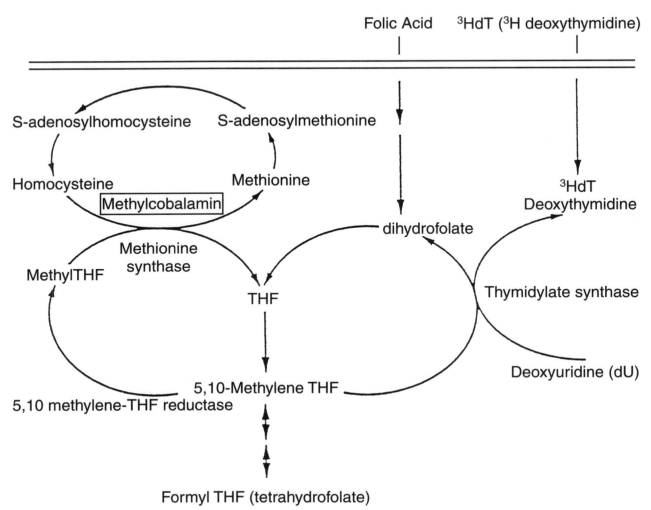

Figure 12.3 The methionine synthase reaction, which is dependent on both vitamin B_{12} (cobalamin) and folate. In the deoxyuridine suppression test (dUST), preincubation of normal bone marrow with deoxyuridine (dU) suppresses the incorporation of ^{3}HdT (tritiated deoxythymidine) into DNA; dU suppression is reduced when vitamin B_{12} and folate are deficient. THF = tetrahydrofolate. Reprinted from Savage and Lindenbaum 1995.

is at the center of the hemoglobin molecule (figure 12.1). Vitamin B_6 deficits impair hemoglobin synthesis by diminishing heme production. Protein is also important for hemoglobin synthesis. Since both hemoglobin and myoglobin are proteins synthesized in the body, adequate dietary protein is required to provide the amino acids necessary to make these proteins.

Rationale for Increased Need for Active People

Because exercise requires delivery of oxygen to and removal of carbon dioxide from working cells, it has been suggested that exercise may increase the need for micronutrients required to make hemoglobin and RBCs. Exercise may also increase the loss of these nutrients. Active people may also require more folate and vitamin B_{12} to build and repair muscle cells on a daily basis, and they may need more iron because of the increased iron losses associated with exercise (see figure 12.2). Theoretically, exercise could increase the need for any of these nutrients in the following ways:

- Alter absorption of the nutrient due to decreased transit time.

- Increase the turnover, metabolism, or loss of the nutrient in urine, feces, or sweat.

- Increase the need due to the biochemical adaptations (e.g., increased concentrations of enzymes that require the nutrient as a cofactor) associated with training.
- Increase the need for the nutrient for tissue maintenance and repair.
- Alter RBC fragility or turnover, which decreases the half-life of the RBC and increases the need for new RBC formation.

In fact, there is some biochemical evidence of poor micronutrient status for these nutrients in active people, although the data for folate, vitamin B_{12}, and copper are limited and equivocal. Some active people may exhibit poor nutritional status due to long-term marginal dietary intakes associated with either poor dietary choices or reduced energy intake. Inconsistencies in these studies may be related to differences in the experimental design. Studies can differ in a number of factors:

- Degree of dietary control
- Type and intensity of exercise used
- Type and number of status indices measured
- Level of regular physical activity in which subjects engage
- Type of subjects included
- Whether or not a control group was included

In summary, exercise may increase the turnover of RBCs, which may in turn increase the total daily needs of iron, copper, folate, and vitamin B_{12} in active people. Even more vitamin B_{12} and folate may be required to help repair and maintain muscle tissue damaged with regular exercise. Finally, exercise appears to increase the losses of iron (figure 12.2). Ideally, if energy intake is adequate to cover energy expenditure, dietary intakes of these micronutrients should be adequate unless dietary food choices are poor or limited.

Assessment of Vitamin and Mineral Status

As mentioned in chapter 11, minerals are different from vitamins in their bioavailability, the length of time required for nutritional status to change, toxicity level, and their storage and turnover within the body. Changing a person's iron or copper status may take much longer and require a different dietary approach than changing the nutritional status of folate or vitamin B_{12}. The following section discusses the most common assessment parameters—including biochemical, dietary intake, and food source data—for iron, copper, folate, and vitamin B_{12}.

Biochemical Assessment of Status

As discussed in chapters 9 and 11, a number of parameters must be measured in order to assess a person's status for a particular vitamin or mineral. These parameters usually include biochemical measures that reflect the body's stores of the nutrient and the amount of the nutrient lost from the body in urine, blood, feces, or sweat. If available, functional measurements should be included—that is, measurements that determine the *availability of the nutrient to function* as a coenzyme within the body. Biochemical measurements can be either direct (measurement of blood, urine, or fecal concentration of the nutrient or its metabolite) or indirect (measurement of an enzyme that requires the nutrient as a cofactor or measurement of that enzyme's functional activity). Finally, the typical dietary intake of the vitamin or mineral should be determined. Since minerals often exhibit poor bioavailability, the form of the dietary mineral needs to be determined, as well as any dietary factors that may alter bioavailability.

Iron

Determination of iron status is done routinely in clinical settings and requires the assessment of blood and hematological parameters (see "How Do You Measure Iron Status in an Active Individual?," page 342), dietary iron intake, other dietary factors that may alter iron absorption, and any factors that may increase iron loss from the body (Gibson 1990). Figure 12.4 outlines the various iron pools within the body and the routes for iron recycling and loss. The body carefully recycles the iron in hemoglobin from old RBCs and uses it to make new RBCs. However, if the loss of iron exceeds the ability to recycle iron or to absorb iron from the diet, iron deficiency can develop.

Table 12.4 describes the stages of iron deficiency and the blood and hematological parameters traditionally assessed. **Iron depletion (stage I)** is characterized by poor serum ferritin concentrations, which indicate that

■ HIGHLIGHT ■

How Do You Measure Iron Status in an Active Individual?

Follow these steps to determine iron status in an active person and to determine the best method of treating iron deficiency if it is present.

1. Measure blood iron status parameters and determine stage of iron deficiency, as outlined in table 12.4. Measure at least one parameter for each stage of iron deficiency. A typical routine blood test for iron status usually measures serum ferritin, serum iron, serum total iron-binding capacity (TIBC), hemoglobin, hematocrit, MCV, and RBC count.

2. Assess total dietary iron intake, and roughly determine intake of heme versus non-heme iron. Is the individual a vegetarian who consumes no heme iron?

3. Assess inhibitors of dietary iron absorption (high tea or coffee consumption, high fiber intake, low vitamin C intake, mineral supplementation, gastrointestinal distress).

4. Determine if there is excess iron loss (fecal, urine, blood losses, blood donations).

5. Determine level and type of physical activity. Has the individual just begun a fitness program, or has he/she been exercising for a long time?

6. Find out if the person has been diagnosed with iron deficiency in the past. Is there a history of iron deficiency in the family?

7. Determine the individual's prior use of iron supplements and if iron supplements cause gastrointestinal distress. Individuals who do not tolerate iron supplements may need to use small doses more frequently during the day and with meals, or increase their intake of heme iron sources, in order to reverse anemia.

iron stores within the body are depleted. A classification of **iron deficiency erythropoiesis (stage II)** is used if serum ferritin and iron concentrations are low, saturation of transferrin with iron is low, and total iron-binding capacity (TIBC) is high (the available sites on transferrin for binding are high). Finally, **iron deficiency anemia (stage III)** is diagnosed by low hemoglobin concentrations, low RBC count, and low hematocrit (the ratio, by volume, of packed red cells and whole blood). It is not unusual for a person (especially an athletic woman) to stabilize at either stage I or II iron deficiency without progressing to stage III iron deficiency anemia. As table 12.4 demonstrates, the development of iron deficiency is slow and progresses through each of the stages. As iron deficiency progresses, the effect on physical activity is more dramatic. The specific effects of stage I or stage II iron deficiency on exercise performance is questionable since research has produced mixed results. The time required to re-

turn a person to good iron status from stage I depletion is much shorter than if the person has progressed to stage III iron deficiency anemia. For this reason, active people, especially females who limit their intake of heme iron, should be routinely assessed for iron status, with *all* assessment parameters being measured (see "How Do You Measure Iron Status in an Active Individual?," above). "Iron Status Assessment Parameters: What Do They Measure? What Do They Mean?" (page 344) explains each of the iron status assessment parameters in more detail.

People who have progressed to stage III iron deficiency anemia have the classic symptoms of fatigue, lethargy, and inability to exercise at previous levels of intensity. Reversing iron deficiency anemia (stage III) usually requires supplemental iron, changes in dietary habits, and reduction of iron losses if they are present. Because iron absorption is low (~10% of dietary iron), it usually takes 4-6 mo or longer before hemoglobin levels are normal. People in stage

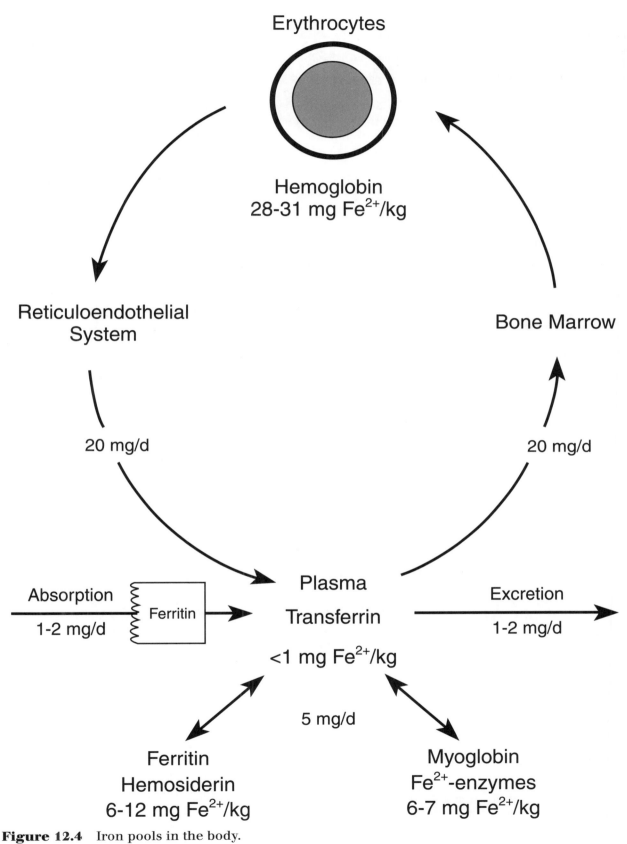

Figure 12.4 Iron pools in the body.

Reprinted from *The Journal of Nutritional Biochemistry* 1991.

Iron Status Assessment Parameters: What Do They Measure? What Do They Mean?

Body iron can be divided into two categories: storage iron and functional iron. Storage iron is that which is stored in the liver, spleen, and bone marrow; functional iron is that found in hemoglobin, myoglobin, and the iron-requiring enzymes of the body. Storage iron represents the balance between the amount of iron taken in or recycled and the amount of iron lost each day. In the United States, males typically have 1000 mg of stored iron while females have 300 mg. Iron can be stored as either **ferritin** or **hemosiderin**. The amount of stored iron can be estimated by measuring serum ferritin concentrations.

Ferritin

Ferritin is a protein that binds iron and stores it within the cells, especially the liver. A small amount of ferritin circulates in the blood. Since circulating ferritin reflects the amount of stored iron within the body, measurement of serum ferritin can be used to estimate iron stores. To estimate iron stores using serum ferritin concentrations, assume that 1 μg ferritin/L = 8 mg stored iron.

Hemosiderin

Hemosiderin is an insoluble form of stored iron that forms large concentrated clusters within the cell.

Serum Iron

Serum iron represents the total amount of iron in the serum, both free iron (usually very little) and iron bound to transferrin (a transport protein in the blood).

Transferrin Saturation

Transferrin is a blood protein that transports minerals, including iron, to the cells. Normally about one-third of transferrin is saturated with iron, with normal saturation ranges from 16-50%.

Total Iron-Binding Capacity (TIBC)

TIBC represents the total capacity for transferrin to bind and carry iron to the cells. If little iron is available, TIBC is high. This is because transferrin has a strong ability to bind iron but none is available to bind. With increasing iron deficiency, TIBC concentration increases while other iron status assessment parameters decrease.

Hemoglobin

Whole blood hemoglobin concentration is a quantitative measure of the amount of hemoglobin in the blood. If this value is low, then the body has insufficient hemoglobin available to make normal RBCs.

Hematocrit

Hematocrit is a proportional measure of the actual volume of red cells in whole blood compared to the total blood volume. A lowered hematocrit means there are fewer red cells in the blood.

Table 12.4 **Stages of Iron Deficiency**

Stage of deficiency	Clinical parameter altered	Effect on exercise performance*
I. Iron depletion (iron stores are low)	• Plasma ferritin <12 µg/L (<12 ng/ml)	Enzymes requiring iron may be inhibited, causing glucose oxidation and lactic acid production to increase.
II. Iron deficiency erythropoiesis (ability to synthesize new RBCs is decreased)	• Plasma ferritin <12 µg/L (<12 ng/ml) • Total iron-binding capacity (TIBC) >4000 µg/L (>400 µg/dL) • Transferrin saturation <16% • Plasma iron <500 µg/L (<50 µg/dL)	Iron available for hemoglobin synthesis is now decreased, and new RBCs will not be made. Delivery of oxygen to the cells may be inhibited, especially in high-intensity exercise.
III. Iron deficiency anemia (number of red cells is decreased because iron is not available)	• Plasma ferritin <12 µg/L (<12 ng/ml) • Total iron-binding capacity (TIBC) >4000 µg/L (>400 µg/dL) • Transferrin saturation <16% • Plasma iron <500 µg/L (<50 µg/dL) • Hemoglobin <120 mg/L (<12 mg/dL) • Hematocrit <36% • RBCs are decreased in number, microcytic, and hypochromic	Ability to do exercise is decreased (especially high-intensity). The following physiological parameters may change: • ↓Oxygen delivery • ↓VO_2max • ↓Endurance exercise • ↓Oxidative capacity • ↑Respiratory quotient, glucose oxidation, and lactic acid production

*The impact of stage I and stage II iron deficiency on exercise performance is equivocal.

Adapted from Weaver and Rajaram 1992; Gibson 1990; Tobin and Beard 1997.

I or stage II deficiency may see improvement in iron status in 3-4 mo if they follow dietary recommendations and minimize iron losses. "Case Studies of Iron Deficiency Anemia" (page 346) describes one case of deficiency caused by blood loss and another that resulted from poor dietary iron intake and increased iron losses.

Copper

Currently, there is no generally acknowledged index of copper status similar to that used for iron (Milne 1998). Assessment of copper status usually involves measuring serum copper and ceruloplasmin concentrations, hair concentrations, and the activities of certain copper enzymes in the blood (superoxide dismutase or cytochrome-c oxidase). Serum copper concentrations are the most routinely measured clinical assessment of severe copper deficiency but are not sensitive enough to use as an index of copper status in healthy people (Gibson 1990; Milne 1998). Serum copper and ceruloplasmin can be artificially increased by many factors such as oral contraceptives, infection, inflammation, stress, and various diseases (leukemia, Hodgkin's disease, collagen disorders, hemochromatosis, inflammation, and myocardial infarctions). Conversely, a number of factors—such as protein-energy malnutrition, malabsorption syndromes, and ulcerative colitis—can decrease serum copper concentrations independent of copper intake. Because numerous factors appear to influence serum copper and ceruloplasmin concentrations, copper-containing enzymes in blood cells, such as RBC superoxide dismutase and platelet cytochrome-c oxidase, may be better indicators of copper status (Milne 1998).

Folate

Assessment of folate status has been well characterized and developed into a four-stage model, similar to the three-stage model used for assessing iron status (Herbert and Das 1994) (see table 12.5). **Negative folate balance (stage I)** is determined by poor folate concentrations, which indicate that folate stores within the body are becoming depleted. Low serum folate concentrations and a decrease in erythrocyte folate concentrations characterize **folate depletion (stage II)**. A classification of **folate deficiency erythropoiesis (stage III)** is used if serum folate and RBC folate concentrations are low, and DNA synthesis is impaired as determined by the deoxyuridine (dU) suppression test. In this test, normal folate must be present for the methylation of dU to thymidine (Gibson 1990). Thus, in stage III folate deficiency, the ability to make RBCs has become impaired, and the signs of anemia will begin to develop if

Case Studies of Iron Deficiency Anemia

Case Study 1: Male Hockey Player With Gastrointestinal Bleeding

A 25-year-old minor league hockey player had been diagnosed with iron deficiency anemia the year before while playing for another team. At that time, his iron deficiency was determined by blood work, and he was started on supplemental iron therapy. No further investigation was done to determine the cause of the deficiency. The player said that he took the supplemental iron whenever he felt fatigued. He could relate no obvious sources of blood loss. He admitted having dark stools but attributed them to the iron therapy. He reported no history of peptic ulcer disease or chronic use of non-steroidal anti-inflammatory drugs (NSAIDs). The player reported occasional bouts of cramping in the lower abdomen but not severe enough to prevent him from playing. He attributed some of his abdominal pain to the iron therapy. He had no family history of inflammatory bowel disease or anemias and no ancestors of Mediterranean descent.

Although the physical exam did not show abdominal tenderness or palpable masses, the rectal exam revealed dark stools that were positive for blood. Blood work indicated significant iron deficiency as evidenced by low iron, percent transferrin saturation, and ferritin.

Iron Status Assessment Parameters for Male Hockey Player With Anemia

	Patient's values	Normal for men[a]
Hemoglobin (g/dL)	13.1	14.0-18.0
Hematocrit (%)	41.0	42.0-52.0
Mean corpuscular volume (μm^3)	80.6	80-100
Serum iron (μg/dL)	20	76-198
Total iron-binding capacity (μg/dL)	312	213-521
Transferrin saturation (%)	6	20-50
Ferritin (ng/ml)[b]	28	30-300

[a] Normal values will depend on the laboratory assessing the parameters.
[b] Ferritin level increases with inflammation, cancer, and liver disease.

The player was referred to a gastroenterologist. Colonoscopy revealed extensive ulceration in the small intestine and deformity of the ileocecal valve. Pathology reports confirmed diagnosis of Crohn's disease. Drugs were used to help control the disease and to stop the gastrointestinal bleeding. After a month of convalescence, he was able to finish the last month of the hockey season. The player was informed of the seriousness of his disease and the risk of increased exacerbations if he continued his hockey career.

Summary: In this case study, the athlete had iron deficiency anemia due to excessive blood loss from the bowel. Although iron supplements helped replace iron lost in the blood, the source of the blood loss needed to be identified before appropriate treatment could begin.

This case study was reprinted with permission from Browne 1996.

Case Study 2: Female Athlete With Poor Dietary Iron Intake

A 21-year-old female athlete and personal trainer complained of fatigue, inability to perform high-intensity workouts, and a decrease in exercise performance. She participated in 23-25 h of exercise per week (running, cycling, strength training, and stair climbing) and competed in local road races and duathlons. Assessment of body composition indicated body fat at 16.6% and a BMI of 19.1 kg/m². Examination of the athlete's diet showed a total energy intake of 2234 kcal/d, iron intake of 10.9 mg/d, calcium intake of 936 mg/d, and zinc intake of 9.1 mg/d. This person generally avoided flesh foods (meat, fish, and poultry) but would occasionally consume tuna or chicken. Most of her dietary iron came from plant foods (whole grains, spinach, and beans) and fortified breakfast cereals (bran cereals).

Iron Status Assessment Parameters for Female Athlete With Anemia

	Patient's values	Normal for women[a]
Hemoglobin (g/dL)	11.3	11.5-15.0
Hematocrit (%)	32	34-43
Mean corpuscular volume (μm³)	93	80-100
Serum iron (μg/dL)	40	60-160
Total iron-binding capacity (μg/dL)	480	250-400
Transferrin saturation (%)	10	20-50
Ferritin (ng/ml)[b]	<5	12-120

[a] Normal values will depend on the laboratory assessing the blood parameters.
[b] Ferritin level increases with inflammation, cancer, and liver disease.

The athlete had never had her iron status measured. She reported no donation of blood or excessive blood losses. Menstrual blood flow was regular and normal. However, she had been limiting her intake of flesh foods over the past 5 years in order to reduce her total fat intake. She agreed to increase daily intake of heme iron (fish and chicken), to add orange juice to meals with cereal or meals high in non-heme iron, and to begin taking an iron supplement daily. Reevaluation of status would be done in 4-6 mo.

Summary: In this case study, the athlete had iron deficiency anemia due to poor iron intake over the last 5 years. She agreed to increase daily intake of heme iron foods (tuna and chicken) and take a daily iron supplement to improve overall iron intake. No sources of the blood loss were identified.

folate intake does not increase. Finally, clinical **folate deficiency anemia (stage IV)** is characterized by the classic anemia symptoms and elevated mean corpuscular volume (MCV) (Herbert and Das 1994). As you can see from table 12.5, the development of folate deficiency is similar to that discussed for iron. As folate intake decreases and less folate is available for metabolic functions, one slowly progresses through each of the stages.

Vitamin B$_{12}$

Assessment of vitamin B$_{12}$ status has also been characterized as a four-stage process (Herbert and Das 1994) (table 12.6). **Negative vitamin B$_{12}$ balance (stage I)** is characterized by a de-

crease in vitamin B$_{12}$ absorption such that the level of vitamin B$_{12}$ transported on serum transcobalamin II (TC II) is decreased. Transcobalamin II is a transport protein for vitamin B$_{12}$. When vitamin B$_{12}$ (cobalamin) is attached to TC II, it is termed holoTC II. **Vitamin B$_{12}$ depletion (stage II)** is characterized in part by a decrease in the percent saturation of the transport protein (TC II) with vitamin B$_{12}$ and a decrease in the absolute amount of holoTC II. Approximately 20% of serum vitamin B$_{12}$ is attached to TC II, and the remainder 80% is bound to other glycoproteins collectively called haptocorrins (Gibson 1990). When vitamin B$_{12}$ is attached to these transport proteins they are called holohaptocorrins

Table 12.5 Stages of Folate Deficiency

Stage of deficiency	Clinical parameter altered	Effect on exercise performance
I. Negative folate balance (folate stores are low)	• Serum folate <3 ng/ml	Enzymes requiring folate may be inhibited.
II. Folate depletion (folate stores are depleted)	• Serum folate <3 ng/ml • RBC folate <160 ng/ml • Serum homocysteine may be elevated	Enzymes requiring folate may be inhibited.
III. Folate deficiency erythropoiesis (ability to synthesize new RBCs is decreased due to defective DNA synthesis)	• Serum folate <3 ng/ml • RBC folate <160 ng/ml • Deoxyuridine (dU) suppression test is abnormal • Liver folate <1.2 µg/g	Ability to produce RBCs is inhibited, and new RBCs will not be made. Delivery of oxygen to the cells may be inhibited, especially in high-intensity exercise.
IV. Folate deficiency anemia (number of red cells is decreased because folate is not available for DNA synthesis)	• Serum folate <3 ng/ml • RBC folate <110 ng/ml • Deoxyuridine (dU) suppression test is abnormal • Liver folate <1.2 µg/g • MCV is elevated and RBCs are macrocytic • Hemoglobin <120 g/L (<12 g/dL) • RBCs low	Ability to do (especially high-intensity) exercise is decreased. RBCs are larger than normal, with poor ability to transport oxygen. The following physiological parameters may change: • ↓Oxygen delivery • ↓$\dot{V}O_2$max • ↓Endurance exercise • ↓Oxidative capacity

RBC = red blood cell; MCV = mean cell volume.

Adapted from Fischback 2000; Gibson 1990; Herbert and Das 1994; Lindenbaum and Allen 1995.

(holohap). Stage II, then, is characterized by (1) low serum holoTC II concentrations, (2) decreased saturation of TC II, *and* (3) decreased holohap levels.

A classification of **vitamin B$_{12}$ deficiency erythropoiesis (stage III)** is used if (1) all the above characteristics are present, (2) RBC folate and serum vitamin B$_{12}$ are low (<100 pg/ml), *and* (3) DNA synthesis is impaired as determined by the dU suppression test (Gibson 1990). Thus, in stage III vitamin B$_{12}$ deficiency, the biochemical function of vitamin B$_{12}$ is impaired, making folate unavailable for RBC synthesis. At this stage of deficiency, the classic signs of anemia will begin to develop if vitamin B$_{12}$ intake does not increase. Finally, the classic anemia symptoms, along with elevated MCV and low hemoglobin (Herbert and Das 1994), characterize clinical **vitamin B$_{12}$ deficiency anemia (stage IV).** As you can see from table 12.6, the development of vitamin B$_{12}$ deficiency is similar to the process described for both iron and folate.

Dietary Intakes of Active Individuals

As discussed in chapters 9 and 14, determination of accurate and typical dietary intakes of micronutrients can be difficult. If you use dietary records, you must rely on clients' abilities to accurately record portion sizes, remember foods consumed, and save and record information from labels and restaurant menus. (Remember also, as you read research articles, pay close attention to how the authors collected the nutrient intake data they reported—shaky data lead to shaky conclusions!) If you use diet records, have your clients report data for a minimum of 3 d. And always consider carefully the energy intake that is required for a given client to maintain his or her current activity level.

Iron

Iron depletion (low serum concentrations of ferritin) is one of the most prevalent nutrient deficiencies in the world as well as in the United States (Yip 1994). It is estimated that 6-11% of females of reproductive age are iron depleted. The number is higher in some subgroups—about 14% of females aged 15-19 years, and 25% of pregnant women (Tobin and Beard 1997). This poor iron status is usually attributed to poor total and heme iron intakes, habitual dieting, or smoking (Houston et al. 1997).

Examination of dietary iron intakes of ac-

Table 12.6 Stages of Vitamin B₁₂ Deficiency

Stage of deficiency	Clinical parameter altered	Effect on exercise performance
I. Negative vitamin B$_{12}$ balance (vitamin B$_{12}$ absorption decreased)	• Serum holo TC II <40 pg/ml • TC II saturation <4%	Enzymes requiring vitamin B$_{12}$ may be inhibited.
II. Vitamin B$_{12}$ depletion (vitamin B$_{12}$ stores are depleted)	• Serum holo TC II <40 pg/ml • TC II saturation <4% • Holohap <150 pg/ml	Enzymes requiring vitamin B$_{12}$ may be inhibited.
III. Vitamin B$_{12}$ deficiency erythropoiesis (ability to synthesize new RBCs is decreased due to defective DNA synthesis)	• Serum holo TC II <40 pg/ml • TC II saturation <4% • Holohap <100 pg/ml • Serum B$_{12}$ <100 pg/ml • Deoxyuridine (dU) suppression test is abnormal • TBBC % sat <15%	Ability to produce RBCs is inhibited, and new RBCs will not be made. Delivery of oxygen to the cells may be inhibited, especially in high-intensity exercise.
IV. Vitamin B$_{12}$ deficiency anemia (number of red cells is decreased because vitamin B$_{12}$ is deficient)	• Serum holoTC II <40 pg/ml • TC II saturation <4% • Holohap <100 pg/ml • Serum B$_{12}$ <100 pg/ml • Deoxyuridine (dU) suppression test is abnormal • MCV = elevated and RBCs are macrocytic • Hemoglobin <120 g/L • Serum homocysteine elevated • Serum methylmalonic acid elevated	Ability to do (especially high-intensity) exercise is decreased. RBCs are larger than normal with poor ability to transport oxygen. The following physiological parameters may change: • ↓Oxygen delivery • ↓ V̇O$_2$max • ↓Endurance exercise • ↓Oxidative capacity

RBC = red blood cell; TC II = transcobalamin II; MCV = mean cell volume; holoTC II = holotranscobalamin II (transcobalamin II with attached cobalamin); TC II saturation = percentage of total TC II with attached cobalamin; holohap = holohaptocorrin with attached cobalamin; TBBC = total B$_{12}$-binding capacity; TBBC % sat = percentage of plasma TBBC with attached B$_{12}$.

Adapted from Fischbach 2000; Gibson 1990; Herbert and Das 1994; Lindenbaum and Allen 1995.

tive people who do not supplement with iron indicates that for males iron intakes are usually well above the RDA of 10 mg/d (Food and Nutrition Board 1989) (table 12.7). This high iron intake is typically due to the higher energy intakes of male athletes since the iron density of their diets is similar to that seen in female athletes and in the typical American diet (6 mg iron/1000 kcal). The iron intake of female athletes is more variable (table 12.7). Studies published in the late 1980s and early 1990s typically report the dietary iron intakes of female athletes to be less than the RDA of 15 mg/d (Haymes and Clarkson 1998). However, more recent studies report higher iron intakes in female athletes from diet alone (Nuviala and Lapieza 1997). For example, Beals and Manore (1998) examined the diets of 24 female athletes classified with subclinical eating disorders and 24 female athlete controls. Although 20-30% of the athletes had low plasma ferritin concentrations (indicating stage I iron depletion), they had mean dietary iron intakes between 17-22 mg/d, well above the RDA of 15 mg/d. However, much of this iron was from non-heme fortified foods such as breakfast cereal, energy and breakfast bars, and fat-free or low-fat snacks. Unfortunately, this type of iron is not very bioavailable. The increased prevalence of fortified foods in the typical American diet, and particularly in the diets of athletes, has increased the intake of many micronutrients, including iron. However, this increased intake of iron did not eliminate the iron deficiency in these athletes.

Copper

Determination of copper intake in active people is limited since most current nutrient databases have poor or limited copper data. For the few studies that have reported copper intake in active individuals (Bazzarre et al. 1993; Lukaski et al. 1990; Lukaski et al. 1996; Worme et al. 1990), mean intakes are reported to be 1.3-2.5 mg/d. Although there is no RDA for copper, the current recommended safe and

Table 12.7 **Incidence of Low or Marginal Iron, Copper, Folate, and Vitamin B$_{12}$ Status in Nonsupplemented Active People**

Study	Assessment indexes	No. subjects	Type of subjects	Low status (%)	Mean dietary intake (mg/d)[1]	(mg/1000 kcal)	Type of diet record
Iron							
Beals and Manore 1998	Ferritin[2,6]	24	Female athletes	21%	21.8	9.1	7-d
Fogelholm et al. 1992	Ferritin[2]	24	SCED female athletes	29%	17.6	8.7	7-d
	Ferritin[2,6]	427	Male athletes	3%	21.6	7.1	FFQ
Gray et al. 1993	Ferritin[2,6]	10	Male triathletes	0%	—	—	none
Manore et al. 1989	Ferritin[2,6]	10	Female runners	50-60%	11.6	5.7	9-d
Matter et al. 1987	Ferritin[2]	85	Female runners	16%	—	—	none
Newhouse et al. 1989	Ferritin[2,6]	155	Female recreational runners	25%	80% of those with low ferritin reported consuming <14 mg/d of iron		
Nuviala and Lapieza 1997	Ferritin	78	Female athletes	18%	13.5-14.1	6.1-6.4	7-d
Singh et al. 1992	Ferritin[5]	11	Active males	0%	23.2	8.3	4-d
Weight et al. 1988	Ferritin[6]	30	Male runners	0%	14.9	6.0	5-d
Copper							
Bazzare et al. 1993	Serum Cu	16	Male athletes[5]	0%	2.7 ± 1.1	1.2	7-d
Lukaski et al. 1990	Serum Cu	13	Male swimmers	0%	1.6 ± 0.1	0.5	7-d
	Serum Cu	16	Female swimmers	0%	1.3 ± 0.1	0.6	7-d
Lukaski et al. 1996	Serum Cu	5	Male swimmers	0%	1.8 ± 0.2	0.5	3-d
		5	Female swimmers	0%	1.3 ± 0.2	0.6	3-d
Weight et al. 1988	Serum Cu	30	Male runners	0%	2.2 ± 0.6	0.9	5-d
Folate							
Matter et al. 1987	Serum folate	85	Female marathoners	33%	—	—	none
Singh et al. 1992	Serum folate	11	Active males	0%	399 ± 90[4]	143[4]	4-d
Telford et al. 1992	Serum folate	44	Athletes[3]	11%	—	—	none
Weight et al. 1988	Serum and RBC folate	30	Male runners	0%	264 ± 100[4]	107[4]	5-d
Vitamin B$_{12}$							
Singh et al. 1992	Whole blood B$_{12}$	11	Active males	0%[5]	4.5 ± 0.9[4]	1.61[4]	4-d
Telford et al. 1992	Serum B$_{12}$	44	Athletes[3]	5%	—	—	none
Weight et al. 1988	Serum B$_{12}$	30	Male runners	0%	4.9 ± 3.2[4]	2.01[4]	5-d

[1]Mean ± SD or range of intake. [2]Ferritin <20 µg/L used to indicate poor status, except that Beals and Manore (1998) and Nuviala and Lapieza (1977) used <12 µg/L to indicate poor status, and Matter et al. (1987) used <40 µg/L. [3]Included both males and females. [4]Units are µg/d and µg/1000 kcal. [5]Data from placebo group only (no supplements); [6]Measured all iron status parameters (ferritin, serum iron, total iron-binding capacity [TIBC], hemoglobin, hematocrit). FFQ = food frequency questionnaire; SCED = athletes with subclinical eating disorders; RBC = red blood cell.

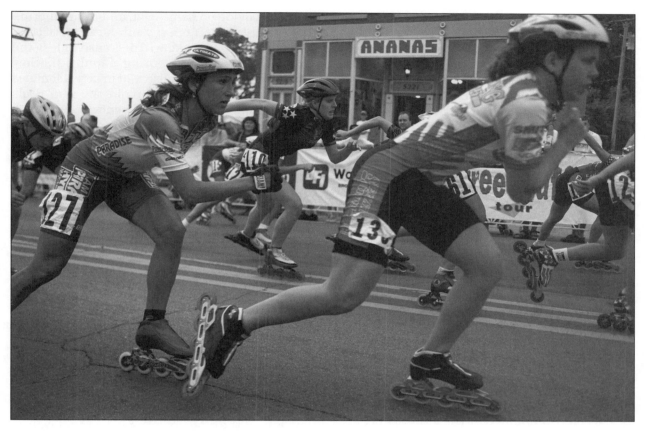

Optimal hemoglobin concentrations are important for delivery of oxygen to the muscles during high-intensity endurance exercise.

adequate range is 1.5-3.0 mg/d (Food and Nutrition Board 1989).

Folate and Vitamin B_{12}

According to large population surveys done in the United States (NHANES II), mean dietary *folate* intake is reported to be 393 µg/d for people 6 years and older—and about 369-411 µg/d for adult women and 387-429 µg/d for adult men (Sauberlich 1995). The median intake of *vitamin B_{12}* from food in the United States is estimated to be 5 µg/d for men and 3.5 µg/d for women (Food and Nutrition Board 1998).

Research examining the folate and vitamin B_{12} intakes of recreationally active adults is limited, with most of the data reflecting the dietary intakes of competitive athletes. In general, studies examining dietary intakes of active males (using at least 3-d diet records and published within the last 10 years) report adequate mean intakes of folate and vitamin B_{12} (Bazzarre et al. 1993; DeBolt et al. 1988; Faber and Benade 1991; Jensen et al. 1992; Nieman

et al. 1989; Niekamp and Baer 1995; Singh et al. 1992; Weight et al. 1988; Worme et al. 1990). These adequate intakes can be attributed to the relatively high-energy diets of these subjects. However, DeBolt et al. (1988) and Faber and Benade (1991) reported that some of their male athletes (5-38%) were consuming less than the RDA for thiamine, riboflavin, vitamin B_6, niacin, and folate. In summary, it appears that the high-energy intake of active males keeps dietary intakes of folate and vitamin B_{12} high, usually 1.5-2.0 times the RDA.

As expected, dietary intakes of folate and vitamin B_{12} are lower in active females than in active males. Folate is the one B-complex vitamin that appears to be consistently low in the diets of active females. The current RDA for folate is 400 µg/d for adult women (Food and Nutrition Board 1998). It is also recommended that, to prevent fetal neural tube defects, women of childbearing age consume an additional 400 µg/d of synthetic folic acid above that found in the diet (Food and Nutrition Board 1998; O'Keefe et al. 1995; Scott et al. 1995).

Currently, there are no studies in active females that report mean folate intakes >400 µg/d. The typical mean folate intakes reported for active young females range from 126-364 µg/d (Baer and Taper 1992; Bazzarre et al. 1993; Beals and Manore 1998; Faber and Benade 1991; Keith et al. 1989; Nieman et al. 1989; Nuviala and Lapieza 1997; Worme et al. 1990). A recent study by Beals and Manore (1998) found that 53% of their female athletes consumed less than 400 µg/d of folate. *These data suggest that many active women do not have adequate folate intakes, even when they use fortified foods.* Two factors may contribute to the low folate intake values in active women reported in the literature. First, early studies on folate intake may have underreported the actual amount of folate in the diet since the folate databases for many foods were incomplete. Second, if the active women surveyed restricted energy intake or made poor food choices, then folate intakes would be low. However, in January 1998, the USDA mandated the fortification of bread, flour, cornmeal, pasta, and rice with folic acid. If female athletes consume these foods, then folate intake should increase compared to their intake before mandated fortification. There are no studies reporting low mean vitamin B_{12} intakes in active females.

Nutritional Status of Active Individuals

The following section discusses the incidence of poor status of iron, folate, and vitamin B_{12} in active people.

Iron

There are three primary reasons to examine iron status in active people:

1. Iron deficiency is one of the most prevalent deficiency problems in the United States, especially in adolescent girls and premenopausal women.

2. Active females appear to have a higher incidence of iron deficiency than that typically found in the general female population. This may be due to weight and health issues since this population frequently avoids foods high in heme iron, such as meat, fish, and poultry. Many female athletes follow vegetarian diets, which provide no heme iron, and/or are dieting for weight loss. If energy intake is restricted, total daily iron intake will decrease unless the individual is supplementing. Finally, the low serum ferritin values observed in active females may represent a mere shift in the iron pools rather than a true iron deficiency.

3. Iron plays an essential role in hemoglobin formation, and active people need adequate RBCs to transport oxygen to working muscles. Moreover, active individuals may have greater iron losses than their sedentary counterparts (figure 12.2).

Iron status is typically determined by measuring blood iron parameters for each of the stages of iron deficiency; however, ferritin is the most common iron assessment index reported. In active males, iron status is typically good, with most studies reporting 0-13% of subjects with low ferritin concentrations (table 12.7) (Haymes and Clarkson 1998). Although iron deficiency anemia is reported in some male athletes (Browne 1996), the incidence is similar to the 2% seen in the general U.S. male population. Only Fogelholm and colleagues (1993) examined the effect of gradual or rapid weight loss in male athletes on iron status. They found that neither gradual weight loss (5% of body weight lost over a 3-week period) or rapid weight lost (6% of body weight lost over a 59-h period) changed serum ferritin concentrations. However, most of the subjects had been supplementing before participating in the study and, even while dieting, were consuming more than the RDA for iron.

Incidence of poor iron status in active females is much more variable and often depends on the type of athlete examined. However, if ferritin concentrations are used as the assessment criterion (either <12 or <20 µg/L are typically used), 15-60% of female athletes are reported to have poor iron stores (table 12.7) (Haymes 1998; Haymes and Clarkson 1998). This number is somewhat higher than the incidence of iron depletion (20-30%) in the general U. S. adolescent and female population (Haymes 1998; Haymes and Clarkson 1998). The number of female athletes with stage III iron deficiency anemia is much lower than those reporting stage I depletion and similar to that seen in the general female U.S. population (5-6%). *Thus, the incidence of stage I iron depletion, which is indicative of poor iron stores,*

What Is Sports Anemia?

In the 1960s and 1970s, the term "sports anemia" was coined to describe the increased red cell destruction reported in active people and to reflect the widespread belief that active people were deficient in iron (Weight 1993). More recently, researchers have reported changes in iron status in athletes who increase their training programs and in sedentary people who begin an exercise program. It was unclear whether the observed changes were signs of iron deficiency or were merely transient changes that occurred with the initiation of a strenuous exercise program. Follow-up research indicated that some individuals with low iron status did not respond to iron supplementation, implying that their poor iron status was due not to poor iron intake but to other metabolic factors such as increased plasma volume or incorporation of iron into muscle. Not everyone who presents with low iron status indexes has an iron deficiency. It appears that exercise—especially in people who are increasing exercise training or who are initiating an exercise program—can cause transient changes in iron status parameters.

If your client has poor iron status, how do you know if it is an artifact due to change in exercise training or intensity, or a real change in iron status? Here are some questions to help you make this determination:

- Is there a history of iron deficiency?
- Does the individual have low iron intakes, especially heme iron?
- Are there dietary factors that decrease iron absorption?
- Has the person just increased his or her exercise training, or initiated an exercise program?
- Was iron status normal before exercise training was increased or initiated?
- Does the person respond to iron supplementation or to increase of iron in the diet?
- Are there increased blood losses?

If people respond to iron supplementation, then their low iron status was most likely due to inadequate iron. If they do not respond, low hemoglobin may be due to other dietary factors or may be a transient change due to physical activity. In the studies reviewed by Haymes (1998) on iron supplementation (18-300 mg/d) in active individuals, only 6 of 16 papers reported increases in hemoglobin concentrations with supplementation, while 11 of 12 studies showed increases in ferritin concentrations. Whether improvement in ferritin concentrations improves exercise performance is equivocal and probably depends on whether the subject's serum ferritin concentrations are low initially (Lamanca and Haymes 1992). For example, Zhu and Haas (1997) reported a significantly lower $\dot{V}O_2max$ in active women with serum ferritin concentrations <12 ng/ml (stage I iron depletion) compared with active women who had serum ferritin concentrations indicating adequate status. Finally, iron status measurements usually improve as people adapt to exercise programs or if exercise training is decreased.

The degree that exercise may influence iron status assessment parameters depends on the following factors:

- Type of sport engaged in (endurance sports appear to change iron status assessment parameters more than other sports)
- Intensity and duration (hours/week) of the sport
- Adaptation to training
- Gender (females involved in endurance sports or aesthetic sports, which require a low body weight, are at much greater risk for iron deficiency than females in strength sports)
- Effect of exercise on menstrual blood losses

is much higher in active females than active males. Because of this, assessment of iron status, including dietary iron intakes, should be routinely done for active females. Care should also be taken to determine if changes in iron status reflect changes in iron stores and are not artificial changes due to the changes in plasma volume that occur with training.

Copper

Assessment of copper status in active people has been limited. Only two laboratories (Bazzarre et al. 1993; Lukaski et al. 1990; Lukaski et al. 1996) have reported both dietary copper intake and serum copper concentrations (table 12.7). According to these studies, copper status appears to be adequate.

Folate and Vitamin B$_{12}$

According to national surveys in the United States (NHANES II), ~10% of the U.S. population have low folate stores, based on low serum folate concentrations (<3 ng/ml). Those at highest risk for poor folate status are women aged 20-44 years: 15% of this subpopulation have low serum folate concentrations (stage I folate deficiency), and 13% have low RBC folate (<140 ng/ml) (stage II folate deficiency) (Sauberlich 1995). Women who smoke have a greater risk of low folate than nonsmokers.

The determination of folate and vitamin B$_{12}$ status in active individuals has been limited (table 12.7). Only four research groups have examined folate status in nonsupplementing active individuals. Singh et al. (1992) and Weight et al. (1988) examined the folate status of active men and reported all subjects with good status, although folate intakes were below the current RDA of 400 μg/d. Two other studies reported poor folate status in active people (men and women combined) and female marathon runners. Matter et al. (1987) reported that 33% of their female marathon runners (n = 85) had poor folate status, while Telford et al. (1992) reported poor status in 11% of their active male and female subjects. Telford and colleagues also reported that 5% of their subjects had poor vitamin B$_{12}$ status. Unfortunately, neither of these reports provided information on dietary folate or vitamin B$_{12}$ intakes. Beals and Manore (1998) examined folate and vitamin B$_{12}$ status in female athletes (~50% re-

ported supplementing) and found 4% of the athletes to be in negative folate balance (plasma folate ≤1.8 nmol/L, or ≤3 ng/ml); none had poor vitamin B$_{12}$ status. These data suggest that active women are at greater risk of poor folate status than active men, primarily due to their low folate intakes. However, the data also suggest that the prevalence of poor folate status is quite low. Based on the limited data available, the risk of poor vitamin B$_{12}$ status is low in active people unless they consume no animal products and do not use supplements.

Chapter in Review

We started this chapter discussing the roles that iron, copper, folate, and vitamin B$_{12}$ play in the synthesis of hemoglobin and production of red blood cells, as well as other metabolic pathways related to exercise. We wanted to find out whether exercise increased the need for these micronutrients. In addition, we wanted to know if supplementation with these nutrients would improve exercise performance. This section summarizes the research available to answer these questions.

Does Exercise Increase the Need for Blood-Building Micronutrients in Active Healthy Individuals and Athletes?

Research examining the need for these micronutrients in active people and athletes is still limited, with most of the work having been done on iron metabolism. It appears that iron requirements increase with strenuous exercise, especially for endurance athletes. This increase in iron requirements appears to be due to increased losses of iron from the body. However, most male athletes consume more than adequate amounts of iron to cover any increased iron losses. Conversely, female athletes are at much greater risk for iron deficiency due to their increased iron losses with menstruation and exercise, their decreased iron intakes, and their decreased intake of heme iron. Since many active women restrict energy intake for weight loss, their intake of dietary iron will also decrease unless they take supplements or eat iron-dense foods. Because active females are at risk for iron deficiency, they should routinely have their iron status assessed. Performance of anemic athletes will improve when they reestablish normal iron status or correct the underlying cause of the anemia.

Our knowledge of the effect of exercise on folate and vitamin B_{12} metabolism is limited. There is not enough information to determine whether exercise increases the need for these vitamins. Available data suggest that, although active men have good folate and vitamin B_{12} status due to their high energy intakes, reported mean folate intakes are still less than recommended (400 µg/d). Active women have a greater risk for folate deficiency because of their low dietary folate intakes. There are few data on vitamin B_{12} status in either men or women. No one has specifically examined whether being physically active increases the need for either folate or vitamin B_{12}. There also are few data on the effect of exercise on copper status. If athletes are anemic due to folate, vitamin B_{12}, or copper deficiency, their exercise performance will improve when they reestablish normal status through diet or supplementation.

Little research has been done on the effect of combining diet and exercise for weight loss on iron, copper, folate, or vitamin B_{12} status. If active people restrict energy intake for weight loss or make poor dietary choices, their intakes of these nutrients will probably be low, and they will increase their risk of poor status.

Does Supplementation With Blood-Building Nutrients Improve Exercise Performance?

In active people who already have good nutritional status, there are no data to demonstrate that vitamin or mineral supplementation improves exercise performance. However, if a person has marginal or poor nutritional status, supplementation may improve performance by providing sufficient cofactors for the synthesis of hemoglobin, for production of new red blood cells, and for activation of enzymes within the energy metabolism pathways.

KEY CONCEPTS

 1. Identify the exercise-related functions, dietary requirements, and food sources of the blood-forming nutrients (iron, copper, folate, and vitamin B_{12}).

The red blood cells (RBCs) deliver oxygen to the working muscles and transport carbon dioxide back to the lungs. Thus, these four nutrients are important to any active person. Iron is required as part of the structural formation of heme in hemoglobin; copper is required for normal iron transport; folate and vitamin B_{12} are important for new red cell production. The RDA for iron is 10 mg/d for adult men and 15 mg/d for premenopausal women. The RDAs for folate and vitamin B_{12} are 400 µg/d and 2.4 µg/d, respectively, for adults. Copper does not have an RDA, but the estimated safe and adequate dietary intake for adults is 1.5-3.0 mg/d. The most bioavailable form of iron is heme iron, which is found only in meat, fish, and poultry. The highest concentrations of copper are found in cooked organ meats and oysters, but meat, seafood, vegetables, and legumes are good sources. Folate is found in many foods but is especially high in brewer's yeast, leafy green vegetables, legumes, and nuts. As of January 1998, breads, cereals, pasta, and rice are fortified with folate in the United States. Vitamin B_{12} occurs only in animal proteins such as milk and dairy products, meat, eggs, fish, and poultry.

 2. Explain the rationale for increased need for the blood-building nutrients in active individuals.

Theoretically, exercise could increase the need for any of these nutrients in the following ways:

- Alter absorption of the nutrient due to decreased transit time
- Increase the turnover, metabolism, or loss of the nutrient in urine, feces, or sweat
- Increase the need due to the biochemical adaptations (e.g., increased concentrations of enzymes that require the nutrient as a cofactor) associated with training

355

- Increase the need for the nutrient for tissue maintenance and repair
- Alter red blood cell fragility or turnover, which decreases the half-life of the RBCs and increases the need for new RBC formation

3. Understand the nutrition assessment methods for iron, copper, folate, and vitamin B_{12}.

Determination of iron status requires the assessment of blood and hematological parameters, dietary iron intake, and other dietary factors that may alter iron absorption; it also requires determination of any factors that may increase iron loss from the body. Poor iron status can be classified into one of three stages: iron depletion, iron deficiency erythropoiesis, and iron deficiency anemia. Since there is no standardized assessment method for copper, assessment is done by measuring various copper concentrations in the blood and the activity of copper-dependent enzymes. Assessment of folate and vitamin B_{12} requires measurement of blood concentrations of the vitamins and of red cell characteristics. Poor folate or vitamin B_{12} status can be classified into one of four stages, similar to iron assessment.

4. Discuss the iron, copper, folate, and vitamin B_{12} status of active individuals.

The incidence of iron deficiency anemia (low hemoglobin concentrations) in active men and women is similar to that seen in the general population. However, active women have an increased incidence of iron depletion (low ferritin concentrations) compared to the general female population. Data on copper and vitamin B_{12} status in active individuals is limited, but what is available indicates good status. In addition, folate status appears to be good in active people.

KEY TERMS

ceruloplasmin
cobalamin
dietary folate equivalent (DFE)
erythrocyte
ferritin
folate deficiency anemia (stage IV)
folate deficiency erythropoiesis (stage III)
folate depletion (stage II)
heme
hemochromatosis (iron toxicity)
hemoglobin
hemosiderin
homocysteine
intrinsic factor
iron deficiency anemia (stage III)
iron deficiency erythropoiesis (stage II)

iron depletion (stage I)
macrocytic anemia
macrocytic red cells
megaloblast
megaloblastic anemia
myoglobin
negative folate balance (stage I)
negative vitamin B_{12} balance (stage I)
pernicious anemia
red blood cell (RBC)
tetrahydrofolate (THF)
transferrin
vitamin B_{12} deficiency anemia (stage IV)
vitamin B_{12} deficiency erythropoiesis (stage III)
vitamin B_{12} depletion (stage II)

References

Baer JT, Taper LJ. Amenorrheic and eumenorrheic adolescent runners: dietary intake and exercise training status. J Am Diet Assoc 1992;92:89-91.

Bazzarre TL, Scarpino A, Sigmon R, Marquart LF, Wu SL, Izurieta M. Vitamin-mineral supplement use and nutritional status of athletes. J Am Coll Nutr 1993;12(2):162-9.

Beals KA, Manore MM. Nutritional status of female athletes with subclinical eating disorders. J Am Diet Assoc 1998;98:419-25.

Benito P, Miller D. Iron absorption and bioavailability: an updated review. Nutr Res 1998;18:581-603.

Browne RJ. Evaluating and treating active patients for anemia. Physician Sportsmed 1996;24(9):79-84.

Clarkson PM. Exercise and the B vitamins. In: Wolinsky I, ed. Nutrition in Exercise and Sport. Boca Raton, FL: CRC Press, 1998:179-95.

Clarkson PM, Haymes EM. Exercise and mineral status of athletes: calcium, magnesium, phosphorus, and iron. Med Sci Sports Exerc 1995;27:831-43.

DeBolt JE, Singh A, Day BA, Deuster PA. Nutritional survey of the US Navy SEAL trainees. Am J Clin Nutr 1988;48:1316-23.

Faber M, Benade AJS. Mineral and vitamin intake in field athletes (discus-, hammer-, javelin-throwers and shot-putters). Int J Sport Med 1991;12:324-7.

Fischback F. A Manual of Laboratory and Diagnostic Test, 6th ed. Baltimore, MD: Lippincott, 2000.

Food and Nutrition Board, Institute of Medicine. Recommended Dietary Allowances, 10th ed. Washington, DC: National Academy Press, 1989.

Food and Nutrition Board, Institute of Medicine. Dietary Reference Intakes: thiamin, riboflavin, niacin, vitamin B_6, folate, vitamin B_{12}, pantothenic acid, biotin, and choline. Washington, DC: National Academy Press, 1998.

Fogelholm GM, Himberg JJ, Alopaeus K, et al. Dietary and biochemical indices of nutritional status in male athletes and controls. J Am Coll Nutr 1992;11:181-91.

Fogelholm GM, Koskinen R, Laakso J, Rankinen T, Ruokonen I. Gradual and rapid weight loss: effects on nutrition and performance in male athletes. Med Sci Sports Exerc 1993;25:371-7.

Gibson RS. Principles of Nutritional Assessment. New York: Oxford University Press, 1990.

Gray AB, Telford RD, Weidemann MJ. The effect of intense interval exercise on iron status parameters in trained men. Med Sci Sports Exerc 1993;25:778-82.

Green R, Jacobsen DW. Clinical implications of hyperhomocysteinemia. In: Bailey LB, ed. Folate in Health and Disease. New York: Marcel Dekker, 1995:75-122.

Haymes EM. Trace minerals and exercise. In: Wolinsky I, ed. Nutrition and Exercise and Sport. Boca Raton, FL: CRC Press, 1998:1997-2218.

Haymes EM, Clarkson PM. Minerals and trace minerals. In: Berning JR, Steen SN, eds.

Nutrition and Sport and Exercise. Gaithersburg, MD: Aspen, 1998:77-107.

Herbert V. Vitamin B-12. In: Ziegler EE, Filer LJ, eds. Present Knowledge in Nutrition. Washington, DC: ILSI Press, 1996:191-205.

Herbert V, Das KC. Folic acid and vitamin B-12. In: Shils ME, Olson JA, Shike M, eds. Modern Nutrition in Health and Disease. Philadelphia: Lea & Febiger, 1994:402-25.

Houston MS, Summers SL, Soltesz KS. Lifestyle and dietary practices influencing iron status in university women. Nutr Res 1997;17:9-22.

Jensen CD, Zaltas ES, Whittam JH. Dietary intakes of male endurance cyclists during training and racing. J Am Diet Assoc 1992;92:986-8.

Johnson MA. Iron: nutrition monitoring and nutrition status assessment. J Nutr 1990;120:1486-91.

Keith RE, O'Keeffe KA, Alt LA, Young KL. Dietary status of trained female cyclists. J Am Diet Assoc 1989;89:1620-3.

Klevay LM, Buchet JP, Bunker VW. Copper in the Western diet. In: Anke M, Meissner D, Mills CF, eds. Trace Elements in Man and Animals. TEMA-8. Gersdorf, Germany: Verlag Media Touristik 1993:207-10.

Lamanca JJ, Haymes EM. Effects of low ferritin concentration on endurance performance. Inter J Sport Nutr 1992;2:376-85.

Lindenbaum J, Allen RH. Clinical spectrum and diagnosis of folate deficiency. In: Bailey LB, ed. Folate in Health and Disease. New York: Marcel Dekker, 1995:43-73.

Lukaski HC, Hoverson BS, Gallagher SK, Bolonchuk WW. Physical training and copper, iron and zinc status of swimmers. Am J Clin Nutr 1990;51:1093-9.

Lukaski HC, Siders WA, Hoverson BS, Gallagher SK. Iron, copper, magnesium and zinc status as predictors of swimming performance. Int J Sports Med 1996; 17:534-40.

Manore MM, Besenfelder PD, Wells CL, Carroll SS, Hooker SP. Nutrient intakes and iron status in female long-distance runners during training. J Am Diet Assoc 1989;89:257-9.

Matter M, Stittfall T, Graves J, Myburgh K, Adams B, Jacobs P, Noakes TD. The effect of iron and folate therapy on maximal exercise performance in female marathon runners with iron and folate deficiency. Clin Sci 1987;72:415-22.

McMartin K. Folate and vitamin B-12. In: Wolinsky I, Driskell JA, eds. Sport Nutrition: Vitamins and Trace Elements. Boca Raton, FL: CRC Press, 1997:85-96.

Milne DB. Copper intake and assessment of copper status. Am J Clin Nutr 1998(suppl.); 67:1041S-5S.

Newhouse IJ, Clement DB, Taunton JE, McKenzie DC. The effects of prelatent/latent iron deficiency on physical work capacity. Med Sci Sports Exerc 1989;21:263-8.

Niekamp RA, Baer JT. In-season dietary adequacy of trained male cross-country runners. Int J Sport Nutr 1995;5:45-55.

Nieman DC, Butler JV, Pollett LM, Dietrich SJ, Lutz RD. Nutrient intake of marathon runners. J Am Diet Assoc 1989;89:1273-8.

Nuviala RJ, Lapieza MG. Disparity between diet and serum ferritin in elite sportswomen. Nutr Res 1997;17:451-61.

O'Keefe CA, Bailey LB, Thomas EA. Controlled dietary folate affects folate status in nonpregnant women. J Nutr 1995;125:2717-25.

Pathways of nutritional biochemistry: iron pools. J Nutr Biochem 1991;2:247.

Reeves PG. Copper. In: Wolinsky I, Driskell JA, eds. Sport Nutrition: Vitamins and Trace Elements. Boca Raton, FL: CRC Press, 1997:175-87.

Sauberlich HE. Folate status of U.S. population and groups. In: Bailey LB, ed. Folate in Health and Disease. New York: Marcel Dekker, 1995:171-94.

Savage DG, Lindenbaum J. Folate-cobalamin interactions. In: Bailey LB, ed. Folate in Health and Disease. New York: Marcel Dekker, 1995:237-85.

Schreiber WE. Iron, porphyrin, and bilirubin metabolism. In: Kaplan LA, Pesce AJ, eds. Clinical Chemistry. St. Louis: Mosby, 1989:496-509.

Scott JM, Weir DG, Kirke PN. Folate and neural tube defects. In: Bailey LB, ed. Folate in Health and Disease. New York: Marcel Dekker, 1995:329-60.

Selhub J, Rosenberg IH. Folic acid. In: Ziegler EE, Filer LJ, eds. Present Knowledge in Nutrition. Washington, DC: ILSI Press, 1996:206-19.

Shane B. Folate chemistry and metabolism. In: Bailey LB, ed. Folate in Health and Disease. New York: Marcel Dekker, 1995:1-22.

Singh A, Moses FM, Deuster PA. Vitamin and mineral status in physically active men: effects of a high-potency supplement. Am J Clin Nutr 1992;55:1-7.

Telford RD, Catchpole EA, Deakin V, McLeay AC, Plank AW. The effect of 7 to 8 months of vitamin/mineral supplementation on the vitamin and mineral status of athletes. Int J Sport Nutr 1992;2:123-34.

Tobin BW, Beard JL. Iron. In: Wolinsky I, Driskell JA, eds. Sport Nutrition: Vitamins and Trace Elements. Boca Raton, FL: CRC Press, 1997:137-56.

Wagner C. Biochemical role of folate in cellular metabolism. In: Bailey LB, ed. Folate in Health and Disease. New York: Marcel Dekker, 1995:23-42.

Wapnir RA. Copper absorption and bioavailability. Am J Clin Nutr 1998(suppl.);67:1054S-60S.

Weaver CM, Rajaram S. Exercise and iron status. J Nutr 1992;122:782-7.

Weight LM. Sports anemia: does it exist? Sports Med 1993;16:1-4.

Weight LM, Noakes TD, Labadarios D, Graves J, Jacobs P, Berman PA. Vitamin and mineral status of trained athletes including the effects of supplementation. Am J Clin Nutr 1988;47:186-91.

Worme JD, Doubt TJ, Singh A, Ryan CJ, Moses FM, Deuster PA. Dietary patterns, gastrointestinal complaints, and nutrition knowledge of recreational triathletes. Am J Clin Nutr 1990;51:690-7.

Yip R. Iron deficiency: contemporary scientific issues and international programmatic approaches. J Nutr 1994;124:1479S-90S.

Zhu YI, Haas JD. Iron depletion without anemia and physical performance in young women. Am J Clin Nutr 1997;66:334-41.

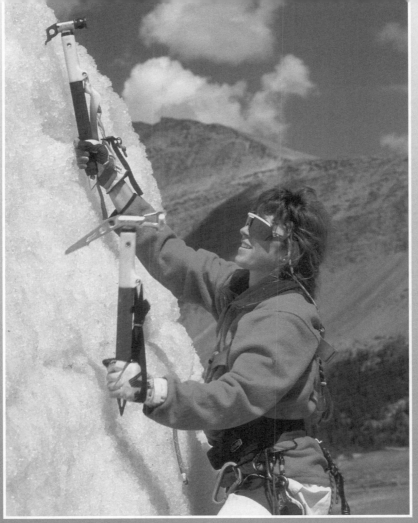

CHAPTER 13

Nutrients for Bone Health

After reading this chapter you should be able to

- describe the stages of bone metabolism, and list the primary nutrients associated with bone health;

- discuss the methods used to assess calcium, identify calcium requirements and intakes of athletes, and identify sources of calcium and related supplementation products;

- describe the methods of assessment, the requirements, and dietary sources of phosphorus;

- discuss magnesium's role in bone health;

- describe the methods of assessment, the requirements, dietary sources, and supplementation products of vitamin D; and

- describe how fluoride, energy, and protein play a role in bone metabolism.

Although we tend to think of bone as a rigid tissue that supports the body, bone is in fact a dynamic tissue that actively participates in serum calcium regulation. A number of nutrients play a critical role in bone metabolism, including calcium, phosphorus, magnesium, fluoride, and vitamin D. Adequate bone development during youth is necessary to achieve a healthy adult skeleton. While it is recognized that early bone development is critical to health, this chapter focuses primarily on the interactions within adults of exercise, certain nutrients, and bone health. We provide a brief review of bone metabolism prior to discussing the specific nutrients related to bone health.

Review of Bone Metabolism

There are three stages of bone development (Dalsky 1990):

1. Growth
2. Modeling
3. Remodeling

The *size* of a bone is determined during its years of growth; its *shape* is determined during the **modeling stage. Remodeling,** also referred to as turnover, is the process of replacing existing bone matrix with new bone matrix (Anderson 1991). Growth, modeling, and remodeling occur in the developing skeleton, while remodeling occurs in adult bone. Remodeling maintains the mineral homeostasis of bone and prevents the accumulation of microfractures (Dalsky 1990).

Figure 13.1 reviews the bone remodeling process. Osteoblasts and osteoclasts are cells involved in this process. Precursor cells in the bone marrow are converted to either osteoblasts or osteoclasts. **Osteoclasts** act to erode the bone surface and form cavities in the bone. This activity is called **resorption. Osteoblasts** act at the site of the cavities to synthesize new bone matrix, a process called **formation.** The new matrix is subsequently mineralized, resulting in new bone tissue. *Appropriate coupling of resorption and formation results in the maintenance of bone tissue. Bone loss results when the rate of resorption exceeds that of formation.*

Many factors regulate bone remodeling, including

- hormones such as estrogen, vitamin D, parathyroid hormone (PTH), and calcitonin;

- nutrient status, particularly calcium bioavailability;
- exercise, especially weightbearing activity; and
- hormonal status.

We discuss each of these factors in detail in subsequent sections of this chapter.

Adult bone comprises two major types of tissue: cortical (or compact) and trabecular (or cancellous) tissue. **Trabecular bone** makes up approximately 20% of the entire skeleton and has a faster turnover rate than cortical bone. No more than 20% of adult trabecular bone is in active remodeling at one time (Frost 1987). **Cortical bone** comprises the remaining 80% of the skeleton, has a slower turnover rate than trabecular bone, and has only 5% of its surfaces in active remodeling at one time. Cortical bone is found primarily in the long bones of the body, while much of trabecular bone is found in the axial skeleton, the flat bones, and the ends of long bones (Baylink and Jennings 1994). Trabecular bone is found at fracture sites in the vertebrae, distal radius, and proximal femur. Due to the faster remodeling rate of trabecular bone, it is more sensitive to changes in hormonal status, and bone loss at these sites is more easily detected than at sites with predominantly cortical bone (Dalsky 1990).

Peak bone mass is generally achieved after adult height has been reached and the bones have gone through the "consolidation phase." On average, females achieve 90% of their bone mineral content by age 16.9 years. In males, bone mass at various sites has been found to increase up to 18 years of age (Bonjour et al. 1991), with peak bone mass most likely occurring between the ages of 20-29 years. It is important to note that while these changes are true for *whole-body* peak bone mass, individual bones attain peak bone mass at different ages. As a person ages, the rate of bone resorption exceeds that of bone formation, which results in a net loss of bone. Bone loss is accelerated during periods of prolonged inactivity or bed rest, following menopause in women, and when there is poor calcium or vitamin D nutrition. As we discuss in chapter 15, amenorrheic athletes may also experience bone loss due to estrogen deficiency.

Calcium

Calcium is the predominant component of bone, being the largest constituent of the **hydroxy-**

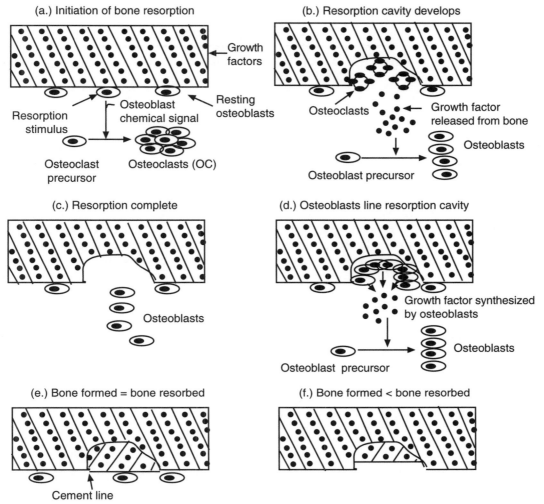

Figure 13.1   The bone remodeling process. (A.) Bone resorption is initiated by a stimulus (e.g., PTH) which acts on resting osteoblasts (OBs) to produce a chemical signal. This chemical signal acts on osteoclast (OC) precursors to increase the number and resorption activity of OCs. (B.) OCs excavate bone, which causes a release of growth factors (GF) from bone. These GFs act on OB precursors to produce OBs. (C.) The resorptive phase is complete and OCs disappear from the surface of the resorptive cavity. (D.) Mature OBs formed during the resorptive phase line up on the cavity surface and begin to fill in the cavity with new bone. The extent that the resorptive cavity is filled in is determined by the amount of GF produced by contemporary OPBs. (E.) The amount of new bone formed in normal individuals is equal to the amount of bone resorbed. (F.) The amount of new bone formed is less than the amount resorbed; this occurs during estrogen or calcium deficiency.

Reprinted from Baylink and Jennings 1994.

---

apatite crystals, or solid particles, of bone. Table 13.1 reviews the distribution of the body's "major minerals" (those present in amounts >5 g— i.e., calcium, phosphorus, and magnesium). Although calcium is recognized primarily for its role in bone health, it has other important functions related to exercise, including

- enzyme activation,
- nerve transmission,
- muscle contraction,
- hormone function, and
- membrane transport.

The body prioritizes maintenance of blood calcium levels over those of bone tissue. When calcium intake is inadequate, blood calcium levels are maintained by withdrawing more calcium from bone, increasing intestinal absorption of calcium, and increasing renal uptake of

Table 13.1 Calcium, Phosphorus, and Magnesium Distribution in a 154-lb (70-kg) Adult

Element	Mass present	Percentage in the skeleton	Percentage in soft tissues
Ca	1200 g	99%	1%
P	900 g	88%	12%
Mg	24 g	60%	40%

Reprinted from Gibson 1990.

calcium. These adaptations occur through the actions of select hormones, such as parathyroid hormone (PTH) and vitamin D. Table 13.2 reviews the hormones associated with calcium metabolism.

Methods of Assessment

There is no satisfactory direct method for assessing calcium status. Serum calcium levels cannot be used to indicate calcium status since these levels are tightly controlled and remain constant under most conditions. Approximately 50% of the serum calcium concentration is ionized and under hormonal control, while the remaining 50% is bound to plasma proteins, primarily plasma albumin. Only the ionized form of serum calcium is physiologically active and can be used for muscular contractions, transmission of nerve impulses, and blood clotting

Table 13.2 Hormones Associated With Bone Metabolism, and Their Actions

Hormone	Actions
Parathyroid hormone (PTH)	Increases resorption of calcium from bone into blood to maintain blood calcium levels.
	Stimulates conversion of the inactive form of vitamin D to its active form (1,25 vitamin D).
	Conserves calcium by acting on distal tubules in the kidney to increase calcium resorption.
Thyroxine	Normal levels are critical to maintaining healthy bone metabolism.
	Hyperthyroidism results in a significant increase in bone resorption, resulting in bone loss.
	Hypothyroidism results in a slowing of bone turnover and diminishes the bone calcium pool.
Insulin-like growth factor I	Regulates bone growth and remodeling through its action on osteoblast differentiation and collagen/matrix synthesis.
Estrogen	Decreases bone resorption, possibly by decreasing the responsiveness of osteoclasts to PTH.
Vitamin D	Increases intestinal absorption of calcium and phosphorus.
	Promotes bone resorption by increasing osteoclast number.
	Increases reabsorption of calcium in the distal tubule of the kidney.
Calcitonin	Conserves bone tissue by inhibiting osteoclast activity and maintaining normal serum calcium levels.
Corticosteroids	Modulate osteoclastic activity.
	Excess levels can inhibit bone formation by impairing synthesis of bone matrix.
	Excess levels stimulate bone resorption.
	Excess levels inhibit active calcium transport in the intestine.

(Gibson 1990). Levels of ionized calcium are monitored during surgery, such as open heart and liver transplants, and are also used to monitor certain renal and thyroid diseases. Normal adult values for ionized calcium are 4.65-5.28 mg/dL (1.16 to 1.32 mmol/L), while normal adult values for total serum calcium are 8.6-10.0 mg/dL (2.15 to 2.50 mmol/L) (Fischbach 1996). Abnormal values for serum and ionized calcium can result from a variety of maladies, including hyper- or hypoparathyroidism, certain cancers, malabsorption disorders, and Paget's disease of bone (Fischbach 1996).

Serum ionized calcium is analyzed using ion-specific electrodes (Wandrup and Kvetny 1985). Since several factors can confound this measurement—a recent meal, high levels of magnesium and sodium, changes in pH of the sample, and the presence of trypsin or heparin (Ladenson and Bowers 1973)—it is important to standardize the measurement process when analyzing serum ionized calcium levels.

Under certain conditions, measurements of urinary calcium are used to assess changes in calcium metabolism. Because urinary calcium levels have a significant, but low, correlation with calcium intake (Weaver 1990), they are of limited use as an indicator of adequate dietary calcium intake. Urinary calcium is affected by recent calcium intake, calcium requirement, urinary output, and dietary protein, making it more variable than plasma calcium. Expressing urinary calcium as a **calcium:creatinine ratio** normalizes calcium excretion values. This ratio corrects for differences among people in lean body mass and also corrects for errors in the timing of urine collections (Weaver 1990).

It is important to interpret urinary calcium values in conjunction with assessments of dietary intake.

The assessment of bone is crucial to evaluating long-term calcium status. Note that although poor calcium nutrition over one's lifetime is thought to have a negative impact on bone, many factors in addition to dietary calcium intake play a role in bone health, including hormonal status, genetic factors, and levels of physical activity. Bone measurements do not reflect recent dietary calcium intakes. See "A Review of Bone Measurement Methods," page 364, for more details about measurements. For a complete description of methods used to assess calcium status and metabolism, refer to Weaver (1990).

Requirements

Dietary calcium intake, intestinal absorption, urinary excretion, and fecal losses play an important role in calcium balance and affect individual calcium requirements. While calcium absorption from food is typically 25-35% (Heaney and Recker 1986), several factors can influence absorption (table 13.3). The impact of many of these factors on bone health in humans is controversial, and their effect on bone in healthy people may be minimal (Anderson 1991). Additional factors that could degrade bone health include consumption of excess aluminum (in antacids), which may result in excess urinary calcium excretion, and use of glucocorticoids (used to treat many inflammatory illnesses such as arthritis, asthma, and inflammatory bowel disease), which can impair calcium absorption.

Table 13.3 **Factors That May Affect Calcium Availability**

Improve availability	Decrease availability
Increased vitamin D levels	Vitamin D deficiency
Dietary fat	High dietary sodium
Acidic environment in intestines	Alkaline environment in intestines
Lactose (with normal lactase activity)	Lactose (with lactase deficiency)
Lysine and arginine (acidic amino acids)	High dietary animal protein
Ingesting calcium with meal	Phytates and oxalates
Calcium deficiency	Dietary fiber
	Aging
	Caffeine
	High dietary phosphate

A Review of Bone Measurement Methods

Measurements of bone status include estimates of bone mineral content (or densitometry) and assessment of markers that indicate bone turnover and skeletal status. Bone densitometry techniques include

- quantitative computed tomography (QCT),
- single- and dual-photon absorptiometry (DPA), and
- dual-energy X-ray absorptiometry (DXA or DEXA).

These techniques can measure the mineral content of specific bones or of the total body. DXA has become more popular than the other methods in recent years due to its greater resolution and precision, more rapid scan time, and lower radiation exposure (Weaver 1990).

A number of biochemical markers in blood and urine can indicate bone turnover. It is important to remember that these markers are degradation products of the metabolism of bone and other tissue and are not necessarily specific to bone. Studies of large populations show an inverse relationship between bone mineral density and markers of bone turnover. The following table lists and describes some of the biochemical markers of bone turnover:

Marker	Description
Total alkaline phosphatase	Originates from bone, liver, intestine, and kidney.
Bone specific alkaline phosphatase	Originates from bone; a product of osteoblasts.
Osteocalcin	Originates from bone; a product of osteoblasts.
Carboxyterminal propeptide of type I procollagen	Originates from bone, soft tissue, skin; product of proliferating osteoblasts and fibroblasts.
Aminoterminal propeptide of type I procollagen	Originates from bone, soft tissue, skin; product of proliferating osteoblasts and fibroblasts.
Hydroxyproline	Originates from bone, cartilage, soft tissue, skin, blood; found in all collagenous proteins.
Pyridinoline	Originates from bone, cartilage, tendon, and blood vessels; found in collagens, with highest concentrations in cartilage and bone.
Deoxypyridinoline	Originates in bone and dentin; found in collagens, with the highest concentrations in bone.
Carboxyterminal crosslinked telopeptide of type I collagen	Originates in bone and skin; found in type I collagen, with the highest contribution from bone.
Aminoterminal crosslinked telopeptide of type I collagen	Originates in bone and skin; found in type I collagen, with the highest contribution from bone.

Although these markers are frequently used to assess skeletal status, they appear to be better markers when used to assess group values than when used for individuals (Lunar Corporation 1994). Although inter-assay variation is low, the most limiting factor in the use of these markers is their relatively high day-to-day variation over the short term, particularly in individuals with high bone turnover (e.g., postmenopausal women). Since daily variability in some of these markers can be as high as 50%, only very dramatic changes in the markers would reveal a change in skeletal status, thus limiting the predictive accuracy of the assays. Another limitation is that bone markers are not predictive of other factors that affect fracture risk, such as peak bone mass, current bone mineral density, bone architecture, and bone stiffness. It is recommended that biochemical markers be used in combination with bone density measures to define a person's skeletal status. At the present time, we do not have a particularly accurate marker for skeletal status.

Determining calcium requirements is a process fraught with difficulty. Epidemiological studies have been used to estimate calcium intake by healthy people. While data from these types of projects can indicate patterns of dietary calcium intake, they do not clearly define calcium requirements. Calcium balance studies have been used to determine the dietary calcium intake required to maintain calcium balance—the assumption being that negative calcium balance indicates bone loss. Limitations of balance methodology result from errors inherent in the collection process, failure to include measures of dermal losses, and the inability of short-term balance studies to accurately predict long-term adaptations to changes in calcium intake (Weaver 1994).

Despite methodological limitations, dietary calcium requirements have been established for men and women across the life span. Both Recommended Dietary Allowances (RDAs) and Dietary Reference Intakes (DRIs) have been established for calcium and the other nutrients

associated with bone metabolism. Both the Food and Nutrition Board (1997) and Yates et al. (1998) have reviewed the development and purpose of DRIs for bone nutrients. The DRIs were established for use in planning and assessing diets for healthy people. While the RDAs represent the average daily intake level that is sufficient to meet the nutrient needs of virtually all healthy people, the DRIs were developed to go beyond the scope of deficiency diseases and to address the nutrient needs for lifelong health. The DRIs include the Estimated Average Requirement (EAR), the RDA, the Adequate Intake (AI), and the Tolerable Upper Intake Level (UL). Chapters 1 and 9 (on RDA vs. DRI) define these terms in detail.

Table 13.4 includes DRI values for calcium, phosphorus, magnesium, vitamin D, and fluoride for various age groups. If no definitive data are available on which to base an EAR or RDA, the AI is a useful goal for individual nutrient intakes (Food and Nutrition Board 1997).

Table 13.4 Dietary Reference Intakes: Recommended Levels for Individuals[a,b]

Age group (years)	Calcium (mg/d)	Phosphorus (mg/d)	Magnesium (mg/d)	Vitamin D[c,d] (µg/d)	Fluoride (mg/d)
Males					
14-18	1300*	**1250**	410	5*	3*
19-30	1000*	**700**	400	5*	4*
31-50	1000*	**700**	420	5*	4*
51-70	1200*	**700**	420	10*	4*
>70	1200*	**700**	420	15*	4*
Females					
14-18	1300*	**1250**	360	5*	3*
19-30	1000*	**700**	310	5*	3*
31-50	1000*	**700**	320	5*	3*
51-70	1200*	**700**	320	10*	3*
>70	1200*	**700**	320	15*	3*

[a]Values are those of the Food and Nutrition Board 1997.

[b]Recommended Dietary Allowances (RDAs) are presented in bold type and Adequate Intakes (AIs) in ordinary type followed by an asterisk (*). RDAs and AIs may both be used as goals for individual intake. RDAs are set to meet the needs of almost all (97-98%) individuals in the group. The AI is believed to cover needs of all individuals in the group, but lack of data or uncertainty in the data prevents being able to specify with confidence the percentage of persons covered by this intake.

[c]As cholecalciferol; 1 µg cholecalciferol = 40 IU vitamin D.

[d]In the absence of adequate exposure to sunlight.

Adapted from Yates et al. 1998.

Intakes of Athletes

Fleming and Heimbach (1994) reported calcium intake and food source data from the 1987-88 USDA Nationwide Food Consumption Survey. The average per capita intake of calcium for the total U.S. population was 737 mg, which is lower than the present AI for calcium (1000 mg/d for ages 19-50 years; 1200 mg/d for ages ≥51 years). Per capita intake was highest for people living in the western United States, for non-Hispanic whites, and for those with the highest income. The lowest per capita intake was in people living in the southern United States, for non-Hispanic blacks, and for those with the lowest income. Milk and milk products supplied over 50% of the total calcium intake; milk as an ingredient in other foods (e.g., cheese on pizza, beef stroganoff) provided approximately 20% of total calcium intake; and grain products provided 12%. As respondents' ages increased, there was a decrease in the percentage contribution of milk and milk products to total calcium intake. *These results show that the U.S. population on average is consuming less than the 1997 AI for calcium.*

Similar results are found among athletes. Self-reported dietary intake records of female athletes show intakes of calcium that are less than the 1997 AI—particularly among participants in aesthetic sports such as gymnastics and among distance runners (Benardot et al. 1989; Loosli et al. 1986; Wiita and Stombaugh 1996). However, *male athletes (ages 19-50 years) reported calcium intakes ranging from 800 to 1200 mg/d, thus consuming 80-120% of the current recommendation of 1000 mg/d* (Guezennec et al. 1998). This discrepancy between the reported calcium intakes of male and female athletes is probably due to the relatively low energy intakes of female athletes and to female athletes' tendency to avoid dairy products because they view them as being high in dietary fat (Manore 1996, 1999). There are many calcium sources available in the U.S. diet. However, it may be necessary for many people, including athletes, to take supplemental calcium because they are unable or unwilling to consume adequate calcium from dietary sources.

Dietary Sources and Supplementation Products

Dairy products are the most regularly consumed sources of calcium in the U.S. diet. Yet

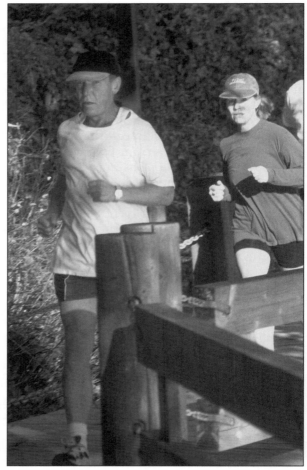

© Oscar C. Williams

Weightbearing activities such as running and walking help maintain or improve bone mineral density.

these products are often avoided by physically active people for two reasons. First, about 30% of adults in the United States (and up to 75% of adults around the world) are lactose intolerant, and consumption of milk products causes gastrointestinal distress. Second, since dairy products are often thought of as being high in dietary fat, people attempting to reduce fat in their diet tend to avoid these products (Manore 1996, 1999). For these reasons, it is important to stress to active people that skim and low-fat dairy sources have calcium contents similar to the regular-fat products. Many people mistakenly assume that reducing the fat in dairy products also lowers the calcium content. Moreover, research shows that people with lactose maldigestion can often use small amounts of milk without adverse effects (Suarez et al. 1998)—and there are now many lactose-free dairy products in the dairy sections of most major grocery stores.

Table 13.5 lists the calcium and phosphorus content of various foods. The significance of the calcium-to-phosphorus ratio (Ca:P) will be discussed later in this chapter. As table 13.5 reveals, dairy products have the highest calcium contents per serving, as do calcium-fortified foods such as tofu and fruit juices. Although spinach contains a relatively high amount of calcium, absorption may be limited by the ox-

alic acid present in spinach; only 5% of the calcium in spinach is absorbed, compared to 27% of the calcium in milk, when equal calcium loads are consumed (Weaver and Heaney 1999). The calcium absorption from kale is similar to that from milk products, but 10 cups would be necessary to meet the current calcium recommendations, which is not practical for most people. Meeting the current calcium recommendations through dietary means is difficult for people who do not regularly consume dairy

Table 13.5 **Food Sources of Calcium, Phosphorus, and Their Corresponding Levels of Fat, Energy (kcal), and Calcium-to-Phosphorus (Ca:P) Ratio**

Food	Serving size	Calcium (mg)	Phosphorus (mg)	Ca:P ratio[a]	Fat (g)	Kcal/ serving
Milk						
2% fat	8 fl oz	298	232	1.28	4	121
1% fat	8 fl oz	300	235	1.28	2	102
Skim	8 fl oz	301	247	1.22	0	86
Ice milk						
Vanilla	1 cup	183	144	1.27	5	183
Soft-serve	1 cup	276	213	1.30	4	222
Cheese						
American	1 slice	129	156	0.83	6	79
Cottage (2% fat)	1 cup	155	341	0.45	4	203
Monterey Jack	1 oz	211	126	1.67	8	106
Cream	1 oz	23	29	0.79	9	99
Cheddar	1 oz	200	145[b]	1.38	5	80
Yogurt						
Low-fat (plain)	8 oz	415	327	1.27	3	144
Dannon nonfat frozen (all flavors)	8 oz	336	257	1.31	0	249
Soft-serve (vanilla)	8 oz	324	293	1.11	12	361
Tofu						
Regular	3 oz	95	83	0.43	3.75	65
w/calcium sulfate	3 oz	581	162	1.35	7.13	123
Juice						
Orange (fresh)	8 fl oz	27	42	0.64	0	112
Orange (w/calcium, Citrus Hill)	8 fl oz	316	20	15.8	0	112
Apple-grape (w/calcium)	8 fl oz	161	15	10.7	0	91

(continued)

Table 13.5 *(continued)*

Food	Serving size	Calcium (mg)	Phosphorus (mg)	Ca:P ratio[a]	Fat (g)	Kcal/ serving
Vegetables						
Spinach (boiled)	1 cup	245	101	2.4	0	41
Kale	1 cup	94[b]	36[b]	2.6[b]	0[b]	42[b]
Kidney beans	1 cup	50[b]	252[b]	0.2[b]	1[b]	225[b]
McDonald's french fries	1 large	20	190	0.1	21	448
Soda pop						
Pepsi Cola (regular)	8 fl oz	0	35	0.0	0	100
Diet Coke	8 fl oz	9	21	0.4	0	2
Fast foods						
Ground beef (16% fat)	3 oz	8	162	0.05	13	225
Taco	1 each	100	146	0.7	11	190
Pizza (cheese, 12 in.)	1 piece	142	113[b]	1.3	7	235
Cereals						
Oatmeal (cooked)	1 cup	19	178	0.1	2	145
Cornflakes	1 cup	0	11	0.0	0	100
Cheerios	1 cup	42	86	0.5	1	83

Values obtained from ESHA Research, Food Processor, Version 7.02, 1997, unless otherwise indicated.

[a]An ideal Ca:P ratio, based on the current RDAs, is considered to be 1.42 (1.0:0.7) to 2.0 (2:1).

[b]Values obtained from Pennington 1994.

products or calcium-containing vegetable products; it is also difficult for people with relatively low energy intakes. Thus, supplementing with calcium may be necessary.

Hundreds of calcium supplements are available. How can one know which supplement to take? Unfortunately, it is difficult for the average consumers to determine which supplement is best for their particular calcium needs. Levenson and Bockman (1994) provide a thorough review of calcium supplements and other forms of preparations (table 13.6). "A Comparison of Calcium Supplements" on page 369 summarizes the calcium content and cost as of 1999 of various calcium supplements. Although there is a significant difference in cost among many supplemental forms of calcium, there is little evidence that one chemical compound of calcium is superior to another in maintaining bone health.

In addition to the factors listed previously in table 13.3, the amount of calcium consumed in one dose also affects its absorption. Absorp-

tion of calcium plateaus at 400-500 mg (figure 13.2), and doses divided over time appear to be better absorbed. People supplementing with calcium should limit individual doses to <500 mg, with the doses spaced throughout the day (Levenson and Bockman 1994).

High calcium intakes, from either supplements or calcium-fortified foods, can affect the nutrient status of other minerals in the body. For example, it has been suggested that calcium supplements decrease the absorption of dietary iron and zinc (Minihane and Fairweather-Tait 1998; Whiting 1995; Wood and Zheng 1997). However, Minihane and Fairweather-Tait (1998) found that long-term calcium supplementation did not reduce plasma ferritin concentrations (a measure of iron status) in iron-replete people who consumed a typical Western diet. Although high calcium intake can reduce zinc absorption, no one has investigated the effect on long-term zinc status. Calcium supplementation can also result in exposure to contaminants (e.g., lead,

Table 13.6 Percentage Calcium in Various Food or Supplement Preparations

Preparation	% Calcium	Comments
Carbonate	40	Insoluble at neutral pH
Tricalcium phosphate*	38	Phosphorus source
Dicalcium phosphate*	31	Insoluble; phosphorus source
Bone meal	31	May contain contaminating metals
Calcium-fortified orange juice	30	Food supplement
Oyster shell	28	May contain contaminating metals
Citrate	21	Soluble, taken in dissolved form

*Formulated for enteral use.

Adapted from Levenson and Bockman 1994.

mercury, and arsenic) which are found in some preparations of bone meal and dolomite. Vitamin D toxicity can occur if one takes large amounts of calcium supplements that include vitamin D. Finally, calcium supplements cause constipation, bloating, and excess gas in some people.

Phosphorus

Phosphorus occurs in bone primarily as calcium phosphate and hydroxyapatite. Approximately 88% of the phosphorus in the human body is found in the skeleton (table 13.1). Apart from bone, phosphorus is found primarily as inorganic

■ HIGHLIGHT ■

A Comparison of Calcium Supplements

A common question posed by the consumer is, "Which calcium supplement should I buy?" As calcium supplements are prepared using different compounds, it is important for consumers to purchase the supplement that will provide them with the most absorbable form of calcium for their money. Table 13.6 shows the percentage of calcium in various preparations. Although it would appear beneficial to take a preparation with the highest percentage calcium, bioavailability and absorbability of the calcium are of paramount concern. For instance, even though the carbonate form has the highest percentage of calcium, it is relatively insoluble, particularly at a neutral pH. Individuals with a condition of low stomach acid content, or **achlorhydria** (common among older people), cannot absorb this form of calcium. Such people more easily absorb the citrate form of calcium. The **absorptive fraction** (the percentage of calcium absorbed by the body) varies among calcium sources. Most forms of calcium have an absorptive fraction of about 26-37%, with the citrate form having the highest absorptive fraction (Levenson and Bockman 1994). To test the absorption of a calcium supplement, place one tablet in 6 oz of white vinegar at room temperature and stir occasionally. The tablet should dissolve in about 30 min (Gossel 1991). While this test illustrates how well the tablet dissolves, it does not guarantee the extent to which your body will absorb the elemental calcium in the tablet (Levenson and Bockman 1994).

Cost of the supplement is also an issue for consumers. We compared the cost of various calcium supplements at a local drugstore. In 1999, the cost of calcium supplements ranged from $2.40 to $26.25/mo. Thus, the amount of calcium, its absorbability, and the cost of the supplement are important factors to consider when purchasing a calcium supplement.

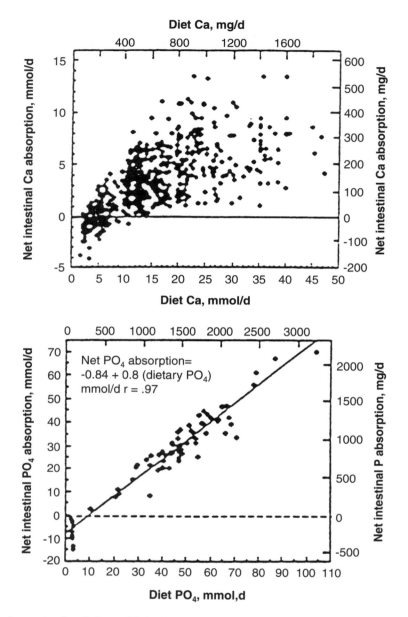

Figure 13.2 Net intestinal calcium (Ca) absorption as measured by the metabolic balance method in relation to dietary Ca intake among healthy adults (top panel); net intestinal phosphate (PO$_4$) absorption in relation to dietary PO$_4$ intake among healthy adults.

Reprinted from Anderson 1991.

phosphate. Important roles of inorganic phosphate related to exercise include its being a part of nucleic acids, proteins, ATP, and lipids. Phosphorus salts act as buffers that maintain acid-base balance and are also important as electrolytes in fluid balance. Inorganic phosphate is also a component of **2,3-diphosphoglycerate (DPG),** which affects the hemoglobin-oxygen dissociation curve. "Phosphorus and Sport Performance" (page 371) reviews the practice of "phosphate loading" among athletes.

Unlike calcium, phosphorus is readily absorbed at an efficiency of 60-70%. While calcium absorption plateaus at an intake of approximately 500 mg, absorption of phosphorus increases linearly with dietary intake (figure 13.2). Calcium and phosphorus absorption are coupled, with low phosphorus absorption linked with reduced calcium absorption. Following a meal, calcium and phosphorus appear to complex and are subsequently transported via passive mechanisms and taken up by soft and bone

■ HIGHLIGHT ■

Phosphorus and Sport Performance

Phosphorous supplementation, or **phosphate loading,** involves consuming high doses (usually 4 g/d) of phosphorus in the form of phosphate salts for several days before competition. This practice has been shown to increase serum phosphorus, 2,3-DPG levels, $\dot{V}O_2$max, and anaerobic threshold, and also to improve performance time (Cade et al. 1984, Kreider et al. 1990; Kreider et al. 1992). Clarkson and Haymes (1995) reviewed the practice of phosphate loading and concluded that it may enhance performance. Although the underlying physiological mechanism is unclear, the practice apparently can

- enhance 2,3-DPG synthesis, which results in better oxygen exchange at a given partial pressure of oxygen;
- improve the body's respiratory and metabolic buffering capacity; and
- improve myocardial and cardiovascular capacity during exercise.

Since phosphorus is widespread in foods, supplementation with phosphorus is unnecessary in healthy individuals. Clarkson and Haymes (1995) caution against using high amounts of phosphorus on a regular basis, as this practice can curb production of the active form of vitamin D, which in turn reduces absorption of calcium.

tissues (Anderson 1991). Phosphorus regulation appears to be less tightly controlled than that of calcium, with phosphorus loss occurring through the urine, skin, and secretions into the gut.

Methods of Assessment

Phosphorus status is usually determined by measuring serum phosphorus levels. The predominant forms of phosphorus in serum are inorganic phosphates, particularly the divalent HPO_4^{2-} and monovalent $H_2PO_4^-$ anions (Gibson 1990). Children have higher serum phosphorus concentrations than adults, with normal values reached by the third decade of life. While the serum phosphorus levels of males decrease with age after the third decade, the levels for women generally decrease between the ages of 20 and 35 years and increase after 40 years of age. People with insulin-dependent diabetes mellitus have fluctuating serum phosphorus levels, as insulin decreases serum phosphorus levels. Normal serum phosphorus values for adults are 2.5-4.5 mg/dL (0.87-1.45 mmol/L) (Fischbach 1996). Serum phosphorus should always be evaluated in relation to calcium levels since levels of the two minerals have an inverse relationship. Serum phosphorus values can be falsely elevated by hemolysis of red blood cells and laxatives containing large amounts

of sodium phosphate can increase serum phosphorus levels (Fischbach 1996).

Requirements

The RDA for phosphorus is 700 mg/d for both men and women (table 13.4). In the U.S. diet, phosphorus deficiencies are rare as phosphorus is readily absorbed and highly abundant in virtually all foods. Deficiencies can occur in people who consume large amounts of aluminum hydroxide antacids or in patients with diabetic keto-acidosis who are treated with insulin without supplemental phosphorus.

A more significant concern than phosphorus deficiency is the potential for bone loss with high dietary phosphorus intakes. Achievement of peak bone mass and the healthy maintenance of bone depend on a proper calcium and phosphorus balance. Excessive phosphorus intake in relation to calcium causes **secondary hyperparathyroidism** and also increases blood levels of 1,25-dihydroxy vitamin D in animals and humans. Since these conditions can cause removal of calcium and phosphorus from bone, it is possible that over long time periods they may result in bone loss (Anderson and Barrett 1994). The effect of a high phosphorus intake on bone status is still controversial in humans, however, and the long-term implications of a low calcium:phosphorus ratio have yet to be definitively determined (Calvo 1993; Food and Nutrition Board 1997).

Dietary Sources and Supplementation Products

Although it is found in most food sources, phosphorus is particularly abundant in dairy foods. Common sources of phosphorus in the U.S. diet include milk products, meats, grains, soda pop, and phosphorus additives to foods (mostly in the form of phosphates). The phosphorus intake of humans appears to be more than adequate, with the U.S. average intake reported to be 136-150% of the RDA (Food and Nutrition Board 1997; USDHHS 1986). In fact, it has been proposed that the phosphorus intake of Americans is even greater than that estimated since the nutrient databases used to estimate phosphorus intakes have not been updated with the levels of phosphorus in food additives. Estimates of additional phosphate intake from additives are 400-500 mg/d (International Food Additive Council [IFAC] 1992); Oenning et al. (1988) found that using only nutrient composition tables to estimate phosphorus content of food underestimates actual phosphorus content by 15-25%.

Table 13.5 lists the phosphorus content and the calcium:phosphorus ratio of select foods. The calcium:phosphorus ratio is low in foods such as cream, french fries, soda pop, ground beef, and cereals. The calcium:phosphorus ratio for the U.S. populations is low according to the new 1997 dietary recommendations for calcium (1000 mg/d) and phosphorus (700 mg/d) (or a recommended calcium:phosphorus ratio of 1.0:0.7, or 1.43). People who consume the recommendation for calcium have a ratio of 1.0:1.4, or 0.7, while people who consume less than the recommendation for calcium have a calcium:phosphorus ratio that is even lower (1.0:2.0, or 0.5 and lower). This low calcium:phosphorus ratio is most likely due to the high abundance of phosphorus in foods, the reduced consumption of milk coupled with an increased intake of soda pop, and the increased use of phosphorus-containing food additives. In light of the normally high intake of phosphorus from food sources, supplementation of phosphorus is not recommended.

Magnesium

Since chapter 11 thoroughly reviewed magnesium, we include here only a brief description of this mineral as it relates to bone. Magnesium is the third most common mineral in bone, with 60% of the body's magnesium found in the skeleton (table 13.1). Magnesium is involved in the bone mineralization process, and the magnesium in bone can act as a reservoir to ensure that adequate magnesium is available for bodily functions. Magnesium also holds calcium in tooth enamel, which assists in preventing dental caries. Magnesium is critical to adult bone health, as serum magnesium and dietary intakes of magnesium are positively correlated with a higher bone mineral content (Angus et al. 1988). Moreover, postmenopausal osteoporotic women tend to have low dietary intakes and serum levels of magnesium (Reginster et al. 1989; Tranquilli et al. 1994); magnesium supplements have beneficial effects in reducing fracture risk and bone loss in postmenopausal women (Stendig-Lindenberg et al. 1993).

Magnesium also plays an important role in substrate metabolism and energy production. Chapter 11 details magnesium's role in energy metabolism, the methods of assessment and requirements for magnesium, dietary sources of magnesium, and the magnesium status of athletes. Due to the abundance of magnesium in foods, deficiency in active and inactive people is rare, and, although magnesium losses increase with exercise, the dietary intake and status of magnesium in athletes are adequate and do not appear to be nutritional concerns. However, magnesium intakes could be jeopardized in athletes with very low energy intakes, and postmenopausal female athletes need to be aware of the critical role that adequate magnesium plays in bone health.

Vitamin D

Vitamin D is a *nutrient* involved in regulating serum calcium. *In addition to being classified as a vitamin, vitamin D is also considered a hormone* (Holick 1994; Combs 1992). The two primary sources of vitamin D are from its synthesis in skin tissue (stimulated by ultraviolet light) and from vitamin D-supplemented food products (primarily milk). Figure 13.3 illustrates the conversion of **7-dehydrocholesterol** to vitamin D_3 in the skin and subsequent conversion of that substance to the biologically active form of vitamin D **(1,25-dihydroxy vitamin D,** or **cholecalciferol).** The primary

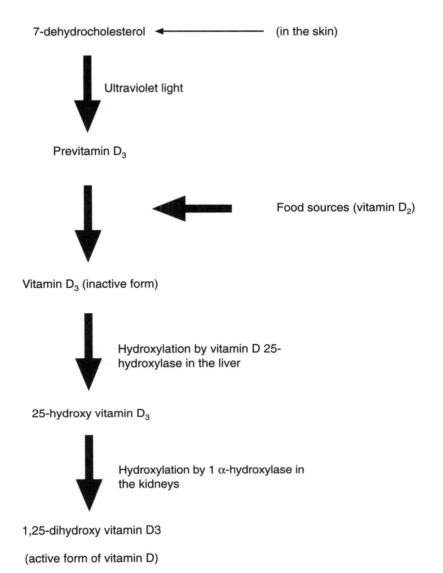

7-dehydrocholesterol ◄─────────── (in the skin)

Ultraviolet light

Previtamin D$_3$

Food sources (vitamin D$_2$)

Vitamin D$_3$ (inactive form)

Hydroxylation by vitamin D 25-hydroxylase in the liver

25-hydroxy vitamin D$_3$

Hydroxylation by 1 α-hydroxylase in the kidneys

1,25-dihydroxy vitamin D3

(active form of vitamin D)

Figure 13.3   Vitamin D synthesis and activation. Cholesterol in the skin is converted to previtamin D$_3$ in the presence of ultraviolet light. Inactive forms of vitamin D, from both the skin and the diet, are activated via two separate hydroxylation reactions to the active form of vitamin D (1,25-dihydroxy vitamin D).

role of vitamin D is to maintain skeletal calcium balance. Vitamin D meets this role by

- promoting absorption of calcium from the intestines,
- promoting bone resorption,
- maintaining adequate quantities of calcium and phosphorus for bone formation by its actions on the kidney and intestines, and
- allowing proper functioning of parathyroid hormone to maintain serum calcium at proper levels.

Methods of Assessment

The most useful index of vitamin D status is serum **total 25-hydroxy vitamin D (25-OH-D),** as this marker reflects the amount of vitamin D in the liver, which is the major area of storage for vitamin D (Gibson 1990). Serum 25-OH-D is measured using competitive protein-binding assays and high-performance liquid chromatography (HPLC). After HPLC separates 25-OH-D from other metabolites, the 25-OH-D can be assayed using the competitive protein-binding technique. It is not yet clear what levels of serum 25-OH-D indicate deficiency or toxicity. Concentrations below 3.0 ng/ml (7.5 nmol/L) seem to be associated with clinical signs of vitamin D deficiency, while levels above 200 ng/ml (500 nmol/L) may indicate toxicity (Haddad and Stamp 1974). A number of factors influence serum concentrations of 25-OH-D:

- **Season:** Highest levels occur in the summer, lowest in the winter.
- **Supplement use:** Higher levels are found in people who take vitamin D supplements.
- **Age and sex:** Levels decrease with age and tend to be lower in women than in men.
- **Latitude:** People living in higher latitudes are exposed to lower levels of solar radiation, decreasing their conversion of vitamin D in the skin.
- **Levels of sun exposure:** People of any latitude who get little or no sun exposure are at risk for low levels of 25-OH-D—a condition common in home-bound elderly, people who work indoors, and those who live in areas where the sky is overcast much of the time, *particularly during the winter months.*

Requirements

Table 13.4 lists the recommended AI values for vitamin D. Requirements for vitamin D increase with age—probably because of age-related changes in vitamin D conversion in the skin, reduced absorption of dietary vitamin D in the intestines, decreased production of 25-OH-D by the kidneys, and reduced exposure to sunlight with age (Baylink and Jennings 1994). No evidence exists to suggest that active people have a higher vitamin D requirement than nonactive people. However, meeting vitamin D requirements may be difficult for athletes who train indoors (e.g., figure skaters, gymnasts), who live at higher latitudes, and who fail to consume vitamin D-supplemented food products.

Dietary Sources and Supplementation Products

The form of vitamin D used as a supplement in foods (e.g., milk, margarine, baked goods, grain products) includes both **vitamin D$_2$ (ergocalciferol)** and **vitamin D$_3$ (cholecalciferol),** while the form metabolized in the skin is **previtamin D$_3$** (Combs 1992). Vitamin D$_2$ is

found in only small amounts in some plants, fungi, molds, and lichens; oily fish products, fish liver, and eggs contain the D$_3$ form. Although scientists traditionally have believed that the D$_2$ and D$_3$ forms were metabolized identically and resulted in the same increase in 25-OH-D in humans, Trang et al. (1998) have challenged this assumption. They found that the D$_3$ form of the vitamin resulted in a 70% greater increase in serum 25-OH-D concentrations than the D$_2$ form. This effect was particularly pronounced in subjects with the lowest serum 25-OH-D levels at baseline, indicating that the D$_3$ form may be most effective in increasing 25-OH-D levels in people with reduced vitamin D status.

Vitamin D supplementation appears effective in preventing hip and spine fractures in the elderly and is an important therapeutic option in treating osteoporosis. Younger people may also need supplements if they have little exposure to the sun and poor dietary intakes of vitamin D. Because vitamin D is fat soluble (and therefore stored in the body), it is important to assess vitamin D status if possible prior to supplementation. If this is not possible, the typical vitamin D intake and extent of exposure to the sun should be determined. Excessive intake of vitamin D supplements can result in vitamin D toxicity and decreased bone mass. Adams and Lee (1997) identified a group of postmenopausal women who had high levels of urinary calcium and elevated serum 25-OH-D concentrations. These women were taking several dietary supplements (ranging from three to eight supplements per day), some of which contained as much as 3600 IU of vitamin D$_3$ per daily dosage (nine times the recommended amount for women ages 51-70 years). The bone mineral density of the women was indicative of osteoporosis. Withdrawal of the supplements resulted in the normalization of urinary calcium and serum 25-OH-D concentrations and an increase in bone mineral density. This study is one example of the deleterious effects of excessive intakes of vitamin D supplements and highlights the fact that unrestricted supplementation can have a significant negative impact on a person's health.

Other Nutrients Involved in Bone Metabolism

In addition to the nutrients already discussed, there are several others that play an important role in bone health.

Fluoride

Fluoride plays a critical role in the strengthening of bones and teeth. Fluoride replaces the hydroxyl portions of the hydroxyapatite crystal after mineralization of the bones and teeth, making them stronger and, in the case of teeth, more resistant to decay. **Fluorapatite** is the stabilized form of the apatite minerals in bone and teeth. The most significant sources of fluoride are fluoridated water, tea, and seafood. Short-term (2-3 years), low-dose fluoride therapy can increase bone mineral density in the spine (Pak et al. 1994). Long-term (5 years) treatment with fluoride is not recommended, as it results in the formation of large, abnormally placed mineral crystals, and long-term therapy may decrease bone strength and quality (Sogaard et al. 1994).

Energy and Protein

Adequate energy intake is critical for everyone, as macro- and micronutrients cannot be consumed in adequate amounts if energy intake is insufficient. Chronically low energy intakes hinder complete bone development and maintenance of healthy bone mass. This relationship between adequate energy and bone health plays an important interactive role in the "female athlete triad" (see "Female Athlete Triad and Osteoporosis," below, and chapter 15).

Bone formation, growth, and maintenance are impossible without adequate protein. Proteins are a part of collagen and of noncollagenous tissues, as well as growth factors involved in bone formation; and they are primary constituents of the bone matrix material. The effect of high dietary protein on bone health is controversial, with claims that high protein intake can increase urinary calcium losses. In reviewing this topic, Spencer and colleagues (1989) concluded that *dietary protein sources that contain phosphorus (e.g., meat, fish, and poultry)* do not result in bone loss. Purified protein sources *such as soy protein, protein powders, and single amino acid supplements*, however, may have a negative impact on calcium balance and bone health. These authors also caution against recommending low-protein diets to elderly people, who are already at risk for low protein (and subsequently phosphorus)

■ HIGHLIGHT ■

Female Athlete Triad and Osteoporosis

Normal menstrual function is vital to the maintenance of bone health. The **female athlete triad** is a condition comprised of *amenorrhea, disordered eating,* and *osteoporosis.* Chapter 15 provides a complete description of this condition. We include a brief discussion here because of the direct links between osteoporosis and inadequate energy intake, low calcium intake, relatively high energy expenditure, and altered menstrual function. The term **osteopenia** generally refers to bone *mass* reduction. **Osteoporosis** is defined as "skeletal *fragility* due to decreased bone mass and to microarchitectural deterioration of bone tissue, with a consequent increase in risk of fracture" (Consensus Development Conference 1991).

Table 13.7 includes the risk factors for development of osteoporosis in elderly women, who appear to be most at risk for developing the condition. A history of athletic menstrual dysfunction and disordered eating increases a woman's risk for developing osteoporosis. Figure 13.4 illustrates a proposed model of the mechanisms that result in bone loss during estrogen deficiency. The low circulating estrogen levels that accompany menopause (or menstrual dysfunction in premenopausal athletes) lead to a decrease in bone formation, an increase in bone resorption, and consequent changes in serum calcium and hormones related to calcium metabolism; the end result is a decrease in calcium absorption and an increase in urinary calcium loss. One major protective factor against osteoporosis in women is maintenance of normal menstrual function during the premenopausal phase of life. Treatment options for osteoporosis include exercise, estrogen, calcium and vitamin D supplementation, **bisphosphonates** (anti-bone-resorbers), and sodium fluoride.

Table 13.7 Risk Factors Associated With Osteoporosis in the Elderly

- Estrogen depletion (in women):

  Postmenopausal state (natural or artificial)

  History of athletic amenorrhea, anorexia nervosa, oligomenorrhea, etc.
- Calcium deficiency
- Diminished peak bone mass at skeletal maturity (varies with sex, race, and heredity)
- Diminished physical activity
- Positive family history of osteoporosis
- Testosterone depletion (in men)
- Aging
- Leanness (adipose tissue is the major source of postmenopausal extragonadal estrogen production)
- Alcoholism
- Smoking
- Excessive dietary protein intake (resulting in increased loss of calcium in the urine)
- Medications (corticosteroids, excessive thyroid hormone, prolonged heparin usage)

Reprinted, by permission, from C.H. Chestnut, 1994, Osteoporosis. In *Principles of Geriatric Medicine and Gerontology*, 3rd ed. (New York: McGraw-Hill), 899. Reproduced with permission of The McGraw-Hill Companies.

intakes; such diets could further compromise bone health in these individuals.

Vitamins K and C

Vitamin K plays an important role in blood coagulation and is required for synthesis of osteocalcin. **Osteocalcin** is produced by osteoblasts in bone tissue and is involved in bone formation. Vitamin K is endogenously produced by bacteria in the digestive tract. Food sources of vitamin K include liver, avocado, green leafy vegetables (e.g., spinach), chili peppers, cruciferous vegetables (cabbage, brussels sprouts, broccoli), and milk. No one has studied vitamin K status in athletes, and few data are available on the use of vitamin K supplements to improve bone health.

The role of vitamin C in bone health is most likely related to its role in the formation of collagen. Epidemiological studies report conflicting results: Gunnes and Lehmann (1995) found that dietary vitamin C was positively related to forearm bone mineral density in children and adolescents, yet Leveille et al. (1997) found no association between dietary vitamin C with bone mineral density in postmenopausal women. However, it makes intuitive sense that a severe vitamin C deficiency would alter collagen, and thus bone, formation. Regular consumption of fruits, juices, and vegetables can easily provide adequate vitamin C.

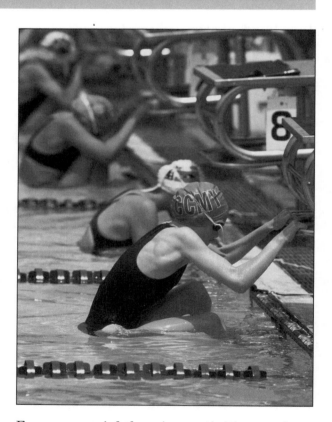

Even nonweightbearing activities such as swimming contribute to bone health because the muscles pull against the bone. Nonweightbearing activities should be combined with weightbearing activities for good bone health.

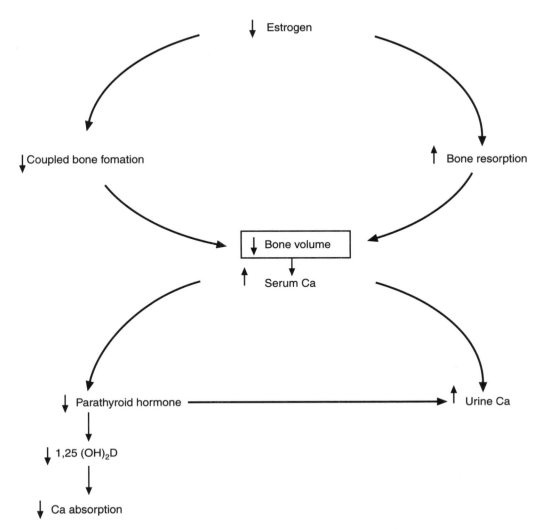

Figure 13.4 Model of mechanisms of bone loss in estrogen deficiency. Estrogen deficiency increases bone resorption and also destroys the usual balance between bone formation and bone resorption. The net result is bone loss. The bone loss stimulates serum calcium counterregulatory mechanisms (i.e., decreased calcium absorption and increased urinary calcium levels), the end result being that the extra calcium released from the bone is constantly removed from circulation and is excreted in the urine.

Reprinted from Baylink and Jennings 1994.

Effects of Exercise on Bone Health

Hundreds of research articles have focused on exercise, physical activity, and bone health. We especially recommend recent review articles by Barr and McKay (1998), Suominen (1993), and Anderson and Metz (1993). Here is what we currently understand about the relationship between exercise and bone health:

- Epidemiological studies show that regular participation in moderate to vigorous weightbearing physical activity is related to a higher bone density (Halioua and Anderson 1989).

- Active people tend to have higher bone density values than do sedentary people (Dook et al. 1997; Suominen 1993).

- Participation in a weightbearing exercise program (resistance training, walking, or running) can result in a modest increase in bone density (Nelson et al. 1991; Snow-Harter et al. 1992).

- Certain male and female athletes are at risk for low bone density (Drinkwater et al. 1990; Hetland et al. 1993). Females with altered menstrual function are most at risk; the mechanism contributing to low bone density in male athletes who participate in non-weightbearing activities (e.g., cyclists) is not clear.

- Participation in impact loading-type sports, such as gymnastics and bodybuilding, results in a higher bone density than in other sports, even in female athletes with compromised menstrual status (Fehling et al. 1995; Robinson et al. 1995).

Thus, it appears that physical activity and exercise can play health-promoting roles in bone formation and maintenance. However, proper hormonal, energy, and nutrient balance is critical to deriving the benefits of exercise on bone.

Chapter in Review

Calcium, phosphorus, magnesium, and vitamin D play critical roles in forming the bone matrix and in maintaining adult bone. Many U.S. adults do not consume the current recommended intake for calcium, and certain people may benefit from calcium supplementation. Vitamin D deficiencies can occur in elderly people who spend little time outdoors, in people who live at high latitudes, and in athletes who train and compete indoors and fail to consume adequate dietary sources of vitamin D. Exercise and weightbearing physical activity appear to have beneficial effects on bone maintenance in adults, but failure of women to maintain regular menstrual function can result in a reduction in bone mass and increase the risk for osteoporosis.

KEY CONCEPTS

 1. Describe the stages of bone metabolism, and list the primary nutrients associated with bone health.

> The three stages of bone metabolism are growth, remodeling, and modeling. Calcium, phosphorus, magnesium, and vitamin D are nutrients associated with bone health.

 2. Discuss the methods used to assess calcium, identify calcium requirements and intakes of athletes, and identify sources of calcium and related supplementation products.

> There is no satisfactory way to assess calcium levels directly. Assessment of bone can indicate long-term calcium status. Although calcium requirements are difficult to determine, DRI values have been established to help plan and assess diets for healthy people. Calcium intakes for some athletes and other people are lower than recommended, with milk and milk products being the most common sources of calcium in the United States. Athletes at risk for low calcium intakes are those with low energy intakes. Calcium supplements vary in absorbability and cost.

 3. Describe the methods of assessment, the requirements, and dietary sources of phosphorus.

> Serum phosphorus levels are a general indicator of phosphorus status. The RDA for adult men and women is 700 mg/d, and phosphorus deficiencies are rare in the United States. Long-term excessive phosphorus intake can result in bone loss. Phosphorus is found in most foods and is particularly abundant in dairy products. The phosphorus intake in the United States is reportedly more than adequate. One key to maintaining bone health is to maintain a healthy calcium:phosphorus ratio, the ideal being 1.42-2.0. Although soda pop has significant amounts of phosphorus, its calcium:phosphorus ratio is 0.0 to 0.4, making it a poor nutritional choice.

 4. Discuss magnesium's role in bone health.

> Magnesium is the third most common mineral in bone. Magnesium is involved in bone mineralization and can act as a reservoir in bone to maintain magnesium for other bodily functions. Magnesium is abundant in food, and deficiencies are rare.

5. Describe the methods of assessment, the requirements, dietary sources, and supplementation products of vitamin D.

Vitamin D is a hormone involved in regulating serum calcium. The best marker of vitamin D status is serum total 25-hydroxy vitamin D (25-OH-D). Vitamin D requirements increase with age. There is no evidence that active people require more vitamin D than sedentary people. Vitamin D is supplemented in food; vitamin D is also synthesized in the skin during exposure to ultraviolet light. Caution should be used when taking vitamin D supplements, as it is fat soluble, and vitamin D toxicity can decrease bone mass.

 6. Describe how fluoride, energy, and protein play a role in bone metabolism.

Fluoride is a part of the hydroxyapatite crystals that strengthen teeth and bone. Significant sources of fluoride are fluoridated water, tea, and seafood. Low energy intakes result in low macro- and micronutrient intakes and prevent development and maintenance of healthy bone. Proteins are a critical part of collagen and noncollagenous tissues and of the growth factors involved in bone formation; they also are part of the bone matrix material.

KEY TERMS

1,25-dihydroxy vitamin D (cholecalciferol)
2,3-diphosphoglycerate (DPG)
7-dehydrocholesterol
absorptive fraction
achlorhydria
bisphosphonates
calcium:creatinine ratio
cortical (or compact) bone
female athlete triad
fluorapatite
formation
hydroxyapatite
modeling stage
osteoblasts

osteocalcin
osteoclasts
osteopenia
osteoporosis
phosphate loading
previtamin D_3
remodeling
resorption
secondary hyperparathyroidism
total 25-hydroxy vitamin D (25-OH-D)
trabecular (or cancellous) bone
vitamin D_2 (ergocalciferol)
vitamin D_3 (cholecalciferol)

References

Adams JS, Lee G. Gains in bone mineral density with resolution of vitamin D intoxication. Ann Int Med 1997;127:203-6.

Anderson JJB. Nutritional biochemistry of calcium and phosphorus. J Nutr Biochem 1991;2:300-7.

Anderson JJB, Barrett CJH. Dietary phosphorus: the benefits and the problems. Nutr Today 1994 (March/April):29-34.

Anderson JJB, Metz JA. Contributions of dietary calcium and physical activity to primary prevention of osteoporosis in females. J Am Coll Nutr 1993;12(4):378-83.

Angus RM, Sambrook PN, Pocock NA, Eisman JA. Dietary intake and bone mineral density. Bone Miner 1988;4:265-77.

Barr SI, McKay HA. Nutrition, exercise, and bone status in youth. Int J Sport Nutr 1998;8:124-42.

Baylink DJ, Jennings JC. Calcium and bone homeostasis and changes with aging. In: Hazzard WR, Bierman EL, Blass JP, Ettinger WH, Halter JB, eds. Principles of Geriatric Medicine and Gerontology. New York: McGraw-Hill, 1994:879-96.

Benardot D, Schwarz M, Heller DW. Nutrient intake in young, highly competitive gymnasts. J Am Diet Assoc 1989;89(3):401-3.

Bonjour JP, Theintz G, Buchs B, Slosman D, Rizzoli R. Critical years and stages of puberty for spinal and femoral bone mass accumulation during adolescence. J Clin Endocrinol Metab 1991;73:555-63.

Cade R, Conte M, Zauner C, et al. Effects of phosphate loading on 2,3-diphosphoglycerate and maximal oxygen uptake. Med Sci Sports Exerc 1984;16:263-8.

Calvo MS. Dietary phosphorus, calcium metabolism and bone. J Nutr 1993;123:1627-33.

Chesnut CH. Osteoporosis. In: Hazzard WR, Bierman EL, Blass JP, Ettinger WH, Halter JB, eds. Principles of Geriatric Medicine and Gerontology. New York: McGraw-Hill, 1994:897-909.

Clarkson PM, Haymes EM. Exercise and mineral status of athletes: calcium, magnesium, phosphorus, and iron. Med Sci Sports Exerc 1995;27(6):831-43.

Combs GF. The Vitamins. Fundamental Aspects in Nutrition and Health. San Diego: Academic Press, 1992:153-4.

Consensus Development Conference. Prophylaxis and treatment of osteoporosis. Am J Med 1991;90:107-10.

Dalsky GP. Effect of exercise on bone: permissive influence of estrogen and calcium. Med Sci Sports Exerc 1990;22(3):281-5.

Dook JE, James C, Henderson NK, Price RI. Exercise and bone mineral density in mature female athletes. Med Sci Sports Exerc 1997;29(3):291-6.

Drinkwater BL, Bruemner B, Chesnut CH. Menstrual history as a determinant of current bone density in young athletes. J Am Med Assoc 1990;263(4):545-8.

Fehling PC, Alekel L, Clasey J, Rector A, Stillman RJ. A comparison of bone mineral densities among female athletes in impact loading and active loading sports. Bone 1995;17:205-10.

Fischbach FA. Manual of Laboratory and Diagnostic Tests, 5th ed. Philadelphia: Lippincott, 1996.

Fleming KH, Heimbach JT. Consumption of calcium in the U.S.: food sources and intake levels. J Nutr 1994;124:1426S-30S.

Food and Nutrition Board, Institute of Medicine. Dietary Reference Intakes: calcium, phosphorus, magnesium, vitamin D and fluoride. Washington, DC: National Academy Press, 1997.

Food Processor (software program), Version 7.02. 1997. ESHA Research, Salem, OR.

Frost HM. Some effects of basic multicellular unit-based remodeling on photon absorptiometry of trabecular bone. Bone Miner 1987;7:47-65.

Gibson RS. Principles of Nutritional Assessment. New York: Oxford University Press, 1990.

Gossel TA. Calcium supplements. U.S. Pharmacist 1991 (April):26-32.

Guezennec CY, Chalabi H, Bernard J, Fardellone P, Krentowski R, Zerath E, Meunier P-J. Is there a relationship between physical activity and dietary calcium intake? A survey in 10,373 young French subjects. Med Sci Sports Exerc 1998;30:732-9.

Gunnes M, Lehmann EH. Dietary calcium, saturated fat, fiber and vitamin C as predictors of forearm cortical and trabecular bone mineral density in healthy children and adolescents. Acta Paediatr 1995;84(4):388-92.

Haddad JG, Stamp TCB. Circulating 25-hydroxyvitamin D in man. Am J Med 1974;57:57-62.

Halioua L, Anderson JJB. Lifetime calcium intake and physical activity habits: independent and combined effects on the radial bone of healthy premenopausal Caucasian women. Am J Clin Nutr 1989;49:534-41.

Heaney R, Recker R. Distribution of calcium absorption in middle-aged women. Am J Clin Nutr 1986;43:299-305.

Hetland ML, Haarbo J, Christiansen C. Low bone mass and high bone turnover in male long distance runners. J Clin Endocrinol Metab 1993;77(3):770-5.

Holick MF. Vitamin D. In: Shils ME, Olson JA, Shike M, eds. Modern Nutrition in Health and Disease, 8th ed. Philadelphia: Lea & Febiger, 1994:308-25.

International Food Additive Council. Disappearance of Phosphorus in the U.S. Food Applications. Atlanta: International Food Additive Council, 1992.

Kreider RB, Miller GW, Schenck D, et al. Effects of phosphate loading on metabolic and myocardial responses to maximal and endurance exercise. Int J Sport Nutr 1992;2:20-47.

Kreider RB, Miller GW, Williams MH, Somma Thomas C, Nasser TA. Effects of phosphate loading on oxygen uptake, ventilatory anaerobic threshold, and run performance. Med Sci Sports Exerc 1990;22:250-6.

Ladenson JH, Bowers GN. Free calcium in serum. I. Determination with the ion-specific electrode, and factors affecting the results. Clin Chem 1973;19:565-74.

Leveille SG, LaCroix AZ, Koepsell TD, Beresford SA, Van Belle G, Buchner DM. Dietary vitamin C and bone mineral density in postmenopausal women in Washington State, USA. J Epidemiol Community Health 1997;51(5):479-85.

Levenson DI, Bockman RS. A review of calcium preparations. Nutr Rev 1994;52(7):221-32.

Loosli AR, Benson J, Gillien DM, Bourdet K. Nutrition habits and knowledge in competitive adolescent female gymnasts. Phys Sports Med 1986;14(8):118-30.

Lunar Corporation. Biochemical markers: variability high, predictive accuracy poor. LunarNews 1994 (December):15-7.

Manore MM. Chronic dieting in active women: what are the health consequences? Women's Health Issues 1996;6:332-41.

Manore MM. Nutritional needs of the female athlete. Clin Sports Med 1999;18(3):549-63.

Minihane AM, Fairweather-Tait SJ. Effect of calcium supplementation on daily nonheme-iron absorption and long-term iron status. Am J Clin Nutr 1998;68(1):96-102.

Nelson ME, Fisher EC, Avraham Dilmanian F, Dallal GE, Evans WJ. A 1-y walking program and increased dietary calcium in postmenopausal women: effects on bone. Am J Clin Nutr 1991;53:1304-11.

Oenning LJ, Voegel J, Calvo MS. Accuracy of methods estimating calcium and phosphorous intake in daily diets. J Am Diet Assoc 1988;88:1076-8.

Pak CYC, Sakhaee K, Piziak V, et al. Slow-release sodium fluoride in the management of postmenopausal osteoporosis. Ann Intern Med 1994;120:625-32.

Pennington JA. Bowes and Church's food values of portions commonly used. 16th ed. Philadelphia: Lippincott, 1994.

Reginster JY, Strause L, Deroisy R, Lecart MP, Saltman P, Franchimont P. Preliminary report of decreased serum magnesium in postmenopausal osteoporosis. Magnesium 1989;8:106-9.

Robinson TL, Snow-Harter C, Taaffe DR, Gillis D, Shaw J, Marcus R. Gymnasts exhibit higher bone mass than runners despite similar prevalence of amenorrhea and oligomenorrhea. J Bone Min Res 1995;10:26-35.

Snow-Harter C, Bouxsein ML, Lewis BT, Carter DR, Marcus R. Effects of resistance and endurance exercise on bone mineral status of young women: a randomized exercise intervention trial. J Bone Min Res 1992;7(7):761-9.

Soogaard CH, Mosekilde L, Richards A, Mosekilde L. Marked decrease in trabecular bone quality after five years of sodium fluoride therapy—assessed by biomechanical testing of iliac crest bone biopsies in osteoporotic patients. Bone 1994;15(4):393-9.

Spencer H, Kramer L, Osis D. Do protein and phosphorus cause calcium loss? Nutr Today 1989 (January/February):33-5.

Stendig-Lindenberg G, Tepper R, Leichter I. Trabecular bone density in a two year controlled trial of peroral magnesium in osteoporosis. Magnes Res 1993;6:155-63.

Suarez FL, Adshead J, Furne JK, Levitt MD. Lactose maldigestion is not an impediment to the intake of 1500 mg calcium daily as dairy products. Am J Clin Nutr 1998;68:1118-22.

Suominen H. Bone mineral density and long term exercise. An overview of cross-sectional athlete studies. Sports Med 1993;16(5):316-30.

Trang HM, Cole DEC, Rubin LA, Pierratos A, Siu S, Vieth R. Evidence that vitamin D_3 increases serum 25-hydroxyvitamin D more efficiently than does vitamin D_2. Am J Clin Nutr 1998;68:854-8.

Tranquilli AL, Lucino E, Garzetti GG, Romanini C. Calcium, phosphorus and magnesium intakes correlate with bone mineral content in postmenopausal women. Gynecol Endocrinol 1994;8:55-8.

U.S. Department of Health and Human Services and U.S. Department of Agriculture. Phosphorus. In: Nutrition Monitoring in the United States: A Progress Report of the Joint Nutrition Monitoring Evaluation Committee. Washington, DC: U.S. Department of Health and Human Services and U.S. Department of Agriculture, 1986:154-8.

Wandrup J, Kvetny J. Potentiometric measurement of ionized calcium in anaerobic whole blood, plasma, and serum evaluated. Clin Chem 1985;31:856-60.

Weaver CM. Assessing calcium and status and metabolism. J Nutr 1990;120:1470-3.

Weaver CM. Age related calcium requirements due to changes in absorption and utilization. J Nutr 1994;124:1418S-25S.

Weaver CM, Heaney RP. Calcium. In: Shils ME, Olsen JA, Shike M, Ross AC, eds. Modern Nutrition in Health and Disease, 9th ed. Baltimore: Williams & Wilkins, 1999:141-55.

Whiting SJ. The inhibitory effect of dietary calcium on iron bioavailability: a cause for concern? Nutr Rev 1995;53(3):77-80.

Wiita BG, Stombaugh IA. Nutrition knowledge, eating practices, and health of adolescent female runners: a 3-year longitudinal study. Int J Sport Nutr 1996;6(4):414-25.

Wood RJ, Zheng JJ. High dietary calcium intakes reduce zinc absorption and balance in humans. Am J Clin Nutr 1997;65:1803-9.

Yates AA, Schlicker SA, Suitor CW. Dietary reference intakes: the new basis for recommendations for calcium and related nutrients, B vitamins, and choline. J Am Diet Assoc 1998;98:699-706.

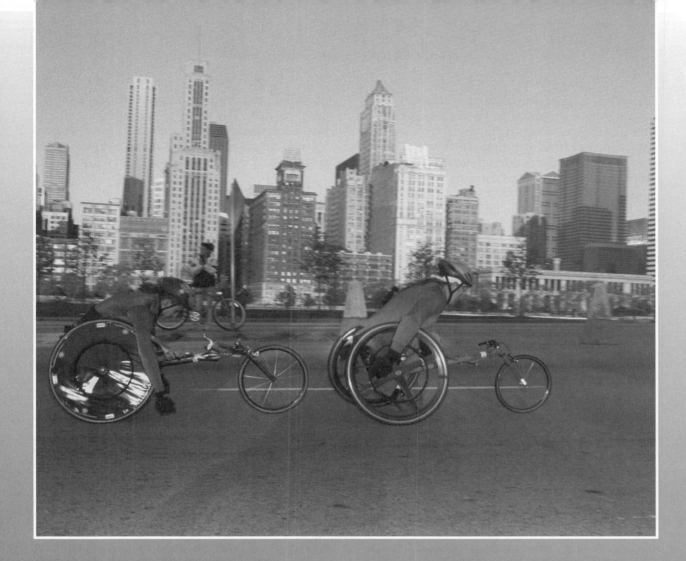

CHAPTER 14

Nutrition and Fitness Assessment

After reading this chapter you should be able to

- describe the characteristics of medical and health history questionnaires;
- discuss the methods used to assess energy and nutrient intakes;
- discuss the methods used to assess energy expenditure; and
- describe specific tests used to assess the components of fitness.

Tammy is a collegiate distance runner, participating in cross-country and track competitions. She is concerned about her performance: she has been very tired at practice and has not been performing her best during competition. (For more information about Tammy's fatigue, see "Case Study: Female Distance Runner Complaining of Fatigue" on page 398.) Tammy wants to maintain a low body weight and a low percentage of body fat since she believes these characteristics will guarantee success in distance running. She wants to find ways to maximize her performance—and avoid body fat or weight gain—by maintaining healthy eating habits. How can you help Tammy maximize her health and performance?

In addition to competitive athletes like Tammy, recreational athletes and untrained people also initiate diet and/or exercise programs and are interested in assessing their current nutrition and fitness status to maximize the benefits of a program. How can you assess a person's present status and design an optimal training program? How can you determine if someone's current program is working? In order to maximize an athlete's performance, you must be able to assess the person's status for health, nutrition, and physical performance.

In this chapter, we review assessment techniques for nutrition and fitness. We briefly describe each technique, including its advantages and disadvantages. Appendixes E.1–E.5 provide samples of some of the assessment techniques reviewed, a table of energy cost values for activities, and a table of recommended values for select laboratory (i.e., blood) tests used to assess health status.

Medical and Health History Questionnaires

The American College of Sports Medicine (ACSM) (1995) has recommended that certain components be included in a medical history and physical examination. These assessments are administered before exercise testing or before beginning an exercise program. The guidelines assist the exercise or nutrition professional in determining a person's level of risk and the extent to which medical evaluation is necessary.

An important component of a medical history is the physical examination. Any untrained or detrained person should have a thorough physical examination before starting an exercise program. The physical examination should be performed by a licensed health professional (physician, nurse practitioner, or physician assistant) and may include the following:

- A 12-lead electrocardiogram
- Laboratory (blood and urine) assessments
- Vital signs (heart rate, blood pressure, temperature, ventilation)
- Heart sounds

The medical professional selects the tests to be conducted based on the client's medical history, risk factors, and disease symptoms. While a young, apparently healthy person does not require a 12-lead electrocardiogram prior to starting an exercise program, a 45-year-old man with elevated blood pressure should have this test.

How often should someone have a thorough physical examination? The answer to this question is not simple, as the frequency of medical assessments should depend on an individual's age and health status. Typically it is recommended that a healthy person <30 years old should have a thorough physical examination every 2-3 years. People aged 30-50 years should have an exam every 1.5-2 years; those >50 years should have an annual examination, including a stress test with a 12-lead electrocardiogram. The frequency of the examination and the screening tests to be conducted depend on the person's current health status and the physician's discretion.

Health history questionnaires help determine the presence of any current or potential health problems. Questionnaires should include the following:

- Demographic information (name, age, height, weight)
- Present medication status (ask for full drug name, dose, and frequency of administration for both prescription and over-the-counter medications) and drug allergies
- Family history of disease
- History of illnesses and injuries
- History of menstrual function (for females)
- Exercise history
- Diet history (including body weight fluctuations and history of eating disorders)

When designing your own health history form or administering a previously published form, always allow extra space for affirmative responses to the questions posed. Review a person's health history, and discuss it with that individual before you initiate any assessment procedures. Figure 14.1 provides an example of a general health history questionnaire appropriate to use with both untrained and active people.

Use the information on the medical examination and health history form to determine a client's level of risk. The American College of Sports Medicine (1995) recommends categorizing an individual into one of three levels of risk:

- ***Apparently healthy:*** Individuals with no symptoms of disease or illness, who are apparently healthy, and who have no more than one major coronary artery disease (CAD) risk factor (see table 14.1 for the CAD risk factors)
- ***Increased risk:*** Individuals who have signs or symptoms of disease and/or who possess two or more risk factors for CAD
- ***Known disease:*** Individuals with known cardiac, pulmonary, or metabolic diseases

Once you determine a client's level of risk, you can use that information to decide the safest course of action for fitness testing. A more de-

tailed discussion of fitness testing is provided later in this chapter.

Assessing Energy and Nutrient Intake

A multitude of techniques is available to assess energy and nutrient intakes. To choose the most appropriate tool(s), first determine the type of information you need to obtain. Do you need to determine only a person's total energy intake, or do you also need to assess all macro- and micronutrient intakes? Is it critical to know the quality of protein and type of carbohydrates and fats the person consumes? Knowing the answers to these questions will help you select the best tool(s). Remember that the techniques discussed in this chapter do not estimate the nutritional *status* of an individual but only nutrient *intake*. To determine nutritional status, you must combine information on nutrient intake with other (e.g., biochemical, anthropometric, body composition) methods.

Collecting energy and nutrient intake involves either *retrospective* methods (e.g., 24-h

Table 14.1 Coronary Artery Disease Risk Factors

Risk factor	Defining criteria
• Age	Males older than 45 years; females older than 55 years or premature menopause without ERT.*
• Family history	A myocardial infarction or sudden death in father or in first-degree male relative before 55 years of age, or in mother or female first-degree relative before 65 years of age.
• Current cigarette smoking	
• Hypertension	Blood pressure ≥ 140/90 mm Hg, confirmed by measurements on at least two separate occasions, or on antihypertensive medication.
• Hypercholesterolemia	Total serum cholesterol > 200 mg/dL or HDL < 35 mg/dL.
• Diabetes mellitus	Persons with insulin dependent diabetes mellitus (IDDM) who are older than 30 years of age or have had IDDM for >15 years.
	Persons with non-insulin dependent diabetes mellitus (NIDDM) who are older than 35 years of age should be classified as patients with disease.
• Sedentary lifestyle/ physical inactivity	Defined by the combination of sedentary job (involving sitting for a large part of the day) and no regular exercise or active recreational pursuits.
• Negative risk factor (protective)	High serum HDL-cholesterol (>60 mg/dL).

*ERT = estrogen replacement therapy.

Adapted from ACSM 1995.

Personal health history questionnaire that can be administered to active or sedentary individuals.

Please complete this as accurately and completely as possible.

Name: _____ Age: _____ Sex: _____

Mailing address: _____

Phone number: (work) _____ (home) _____

Today's date: _____

Ethnic background (circle)
African-American
Asian-American
Caucasian
Hispanic-American
Other _____

1. General Medical History

Circle one

Do you currently have any medical complaints?   Yes   No
(Please specify) _____

_____

Are you on any prescribed or over-the-counter   Yes   No
medication? (Please specify) _____

_____

2. Dietary History

What is the length of time you have maintained your present weight?

_____

Please describe any long-term weight changes you have experienced (e.g., lost 50 lb. in 1982):

_____

Please describe your diet history. Make sure to specify if you participated in bingeing, crash diets, cyclic dieting, or were anorexic and/or bulimic: _____

_____

3. Exercise History

Do you participate in any form of regular exercise?   Yes   No

a. What form of exercise?
b. How many times per week?
c. How long each session?
d. How intensely do you exercise?
e. How long have you been regularly training?

(continued)

Figure 14.1   Personal health history questionnaire that can be administered to active or sedentary individuals.

4. Cardiorespiratory history

Do you have heart disease now?	Yes	No
Have you ever had heart disease?	Yes	No
Do you have family history of heart disease?	Yes	No
Do you have a heart murmur?	Yes	No
Do you have occasional chest pains?	Yes	No
Have you ever fainted?	Yes	No
Do you have high blood pressure?	Yes	No
Do you have asthma or allergies?	Yes	No
Do you have any pulmonary (lung) problems?	Yes	No

Explain any Yes response _____

5. Musculoskeletal History

Do you have any muscle injuries now?	Yes	No
Have you had any muscle injuries in the past year?	Yes	No
Do you have muscle pains when you exercise?	Yes	No
Do you have any bone or joint injuries now?	Yes	No
Have you had any bone or joint injuries in the past?	Yes	No
Have you ever had swollen joints?	Yes	No

Explain any Yes response _____

6. General History

Have you had or do you have:

Adrenal disease	Yes	No
Hypoglycemia (low blood sugar)	Yes	No
Seizures	Yes	No
Diabetes	Yes	No
Kidney or bladder problems	Yes	No
Stomach ulcers	Yes	No
Menstrual irregularities (women only)	Yes	No

Explain any Yes response _____

Figure 14.1   *(continued)*

diet recalls, food frequency questionnaires, diet histories) or *prospective* methods (e.g., diet records, weighed food records, or direct observation of food intake). A combination of methods may provide the best picture of a person's typical diet. For example, you may want to use a diet history or food frequency questionnaire to give you an idea of an individual's dietary habits, plus a diet record of current dietary practices.

Diet History

The diet history is often used with one of the diet assessment methods outlined in table 14.2. This table also lists advantages and limitations of the most commonly used assessment methods. The **diet history** is usually gathered through a questionnaire or an interview process. Table 14.3 suggests an outline for an interview format. The process is intended to help identify a client's nutrition problems or unique situations. It is especially important that you learn about the type, duration, and intensity of the activity in which the person is engaged. You may even want to have the individual keep 24-h activity records (see appendix E.2 for a sample form). This information will help you assess any energy or nutrition problems that may be associated with this person's activity level.

Twenty-Four-Hour Dietary Recall

The **24-hour recall** is a quick and easy way to assess recent food intake. It requires that a person recall *in detail* all of the foods and beverages consumed during the previous 24-h period. The individual needs to know the serving sizes, preparation methods, and brand names of convenience foods or fast foods consumed. This method has serious limitations in that it does not give a picture of a person's "typical intake" unless repeated measures are done on different days of the week. This method is acceptable only when repeated 24-h recalls are done over a period of time. While Basiotis et al. (1987) found that energy intake can be reasonably assessed in *groups* of men and women over 3 d, an accurate assessment of the energy intake of *individuals* requires 27-35 d of data. An even longer period is required to accurately assess intake of nutrients, and many nutrients require records to be taken over 100 d—which is obviously prohibitive for both the client and the practitioner. Moreover, because this approach relies heavily on memory, it is not acceptable for young children or anyone with memory problems. Another source of error is that, during the assessment period, subjects may minimize poor food choices while emphasizing good food choices.

The 24-h recall method is best used with large populations or as a quick check to deter-

Table 14.2 Common Diet Assessment Methods and Their Advantages and Disadvantages

Type of method	Major advantages	Major disadvantages
24-h recall	• Low respondent burden. • Low cost. • Easy to administer.	• Does not provide a good picture of an individual's dietary patterns. • Relies on memory. • May require a trained interviewer.
Food frequency questionnaire	• Low respondent burden. • Low cost. • Easy to administer. • Past dietary habits can be examined.	• Analysis is difficult. • Relies on memory. • Questionnaire needs validation.
Food records, weighed food records, tape-recorded food records, photographed or videotaped food records, telephone food records	• Provide a record of all foods consumed over the designated period. • Give a better picture of current dietary habits and nutrient intakes.	• High respondent burden. • Require that individuals estimate measurements of food consumed. • Individuals can change what they eat during the recording period. • Analysis can be costly. • Require a trained interviewer or data recorder. • May require that scales, camera, or tape recorder be provided.

Table 14.3   Guidelines for Doing an In-Depth Diet History Interview

1. *Weight:* Current weight, usual weight, weight goal for sport and/or weight suggested by coach or trainer, recent weight loss or gain, percent body fat, goal body fat, and frequency of dieting for weight loss.

2. *Appetite/intake:* Appetite changes and factors affecting appetite/intake. Includes such things as food preferences, training routine, activity level, anorexia, stress, allergies, medications, chewing/swallowing problems (bulimia, oral health), gastrointestinal problems (gastritis, laxative abuse, constipation).

3. *Eating patterns:* Typical patterns (weekdays/weekends) (see appendix E.1 for a sample food intake recording form); primary eating place (dormitory, home, cafeteria, training table); primary food shopper at home; dietary restrictions (understanding of and compliance with these restrictions); frequency of eating out; effect of training, precompetition, competition, and travel on typical eating patterns; ethnicity of diet; and food preferences.

4. *Psychological/eating disorder data:* How do they feel about their bodies? Is food intake restricted for any reason? If yes, how does this make them feel?

5. *Psychosocial data:* Economic status, occupation, educational level, living/cooking arrangement, and mental status.

6. *Medication and/or supplement use:* Current medications and supplements used, including amounts and reason for use. Drug-nutrient or nutrient-nutrient interactions may necessitate special dietary considerations. Effect of medication on physical performance and eating habits (some medications are taken with food; others, without food).

7. *Other:* Age; sex; level (minutes per day, miles per week) and types of physical activity engaged in during competition, training, and nontraining periods; fitness level (VO_2max; strength tests; and flexibility).

mine if an individual is following suggested dietary recommendations.

Food Frequency Questionnaires

Food frequency questionnaires allow you to assess the typical dietary pattern in an athlete's life over a predefined period of time. The questionnaires contain lists of foods with questions regarding the number of times the foods are eaten during the specified period of time. *The primary use of food frequency questionnaires is to rank individuals according to energy and nutrient intake (e.g., high vs. low intakes).* Since food frequency questionnaires rely on self-assessments, they are not generally used to provide an *accurate* estimate of nutrient intakes. Both qualitative and semiquantitative questionnaires are available. **Qualitative** information includes only a list of typical foods that are eaten—information that provides a general indication of an athlete's dietary pattern or that helps you compare the consumption of certain types of food before and after a dietary intervention. **Semiquantitative** questionnaires are useful in determining the typical foods eaten and the quantity consumed. You can address concerns about specific nutrients (fats, carbohydrates, etc.) by using these types of questionnaires. It is important to use a questionnaire that has been demonstrated to be reliable. As there are no validated questionnaires designed specifi-

cally for athletes or highly active people, the accuracy of using existing questionnaires for these groups may be limited. Appendix E.3 provides an example of a validated food frequency questionnaire.

Diet Records

The diet record is probably the most frequently used method for assessing the energy and nutrient intakes of individuals. A food or **diet record** is a list of all foods and beverages consumed over a specified time, typically 3-7 d. To more accurately predict energy and nutrient intakes, it is best if foods consumed are first weighed or measured, labels of convenience foods are saved, and labels of all supplements are copied. This method also allows the gathering of more in-depth information such as the times, places, feelings, and behaviors associated with eating. The dietitian or health care professional working with the individual should review the diet record to assure its accuracy. A primary drawback of this method is the tendency for individuals to change their "typical" eating habits on the days when they record food intake. Because this approach is also more time-consuming than 24-h recalls, its accuracy depends on the individual's cooperation and skill in properly recording foods.

How many days' consumption should be followed? Diet records of 3-14 d generally provide good estimates of energy and nutrient intakes

(Schlundt 1988). Within this range, reliability and accuracy appear to increase with each additional day up to 7 d. Thus, *a 7-d diet record during a period of typical food intake should give accurate data for energy, macronutrients, and most micronutrients.* For most nutrients, there appears to be little advantage to recording diet records for >2-3 weeks. One advantage to the 7-d diet record is that it encompasses all the days of the week, including the dietary changes that frequently occur on weekends. The main disadvantage is that as the number of days increases, so does the respondent's burden. Note that, for information on energy intake alone, at least 3 d of records are required to get an accurate estimate for a *group* of people; *individuals* may need to record their intake over many more days. Discuss frankly with your client the limitations of recording dietary intake over an entire week.

Provide specific instructions to people before they use the 24-h recall or diet record method. The days chosen to be recorded should represent the clients' typical dietary and activity patterns. People may have to be trained to measure food portions or may need to practice using a diet scale. Table 14.4 provides guidelines for achieving accurate diet records. Cli-

ents should follow certain criteria when reporting dietary assessment data, as outlined in tables 14.5 and 14.6. A good rule of thumb: *see that the methods are described to clients in sufficient detail that another researcher could duplicate the study design* (Wheeler and Buzzard 1994).

Assessing Daily Energy Expenditure

A plethora of methods are available to assess energy expenditure. These methods vary in their degree of accuracy, cost, and convenience. Unfortunately, the most accurate methods also tend to be the most costly and/or time- and labor-intensive. As with the selection of any assessment tool, you must decide on the type of information you need in order to choose the most appropriate method. This section reviews several of the tools used to assess energy expenditure.

Behavioral Observation Records

Behavioral observation involves the recording of an individual's activity patterns by an

Table 14.4 Instructions for Doing an In-Depth Diet Record

Specific guidelines for keeping diet records should be included in the instruction sheet given to the client, and these instructions should also be reviewed verbally. The following are guidelines for clients who are recording foods in a food record:

1. Record items immediately after they are consumed. Use common measures, such as cups and tablespoons, to describe the amount consumed; and whenever possible, measure or weigh the food items being consumed.

2. Record all beverages and all items added to them, such as sugar and cream added to coffee. Include all sport beverages (Gatorade, Powerade, etc.) and the beverages (e.g., water, soda) taken with medications.

3. Include condiments, such as butter, margarine, mustard, mayonnaise, and salad dressing, even if they are low-fat or fat-free.

4. Completely describe the goods consumed (e.g., "whole wheat bread," "white turkey meat without skin," and "meatless spaghetti sauce").

5. Indicate how the food was prepared (e.g., "fried chicken, broiled beef steak, and steamed vegetables").

6. Record all foods and beverages consumed as snacks, including brand names if possible.

7. Keep the food record diary sheet(s) accessible at all times so the items can be recorded immediately.

8. Write down any nutritional supplements (e.g., vitamins, minerals, food supplements) as well as any sport products (PowerBar, Gatorlode, Gatorbar, etc.) consumed during training or a race. Keep the labels of these products and return with completed diary.

9. When using convenience foods, save the food labels and return them with the completed food diary.

10. Whenever possible, note the brand names of food items (e.g., canned foods, convenience foods, deli items).

11. If food is consumed at a restaurant or fast-food establishment, record the name of the restaurant and the product purchased. The more specific you can be, the better (e.g., "a McDonald's Big Mac with regular fries and regular Diet Coke").

12. Record all medications used, both over-the-counter and prescription.

Table 14.5 Checklist for Reporting Dietary Intake Methodology: Guidelines for Specific Assessment Methods

1. Food records and 24-h recalls

   - Designate the number of days recorded, which days, and whether days were consecutive; describe any weighing algorithms used to account for day-of-the-week differences.

2. Food frequency methods (list-based diet histories)

   - Explain the purpose of the questionnaire (e.g., to rank individuals according to their intake of individual foods, food groups, or nutrients) and identify the nutrients of interest.

   - Identify the population group (e.g., ethnicity and age range) used to develop and validate the questionnaire.

   - Explain how the food list was developed.

   - Indicate the number of foods and food groups in the food list.

   - Indicate the level to which food consumption was quantified.* If relevant, comment on respondent's ability to designate small, medium, or large servings.

   - Describe the options available for specifying frequency of consumption.

   - Indicate the average length of time required to complete the questionnaire.

   - Describe any calibration studies designed to facilitate interpretation of the food frequency data.

3. Diet history methods (meal-based diet histories)

   - Indicate whether questions were open-ended or structured.

   - Indicate the number of "typical" days accounted for as well as the extent of probing for variations in the usual eating pattern.

   - Describe methods used to cross-check the history, such as a 24-h recall or food frequency checklist.

*Food frequency questionnaires can be unquantified, semiquantified, or completely quantified. An unquantified method does not specify serving sizes; instead, the respondent indicates how many times the food is consumed per period of time (day, week, month). For example, a respondent may be asked, "How often do you consume milk?" A semiquantified method provides typical serving sizes as the reference amount for determining frequency of consumption. For example, "How often do you consume an 8-oz glass of milk?" A completely quantified method allows the respondent to indicate any amount of food typically consumed as well as how often the food is consumed; amounts are obtained through open-ended questions, usually prompted by an interviewer. For example, "When do you drink milk, and how much do you usually consume?"

Adapted from Wheeler and Buzzard 1994.

observer. Recording forms have been developed that a trained observer can use to document various behaviors, types and levels of activities, and the time spent performing each activity (Baranowski et al. 1984; Hovell et al. 1978; Torún 1984; Wallace et al. 1985). Figure 14.2 includes an example of a recording form for a child's activities. Once the recording forms are completed, energy expenditure can be calculated using estimated energy cost values (Ainsworth et al. 1993).

Table 14.7 lists the advantages and limitations of behavioral observation records and other assessments of energy expenditure (Montoye et al. 1996). Although they are time-consuming and cumbersome, behavioral observation records are useful for studying activity levels of children and adults at work sites.

Motion Assessment Devices

The most commonly used **motion assessment devices** (instruments used to detect movement) are the pedometer and accelerometer. **Pedometers** typically are worn on the ankle or clipped to a belt at the waist and are used to count the number of steps people take or to estimate the distance they walk. The devices are designed to count steps in response to vertical oscillations of the body and are not capable of measuring other types of movement or energy expenditure. A recent study found that, while different brands of pedometers provide acceptably accurate estimations of steps taken and distance walked, they can vary significantly across walking speeds (Bassett et al. 1996).

Accelerometers detect accelerations and

Table 14.6 Checklist for Reporting Dietary Intake Methodology: Guidelines for All Assessment Methods

1. Describe the time frame of interest. Examples:
   - Usual intake over the last year, including any seasonal variations.
   - Defined period preceding disease incidence.
   - Current intake (e.g., during the last week or month).

2. Provide rationale for selecting the method used to collect dietary data.
   - If an existing method was used, cite published articles that describe the method, and document its validity and reliability.
   - If an existing method was modified, describe key points of the original method and all modifications. Cite references to the original method, including validation and reliability studies.
   - If a new method was developed, describe the procedures used to develop and evaluate the new tool.

3. Describe the results of pretests of the selected assessment method conducted with either the target subjects or a similar population.

4. Describe procedures used to quantify portion sizes of foods eaten.
   - Detail the use of food scales, household measuring cups or spoons, rulers, food pictures, food models, or geometric shapes.

5. Describe procedures used to analyze dietary data. If nutrients were calculated:
   - Identify the food composition database used by name, version number, and release date, and provide the name and location (city and state) of the database developer.
   - Evaluate the completeness of the database for the nutrients of interest.
   - Describe any modifications to the database.
   - Describe procedures for coding the data.
   - Describe quality-control procedures for ensuring accurate calculations.

6. Indicate whether the assessment tool was administered by an interviewer or self-administered by respondents.

When interviewer-administered methods are used:
   - Describe the minimum qualifications of interviewers (e.g., registered dietitian, graduate degree in health science field).
   - Describe training and certification procedures for interviewers.
   - Indicate whether interviews were conducted in person or by telephone.
   - Report the approximate length of the interview.
   - Describe the level of detail solicited about food descriptions (e.g., type or brand of food; processing method, such as canned or dried; eating practices, such as trimming of meat or use of table salt; specification of recipe ingredients and other food preparation methods).
   - Indicate whether the method used to query respondents for details about food intake was automated (interactive computer software that prompts for descriptive detail) or manual; describe any aids used for manual probing, such as a checklist of details required for each food category.

When self-administered methods are used:
   - Describe instructions or training provided to subjects on keeping good records or completing dietary questionnaires.
   - Describe materials provided to help subjects describe foods (e.g., checklist of details required for each food category) or estimate portion sizes (e.g., food scales, household measures, or food models).
   - Describe procedures used to collect additional information after the food records or questionnaires are completed.

Adapted from Wheeler and Buzzard 1994.

decelerations of the body. The accelerations of the body during movement are theoretically in proportion to the forces generated by the muscles and are related to energy expenditure (Montoye et al. 1996). **Single-plane (or axis) accelerometers** detect acceleration exclusively in the vertical plane. The Caltrac is an example of a single-plane accelerometer. This device is worn on a belt that is attached firmly around the waist. Data output is in either kilocalories or movement counts. While the reliability of the Caltrac is good under controlled laboratory conditions, results are poorly reproduced in the field. The validity of the Caltrac is limited; its estimation of energy expenditure during horizontal walking, running, and cycling is acceptable in many situations, but it does not accurately represent the energy cost of activities such as uphill or downhill running. **Triaxial accelerometers** detect acceleration in three dimensions. The reliability of these devices is good, and their output correlates highly with energy expenditure for activities such as level walking, running, and stepping. However, they may underestimate energy expenditure during free-living situations

Activity Comparison

Name *Jan Doe*   Day *Thurs*   *7*

Activity		Time	
Counselor	Camper	Counselor	Camper
Sleep		*8.25 hrs.*	*9.0 hrs.*
Easy			
Moderate			
warm-ups	*warm-ups*	*15 min*	*15 min*
weight training		*30*	
new games		*15*	
	basketball		*30*
Hard			
aerobics		*45*	
swimming	*swimming*	*45*	*45*
	tennis	*45*	*45*
run		*15*	
	basketball		*45*
	dance		*60*
Very Hard			
dance		*60*	
	aerobics		*45*
	games		*45*

(continued)

Figure 14.2 A form to record physical activities of a child.
Reprinted from Wallace et al. 1985.

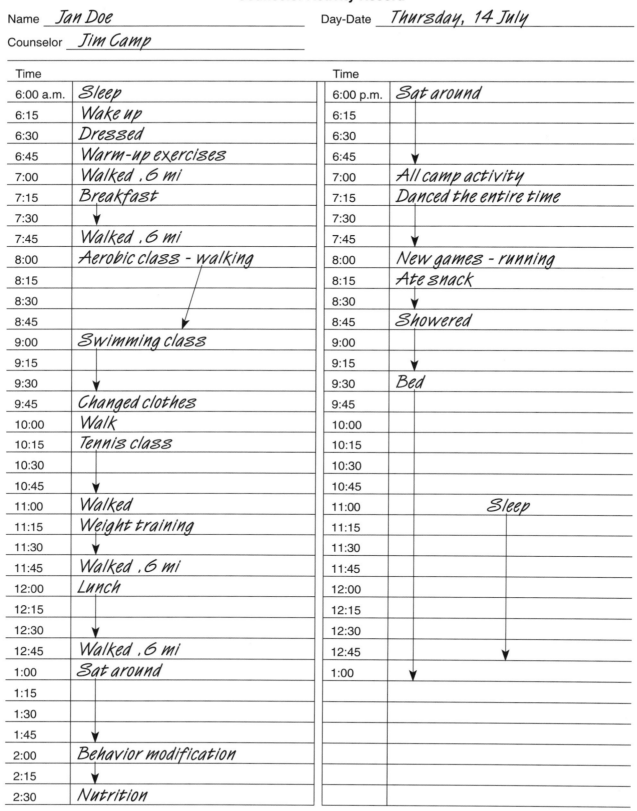

Counselor Activity Record

Name _Jan Doe_   Day-Date _Thursday, 14 July_

Counselor _Jim Camp_

Time		Time	
6:00 a.m.	Sleep	6:00 p.m.	Sat around
6:15	Wake up	6:15	
6:30	Dressed	6:30	
6:45	Warm-up exercises	6:45	
7:00	Walked .6 mi	7:00	All camp activity
7:15	Breakfast	7:15	Danced the entire time
7:30		7:30	
7:45	Walked .6 mi	7:45	
8:00	Aerobic class - walking	8:00	New games - running
8:15		8:15	Ate snack
8:30		8:30	
8:45		8:45	Showered
9:00	Swimming class	9:00	
9:15		9:15	
9:30		9:30	Bed
9:45	Changed clothes	9:45	
10:00	Walk	10:00	
10:15	Tennis class	10:15	
10:30		10:30	
10:45		10:45	
11:00	Walked	11:00	Sleep
11:15	Weight training	11:15	
11:30		11:30	
11:45	Walked .6 mi	11:45	
12:00	Lunch	12:00	
12:15		12:15	
12:30		12:30	
12:45	Walked .6 mi	12:45	
1:00	Sat around	1:00	
1:15			
1:30			
1:45			
2:00	Behavior modification		
2:15			
2:30	Nutrition		

Figure 14.2 *(continued)*

Table 14.7 **Common Energy Expenditure Assessment Methods and Their Advantages and Disadvantages**

Method	Major advantages	Major disadvantages
1. Behavioral observation records	• Allow recording of various behaviors, activities, frequency of activities, etc. • Permit estimates of energy expenditure for brief periods of time.	• Validity may be inadequate. • Subjects may alter activity when they know they are being watched. • Tedious. • Time-consuming. • Accuracy decreases as observation time increases. • Expensive to employ observer(s). • Not practical to use with large groups of subjects or over long periods of time.
2. Motion assessment devices: *Pedometer*	• Inexpensive. • Can be worn for long periods. • Noninvasive. • Gives a general idea of activity level. • Portable.	• Only detects vertical displacements of the whole-body center of gravity. • Does not provide an accurate estimate of energy expenditure. • Reliability and validity can be poor and brand specific.
Single-axis accelerometer	• Relatively inexpensive. • Can be worn for long periods. • Noninvasive. • Provides reasonable estimate of energy cost of certain activities. • Good reliability in the lab.	• Only detects acceleration in the vertical plane. • Poor reliability in the field.
Triaxial accelerometer	• Detects acceleration in three planes. • Can be worn for long periods. • Noninvasive. • Most accurate of the movement devices. • Portable. • Reliable.	• May underestimate free-living energy expenditure. • Relatively expensive.
3. Physical activity questionnaires	• Noninvasive (respondents can maintain current activities). • Can assess energy expenditure and physical activity patterns. • Convenient for subjects. • Inexpensive. • Can assess activity over different time frames. • Available for many populations. • Can be reliable and valid.	• Subject to errors of energy cost values. • Longer time frames rely on memory. • Shorter time frames don't account for seasonal variations or illness. • Activities listed may be biased toward men or younger subjects.
4. Activity records	• Very detailed information can be obtained. • Inexpensive. • No observer required. • May accurately represent energy expenditure in large groups.	• Time-consuming, tedious for subjects. • Can alter activity pattern of subjects. • Processing of records is very time- and labor-intensive. • Need complete cooperation of subjects. • Accuracy diminishes with longer data collection periods. • Inappropriate to use with children. • Subject to errors of energy cost values.
5. Doubly labeled water	• Accurate in controlled settings. • Can also be accurate in the field. • Assesses energy expenditure over a 1–3-week period. • Safe. • Reliable. • Doesn't affect activity patterns of subjects.	• Accuracy may be limited in subjects with metabolic disorders and those consuming an abundance of alcohol and/or "atypical" diets. • Expensive. • Cannot obtain energy expenditure values for specific activities.

(Matthews and Freedson 1995) and during activities such as walking uphill, weight lifting, and stationary cycling (Montoye et al. 1983). Chen and Sun (1997) developed two simple mathematical models that can significantly improve the estimation of energy expenditure over a wide range of activities using triaxial accelerometers.

Table 14.7 lists the advantages and disadvantages of motion assessment devices. For a more detailed description of their reliability, validity, and mechanism of action, refer to Montoye et al. (1996). While pedometers and the Caltrac may be limited in their ability to accurately assess energy expenditure, they can be useful for indicating gross changes in activity level over time. Triaxial accelerometers show promise of accurate assessments of energy expenditure through ongoing modifications of the devices and through use of mathematical models used in calculations.

Published Activity Questionnaires

Several **activity questionnaires** have been designed to assess physical activity and energy expenditure. The simpler ones include single-item questions, while more complex questionnaires involve in-depth surveys done by an interviewer. Different questionnaires are designed to address activity over various time frames (e.g., single day, one month to one year, and as long as a lifetime). Kriska and Caspersen (1997) published an extremely useful review of activity questionnaires. This review includes the original reference, the actual questionnaire, reliability and validity data available for each questionnaire, instructions on administering the questionnaire, and sample calculations.

How do you know which questionnaire to use? First decide what information you want to obtain, and then find a questionnaire that can access this information with a tool *that applies as specifically as possible to the group or individual you are assessing.* Questionnaires are available to assess energy expenditure in males, females, adolescents, adults, older adults, and various ethnic groups. For instance, you may have an older female client who wants to build lean mass and maintain bone. Since it is critical that she concentrate more on weightbearing activities than on energy expenditure, you would look for a questionnaire that could assess these types of activities. For another example: if you work with many female clients, finding a questionnaire that documents household and childcare activities may signifi-

■ HIGHLIGHT ■

Energy Expenditure Values: Where Do They Come From?

A multitude of energy cost values are published in the research literature. How do you decide which values are most accurate and appropriate to use? Many researchers and practitioners use either their own laboratory values or values from a variety of sources in the literature. Until recently there was no standardized, comprehensive list of energy cost values. Ainsworth et al. (1993) published a compendium of physical activities to assist researchers and practitioners with coding and estimating the energy cost of a wide variety of activities. Appendix E.4 illustrates the use of this compendium. Ainsworth et al. (1993) reported energy cost values in **metabolic equivalents (METs)** (see "What Is a Metabolic Equivalent, or MET" on page 397); however, the data in appendix E.4 are expressed in kilocalories per kilogram of bodyweight per minute (kcal/kg BW/min), and we also provide values for a given body weight to assist you with the calculations. While most of these energy cost values were derived using indirect calorimetry to measure oxygen consumption, some of the data were derived using imputed values. Note also that these data were derived from predominantly young adult subjects, limiting their usefulness for children or elderly people (Montoye et al. 1996). While the data are extremely useful to the researcher and practitioner, it is important to understand that these energy cost values will always introduce some degree of error into an estimation of energy expenditure.

What Is a Metabolic Equivalent, or MET?

The abbreviation MET represents a **metabolic equivalent,** a unit of measurement that represents work rate, or oxygen uptake ($\dot{V}O_2$). One MET is equal to a $\dot{V}O_2$ of 3.5 ml/kg/min. The MET unit is generally used in referring to an individual's functional capacity. For instance, an individual with a maximal oxygen uptake ($\dot{V}O_2$max) of 60 ml/kg/min would have a functional capacity of 17 METs (60/3.5 = 17.1). The MET unit is also used to prescribe exercise intensity for training. If an individual with a $\dot{V}O_2$max of 17 METs wishes to train at 80% of his $\dot{V}O_2$max, the training intensity would be 13.6 METs. One can design specific training intensities by referring to *ACSM's Guidelines for Exercise Testing and Prescription* (1995) and to Swain and Leutholtz (1997).

cantly improve the estimation of energy expenditure for these people.

To accurately represent energy expenditure, a questionnaire must provide the following information (Kriska and Caspersen 1997):

- Type of activity, including leisure, occupational, sport, and household activities
- Frequency, or the average number of sessions per time frame of interest
- Intensity of activities being performed
- Duration, or the average number of minutes per session during the time frame of interest

Table 14.7 lists the advantages and disadvantages of using questionnaires. Questionnaires are useful tools to determine energy expenditure and are helpful in classifying an individual's physical activity patterns. While the questionnaires available can be reliable and valid, the representation of energy expenditure obtained is always subject to some degree of error due to the use of standardized energy cost values. While there are no published questionnaires designed specifically for athletes or highly active people, several assess both occupational and leisure activities and provide information on high-intensity and sport-related activities.

Activity Records

Activity records can be used to estimate total daily energy expenditure or to estimate the energy expended during specified activities (see appendix E.2 for sample activity record form). Chapter 5 discussed use of the factorial method or activity records to estimate energy expenditure. Table 14.7 lists the advantages and disadvantages of using activity records to estimate energy expenditure. The energy expenditure values tabulated by Ainsworth et al. (1993) can be used to estimate energy expenditure for selected activities or for all activities performed over a 24-h period. Note that the accuracy of these methods is influenced by people's ability to record their activities correctly and by the degree to which the energy values used represent the actual energy expended (see "Energy Expenditure Values: Where Do They Come From?" on page 396).

Doubly Labeled Water

We discussed the doubly labeled water technique in chapter 5. Table 14.7 reviews the advantages and disadvantages of this technique to allow for comparison with the other methods used to assess energy expenditure.

Fitness Assessment

How do we define fitness? While many people view being "fit" as having good cardiovascular endurance, this is only one of many components of physical fitness. The concept of "metabolic" or "health-related" fitness has recently become a focus of much research. While some researchers consider metabolic fitness to be represented by glucose and lipid metabolism (Bouchard and Shephard 1993), Skinner and Oja (1994) emphasize that there is at this time no clear conceptual definition of metabolic fitness. No protocols exist that allow us to quantitatively define metabolic fitness. The components of fitness we discuss in this section include

Case Study: Female Distance Runner Complaining of Fatigue

The case of Tammy was introduced in the beginning of this chapter. Tammy has been complaining of fatigue and lackluster performance, and wants to maintain a low body weight and percentage body fat while concentrating on healthy eating habits. This case study is provided to illustrate how nutritional and energy expenditure assessment tools can be used with athletes and other clients. Tammy is a distance runner, competing in both cross-country and track. Her descriptive characteristics are as follows:

Age	19 years
Weight	107 lb (48.5 kg)
Height	59 in. (150 cm)
Body fat percentage (derived using hydrostatic weighing)	15.2%
Resting metabolic rate (measured using indirect calorimetry)	1200 kcal/d
Resting heart rate	42 bpm
Resting blood pressure	108/60 mm Hg

Tammy has had problems with anemia in the past. Fasting blood samples were taken to assess her present iron status, and general chemistry screening and lipid panels were also completed at her request. The following table shows the results of those tests.

	Tammy's values	Normal values*
Hemoglobin	12.5 g/dL	12.0-16.0 g/dL
Hematocrit	38%	36-48%
Transferrin	300 mg/dL	200-400 mg/dL
Transferrin (% saturation)	38%	15-50%
Total iron-binding capacity	400 μg/dL	240-450 μg/dL
Ferritin	42 ng/ml	18-270 ng/ml
Glucose	75 mg/dL	65-110 mg/dL
Total cholesterol	146 mg/dL	140-199 mg/dL
LDL-cholesterol	92 mg/dL	<130 mg/dL
HDL-cholesterol	55 mg/dL	40-85 mg/dL
Triglycerides	75 mg/dL	39-124 mg/dL

* Adapted from Fischbach 1996.

Appendix E.5 provides a detailed list of typical clinical laboratory values. These results do not indicate any abnormal values for Tammy. Although Tammy complains of fatigue, neither anemia nor iron deficiency appears to be the culprit. Tammy completed weighed food records and activity diaries over a 3-d period (representing 2 weekdays and 1 weekend day). Appendix E.6 provides examples of one day of each of these records with their corresponding calculation sheets. Tammy's diet was analyzed using the Food Processor Plus nutrient analysis software (version 6.0, ESHA Research, Salem, OR); her total daily energy expenditure was estimated using the energy cost values reported by Ainsworth et al. (1993).

Analysis of her activity records shows that Tammy requires approximately 2300 kcal/d to maintain her current weight. Her diet records show that her average energy intake for the 3-d recording period was 2195 kcal/d. Tammy's total energy intake appears inadequate, providing 105 kcal/d less than necessary to cover her energy expenditure. This discrepancy is within the margin of error of the diet and activity assessment methods (see chapter 5), however, and since she is maintaining her body weight, it is assumed that her energy intake is adequate to meet energy demands. If this discrepancy were maintained over a prolonged period, it is possible that her body weight would drop, and her performance would suffer due to inadequate energy intake.

Tammy's average intakes of carbohydrate, protein, and fat are 58%, 16%, and 26% of total energy intake (kcal/d), respectively. While these percentages are the recommended values for a competitive athlete, she consumes an average of only 282 g of carbohydrate. This is less than the recommended carbohydrate intake for endurance athletes and is probably a major contributor to her sluggish performance. An interview with Tammy also revealed that on race days she is nervous, is often nauseated, and does not eat well. She skips breakfast and consumes only 800-1000 kcal during a typical race day. After addressing these issues, Tammy was able to improve her performance and reduce fatigue by eating more complex carbohydrates on a regular basis and by consuming glucose polymer beverages on race days.

- flexibility,
- muscle strength (isometric, dynamic, and isokinetic),
- muscle endurance,
- cardiorespiratory fitness (also referred to as aerobic fitness), and
- anaerobic fitness (also referred to as power).

The extent to which people can maximize each component of fitness depends on the sport or activity in which they are engaged. A variety of tests are available to assess the level of fitness for each component listed above, and there are standards available for comparison of an individual's performance with that of the general population. It is important to stress that these standards have been developed on groups of individuals with heterogeneous fitness levels, which may limit the application of these standards to clients who deviate significantly from that population. While these tests are extremely useful for assessing the fitness level of the general population, their applicability to certain groups (e.g., athletes or individuals with limited mobility) needs to be determined on an individual basis. Excellent resources are available that describe the tests used in fitness assessment, the normative performance values for each test, and exercise prescription suggestions for each component of fitness (Heyward 1998; Howley and Franks 1997). The purpose of the following section is simply to familiarize you with the components of fitness and provide guidance in accessing information about the tests used in fitness assessment.

Flexibility Tests

Flexibility is defined as "the ability of a joint, or series of joints, to move fluidly thorough a full range of motion" (Heyward 1998, p. 203). Achieving and maintaining appropriate flexibility is critical for optimal performance and for preventing injury. Flexibility is affected by many factors, including

- age;
- fitness level;
- excessive fatty or muscular tissue; and
- tightness of the joint capsule, muscles, tendons, and ligaments.

Flexibility tends to decrease with age due to structural and functional changes in the tissues surrounding the joint capsule. Excess body fat or very large muscles can also hinder flexibility. Inactivity leads to a shortening and tightening of connective and muscle tissues. While flexibility is an extremely important component of fitness, it is often neglected or ignored by people involved in fitness programs: people feel rushed due to time constraints, leading them to minimize the time spent performing flexibility/stretching exercises. Many people, furthermore, are not properly trained to perform such exercises, which can lead to ineffective stretching and potential injury.

Heyward (1998) and Liemohn (1997b) describe tests to assess flexibility about the major joints in the body. Liemohn (1997a, pp. 325-329) also reviews exercise prescription for flexibility and low-back pain. Flexibility is joint specific, and no measure exists for assessing whole-body flexibility. It is important to stress that the proper applications of these tests are critical to ensure the safety of the client being tested. For instance, stretching exercises in which body position or limb movement causes excessive blood flow to the head and upper chest may be contraindicated in clients with hypertension.

Tests of Muscle Strength

Muscle strength is defined as the maximum amount of force exerted by a group of muscles. Muscle strength can be further delineated into three categories:

- *Isometric (or static) strength:* generation of force with no movement about a joint.
- *Dynamic (or isotonic) strength:* generation of force with movement about a joint. Isotonic contractions are further characterized as *concentric* (shortening of the muscle as it exerts tension) or *eccentric* (lengthening of the muscle as it exerts tension).
- *Isokinetic strength:* generation of force at a constant speed throughout the entire range of motion (also a component of dynamic strength).

Dynamometers are devices used to measure static strength. The common muscle groups tested include those involved in hand gripping and the leg and back muscles (figure 14.3). These tests and normative values for static strength are described by Heyward (1998, pp. 107-109) and Bond (1997, pp. 237-242).

Dynamic strength is measured using equipment that provides constant or variable resistance. Weight equipment (both machines and free weights) provides constant resistance. The **1-RM test** (or 1-repetition maximum test) assesses the maximum weight a person can lift for one repetition of a particular movement. The maximum weight lifted is recorded and divided by the individual's body weight in pounds. Stan-

dard values are available for 1-RM tests using the bench press (for upper-body strength) and the leg press (for lower-body strength) and are listed in Heyward (1998, p. 111) and Bond (1997, pp. 243-244). Variable resistance machines include isokinetic dynamometers manufactured by Cybex (including the Cybex II and Orthotron machines) and Hydra-Fitness (the Omni-tron Total Power machine). Heyward (1998, pp. 263-264) has reviewed the average strength values for tests using the Omni-tron machine.

Tests of Muscle Endurance

Muscle endurance is defined as the ability of a group of muscles to exert force repeatedly over a period of time. Tests used to assess muscle endurance include measuring the maximal number of sit-ups, push-ups, chin-ups, and bar-dips one can perform. The American College of Sports Medicine (1993) and Howley and Franks (1997) have published detailed descriptions of test protocols and performance values for these exercises.

For a list of factors to consider about muscle strength and endurance assessments, see "Us-

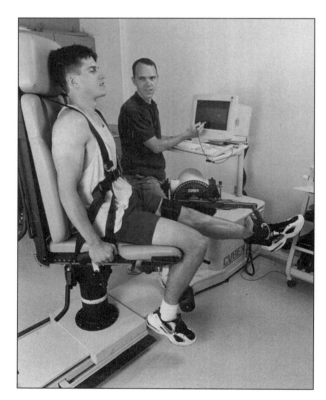

Figure 14.3 Muscle strength can be tested using an isokinetic testing device that provides a constant speed throughout the entire rance of motion.

■ HIGHLIGHT ■

Using Muscular Strength and Endurance Tests

A number of factors must be considered when performing tests to assess muscular strength and endurance. While many tests are simple to perform and score, each test should be selected not only for its convenience but also for its specific application to the client's activities. The following is a list of factors to consider when performing muscle strength and endurance assessments:

- Be familiar with the advantages and limitations of the test and any related equipment. Muscle fitness testing is not completely reliable, and equipment often must be modified. Test results must be carefully interpreted in light of the tests' limitations.

- Muscle fitness tests are specific to a given muscle group and type of contraction being performed. There is no single test of whole-body muscle strength or endurance.

- The test results should be expressed in relative terms (e.g., relative to body weight or amount of lean body mass), as muscle fitness is related to both body weight and the amount of muscle mass. Expression of the results in relative terms also allows for comparison with other people performing the test.

- As tests of muscle fitness involve a maximal effort by the person being tested, every attempt should be made to control factors that affect maximal performance. This includes factors such as physical environment (e.g., temperature, humidity), time of day, the subject's motivation, medications that may affect performance, nutritional and hydration status, and amount of sleep.

- Select tests that the person is able to perform. For instance, some individuals may not be capable of lifting the lightest weight on a Universal machine when performing the 1-RM (repetition maximum) bench press test. Another test may be needed, or modifications of the test may need to be developed.

- The standard values published for most tests of muscular fitness are outdated, and few if any data exist for individuals >25 years of age. Thus, these values may be invalid, unreliable, and inappropriate to use with many individuals.

Adapted from ACSM 1995; Heyward 1998.

ing Muscular Strength and Endurance Tests," above.

Cardiorespiratory Fitness Tests

Assessing **cardiorespiratory fitness** encompasses testing the ability of the respiratory, cardiovascular, and skeletal muscle tissues to take in, deliver, and utilize oxygen while performing prolonged exercise of moderate to high intensity. **Maximal oxygen uptake** (or $\dot{V}O_2$max) is considered the most valid measure of cardiorespiratory fitness. (For a discussion on the limitations of $\dot{V}O_2$max to predict athletic performance, see "$\dot{V}O_2$max and Athletic Performance," page 403.) **$\dot{V}O_2$max** is defined as the maximal amount of oxygen the body can use during a given period of time. $\dot{V}O_2$max is measured during an exercise test to volitional

fatigue using indirect calorimetry. However, it is not always possible or appropriate to measure the $\dot{V}O_2$max of every client. The equipment needed to perform indirect calorimetry is usually available only in exercise physiology laboratories. Also, it may not be safe to have a client with multiple risk factors perform maximal exercise.

Tests have been developed to overcome these obstacles to assessing $\dot{V}O_2$max. $\dot{V}O_2$max can be predicted from submaximal exercise heart rates and from maximal and submaximal exercise performance. Numerous protocols have been designed to predict $\dot{V}O_2$max using a treadmill and bicycle ergometer; and field tests using walking, stepping, and running can be used to test large groups of people. See Heyward (1998, pp. 56-76) and Howley and Franks (1997, pp. 206-227) for descriptions of specific testing protocols and normative values. Table 14.8 shows the $\dot{V}O_2$max values reported for populations ranging from highly fit (cross-country skiers) to those limited by disease (pulmonary disease patients).

How do you decide whether it is safe to perform maximal or submaximal testing, and when is it necessary to have medical supervision during exercise testing? The American College of Sport Medicine (1995) has published guidelines to help answer these questions. Certain conditions have been identified as either **absolute** or **relative contraindications** to exercise testing (table 14.9). If an individual

Table 14.8 Maximal Oxygen Uptake Measured in Healthy and Diseased Populations

Population	$\dot{V}O_2$max (ml/kg/min)	
	Men	Women
Cross-country skiers	82	66
Distance runners	79	62
College students	45	38
Middle-aged adults	35	30
Postmyocardial infarction patients	22	18
Patients with severe pulmonary disease	13	13

Table 14.9 Contraindications to Exercise Testing

Absolute contraindications

1. A recent significant change in the resting electrocardiogram, suggesting infarction or other acute cardiac event
2. Recent complicated myocardial infarction (unless patient is stable and pain free)
3. Unstable angina
4. Uncontrolled ventricular arrythmia
5. Uncontrolled atrial arrhythmia that compromises cardiac function
6. Third-degree atrio-ventricular heart block without pacemaker
7. Acute congestive heart failure
8. Severe aortic stenosis
9. Suspected or known dissecting aneurysm
10. Active or suspected myocarditis or pericarditis
11. Thrombophlebitis or intracardiac thrombi
12. Recent systemic or pulmonary embolus
13. Acute infection
14. Significant emotional distress (psychosis)

Relative contraindications

1. Resting diastolic blood pressure >115 mm Hg or resting systolic blood pressure >200 mm Hg
2. Moderate valvular heart disease
3. Known electrolyte abnormalities (hypokalemia, hypomagnesemia)
4. Fixed-rate pacemaker (rarely used)
5. Frequent or complex ventricular ectopy
6. Ventricular aneurysm
7. Uncontrolled metabolic disease (e.g., diabetes, thyrotoxicosis, or myxedema)
8. Chronic infectious disease (e.g., mononucleosis, hepatitis, AIDS)
9. Neuromuscular, musculoskeletal, or rheumatoid disorders that are exacerbated by exercise
10. Advanced or complicated pregnancy

Adapted from ACSM 1995.

exhibits one or more absolute contraindications, exercise testing should not be performed for any reason until the condition(s) is stabilized. For people exhibiting relative contraindications to exercise, the potential benefits of exercise testing must be weighed against the potential risks.

Physician supervision during exercise testing is recommended under certain conditions. It is *always* recommended during both submaximal and maximal testing of

- men older than 39 years,
- women older than 49 years,
- individuals with known disease, and
- individuals at increased risk (refer to table 14.1) who have one or more signs or symptoms of cardiopulmonary disease (table 14.10).

A physician need not be present during submaximal testing of apparently healthy individuals or for those at increased risk who

Table 14.10 Major Symptoms or Signs Suggestive of Cardiopulmonary Disease*

1. Pain or discomfort (or other anginal equivalent) in the chest, neck, jaw, arms, or other areas that may be ischemic in nature

2. Shortness of breath at rest or with mild exertion

3. Dizziness or syncope

4. Orthopnea or paroxysmal nocturnal dyspnea

5. Ankle edema

6. Palpitations or tachycardia

7. Intermittent claudication

8. Known heart murmur

9. Unusual fatigue or shortness of breath with usual activities

*These symptoms must be interpreted in the clinical context in which they appear since they are not all specific for cardiopulmonary or metabolic disease.

Adapted from ACSM 1995.

■ HIGHLIGHT ■

$\dot{V}O_2$max and Athletic Performance

While $\dot{V}O_2$max is a good indicator of cardiorespiratory fitness, it is limited in its ability to predict athletic performance. In a heterogeneous group of individuals with variable activity levels, $\dot{V}O_2$max is highly correlated with cardiorespiratory fitness level and endurance athletic performance. However, in a group of highly trained athletes with homogeneous $\dot{V}O_2$max values, a variety of factors influence athletic performance. Some of these factors include

- economy of movement (e.g., running economy) (Conley and Krahenbuhl 1980),
- turnover of lactate (Costill et al. 1973; Messonnier et al. 1997),
- sport-specific biomechanical factors (e.g., push-off angle and trunk position in speed skating) (van Ingen Schenau et al. 1996),
- ability to perform exercise for a longer duration at a higher percentage of $\dot{V}O_2$max (Costill et al. 1973), and
- ability to perform various skills and precision techniques specific to a given sport (e.g., soccer, basketball, synchronized swimming).

have no signs or symptoms of cardiopulmonary disease. Maximal exercise testing also can be performed without physician supervision in apparently healthy men younger than 40 years and women younger than 50 years.

Anaerobic Fitness Tests

Of all the components of fitness, the most difficult to assess may be anaerobic fitness. While many available tests are simple to perform, there is disagreement as to what the tests are actually measuring (Inbar et al. 1996). **Anaerobic fitness** is defined as the ability to perform very-high-intensity exercise for relatively short periods of time (from a few seconds up to a few minutes). Anaerobic fitness tests are classified according to their intensity and duration. Table 14.11 lists tests that are "very brief," lasting 1-10 s. Table 14.12 lists tests that are classified as "brief," lasting 20-60 s.

Table 14.11 Very Brief (1-10 s) Anaerobic Tests

Test	Approximate duration (seconds)
Margaria step test	2-4
Vertical jump	<1
Leg extensor force	1-2
Short sprints	3-10
Cycle ergometer (max RPM)	
Resistance:[a]	
4-7 kg	2-5
4 kg	4 s max (40-s test)
75 gm/kg body mass	5 s max (30-s test)

[a]These values are true for the Monark (or any other ergometer where the flywheel moves 6 m per pedal revolution) but not for the Fleisch ergometer.

Reprinted from Inbar et al. 1996.

Table 14.12 Brief (20-60 s) Anaerobic Tests

Test	Duration (s)
Cycle ergometer (arms)	
50 gm/kg body mass at max RPM[a]	30
Cycle ergometer (legs)	
To exhaustion	
350-400 W at 104-128 RPM	40-45
Fixed duration	
$1.5 \times \dot{V}O_2$max at max RPM	20
$0.75 \times \dot{V}O_2$max at max RPM	20
75 gm/kg body mass at max RPM[a]	30
4-6 kg at max RPM[a]	30-40
Treadmill run to exhaustion	
7-8 mph at 20% grade	30-60
10 mph at 15% grade	35-45
Individually designed to elicit exhaustion in 45 s	35-60

[a]These values are true for the Monark (or any other ergometer where the flywheel moves 6 m per pedal revolution) but not for the Fleisch ergometer.

Reprinted from Inbar et al. 1996.

The **Wingate Anaerobic Test (WAnT)** is an example of a very brief test. Inbar et al. (1996) have published an entire book about the WAnT: what it measures, the equipment needed and procedures involved, factors that can influence the test, and normative values for various populations. One disadvantage of the WAnT is that it cannot assess the performance of a specific muscle or muscle groups— it is capable of assessing only the performance of combined muscle groups. Yet there are several advantages to using the WAnT to assess anaerobic fitness (Inbar et al. 1996):

- The test is highly reliable.
- The score is a valid indicator of supramaximal anaerobic capacity.
- The test is sensitive to changes in anaerobic fitness over time.
- It can provide information about peak power, muscle endurance, and muscle fatigability.

- It is simple to administer.
- It is inexpensive.
- It is noninvasive and can be used on many types of people, including those with disabilities.
- It can assess the performance of both upper and lower limbs.

Chapter in Review

Many techniques are available to assess the nutritional and fitness status of an individual. The examples provided in this chapter are not exhaustive; we encourage you to thoroughly search the literature for the most appropriate test for a specific client or population. All tests have advantages and limitations that must be taken into account when you review test results and when you explain the results to a client.

KEY CONCEPTS

1. Describe the characteristics of medical and health history questionnaires.

One important component of the medical history is a physical examination. The physical exam is particularly important for people who are untrained or detrained or who may have risks or symptoms for cardiovascular or metabolic diseases. A licensed health professional should select the tests to be performed during a physical exam. Health history questionnaires help to uncover current or potential health problems. The questionnaires should include questions about medication status, family history of disease, history of illness and injuries, menstrual history (of females), and diet and exercise history. Select fitness tests and prescribe exercises in light of a person's risk classification for coronary artery disease.

2. Discuss the methods used to assess energy and nutrient intakes.

Energy and nutrient intakes can be assessed with a variety of methods including retrospective methods (e.g., 24-h recall, food frequency questionnaires, and diet histories) or prospective methods (e.g., diet records, weighed food records, and direct observation). Each method has its advantages and weaknesses. Validity and reliability of these methods depend on a client's ability to accurately report dietary intake.

3. Discuss the methods used to assess energy expenditure.

Daily energy expenditure can be assessed using questionnaires, observation, self-report records, motion detection devices, and doubly labeled water. The accuracy of most methods depends on the applicability of published energy expenditure values to the actual activities reported. While doubly labeled water does not depend on the ability of the client or observer to accurately report activity or on the use of published energy values, this method is relatively expensive, requires highly specialized equipment, and cannot give an estimation of energy expenditure for a period of time less than 1 week.

4. *Describe specific tests used to assess the components of fitness.*

There are many components of fitness, and no single test can measure total-body fitness. Components of fitness include flexibility, muscle strength, muscle endurance, cardiorespiratory fitness, and anaerobic fitness. "Metabolic fitness" currently is equated with glucose and lipid metabolism, but no protocols exist to assess metabolic fitness at this time. While cost and convenience are important considerations, the reliability, validity, and applicability of assessment methods should also be critical concerns.

KEY TERMS

1-RM test	increased risk
24-hour recall	isokinetic strength
absolute contraindication	isometric (static) strength
accelerometer	known disease
activity questionnaire	maximal oxygen uptake ($\dot{V}O_2$max)
activity records	metabolic equivalent (MET)
anaerobic fitness	motion assessment devices
apparently healthy	muscle endurance
behavioral observation	muscle strength
cardiorespiratory fitness	pedometer
diet history	qualitative questionnaire
diet record	relative contraindication
dynamic (isotonic) strength	semiquantitative questionnaire
dynamometer	single-plane (or axis) accelerometers
flexibility	triaxial accelerometers
food frequency questionnaire	Wingate Anaerobic Test (WAnT)
health history questionnaire	

References

Ainsworth BE, Haskell WL, Leon AS, Jacobs DS Jr., Montoye HJ, Sallis JF, Paffenbarger RS Jr. Compendium of physical activities: classification by energy costs of human physical activities. Med Sci Sports Exerc 1993;25:71-80.

American College of Sports Medicine. Resource manual for guidelines for exercise testing and prescription, 2nd ed. Philadelphia: Lea & Febiger, 1993.

American College of Sports Medicine. ACSM's guidelines for exercise testing and prescription, 5th ed. Baltimore: Williams & Wilkins, 1995.

Baranowski T, Dworkin RJ, Cieslik CJ, et al. Reliability and validity of self report of aerobic activity: Family Health Project. Res Q Exerc Sport 1984;55:309-17.

Basiotis PP, Welsh SO, Cronin FJ, Kelsay JL, Mertz W. Number of days of food intake records required to estimate individual and group nutrient intakes with defined confidence. J Nutr 1987;117:1638-41.

Bassett DR Jr., Ainsworth BE, Leggett SR, Mathien CA, Main JA, Hunter DC, Duncan GE. Accuracy of five electronic pedometers for measuring distance walked. Med Sci Sports Exerc 1996;28:1071-7.

Bond V. Muscular strength and endurance. In: Howley ET, Franks BD, eds. Health Fitness Instructor's Handbook. Champaign, IL: Human Kinetics, 1997: 237-44.

Bouchard C, Shephard RJ. Physical activity, fitness and health: the model and key concepts. In: Bouchard C, Shephard RJ, Stephens T, eds. Physical Activity, Fitness, and Health: Consensus Statement. Champaign, IL: Human Kinetics, 1993:11-23.

Chen KY, Sun M. Improving energy expenditure estimation by using a triaxial accelerometer. J Appl Physiol 1997;83:2112-22.

Conley DL, Krahenbuhl G. Running economy and distance running performance of highly trained athletes. Med Sci Sports Exerc 1980;12:357-60.

Costill DL, Thomason H, Roberts E. Fractional utilization of the aerobic capacity during distance running. Med Sci Sports Exerc 1973;5:248-52.

Fischbach F. A manual of laboratory and diagnostic tests, 5th ed. Philadelphia: Lippincott, 1996.

Heyward VH. Advanced Fitness Assessment and Exercise Prescription, 3rd ed. Champaign, IL: Human Kinetics, 1998.

Hovell MF, Bursick JH, Sharkey R, McClure J. An evaluation of elementary students' voluntary physical activity during recess. Res Q Exerc Sport 1978;49:460-74.

Howley ET, Franks BD. Health Fitness Instructor's Handbook, 3rd ed. Champaign, IL: Human Kinetics, 1997.

Inbar O, Bar-or O, Skinner JS. The Wingate Anaerobic Test. Champaign, IL: Human Kinetics, 1996.

Kriska AM, Caspersen CJ. A collection of physical activity questionnaires for health-related research. Med Sci Sports Exerc 1997;29:S3-S205.

Liemohn W. Exercise prescription for flexibility and low-back function. In: Howley ET, Franks BD, eds. Health Fitness Instructor's Handbook. Champaign, IL: Human Kinetics, 1997a:325-9.

Liemohn W. Flexibility and low-back function. In: Howley ET, Franks BD, eds. Health Fitness Instructor's Handbook. Champaign, IL: Human Kinetics, 1997b:252-62.

Matthews CE, Freedson PS. Field trial of a three-dimensional activity monitor: comparison with self report. Med Sci Sports Exerc 1995;27:1071-8.

Messonnier L, Freund H, Bourdin M, Belli A, Lacour J-R. Lactate exchange and removal abilities in rowing performance. Med Sci Sports Exerc 1997;29:396-401.

Montoye HJ, Kemper HCG, Saris WHM, Washburn RA. Measuring Physical Activity and Energy Expenditure. Champaign, IL: Human Kinetics, 1996.

Montoye HJ, Washburn R, Servais S, Ertl A, Webster JG, Nagle FJ. Estimation of energy expenditure by a portable accelerometer. Med Sci Sports Exerc 1983;15:403-7.

Schlundt DG. Accuracy and reliability of nutrient intake estimates. J Nutr 1988;118:1432-5.

Skinner JS, Oja P. Laboratory and field tests for assessing health-related fitness. In: Bouchard C, Shephard RJ, Stephens T, eds. Physical Activity, Fitness, and Health. Champaign, IL: Human Kinetics, 1994:160-79.

Swain DP, Leutholtz BC. Metabolic Calculations Simplified. Baltimore: Williams & Wilkins, 1997.

Torún B. Physiological measurements of physical activity among children under free-living conditions. In: Pollitt E, Amante P, eds. Energy Intake and Activity. New York: Alan R. Liss, 1984:159-84.

van Ingen Schenau GJ, De Koning JJ, Bakker FC, De Groot G. Performance-influencing factors in homogeneous groups to top athletes: a cross-sectional study. Med Sci Sports Exerc 1996;28:1305-10.

Wallace JP, McKenzie TL, Nader PR. Observed versus recalled exercise behavior: a validation of a seven day exercise recall for boys 11 to 13 years old. Res Q Exerc Sport 1985;56:161-5.

Wheeler ML, Buzzard IM. How to report dietary assessment data. J Am Diet Assoc 1994;4:1255-6.

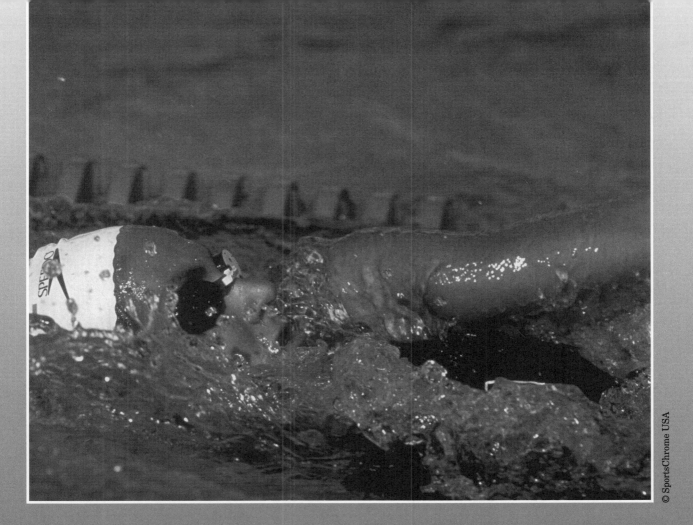

© SportsChrome USA

CHAPTER 15

Nutrition and the Active Female

After reading the chapter you will be able to

- understand the energy and nutrient requirements of active women; and
- identify the components of the female athlete triad, and discuss its treatment.

For most active females, including athletes, every day is a balancing act:

- What to eat? How much to eat?
- Should I supplement? If so, which supplement or supplements? How much?
- How much should I exercise to maintain body weight or increase my competitive edge?
- When I am training harder, do I need more micronutrients?

Active women need to eat enough energy to maintain their fitness level and health; female athletes, moreover, need additional energy to maintain their competitive edge for training and competition. Yet many of these same women want to lose weight. In addition to the body weight issues these women deal with, they are bombarded with advertisements that tell them they need a host of other nutrients, supplements, and herbal preparations. How does one sort fact from fiction? What are the energy and nutrient needs of the active female? What nutritional factors are of greatest concern? This chapter tries to put into perspective the nutritional needs of active females, including female athletes. First, we address the energy requirements of active females and the importance of eating adequate energy for good health and performance. Second, we discuss the health consequences of restricting energy intake too dramatically. Next, we briefly address the major vitamin and mineral concerns for the active female. Finally, we discuss the components of the female athlete triad (eating disorders, amenorrhea, and osteoporosis) and ways to detect and prevent this set of disorders.

Energy and Nutrient Requirements

In order to maintain body weight, female athletes of any age must consume enough kilocalories (kcal) to cover the energy costs of daily living, the energy costs of their sport, and the energy costs associated with building and repairing muscle tissue. Females of reproductive age must also cover the costs of menstruation and reproductive function, while younger females must cover the additional energy costs of growth.

Active females, like most women in our society, are often preoccupied with their body weights and shapes. Although their weights are often normal or even below normal by all medical or health standards, they still want to lose that extra 5-10 lb (2.3-4.5 kg). In addition, female athletes are frequently pressured by coaches, parents, peers, and themselves to weigh less. What are the health consequences of this type of dieting in the active female or the competitive female athlete? What are the potential health consequences if these behaviors are followed into the third, fourth, and fifth decades of life? What strategies can you use to help the active female identify and maintain a healthy body weight for her sport and throughout life? This section reviews the possible health consequences of chronic dieting or energy restriction in active females. Although these women usually do not have a clinical eating disorder, they nevertheless frequently engage in maladaptive dieting behaviors. Finally, we offer strategies for helping female athletes iden-

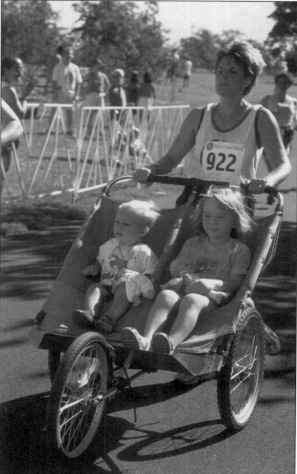

© Dennis Light

Exercise contributes to good health and weight maintenance across the lifecycle.

tify and maintain a healthy body weight throughout their athletic careers and their lives.

Health Consequences of Chronic Dieting

For most healthy women, "going on a diet" for a designated time should present few nutritional or long-term health problems. However, serious health problems may arise for the active female or the female athlete who *chronically* diets or restricts energy intake while expending high amounts of energy in exercise. In fact, the female athlete triad (discussed later in this chapter) is one example of a serious health consequence that can arise from chronic energy restriction in active females.

Poor Energy and Macronutrient Intakes

If an active female constantly restricts energy intake to less than 1800 kcal/d, it is almost impossible to get adequate nutrients (protein, carbohydrate, vitamins, and minerals). Recreational athletes who exercise 6-10 h/week require 2200-2500 kcal/d for weight maintenance; competitive female athletes who exercise 10-20 h or more per week need at least 2500-2800 kcal/d to maintain body weight. Women involved in high-endurance sports (e.g., training for a marathon or triathlon) may need as much as 4000-4500 kcal/d.

Active females with low energy intakes have protein and carbohydrate intakes below those recommended for active people (Coyle 1995; Lemon 1995). They do not eat enough protein to maintain and repair muscle tissue and to cover the cost of any protein used for energy during exercise. As mentioned in chapter 4, active females engaged in endurance activity need more protein (1.2-1.4 g protein/kg body weight) (Lemon 1995) than the **Recommended Dietary Allowance (RDA)** (0.8 g protein/kg body weight) (Food and Nutrition Board 1989). When energy intake is low, moreover, carbohydrate levels are inadequate to replenish glycogen stores used during exercise. Most female athletes in training need ≥5 g carbohydrate/kg body weight to maintain glycogen stores. If activity is exceptionally high and training occurs on a daily basis, carbohydrate needs may be ~6-8 g of carbohydrate/kg body weight (Coyle 1995). Many active females avoid fat either for weight loss or because they think fat is bad for their health. If fat intake is too low (<10-15% of energy intake), the intake and absorption of the fat-soluble vitamins and es-

sential fatty acids may also be low. Finally, many female athletes with poor energy intakes complain of fatigue, frequent injuries, irritability, and poor athletic performance (Dueck, Manore, and Matt 1996). You often can reverse these complaints by having such a client follow two simple guidelines:

- She should increase her total daily energy intake (kcal/d) and/or decrease total energy expenditure (maybe add a rest day to her training routine).
- She should be certain that she is in a state of positive energy balance before beginning any physical activity.

This means that she should be well fed *before* her daily workout. If she has a 3 P.M. workout, she may need to eat a 2 P.M. snack before coming to the track or the gym. This snack helps provide the body with enough energy to fuel both the brain and the muscles during exercise. People who diet frequently tend to restrict energy intake during the day and eat most of their kilocalories at the end of the day. An athlete who follows this pattern will come to her workout fatigued and unable to perform her best. Table 15.1 outlines some of the symptoms of low energy intakes in active women.

Poor Micronutrient Intakes

Active females with poor energy intakes frequently have poor vitamin and mineral intakes—especially calcium, iron, magnesium, zinc, and B-complex vitamins (Beals and Manore 1998; Manore 1999; Manore, in press). These micronutrients are especially important for active individuals and play an important role in energy production, hemoglobin synthesis, maintenance of bone health, and adequate immune function. Prolonged energy restriction combined with poor micronutrient intakes can place the female athlete at risk for poor nutritional status. This can result in decreased bone density, impaired immune response, menstrual dysfunction, anemia, poor exercise performance, and increased recovery time from injury. Which micronutrients are most likely to be deficient? What vitamin and mineral recommendations can you give to the active female?

Table 15.2 suggests intakes of vitamins and minerals for active women and compares them to the current RDAs or to **Dietary Reference Intakes (DRIs)** (Food and Nutrition Board [FNB] 1989, 1997, 1998). (See chapters 9-13 for

411

Table 15.1   How Do You Know If an Active Female Is Not Eating Enough?

If a female athlete is not eating enough food, she may experience some of the following symptoms:

- Hungry, irritable, and may have a difficult time concentrating before or during her exercise routine. Sometimes she may even get shaky and light-headed. This may be especially true if she exercises around 3-4 P.M. and has not eaten since lunch, or if she exercises before breakfast.

- Poor growth rates for young and adolescent female athletes. The diet must provide enough fuel for growth and menstruation, building and repair of muscle tissue, and exercise.

- She may stop having her menstrual periods. This may be a sign that the body does not have enough energy to fuel both exercise and the reproductive functions of the body. An athlete does not have to have an eating disorder to stop having her period. Many female athletes stop menstruating if they are exercising hard and not eating enough food and kilocalories, even if they are making good food choices.

- She is losing weight. This means she is not providing enough fuel for both exercise and weight maintenance. If she is restricting energy intake and exercise intensity is high, both muscle tissue and fat are being used for fuel.

Adapted from Manore 1997.

detailed treatment of each of these nutrients.) Adequate intakes of B-complex vitamins are necessary for energy production during exercise and for the prevention of anemia. About 10-60% of female athletes do not consume the RDA for the B-complex vitamins, the most common deficiencies being in riboflavin, vitamin B_6, and folate (Manore 1994; Manore, in press). No researchers have reported adequate mean intakes of folate in active women. *According to current research, active females should consume at least twice the RDA for riboflavin and vitamin B_6 and at least the RDA for folate.* If adequate intakes for these three B-complex vitamins are achieved, intake should be adequate for the other B-complex vitamins (thiamine, niacin, biotin, and pantothenic acid). Vitamin B_{12} is usually of concern only for people who avoid animal foods or if gastrointestinal problems prevent absorption of the vitamin.

Antioxidant micronutrients (vitamins C, A, and E; β-carotene; and selenium) help main-

tain cellular integrity and prevent tissue damage from the many pollutants in our environment as well as from internal sources of free radicals. Exercise increases the potential for tissue oxidation due to the higher oxygen consumption that occurs during exercise. Athletes who restrict intake of energy or fat may also be reducing their intake of fat-soluble vitamins—especially vitamin E, which is found in the fatty portion of foods and in many vegetable cooking oils. Vitamin C is found in citrus fruits and in some vegetables (e.g., tomatoes, broccoli, or green and red peppers), while vitamin A and β-carotene are found in green, yellow, and dark green vegetables. If these foods are limited in the diet, the probability is high that the intake of these antioxidant vitamins will be low. Keith (1997) reviewed the research literature and found that 10-25% of female athletes consume less than the current 60 mg/d RDA for vitamin C. Intakes of antioxidant nutrients above the current RDA may be necessary for women who perform high-intensity exercise or who exercise in a highly polluted environment (see table 15.2) (Kanter 1998; Keith 1997).

Chapters 11 and 12 discuss in detail the mineral requirements of active people. In this section we highlight the minerals that are of specific concern to active women, who generally are at increased risk for poor intakes of iron, calcium, magnesium, and zinc. This is due in part to the restriction of meat and dairy from the diets of many active women, especially those who restrict energy intake for weight loss. In fact, the reported incidence of iron depletion (stage I) in active females is quite variable and ranges from 15-60%, while only 20-30% in the general female population. Iron is important for hemoglobin synthesis, and exercise may increase the need for this mineral. Thus, female athletes should consume at least the 15 mg/d RDA for iron; if possible, some of this iron should be from heme iron sources (meat, fish, and poultry). If the diet is low or absent in heme iron, higher amounts of daily iron may be required. Iron status should be checked periodically and supplementation used only if warranted.

Calcium intake is also typically low in the diets of active women. Calcium is required for good bones, along with adequate intakes of vitamin D. The new DRI for calcium reflects the increased need for this nutrient in women of

Table 15.2   Recommended Daily Vitamin and Mineral Intakes for Active premenopausal Women

Vitamin or mineral	Suggested intake or range of intakes for active women[1]	Current Recommended Dietary Allowance (RDA) or Dietary Reference Intake (DRI)[2]
Vitamins:		
Thiamine	1.5-2.0 mg/d	1.1 mg/d (19–50 years)
Riboflavin	2.4-3.0 mg/d	1.1 mg/d (19-70 years)
Vitamin B_6	1.5-3.0 mg/d	1.3 mg/d (19-50 years)
Folate (FE)	400 µg/d	400 µg/d (19-50 years)
Vitamin B_{12}	2.4 µg/d	2.4 µg/d (19-50 years)
Vitamin C	200-400 mg/d	60 mg/d (15-51+ years)
Vitamin E	200-400 IU/d	8 mg/d α-TE (11-51+ years)
Vitamin D	10-20 µg/d (400-800 IU/d) if dietary intakes are low or exposure to sunlight is limited	5 µg/d (200 IU/d) (9-50 years) or 10 µg/d (400 IU/d) (50-70 years)
Minerals:		
Iron	15 mg/d	15 mg/d (15-50 years)
Calcium	1300-1500 mg/d, especially for young athletes between the ages of 11-24 years and athletes with exercise-induced amenorrhea	1000 mg/d (19-50 years)
Zinc	12 mg/d	12 mg/d (15-50 years)
Magnesium	350-400 mg/d	280 mg/d (19-50 years)

FE = folate equivalents; TE = α-tocopherol equivalents. 1 mg/d α-tocopherol = 1 α-TE = 1 IU.

[1]Anderson et al. 1998; Anderson 1996; Kanter 1998; Joy et al. 1997; Manore in press.

[2]Food and Nutrition Board 1989, 1997, 1998.

all ages (see chapter 13). Active women should strive to consume at least the DRI for calcium every day (table 15.2). If the diet is limited in dairy products, it is much more difficult to consume the required amounts of calcium from foods unless a person uses fortified foods. Milk is frequently fortified with vitamin D, which stimulates intestinal calcium absorption. Vitamin D levels are often low for people who consume little milk and who have limited exposure to the sun. For female athletes who participate primarily in indoor sports (e.g., figure skating, hockey, volleyball, basketball, and gymnastics), exposure to the sun may be quite limited. This is especially true for people in northern climates where winter months may dramatically limit exposure to sunlight. For these people, dietary vitamin D supplementation or fortification in foods may be very important to maintain good bone density. Remember that adequate calcium and vitamin D intakes are very important for young females who are still laying down new bone. *More than 90% of total **bone mineral density (BMD)***

occurs by 17 years of age, with peak bone density occurring between the ages of 25-30 years (figure 15.1). *It is imperative that all the micronutrients necessary for optimal bone growth are provided during this time.* See "Calcium and Vitamin D Requirements of Active Women" on page 414 and table 15.2 for more specific recommendations concerning calcium and vitamin D intake for active females.

If meat products are limited in a diet or if the diet is high in refined foods, zinc and magnesium intakes may be low. Zinc is especially important for building and repairing tissue, while magnesium is important for energy production during exercise. Active females should strive to consume at least the RDA for these nutrients (table 15.2). They should be careful not to oversupplement with minerals since mineral-mineral interactions may cause one mineral to block the absorption or transport of another. A good rule to follow is always to consume minerals at or near the RDA or DRI level unless a particular deficiency dictates otherwise.

■ HIGHLIGHT ■

Calcium and Vitamin D Requirements of Active Women

Females aged 9-18 years need to consume 1300 mg/d of calcium, while women aged 19-50 years need to consume 1000 mg/d. Women >51 years of age need 1200 mg/d of calcium to help maintain bone density during the menopausal years. Since milk and other dairy products are the primary source of calcium in the American diet, an athlete who does not use dairy products may need to supplement or use fortified foods, such as fortified soy milk or orange juice. Active females who already have poor bone density may need higher calcium intakes (1500 mg/d).

Vitamin D is necessary for optimal intestinal absorption of calcium. Vitamin D is obtained in the diet and/or synthesized in the skin through exposure to sunlight. Sun exposure to hands, arms, and face for 5-15 min/d is thought to be adequate to provide sufficient amounts of vitamin D. For active females who train or exercise primarily indoors and/or who live in northern climates, where exposure to sun is limited in the winter months, vitamin D intakes may be poor. These individuals may need to supplement with 400-800 IU (10-20 μg/d) of vitamin D or use vitamin D-fortified milk. Massive doses of vitamin D are not recommended.

Decreased Resting Metabolic Rate and Total Daily Energy Expenditure

One effect of dieting is that it reduces **resting metabolic rate (RMR).** During the dieting period, RMR declines to a greater extent than that predicted based on decreases in total body weight and **fat-free mass (FFM).** This means that total daily energy expenditure is reduced in people who chronically restrict energy intake. This decrease is compounded when heavy physical activity is combined with low energy

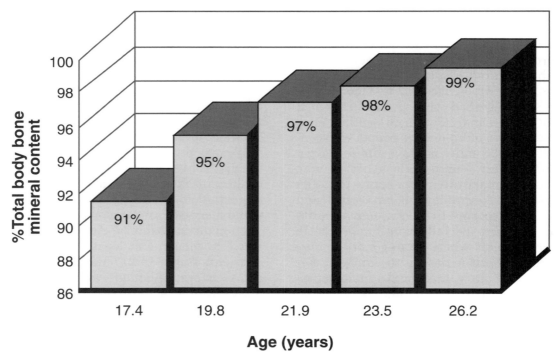

Figure 15.1 Total bone mineral content adjusted for age in young women.
Adapted from Teegarden et al. 1995.

intakes (Thompson et al. 1996). Moreover, the energy cost of digesting and metabolizing food declines when energy intake is restricted, thus further decreasing the total energy needs for the day. The end result of chronic energy restriction and high physical activity is that fewer kilocalories are required to maintain body weight in the dieting athlete than in a nondieting person of similar size and activity level.

The above point is illustrated by Donnelly and colleagues (1994), who examined the effect of severe dieting (520 kcal/d) and exercise on RMR and FFM. Although this study was done in obese women, the results are applicable to nonobese people—especially active females of any size. This study is unique in that it used both aerobic and weight training exercise treatments. Sedentary women (n = 115) were randomly assigned to one of six dieting groups for a 12-week period. Each group was fed the same low-energy diet (520 kcal/d) for the entire 12 weeks, and the researchers monitored all the exercise. The treatments were as follows:

1. ***Diet-only group (control group):*** Did not exercise.

2. ***Diet + endurance exercise:*** Did treadmill walking or cycling at 70% heart rate reserve, 4 d/week; exercise progressed from 20 to 60 min/d.

3. ***Diet + weight training:*** Performed six to eight repetitions at 70-80% of 1-RM using five different weight lifting exercises, 3 d/week.

4. ***Diet + endurance exercise (same as above) + weight training (same as above):*** Performed same weight training as group 3 and same endurance (aerobic) exercise as group 2.

5. ***Diet only for the first 4 weeks, with endurance exercise (same as above) added for the last 8 weeks:*** For the first 4 weeks, did not exercise; for weeks 5-12, they performed the same endurance (aerobic) exercise as group 2.

6. ***Diet + weight training (same as above) for the first 4 weeks, with endurance exercise (same as above) added for the last 8 weeks:*** For the first 4 weeks, performed same weight training as group 3; for weeks 5-12, they continued the strength training but added the same endurance (aerobic) exercise as group 2.

All the groups lost weight, but total weight loss did not differ between the groups and ranged from 16.7-22.3% of baseline body weight. In addition, changes in body fat were similar for all groups, ranging from 6.9-9.3%. Relative RMR (kcal/kg FFM/d) also decreased 1.6-9.3% over the treatment periods, but there were no significant differences between the groups. The greatest absolute decrease in RMR (down 240 kcal/d, which represented a 13.5% decrease) occurred in group 4—the dieters who did both endurance exercise and weight training ($p < 0.05$) (figure 15.2). However, the amount of FFM lost in this group was similar to that lost in the other five groups (9 lb or ~4 kg). These results illustrate that, *in the presence of severe energy restriction, exercise does not increase weight loss or slow the decrease of FFM or RMR compared to dieting without exercise.* The group (group 4) with the highest exercise energy expenditure had the greatest absolute decrease in RMR during the 12-week dieting period. The body decreases RMR to conserve energy in the presence of severe negative energy balance (low energy intake and high energy expenditure).

A more reasonable approach to weight loss is to increase energy expenditure (~300-500 kcal/d, 4-5 d/week) using both endurance and strength training while making only moderate decreases in energy intake (~300-500 kcal/d). The actual decrease in energy intake should depend on age, sex, health, body size, and current energy intake/expenditure and can usually be achieved by altering food choices and serving sizes without counting kilocalories. This more moderate approach minimizes decreases in FFM and RMR—while most of the weight lost is fat.

If a female athlete needs to lose weight, she should closely examine her current energy expenditure and intake. If she is already training hard, she should not increase her exercise and should attempt only small decreases in energy intake. If energy restriction is too severe, she will be fatigued, irritable, have poor exercise performance and concentration, and be at increased risk of injury. She should be able to achieve small to moderate decreases in energy intake by altering food choices and serving sizes. Chapter 6 provides more detailed information on weight loss in athletes.

Poor Exercise Performance

The effect of chronic dieting on exercise performance has been examined in female athletes

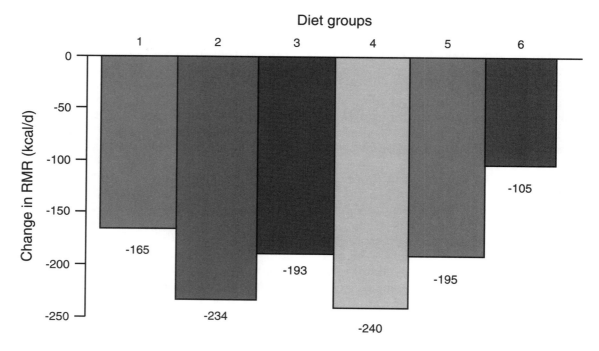

Figure 15.2 Changes in absolute resting metabolic rate (RMR) before and after a 12-week diet or diet-plus-exercise program. All groups followed a highly restrictive diet (520 kcal/d) for the entire 12 weeks. Group 1 = diet only; Group 2 = diet + endurance exercise; Group 3 = diet + weight training; Group 4 = diet + endurance exercise + weight training; Group 5 = diet only for first 4 weeks + endurance exercise for last 8 weeks; Group 6 = diet + weight training for first 4 weeks + endurance exercise for the last 8 weeks. Differences from baseline were statistically significant for each group, but *differences between groups were not statistically significant.*
Adapted from Donnelly et al. 1994.

involved in aesthetic or lean-build sports (e.g., dancers, gymnasts, and figure skaters) (Sundgot-Borgen 1993, 1994). These individuals are constantly pressured to maintain a lean body for their sport, and many chronically diet to maintain a competitive weight. They are thinner and typically report higher incidence of maladaptive dieting behaviors than athletes participating in sports allowing more normal builds, such as basketball, volleyball, or downhill skiing (Beals and Manore 1994, 1998). Participants in lean-build sports report poorer energy intakes, higher rates of injury, less ability to concentrate, and longer recovery times from injuries as compared with athletes in normal-build sports (Beals and Manore 1994, 1998; Sandri 1993). Poor physical performance can have a devastating psychological effect, especially if it is tied to team eligibility or scholarships. A number of psychological stresses are reported with severe dieting in athletes, including increased depression, obsession with food and body weight, increased incidence of binge-purge eating behaviors, increased stress of con-

stantly trying to make weight or maintain an unrealistic body weight, and increased risk of developing an eating disorder (Beals and Manore 1994, 1998; Brownell et al. 1992).

Strategies for Maintaining a Healthy Body Weight

The goal of the health professional is to help active females and female athletes to achieve and maintain a healthy body weight for their sport and for good health. The process begins by identifying what constitutes a realistic, healthy body weight based on genetic, physiological, social, sport, and psychological factors. A healthy weight is one that can be realistically maintained, allows for involvement in physical activity, and reduces risk factors for chronic disease. Table 15.3 gives strategies for helping active females identify and maintain a healthy body weight throughout the life cycle.

Research shows that when pressure to achieve a weight goal is high, women attempt any weight-loss method to achieve success, re-

Table 15.3 **Techniques to Help an Active Individual Identify and Maintain a Healthy Body Weight Throughout the Life Cycle**

I. Emphasize personal health and well-being, not weight.
- Focus less on the scale and more on healthy habits such as regular exercise, stress management, and making good food choices.
- Set realistic weight goals: What is the maximum weight for your height that would be acceptable? What is the maximum weight that will reduce the risk of chronic disease? What was the last weight you could maintain without constantly dieting?
- Mark progress by measuring changes in fitness level, health parameters (positive changes in blood pressure, glucose, lipids, etc.), and general well-being.
- Make lifestyle changes that help you maintain a healthy weight for yourself—not for your job, for your spouse, for your friends, or to prove a point.

II. Change diet and eating behaviors.
- Do not constantly deprive yourself of favorite foods or set unrealistic dietary rules or guidelines.
- Make basic dietary changes that reduce energy intake, that fit into your lifestyle, and that you know you can achieve.
- Reduce fat intake, but remember that a lower-fat diet will not guarantee weight loss if you do not achieve a negative energy balance (reduced energy intake and increased energy expenditure).
- Eat more whole grains, cereals, fruits, and vegetables.
- Make sure you consume adequate dietary fiber (>25 g/d)
- Do not skip meals or do not let yourself get too hungry.
- Eat something for breakfast. This will prevent you from being too hungry and overeating at lunch.
- Plan ahead and be prepared for when you might get hungry. Always have good food available when and where you get hungry.
- Identify your own dietary weaknesses and plan a strategy for dealing with them.
- Remember you are making life-long dietary changes that will result in weight loss. You are not going on a diet that you will some day go off of.

III. Change exercise behaviors.
- Start and maintain a regular exercise program. *This is an absolute requirement for the maintenance of a healthy body weight.*
- Pick an activity or activities that you enjoy, including some that you can do on your own.
- Pick an activity that is inexpensive and does not require fancy equipment. This means you will maintain your fitness program even when you are traveling and away from home.
- Find an exercise partner or exercise class to help you get started and motivate you. It will also help you get through the difficult days until exercise is a part of your lifestyle.
- Participate in group exercise activities whenever possible.
- Plan regular exercise into your day: add additional exercise by walking instead of driving or use stairs instead of the elevator.

Realize that you are making a lifetime change and a lifetime commitment to yourself for good health and weight management.

Adapted from Manore 1996.

gardless of health consequences. Any successful weight-loss or weight-maintenance program must address *changes in lifestyle* that can help athletes achieve and maintain a healthy weight for their sport without constantly dieting.

Female Athlete Triad

The **female athlete triad** is a serious syndrome that comprises three medical disorders frequently seen in female athletes: disordered eating, amenorrhea, and osteoporosis. These components are interrelated in etiology, pathogenesis, and consequences (Otis et al. 1997). The American College of Sports Medicine takes this syndrome quite seriously—see "American College of Sports Medicine (ACSM) Position Statement on the Female Athlete Triad," page 418.

Active women, like most women in our society, are often concerned or even preoccupied with their body weight and shape. Their source of pressure is twofold: not only are they burdened by the general sociocultural demands placed on women to be thin, but they are also expected to meet weight standards or body size

■ HIGHLIGHT ■

American College of Sports Medicine (ACSM) Position Statement on the Female Athlete Triad

"The Female Athlete Triad is a syndrome occurring in physically active girls and women. Its interrelated components are disordered eating, amenorrhea, and osteoporosis. Pressure placed on young women to achieve or maintain unrealistically low body weight underlies development of the Triad. Adolescents and women training in sports in which low body weight is emphasized for athletic activity or appearance are at greatest risk. Girls and women with one component of the Triad should be screened for the others.

"Alone or in combination, Female Athlete Triad disorders can decrease physical performance and cause morbidity and mortality. More research is needed on its causes, prevalence, treatment, and consequences. All individuals working with physically active girls and women should be educated about the Female Athlete Triad and develop plans to prevent, recognize, treat, and reduce its risks." (Otis et al. 1997)

expectations for their sport. Failure to meet these weight standards can result in severe consequences, such as being cut from the team, being given less participation with the team, or even being eliminated from competition. As the pressure to be thin mounts, active women may engage in disordered eating behaviors. This in turn may disrupt the menstrual cycle and result in amenorrhea. Without a normal menstrual cycle and adequate reproductive hormones, which play an important role in bone health, a woman can experience decreases in bone mineral density. The most severe cases lead to osteoporosis. Thus, for many female athletes, disordered eating is the event that leads to the absence of menstruation (amenorrhea) and poor bone mineral density. Sports that emphasize leanness or a thin body build may place young girls or women at risk for the female athlete triad. The American College of Sports Medicine has identified these sports as follows (Otis et al. 1997):

- Sports that have subjective performance scoring, such as dance, skating, diving, and gymnastics

- Endurance sports that emphasize a lean build and/or a low body weight, such as long-distance running, cycling, and cross-country skiing

- Sports that require the athlete to wear body-contouring or body-revealing clothing, such as gymnastics, swimming, volleyball, aerobics, track, and dance

- Sports that require athletes to weigh in or that use weight-specific sport categories for participation, such as horse racing, martial arts, and rowing

- Sports that emphasize a preadolescent body build for success, such as gymnastics, figure skating, and diving

Although participants in the above sports may have an increased risk for developing one or more of the symptoms of the female athlete triad, it is important to remember that no sport is immune to this disorder.

The following sections outline each of the components of the female athlete triad and the serious health consequences associated with this syndrome.

Eating Disorders

The pressure to be thin is so pervasive in our society that it is difficult to differentiate normal from abnormal eating behavior. One fact on which eating disorder specialists agree is that dieting can lead to more severe forms of disordered eating. Thus, the pressure to be thin at any cost can lead some active females to develop disordered eating behaviors (Johnson 1994; Peterson et al. 1995). Eating behaviors form a continuum that ranges from normal to subclinical disorders to clinically diagnosed abnormal behaviors such as anorexia nervosa or bulimia nervosa (Thompson and Sherman 1993; Tuschl et al. 1990). To be diagnosed with a clinical eating disorder, one must meet the criteria outlined

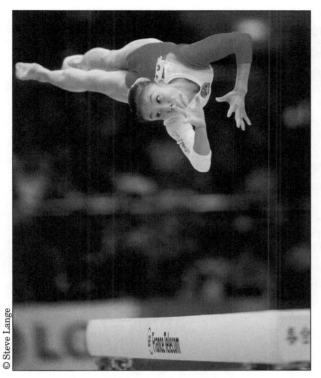

© Steve Lange

Female athletes in "thin-build" sports, such as gymnastics, distance running, or dance, are at risk for developing one or more components of the female athlete triad.

by the American Psychiatric Association's (APA) *Diagnostic and Statistical Manual of Mental Disorders* (DSM-IV) (1994) and outlined in "Diagnostic Criteria for Anorexia Nervosa and Bulimia Nervosa" on page 420.

The factors that trigger **anorexia nervosa** in a female athlete may differ from those that lead to the disorder in a nonathlete, and the early symptoms may differ from those in sedentary people since the disorder affects exercise performance early on. But the diagnostic symptoms are the same for everyone: (1) People with anorexia nervosa have a "drive for thinness" and a "need for weight loss" that must be present for diagnosis, yet the amount of weight loss required for diagnosis is variable (Garfinkel 1995). Because many female athletes are already lean and have low body mass indexes (BMI), the amount of weight they lose may be less than that observed in the nonathlete. (2) Individuals with anorexia nervosa have an intense fear of gaining weight or of becoming fat; even small amounts of weight gain trigger high stress and anxiety. (3) Amenorrhea is a criterion for diagnosis of anorexia nervosa and is due to hypo-

thalamic dysfunction, which results from malnutrition.

Like anorexia nervosa, **bulimia nervosa** has specific characteristics that must be present for diagnosis: (1) There is an uncontrollable desire to overeat or binge on food; however, the quantity of food that constitutes a binge is much more difficult to define. For practical purposes, a "binge" is usually determined on an individual basis. For a small active female, what constitutes a binge might be quite different than what would constitute a binge for a larger, less active person. (2) Binge eating must also be characterized by a subjective sense of loss of control (Garfinkel 1995). This means that the person feels she cannot control the situation or prevent the binge once it has started. (3) The binge must occur within a discrete time period. This criterion is included to remove the classification of "continual snacking" or "grazing" from qualifying as a binge episode. It is less clear, however, how frequently a binge must occur before an individual is classified as bulimic. The DSM-IV criteria designate that the binge must occur on average at least twice a week for 3 mo (APA 1994). An individual need not purge after the binge to be diagnosed with bulimia nervosa.

For the female athlete who is pressured to maintain a lean body weight, purging often follows a binge episode. This pattern of disordered eating may begin as an infrequent occurrence in which the athlete must deal with unwanted food in a social situation. For example, the team is having a pizza party, and the athlete wants to join in the fun but feels guilty about eating so much food. Thus, what may begin as an isolated incident can develop into a daily event until the athlete is frequently purging after eating, regardless of the volume. Bingeing and purging behaviors can also be triggered by periods of dieting where the athlete has deprived herself of adequate food and energy for a period of time or engaged in some other destructive weight-loss behaviors (table 15.4). Whatever the factors that trigger the bingeing and purging, the athlete can quickly lose control of her ability to deal with food rationally. Not all athletes engage in vomiting to purge unwanted foods. They may use excessive exercise, laxatives, enemas, diuretics, or fasting to purge the unwanted kilocalories consumed in a binge. For example, after a binge, athletes may increase their daily mileage to equal the "calculated"

419

■ HIGHLIGHT ■

Diagnostic Criteria for Anorexia Nervosa and Bulimia Nervosa

Anorexia Nervosa

- Refusal to maintain body weight at or above a minimally normal weight for age and height (e.g., weight loss leading to maintenance of body weight less than 85% of that expected; or failure to make expected weight gain during period of growth, leading to body weight less than 85% of that expected).

- Intense fear of gaining weight or becoming fat, even though considered underweight by all medical criteria.

- Disturbance in the way in which one experiences his or her body weight or shape; undue influence of body weight or shape on self-evaluation; or denial of the seriousness of the current low body weight.

- In postmenarchal females, amenorrhea (the absence of at least three consecutive menstrual cycles). (A woman is considered to have amenorrhea if her periods occur only when given hormones, e.g. estrogen.)

Bulimia Nervosa

- Recurrent episodes of binge eating.

- Recurrent inappropriate compensatory behavior in order to prevent weight gain, such as self-induced vomiting; misuse of laxatives, diuretics, enemas, or other medications; fasting; or excessive exercise.

- Binge eating occurs on average at least twice a week for 3 mo.

- Body shape and weight unduly influence self-evaluation. (The disturbance does not occur exclusively during episodes of anorexia nervosa.)

Adapted from APA 1994.

---

energy content of the binge, or they may fast for a day or two until they feel they have purged the extra kilocalories (Garfinkel 1995). These destructive behaviors can have long-term health consequences; thus, female athletes need to be taught healthy weight-loss and/or weight-maintenance skills to prevent the development of this eating disorder. See table 15.3 for guidelines in helping an athlete identify and maintain an ideal body weight for good health and exercise performance.

Peterson and colleagues (1995) demonstrated how dieting and severe energy restriction in active people can increase the incidence of disordered eating behaviors. They examined the presence of bulimic weight-loss behaviors in individuals enrolled in three weight-management programs:

1. A military weight-management program (n = 51)

2. A civilian weight-management program (n = 53)

3. A comparison military (normal-weight) group (n = 51)

The military weight-management group consisted of United States Air Force (USAF) members who were mandated to enroll and required to lose weight or face possible administrative action or discharge. People in the civilian weight-management group were volunteers. The study included both males (n = 78) and females (n = 77). Results showed that the military weight-management group engaged in bulimic weight-loss behaviors two to five times more often than the comparison groups. They engaged in vomiting, strenuous exercise, and the use of the sauna/steam room for weight loss four times as often as the civilian weight-management group. There was no statistically significant difference between men and women

420

Table 15.4 **Disordered Eating Behaviors and Weight-Loss Practices Frequently Used by Female Athletes and the Resulting Health Consequences**

Dieting behavior	Health consequences
Fasting/starvation	Loss of lean body mass and bone density; lower metabolic rate; increased risk of poor nutritional status; poor exercise performance.
Diet pills	Medical side effects such as rapid heart rate, anxiety, inability to concentrate, nervousness, inability to sleep, and dehydration. Any weight lost is quickly regained.
Diuretics (increase water loss from body)	Weight loss is primarily water, and weight is quickly regained once medication is stopped. Dehydration and electrolyte imbalance can be problems. Little fat is lost.
Laxatives (increase water loss from body and increase gastrointestinal mobility)	Weight loss is primarily water, and weight is quickly regained once laxatives are stopped. Dehydration and electrolyte imbalance can be problems. Little fat is lost. Laxatives can be addictive.
Fat-free diets	May be lacking in essential nutrients, especially fat-soluble vitamins and essential fatty acids. Total energy intake must still be reduced to produce weight loss. Many fat-free convenience foods are highly processed, with a high sugar content and few micronutrients unless the foods are fortified. Diet is difficult to follow.
Self-induced vomiting	Dehydration and electrolyte imbalances; gastrointestinal problems, especially irritation of the stomach and esophagus; erosion of dental enamel.
Saunas	Dehydration and electrolyte imbalances; weight regained quickly.
Enemas	Dehydration and electrolyte imbalances; gastrointestinal problems.
Excessive exercise	Increased risk of overuse injuries.

Adapted from Otis 1998.

within the military weight-management group in the bulimic weight-loss behaviors. For overeating behaviors, however, women engaged in binge eating twice as often as men (males = 42%; females = 81%). Finally, more people (53%) in the military weight-management group reported losing at least 10 lb (4.5 kg) in a month compared to the other groups (18%); yet more people from this group also regained at least 5 lb (2.3 kg) in the first week after the diet was over. At least 41% of the military weight-management group reported such a gain, compared to only 27% in the civilian weight-management group and 14% in the control group. The authors concluded that bulimic weight-loss behaviors might develop in people who feel extreme pressure to lose weight. Thus, under pressures to lose weight or face possible discharge, these USAF soldiers resorted to excessive and unhealthy weight-loss measures. This study can easily be applied to the female athlete who is required to lose weight to make the team or to please a coach or parent. When the pressure and stakes are high for weight loss to occur, female athletes frequently turn to harmful dieting practices to achieve their goal.

It appears that many active women have atypical or subclinical eating disorders as evidenced by their preoccupation with food, kilocalories, body shape, and weight (Beals and Manore 1994, 1998, 1999; Fairburn and Walsh 1995). However, these women do not meet all the criteria necessary to classify them with a clinical eating disorder such as anorexia nervosa or bulimia nervosa (Sundgot-Borgen 1993, 1994; Tuschl et al. 1990; Wilmore 1991). How do you know if a person has an atypical or subclinical eating disorder? The American Psychiatric Association recognizes certain atypical eating disorders, whose diagnostic criteria are listed in "Criteria for an Atypical or Subclinical Eating Disorder," page 422. Women with an atypical eating disorder may or may not develop a clinical eating disorder, but they need to realize that their dieting behaviors can be harmful to their health (Fairburn and Walsh 1995). The trigger factors that may predispose an active woman to an eating disorder can include the following (Beals and Manore 1999, in press; Peterson et al. 1995; Sundgot-Borgen 1994):

• Prolonged periods of dieting

421

- Frequent weight fluctuations
- A sudden increase in training volume
- A traumatic stressful event
- Pressure placed on the female to maintain or achieve a low body weight

These trigger factors can be a warning to health professionals, coaches, and parents that an athlete is struggling with body image issues or may have a subclinical eating disorder that could progress to a more serious eating disorder. Active females with subclinical or atypical eating disorders are at risk for poor nutritional status since they generally restrict energy intake, frequently avoid animal products, and strictly limit their fat intake. Beals and Manore (1998) examined nutritional status in 24 female athletes classified as having a subclinical eating disorder, compared to 24 control female athletes. Athletes with subclinical eating disorders had significantly lower energy, protein, and fat intakes, and many consumed less than 66% of the RDA for 8 (calcium, iron, magnesium, zinc, folate, niacin, vitamin B_6, and B_{12}) of the 11 micronutrients examined. Approximately half of the athletes with a subclinical eating disorder had one or more parameters indicating low iron status and had iron intakes that were less than the RDA. None of the control group had low iron intakes, yet some still presented with poor iron status. Five of the control athletes were in stage I iron depletion (low serum ferritin), compared to seven of the subclinical eating disordered athletes. Supplementation and fortified foods (sport foods and cereals) contributed significantly to the total micronutrient intakes of all the athletes, helping to improve overall nutritional status in spite of poor dietary intakes—yet the athletes with subclinical eating disorders were still not getting adequate energy and protein intakes to sustain their high level of physical activity. Low energy intake levels in some female athletes become even more harmful if the athletes use excessive exercise to purge the body of unwanted energy intake.

Menstrual Dysfunction

Diet and exercise can significantly impact reproductive hormones and function with the most severe consequence being amenorrhea, where reproductive hormones are severely sup-

---

■ HIGHLIGHT ■

Criteria for an Atypical or Subclinical Eating Disorder

In 1994, the American Psychiatric Association added a new category of disordered eating called **eating disorders not otherwise specified (EDNOS).** This category is for disorders of eating that do not meet the criteria for any specified eating disorder, such as anorexia nervosa or bulimia nervosa. It is also frequently referred to as **subclinical eating disorders.** The criteria for EDNOS are as follows:

- For females, all the criteria for anorexia nervosa are met except that the individual has regular menses.
- All the criteria for anorexia nervosa are met except that, despite significant weight loss, the individual's current weight is in the normal range.
- All the criteria for bulimia nervosa are met except that the binge eating and inappropriate compensatory mechanisms occur at a frequency of less than twice per week or for a duration of less than 3 mo.
- There is regular use of inappropriate compensatory behavior by an individual of normal body weight after eating small amounts of food (e.g., self-induced vomiting after eating two cookies).
- The individual repeatedly chews and spits out, but does not swallow, large amounts of food.
- There are recurrent episodes of binge eating in the absence of the regular use of inappropriate compensatory behaviors characteristic of bulimia nervosa.

Adapted from APA 1994.

pressed. In the amenorrhea associated with anorexia nervosa, starvation is severe enough to shut down reproductive capabilities. Note, however, that an athlete need not have an eating disorder to sustain exercise-induced changes in her menstrual cycle. See "Normal Menstrual Cycle" below for a description of a normal menstrual cycle and the hormonal changes that occur over a typical cycle.

There is a growing body of evidence suggesting that exercise-induced amenorrhea, as well as other reproductive hormone abnormalities seen in active women, may be due in part to periods of energy deficiency (Dueck, Manore, and Matt 1996; Loucks 1994; Williams et al. 1995). Three factors contribute to negative energy balance in active females:

- High energy expenditure
- Low energy intake compared to energy expenditure
- High psychological and physical stress

Exercise-induced changes in the menstrual cycle may be an energy-conserving strategy to protect more important biological and reproductive processes (Dueck, Manore, and Matt 1996; Dueck, Matt et al. 1996). The prevalence of exercise-induced menstrual dysfunction may be as high as 50% in female athletes. Thus, the possibility that a female athlete may have some type of menstrual dysfunction should not be ignored (Beals and Manore 1998; Dueck, Manore, and Matt 1996). See "Common Types of Menstrual Dysfunction Seen in Active Women" on page 424.

Researchers examining the effect of negative energy balance on the menstrual cycle and reproductive hormones have asked the following research questions:

- What is the role of dieting (energy restriction) alone on menstrual status?
- What is the role of exercise alone on menstrual status?
- What is the combined role of diet and exercise on menstrual status?

Energy deprivation can alter the hormonal profiles and the menstrual cycles of healthy women. The degree of menstrual dysfunction that occurs with dieting appears to depend on the magnitude of the energy restriction, the body's level of energy reserves, and the initial

◼ HIGHLIGHT ◼

Normal Menstrual Cycle

The normal menstrual cycle is typically characterized by two phases that are separated by ovulation at midcycle (figure 15.3). The beginning phase, or the **follicular phase,** is marked by the onset of menstruation. During this phase of the cycle, **follicle stimulating hormone (FSH)** plays an integral role in the recruitment of a single follicle. As the follicle grows, it begins to secrete **estradiol,** which acts in a positive feedback loop to stimulate the release of **luteinizing hormone (LH).** The end of the follicular phase is marked by ovulation, which typically occurs on days 15-18 and is characterized by a large increase in LH. The hormonal events associated with the follicular phase serve to ensure that ovulation and fertilization take place. After ovulation, the second phase of the cycle begins. This stage, called the **luteal phase,** is characterized by increases in ovarian production of estradiol and **progesterone,** which act in a negative feedback loop to inhibit LH and FSH release. After ovulation, the cells remaining after the egg is released from the follicle are called the **corpus luteum,** which produces estradiol and progesterone. These ovarian steroids play an integral role in preparing the uterus for implantation, if fertilization occurs. Without fertilization, there is a rapid decrease in estradiol and progesterone as the corpus luteum becomes atrophied. The intricate series of hormonal events associated with normal menstrual function can be easily disrupted by physiological, metabolic, and/or physiological stress. Furthermore, the intensity of the stressor can have variable effects on the level and magnitude of disruption.

Reproduced from Dueck, Manore, and Matt 1996.

■ HIGHLIGHT ■

Common Types of Menstrual Dysfunction Seen in Active Women

Luteal Phase Deficiency

Luteal phase deficiency is usually characterized by insufficient progesterone production with or without a shortened luteal phase length. Since the total menstrual cycle length may be normal, however, many women do not notice a change in menstrual status and report that they have normal menstrual cycles (Dueck, Manore, and Matt 1996).

Anovulation

Anovulation is the absence of ovulation, which can occur in the presence of menstrual bleeding; however, the menstrual cycle can be shorter (less than 21 d) or longer (35-50 d) than normal. Longer menstrual cycles are usually referred to as oligomenorrhea.

Oligomenorrhea

Oligomenorrhea refers to irregular, longer menstrual cycles—for instance, a woman may have only 6 cycles per year instead of 12. Many active women have irregular cycles during periods of strenuous exercise training but return to more normal cycles when they reduce training levels. These individuals may ovulate infrequently or not at all, and reproductive hormones are usually suppressed.

Amenorrhea

Amenorrhea is the absence of menstrual periods. **Primary amenorrhea** is the absence of menstruation by the age of 16 in a girl who has secondary sex characteristics, while **secondary amenorrhea** is the absence of the menstrual period for ≥ 3 mo after menarche (Otis et al. 1997). These individuals do not ovulate, have low levels of estrogen, and lack the spike in luteinizing hormone (LH) that results in ovulation (Dueck, Manore, and Matt 1996). The most common causes of amenorrhea are pregnancy and menopause. Both exercise-induced and anorexia-induced amenorrhea are forms of **hypothalamic amenorrhea.** This type of amenorrhea is characterized by a decrease in **gonadotropin releasing hormone (GnRH)** from the hypothalamus. GnRH stimulates the pituitary gland to release LH, which in turn signals the ovaries to produce estrogen and progesterone. The result of depressed GnRH concentrations is that no ovulation or menstrual bleeding occurs.

hormonal status before dieting begins. In other words, if an individual already has some type of menstrual dysfunction, dieting may lead to amenorrhea more quickly than in someone who begins a diet with normal menstrual function. Kurzer and Calloway (1986) fed six healthy women (104-130% of ideal body weight) two diets differing only in energy intake. All subjects reported normal menstrual cycles during the 9 mo before beginning the study. The first diet provided a typical energy intake (40 kcal/kg body weight); the second provided 41% of the

first diet (17 kcal/kg body weight). Both diets lasted the length of the menstrual cycle plus 1 week; all subjects received their food daily from a metabolic unit. Weight loss on the low-energy diet ranged from 7.0-14.5 lb (3.2-6.7 kg) during the study. The two leanest women lost the most weight and became anovulatory and amenorrheic during this period. Thus, in this study *the leanest subjects displayed the greatest menstrual dysfunction when placed on an energy restrictive diet*. Their bodies appeared to respond to low energy reserves in the presence of energy

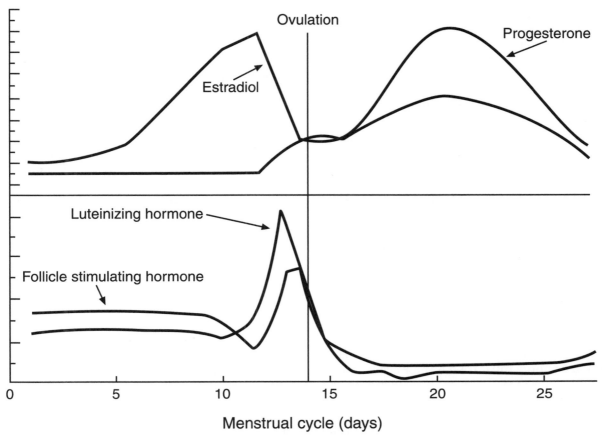

Figure 15.3 Normal menstrual cycle showing changes in plasma levels of hormones. Days 1-15 represent the follicular phase; days 15-28 represent the luteal phase; they are divided by ovulation at the midpoint of the cycle.

Reprinted from Dueck, Manore, and Matt 1996.

restriction by suppressing the ability for reproduction. This is supported by data showing that amenorrhea becomes more common during times of starvation.

Research also shows that energy restriction plus exercise regimens severe enough to produce significant weight loss produce the greatest changes in menstrual function. Increasing energy expenditure while decreasing energy intake creates a negative energy balance, requiring the body to draw on energy reserves to cover the cost of exercise. This combination has a more negative effect on menstrual status than just exercise alone. Williams and colleagues (1995) illustrated this point while examining the effect of exercise—with and without energy restriction—on luteinizing hormone secretion. They studied four moderately trained normally menstruating women over three consecutive menstrual cycles during the follicular phase (refer to "Normal Menstrual Cycle" on page 423 and to figure 15.3). Subjects experienced the greatest decrease in luteinizing hormone during the period of diet plus high exercise, as compared to the other two periods (control period, high-exercise period). These results suggest that abrupt increases in training volume lead to a disruption in luteinizing hormone secretion if subjects are restricting energy and are in negative energy balance. Furthermore, only the period of diet plus high exercise produced significant weight loss, while weight was maintained in the high-exercise-only period. These results support the earlier work of Bullen and colleagues (1985), who reported that abrupt increases in physical activity that result in weight loss (i.e., negative energy balance) are accompanied by a higher incidence of menstrual abnormalities than when exercise is accompanied by weight maintenance. To summarize: *the combined effect of diet and exercise appears to have a more negative effect on menstrual status than just exercise alone or diet alone.*

We now know that the menstrual dysfunction associated with sports is multifaceted, and that for any one individual a number of factors may be involved. Several lifestyle stressors have been identified as predisposing factors for the onset of menstrual dysfunction—including inadequate dietary habits, a history of weight fluctuations, a rigorous training regimen, and the social pressures associated with competition. The primary endogenous stressor most commonly associated with amenorrhea is an inadequate level of body fat (Frisch and McArthur 1974). Although there is no critical level of body fat required of all women for the maintenance of menstruation, one's level of body fat stores cannot be totally ignored. Body fat is only one component of the body's total energy reservoir, but this particular reservoir may be an important determinate in the etiology of athletic menstrual dysfunction. The total energy reservoir includes the amount of energy stored in glycogen and body fat and the energy consumed daily through food. This available energy must then be balanced against the daily energy expenditure. Athletes with the lowest energy reserves may have less tolerance for chronic negative energy balance and be at greater risk for developing menstrual dysfunction. Figure 15.4 outlines a model demonstrating the effect low energy reserves may have on the development of menstrual dysfunction in active women. This figure also outlines some of the suggested health consequences that may arise from prolonged decreases in reproductive hormones.

To more clearly demonstrate the effect strenuous exercise has on menstrual function, read "Case Study: Exercise-Induced Amenorrhea" on page 428. Although the athlete in this study was not purposely restricting energy intake, her energy intake was not adequate to cover her high exercise energy expenditure. If an athlete presents exercise-induced amenorrhea, one of the first steps in treating the disorder is to improve her energy balance by increasing her energy intake (250-350 kcal/d) and decreasing energy expenditure by 10-20% (Otis 1998).

Osteoporosis

The final component of the female athlete triad is **osteoporosis.** If amenorrhea is allowed to persist, the resulting low levels of reproductive hormones can lead to loss of bone mineral density (BMD). This in turn increases the risk of osteoporosis, both when the athlete is young and later in life. Reduced BMD also increases the risk of musculoskeletal injuries such as stress fractures. Figure 15.4 outlines some other potential health problems associated with long-term amenorrhea. See chapter 13 for more detailed definitions and descriptions of osteoporosis. Note that in the context of the female athlete triad, the term "osteoporosis" is used loosely to represent the loss of bone mass or the decrease in bone deposition rather than the strict definitions for osteoporosis given in chapter 13.

Amenorrheic athletes typically display reduced levels of estradiol and progesterone and have hormonal profiles more like those of postmenopausal women than those of their age-matched eumenorrheic counterparts (Drinkwater et al. 1984; Loucks 1994). Thus, despite the established positive effects of exercise training on bone, exercise may not be able to compensate wholly for the negative effects of estrogen and progesterone deficiency (Dalsky 1996). During estrogen deficiency, bone becomes more sensitive to the calcium-mobilizing effect of parathyroid hormone. As a result, a greater number of resorptive sites are established and a gradual loss of bone mass occurs. Research shows that lumbar BMD is reduced ~14% in amenorrheic athletes compared to eumenorrheic athletes (Dueck, Manore, and Matt 1996) and as much as 27% compared to normal cycling sedentary women (Cann et al. 1984). However, not every amenorrheic athlete experiences decreased BMD. The effect of estrogen deficiency on an athlete's BMD may depend in part on the workloads placed on the bone and on how long she has been amenorrheic. With sufficiently high exercise stress, amenorrheic athletes may still be able to maintain BMD similar to or even higher than age-matched norms (see "Case Study: Exercise-Induced Amenorrhea," page 428). The degree to which exercise-induced amenorrhea influences BMD depends on a number of factors, as listed below:

- Current age
- Age when amenorrhea occurred
- Length of time an individual has been amenorrheic
- Current body size and composition
- Type of exercise engaged in

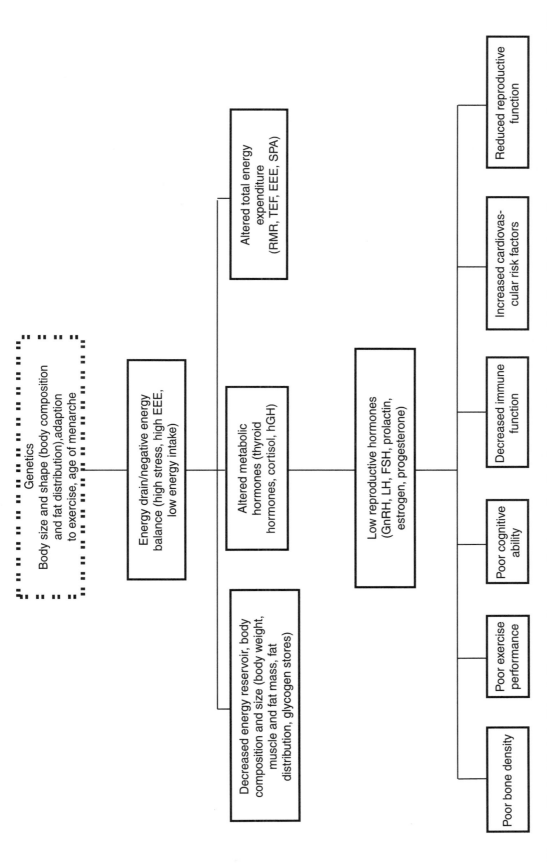

Figure 15.4 Model of the influence of energy drain on the development of menstrual dysfunction in active women, and potential health and performance outcomes due to low reproductive hormones. EEE = exercise energy expenditure; FSH = follicle stimulating hormone; GnRH = gonadotropin releasing hormone; hGH = human growth hormone; LH = luteinizing hormone; RMR = resting metabolic rate; SPA = spontaneous physical activity; TEF = thermic effect of food.

Adapted from Dueck, Manore, and Matt 1996.

Case Study: Exercise-Induced Amenorrhea

A 19-year-old amenorrheic runner reported the loss of menstrual function a year ago when she switched from sprinting to distance events. After switching sports, she reported difficulty maintaining weight and had lost 6.5 lb (3 kg) during the previous track season. She complained of chronic fatigue, poor performance, and high frequency of illness and injury. She had been amenorrheic for 14 consecutive months before seeking help and participating in a research project designed to improve energy balance. Her running schedule at that time included morning and afternoon runs 4 d/week, and she lifted weights 3 d/week. She then began a 15-week nutrition and exercise intervention program designed to increase energy intake by 360 kcal/d (one can of GatorPro per day) and reduce energy expenditure by adding 1 d of rest per week.

Body Weight, Composition, and Energy/Nutrient Intakes of an Amenorrheic Runner

	Before intervention	After intervention (15 weeks)
Weight (kg)	48.2	50.9
Body mass index (kg/m²)	19.1	20.1
Body fat (%)	8.2	14.4
Energy intake (kcal/d)[a]	3045	3683
Energy expenditure (kcal/d)[a]	3200	3000
Energy balance (kcal/day) (intake-expenditure)[a]	−155	+683
Bone density (% of age-matched norm for lumbar spine)[b]	111	113
Menstrual status[c]	Amenorrheic	Amenorrheic

[a] Estimates based on 7-d diet records and activity logs.
[b] Body composition and bone mineral density measured by dual-energy X-ray absorptiometry (DXA).
[c] Normal menstrual status returned after the athlete had followed the intervention program for an additional 3 mo.

Although the intervention program improved the young woman's energy balance, menstrual function did not return until she had followed the intervention program for an additional 3 mo after the 15-week intervention. Hormonal changes during the 15-week intervention revealed increased fasting levels of luteinizing hormone and decreased cortisol. *The athlete reported dramatic increases in performance and set personal best times in some of her events.* She went on to receive a track scholarship from a major university.

Summary: This young woman had exercise-induced amenorrhea. She did not have an eating disorder, and her amenorrhea had not yet resulted in significant reductions in bone loss. Although her bone mineral density was higher than age-matched norms, we do not know what her bone mineral density could have been had she not been amenorrheic for 14 mo. The athlete complained of weight loss and poor exercise performance. Improvement in energy balance and a small increase in body weight during a 15-week intervention period began to improve her reproductive hormonal profile. She reported improved exercise performance and reduced fatigue as a result of the intervention; however, an additional 3 mo on the intervention program was required to bring about menses. This case study demonstrates that nonpharmacological treatment of exercise-induced amenorrhea can be successful if the athlete is willing to eat more, gain small amounts of weight, and reduce exercise training.

Reprinted from Dueck, Matt et al. 1996.

- Dietary intakes of bone-building micronutrients
- Dietary and drug factors that decrease total-body calcium levels
- Total energy intake
- Baseline blood cortisol concentrations
- Genetics

Thus, despite the positive stimulus of exercise on bone, the hormonal changes associated with menstrual dysfunction compromise BMD and increase the risk for fracture. Brukner and Bennell (1997) reviewed 11 studies comparing stress fractures in female athletes with and without menstrual dysfunction. They found the risk of stress fracture was much higher in athletes with menstrual dysfunction (52%) than in their eumenorrheic counterparts (28%) (figure 15.5). This increased risk of stress fracture not only jeopardizes a woman's athletic career but also increases her risk for bone fracture after menopause.

As mentioned above, not all data have shown reduced bone mineral density in amenorrheic athletes compared to active eumenorrheic females. Wilmore et al. (1992) found no differences in lumbar spine BMD between amenorrheic and eumenorrheic runners. Dueck, Matt et al. (1996) even reported a higher BMD in the femoral neck of an endurance amenorrheic athlete compared to her eumenorrheic teammates. These discrepancies illustrate the need to consider several important issues when interpreting bone density data. The development of peak bone mass is not determined solely by the levels of estrogen and progesterone during puberty and the ensuing 10-15 years of musculoskeletal growth and development. Bone mineral density is greatly influenced by genetics and dietary factors. For example, adequate intakes of calcium, vitamin D, and energy are important for bone formation, while high intakes of alcohol, caffeine, and sodium increase calcium losses from the body (Beatty and Finn 1995).

The duration and type of sport in which an individual has participated may also affect the accretion of bone mass. Sports that significantly load the bones, such as gymnastics, stimulate BMD. Gymnasts appear to have significantly higher BMD than matched controls and other female athletes participating in endurance sports (Kirchner et al. 1995; Robinson et al. 1995)—even when the gymnasts report menstrual dysfunction (Robinson et al. 1995). The actual BMD that these athletes *could* have achieved if menstrual dysfunction had not occurred is unknown. Remember, however, that even gymnasts can lose bone mass if amenorrhea persists for an extended period of time.

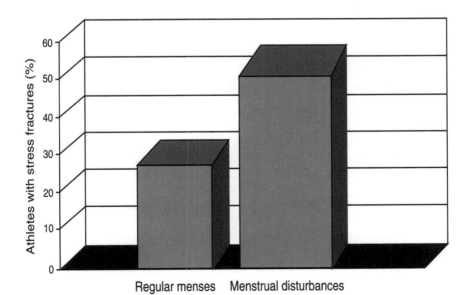

Figure 15.5   Comparison of stress fractures in athletes with and without menstrual disturbances in 11 cross-sectional studies.

Adapted from Brukner and Bennell 1997.

Treatment

Recognition and treatment of an athlete with one or more of the syndromes that comprise the female athlete triad (anorexia nervosa, amenorrhea, osteoporosis) can be difficult, especially if the athlete is less than candid when questioned about the symptoms. For this reason, treating an athlete requires a multidisciplinary approach; the sports medicine team, nutritionist, exercise physiologist, psychologist, coach, trainer, parents, friends of the athlete, and the athlete all must work together. If the athlete is having trouble with weight and body shape issues, take care to deal with these issues before they develop into something more serious. Table 15.4 outlines some of the dieting practices and disordered eating behaviors that may precede the development of an eating disorder. You should learn to look for these symptoms in female athletes. Table 15.5 lists some of the warning signs that a female athlete may be at risk for developing one or more of the components of the female athlete triad.

If someone has one or more of the components of the female athlete triad, her level of participation in her sport should be determined

Table 15.5 Warning Signs of the Female Athlete Triad

1. Excessive dieting for weight loss, large fluctuations in body weight, or too much weight loss
2. Irregular or absent menstrual periods
3. Stress fractures, especially recurrent stress fractures
4. Self-esteem and mood that appear to be dictated by body weight and shape
5. Compulsive overexercise

Adapted from Otis 1998.

by the treating health professional team and should be supported by the coach, the family, and the athlete. *Every sports medicine team should have a standard procedure for preventing and treating disorders of the female athlete triad.* "Case Study: Team Management Approach to Treatment of the Female Athlete Triad" (below) outlines a **team management** approach to treating an athlete suffering from an eating disorder that has become

■ HIGHLIGHT ■

Case Study: Team Management Approach to Treatment of the Female Athlete Triad

A 20-year-old female gymnast returns from summer break, having lost 15 lb (6.8 kg) to reach a current weight of 85 lb (38.6 kg). Current body mass index (BMI) (kg/m²) is 15.6, well below the typical BMI of gymnasts, which is 19-20 kg/m². She has not menstruated for 4 mo. After 2 weeks of preseason conditioning work, she comes to the training room with right shin pain. She reveals that she has been restricting her energy intake to 500-800 kcal/d and thinks the ideal body weight for her 62-in. (157.5-cm) frame is 75 lb (34.1 kg) (BMI = 13.75 kg/m²). Her coach, trainer, and team physician, however, believe that her ideal body weight is closer to 100-105 lb (45.5-47.7 kg). She reports that she had menarche at the age of 15 and has had fairly regular menstrual periods from age 16 until 4 mo ago. She has no history of bone or overuse injury.

Her physical exam reveals she is quite thin, but she has stable vital signs and facial and body lanugo (fine, soft hair that often appears in anorexia nervosa/starvation). An extremity exam reveals local tenderness to palpation on the midshaft of the tibia. Her laboratory results are normal except for low follicle stimulating hormone (FSH) and low estradiol, which are consistent with hypothalamic amenorrhea. A bone scan is positive for a tibia stress fracture.

Treatment: Proposed Role of a Sports Medicine Physician

First, obtain a more detailed history regarding the athlete's recent weight loss and psychological well-being, as well as her insight into the problem. After establishing a relationship with the athlete, confront her with the problem and facilitate getting her into a program involving a psychologist and nutritionist who have expertise in working with disordered eating in athletes. Help her understand and agree to a *written contract* that details the steps she must take for continued participation in her sport. The focus of the contract is on optimal health and on helping the athlete to compete in a safe and healthy manner. For example, the contract may include specific increment goals for weight increases, such as 1/2 to 1 lb per week until she achieves the goal of an established healthy weight range.

Perform a more detailed physical exam and pelvic exam if the athlete has not had one recently. If the results of the medical exam are consistent with hypothalamic, hypoestrogenic amenorrhea, you might recommend oral contraceptive pills. You might recommend a calcium intake of 1500 mg/d and a vitamin D intake of 400-800 IU/d, and you should continue to monitor the progress of the athlete regarding her contract and her interactions with the nutritionist and psychologist. Her training will need to change to non-weightbearing activities because of her stress fracture, and her daily exercises will need to be monitored to assure that her energy expenditure does not exceed her energy intake.

Treatment: Proposed Role of a Nutritionist

First, discuss with the athlete her weight history, her current weight, and what she wants to weigh. Since the optimal weight for a 62-in. gymnast is typically around 100-105 lb (45.5-47.7 kg), remind the athlete that her current weight of 85 lb (38.6 kg) is too low. Show her pictures of anorexic people and point out the muscle wasting that occurs with this disease. Also show pictures of healthy athletes and emphasize that the goal of treatment is to help her be lean, fit, healthy, and at peace with food. It is important to assure her that you are *not* trying to "fatten her up." You might want to take baseline body composition measurements to be used for future reference to show improvements in body composition as the woman rebuilds her body. It is important to discuss with her how she feels about her body and assure her that she is not fat, based on her body composition data. Discuss how food is not the problem but rather a symptom of some unhappiness in her life. Emphasize the importance of food to fuel the body and to provide adequate energy to cover the energy costs of daily living (e.g., 1200 kcal/d for sleep, 500 kcal/d for daily activities, 500 kcal/d for gymnastics). This should help her understand that her current energy intake of 500-800 kcal/d is far below her body's needs. Calculate with her the adequate grams of protein, fat, and carbohydrate she requires per day and design a healthy eating plan. This eating plan should *gradually* increase the athlete's energy intake to accommodate total energy expenditure and to improve weight gain. The initial amount of energy added per day may vary from as little as an extra 100 kcal/meal (e.g., a yogurt for breakfast, a banana for a pre-exercise snack, etc.) to an additional 400-500 kcal/meal.

One goal of nutrition counseling is to move the athlete away from the fear that food is the fattening enemy and to help her see food as a fuel for her muscles so she can become a better athlete. You might ask her, "Are you training to improve your performance or to burn off kilocalories? What are you invested in? What are your goals? Do you think that you are ready to let go of the anorexia and be a healthy athlete?"

Another goal of nutrition counseling is to educate the athlete about the best ways to fuel her body. Make it clear that you can provide information, but she must choose to put the information into practice. For example, if an anorexic athlete only feels safe eating broccoli, bagels, pretzels, and rice cakes, point out that there is little protein, calcium, iron, or zinc in these foods. All nutrients are important for top performance, and a balanced diet, complete with protein-rich foods and dairy products, can provide these nutrients.

(continued)

Subsequent visits should discuss the athlete's fear of food and her drive to eat the perfect diet and have a perfect body. Make it clear to the athlete that she should discuss these issues in her sessions with the psychologist. Monitor the gradual increase in energy intake and food choices. Emphasize all the benefits of better eating habits—improvements in her energy level, health, sleeping ability, ability to concentrate, body warmth, and better workouts. Although the approach used in nutrition counseling will vary from person to person, remember that many anorexic athletes are preoccupied with energy intake (kcal/d). Encourage the athlete to eat a variety of foods including some fat. You might also encourage her to eat with others. If she eats alone, she is more likely to talk herself out of eating enough food. If she is with a supportive friend she trusts, she may feel safer eating all the food.

Treatment: Proposed Role of a Psychologist

First, it is important to find out what the athlete is struggling with in her life, such as relationships, career choices, or values. It is also helpful to identify the sources of stress in her life. Next, it is important to identify her motivation for treatment. Does she see a problem? Is she concerned? Or is she seeking treatment only because a coach, parent, or physician is forcing the issue? Does she see the treatment team members as resources or simply as authority figures? These are important questions that need to be addressed since her view of the treatment and of the health care team can affect her compliance. For example, if she sees the physician or dietitian as authority figures, she may be very passive-aggressive toward them. The physician needs to know that the patient may not be motivated for treatment even if she is smiling in the office. She may have every intention of doing what she promises, but when she is by herself she may not eat as she's supposed to, or she may not report the times she's purging. She may do a lot of different things to cloak her behavior, like water-binge before an appointment at which she is being weighed. Anorexic athletes generally are not deceitful, but they can feel extremely threatened and may therefore hide maladaptive weight-control behaviors. Treat each client uniquely, and develop individualized plans. Final note: the medical management team needs to communicate regarding the treatment of the athlete so that all are in agreement.

Return to Play

The athlete can return to team play or competition only after she has received clearance from the medical management team. Even after the stress fracture is healed, the athlete may need to continue cross-training with a gradual return to weightbearing activities. The physician should continue to monitor the athlete's medical care and make sure that the athlete is continuing to see the nutritionist and the psychologist.

Adapted from Joy et al. 1997.

severe enough to disrupt normal menstrual function and decrease bone density.

The decision to use hormone replacement treatment with a female athlete who presents poor BMD is controversial but may help prevent further bone loss if she is unwilling to change lifestyle factors that will resume menstrual function (Cumming 1996). As with any health problem, prevention is the best treatment. It is imperative that the sports medicine team learn to recognize the risk factors of the female athlete triad and then begin to educate athletes, coaches, and parents about those risk factors.

Chapter in Review

There is increasing pressure on American women to be thin or thinner. This pressure to achieve and maintain a low body weight leads to potentially harmful patterns of chronic dieting, which can affect long-term health. Some of the health consequences of chronic dieting may include the following: poor energy and nutrient intakes, poor nutritional status, decreased RMR and total daily energy expenditure, increased psychological stress, increased risk of developing a clinical eating disorder, and increased risk of exercise-induced amenorrhea. If the pressures to be thin are high, a female athlete may develop the syndromes of the female athlete triad (disordered eating, amenorrhea, osteoporosis). Strategies to help active women get off the dieting bandwagon require the identification of an appropriate and healthy body weight, good eating and exercise habits, and techniques for maintaining these habits throughout the life cycle.

Female athletes need to be educated regarding the adverse effects of the female athlete triad. Athletes also need to know that a menstrual dysfunction can occur without having an eating disorder and that treatments are available. The most successful way to treat exercise-induced menstrual dysfunction or the health problems of the female athlete triad is to prevent them.

KEY CONCEPTS

 ### 1. *Understand the energy and nutrient requirements of active women.*

In active women, energy intake must cover the energy demands of daily living, exercise energy expenditure, reproductive function, building and repair of muscle tissue, and growth in young women. Active women frequently restrict energy intake to achieve a lean body for their sport or for social acceptance. If female athletes restrict energy intake too severely (especially in the presence of high energy expenditure), they increase their risks for one or more of the following health problems: poor macro- and micronutrient intakes, decreased metabolic rate, poor bone mineral density, poor exercise performance, and one or more of the disorders of the female athlete triad.

 ### 2. *Identify the components of the female athlete triad, and discuss its treatment.*

The female athlete triad is a serious syndrome that consists of three medical disorders frequently seen in active females: disordered eating, amenorrhea, and osteoporosis. Each of these disorders exists on a continuum ranging from normal to severe. An athlete who has one disorder of the triad should be screened for the others. Treatment of the female athlete triad requires a multidisciplinary approach since it generally involves medical, nutritional, and psychological interventions plus changes in training and sports participation. Thus, depending on the severity of the problem, one or more of the following individuals or groups may be involved in the treatment: sports medicine team, nutritionist, exercise physiologist, psychologist, coach, trainer, physical therapist, parents, and friends of the athlete. As with any health problem, prevention is the best treatment; thus, screening for the triad in active females is imperative.

KEY TERMS

amenorrhea
anorexia nervosa
anovulation
bone mineral density (BMD)
bulimia nervosa
corpus luteum
Dietary Reference Intake (DRI)
eating disorders not otherwise specified
(EDNOS)

estradiol
fat-free mass (FFM)
female athlete triad
follicle stimulating hormone (FSH)
follicular phase
gonadotropin releasing hormone (GnRH)
hypothalamic amenorrhea
luteal phase
luteal phase deficiency

(continued)

luteinizing hormone (LH)
oligomenorrhea
osteoporosis
primary amenorrhea
progesterone

Recommended Dietary Allowance (RDA)
resting metabolic rate (RMR)
secondary amenorrhea
subclinical eating disorders
team management

References

American Psychiatric Association. Diagnostic and Statistical Manual of Mental Disorders (DSM-IV), 4th ed. Washington, DC: American Psychiatric Association, 1994.

Anderson JJB. Diet and osteoporosis. In: Wolinsky I, Klimis-Tavantzis D, eds. Nutritional Concerns of Women. Boca Raton, FL: CRC Press, 1996:35-59.

Anderson JJB, Stender M, Rondano P, Bishop L, Duckett AB. Nutrition and bone in physical activity and sport. In: Wolinsky I, ed. Nutrition in Exercise and Sport. Boca Raton, FL: CRC Press, 1998:219-44.

Beals KA, Manore MM. The prevalence and consequences of subclinical eating disorders in female athletes. Int J Sport Nutr 1994;4:175-95.

Beals KA, Manore MM. Nutritional status of female athletes with subclinical eating disorders. J Am Diet Assoc 1998;98:419-25.

Beals KA, Manore MM. Subclinical eating disorders in physically active women. Clin Sport Med 1999;14(3):14-29.

Beals KA, Manore MM. Behavioral, psychological and physical characteristics of female athletes with subclinical eating disorders. Int J Sport Nutr (in press).

Beatty D, Finn SC. Position of the American Dietetic Association and the Canadian Dietetic Association: women's health and nutrition. J Am Diet Assoc 1995;95:362-6.

Brownell KD, Robin J, Wilmore JH. Eating, Body Weight and Performance in Athletes: Disorders of Modern Society. Philadelphia: Lea & Febiger, 1992.

Brukner P, Bennell K. Stress fractures in female athletes: diagnosis, management and rehabilitation. Sports Med 1997;24:419-29.

Bullen BA, Skrinar GS, Beitins IZ, Von Mering G, Turnbull BA, McArthur JW. Induction of menstrual disorders by strenuous exercise in untrained women. N Engl J Med 1985;1312:1349-53.

Cann CE, Martin MC, Genant HK, Jaffe RB. Decreased spinal mineral content in amenorrheic women. J Am Med Assoc 1984;251:626-9.

Coyle EF. Substrate utilization during exercise in active people. Am J Clin Nutr 1995;61(suppl):968S-79S.

Cumming DC. Exercise-associated amenorrhea, low bone density, and estrogen replacement therapy. Arch Intern Med 1996;156:2193-5.

Dalsky GP. Guidelines for diagnosing osteoporosis. Phy Sportsmed 1996;24:1-5.

Donnelly JE, Jacobsen DJ, Jakici JM, Whatley JE. Very low calorie diet with concurrent versus delayed and sequential exercise. Int J Obesity 1994;18:469-75.

Drinkwater BL, Nilson K, Chestnut CH III, Bremner WJ, Shainholtz S, Southworth MB. Bone mineral content of amenorrheic and eumenorrheic athletes. N Engl J Med 1984;311:277-81.

Dueck CA, Manore MM, Matt KS. Role of energy balance in athletic menstrual dysfunction. Int J Sport Nutr 1996;6:90-116.

Dueck CA, Matt KS, Manore MM, Skinner JS. Treatment of athletic amenorrhea with a diet and training intervention program. Int J Sport Nutr 1996;6:24-40.

Fairburn CG, Walsh TB. Atypical eating disorders. In: Brownell KD, Fairburn DG, eds. Eating Disorders and Obesity: A Comprehensive Handbook. New York: Guilford Press, 1995:135-40.

Food and Nutrition Board, National Research Council. Recommended dietary allowances. 10th ed. Washington, DC: National Academy Press, 1989.

Food and Nutrition Board, National Research Council. Dietary Reference Intakes: Calcium, phosphorus, magnesium, vitamin D and fluoride. Washington, DC: National Academy Press, 1997.

Food and Nutrition Board, National Research Council. Dietary Reference Intakes: Thiamin, riboflavin, niacin, vitamin B-6, folate, vitamin B-12, pantothenic acid, biotin, and choline. Washington, DC: National Academy Press, 1998.

Frisch RE, McArthur JW. Menstrual cycles: fatness as a determinant of minimum weight for height necessary for their maintenance or onset. Science 1974;185:949-51.

Garfinkel PE. Classification and diagnosis of eating disorders. In: Brownell KD, Fairburn DG, eds. Eating Disorders and Obesity: a comprehensive handbook. New York: Guilford Press, 1995;125-34.

Johnson MD. Disordered eating in active and athletic women. Clin Sports Med 1994;13:355-69.

Joy E, Clark N, Ireland ML, Martie J, Nattiv A, Varechok S. Team management of the female athlete triad. Part 2: Optimal treatment and prevention tactics. Phy Sportsmed 1997;25(4):55-69.

Kanter MM. Nutritional antioxidants and physical activity. In: Wolinsky I, ed. Nutrition in Exercise and Sport. Boca Raton, FL: CRC Press, 1998:245-55.

Keith RE. Ascorbic acid. In: Wolinsky I, Driskell JA, eds. Sport Nutrition: Vitamins and Trace Minerals. Boca Raton, FL: CRC Press, 1997:29-45.

Kirchner EM, Lewis RD, O'Conner PJ. Bone mineral density and dietary intake of female college gymnasts. Med Sci Sports Exerc 1995;27:543-9.

Kurzer MS, Calloway DH. Effects of energy deprivation on sex hormone patterns in healthy menstruating women. Am J Physiol 1986; 251:E483-E488.

Lemon PWR. Do athletes need more protein and amino acids? Int J Sport Nutr 1995;5:S39-S61.

Loucks AB. Physical activity, fitness, and female reproductive morbidity. In: Bouchard C, Shephard RJ, Stephens T, eds. Physical Activity, Fitness, and Health. Champaign, IL: Human Kinetics, 1994:943-54.

Manore MM. Vitamin B6 and exercise. Int J Sport Nutr 1994;4:89-103.

Manore MM. Chronic dieting in active women: what are the health consequences? Women Health Iss 1996;6:332-41.

Manore MM. How do you know when you are eating enough? USA Gymnastics 1997;26(6):8-9.

Manore MM. Nutritional needs of the female athlete. Clin Sports Med 1999;18(3):549-63.

Manore MM. The effect of physical activity on thiamin, riboflavin, and vitamin B-6 requirements. Am J Clin Nutr (in press).

Otis CL. Too slim, amenorrheic, fracture-prone: the female athlete triad. ACSM's Health Fitness J 1998;2(1):20-5.

Otis CL, Drinkwater B, Johnson M, Loucks A, Wilmore J. The female athlete triad. Med Sci Sports Exerc 1997;29:i-ix.

Peterson AL, Talcott W, Kelleher WJ, Smith SD. Bulimic weight-loss behaviors in military versus civilian weight-management programs. Military Med 1995;160:616-20.

Robinson TL, Snow-Harter C, Taffee DR, Gillis D, Shaw J, Marcus R. Gymnasts exhibit higher bone mass than runners despite similar prevalence of amenorrhea and oligomenorrhea. J Bone Miner Res 1995;10:26-35.

Sandri SC. On dancers and diet. Int J Sport Nutr 1993;3:334-42.

Sundgot-Borgen J. Nutrient intake of elite female athletes suffering from eating disorders. Int J Sport Nutr 1993;3:431-42.

Sundgot-Borgen J. Risk and trigger factors for the development of eating disorders in female elite athletes. Med Sci Sports Exerc 1994;26:414-9.

Teegarden D, Proulx WR, Martin BR. Peak bone mass in young women. J Bone Min Res 1995;10:711-5.

Thompson JL, Manore MM, Thomas JR. Effects of diet and diet-plus-exercise programs on resting metabolic rate: a meta-analysis. Int J Sport Nutr 1996;6:41-61.

Thompson RA, Sherman RT. Helping Athletes With Eating Disorders. Champaign IL: Human Kinetics, 1993.

Tuschl R, Platte P, Laessle R, Stichler W, Pirke K. Energy expenditure and everyday eating behaviors in healthy young women. Am J Clin Nutr 1990;52:81-6.

Williams NI, Young JC, McArther JW, Bullen B, Skrinar GS, Turnbull B. Strenuous exercise with caloric restriction: effect on luteinizing hormone secretion. Med Sci Sports Exerc 1995;27:1390-8.

Wilmore JH. Eating and weight disorders in the female athlete. Int J Sport Nutr 1991;1:104-17.

Wilmore JH, Wambsgans, KC, Brenner M, et al. Is there energy conservation in amenorrheic compared with eumenorrheic distance runners? J Appl Physiol 1992;72:15-22.

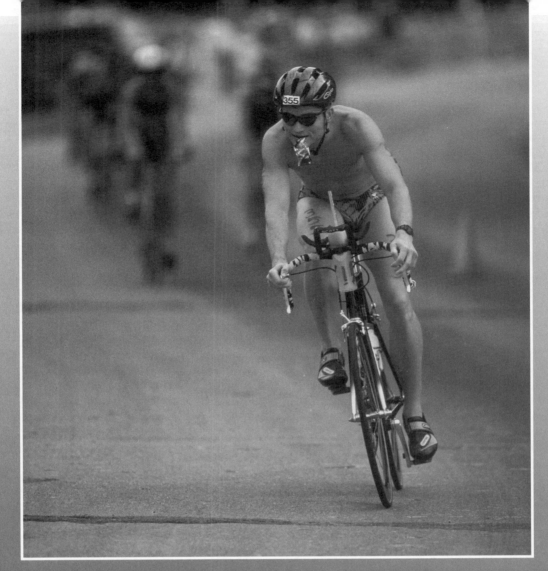

CHAPTER 16

Ergogenic Substances: Evaluating Sport Nutrition Products

After reading this chapter you will be able to

- describe the issues surrounding the use of ergogenic substances;
- understand how to evaluate currently available ergogenic substances; and
- discuss two popular ergogenic aids.

Many people involved in fitness activities are familiar with various ergogenic substances. They have received extensive media attention over the last 20 years and include products such as anabolic steroids, ephedrine, caffeine, and creatine—or even practices such as blood doping. The use of ergogenic aids is widespread in the professional athletic community and is increasingly popular with youth and recreational athletes.

Why do people use ergogenic substances? How can the sport nutrition professional properly evaluate ergogenic substances? This chapter is not designed to review the ergogenic substances now available as many books and research articles offer such information (e.g., Bucci 1993; Clarkson 1996; Grunewald and Bailey 1993; Kreider et al. 1993; Williams and Branch 1998). In this text, we have briefly reviewed a number of ergogenic aids (chapters 2, 3, 4, 8, and 11). The primary goals of this chapter are to review basic definitions of ergogenic substances and to address the following questions:

1. How prevalent is the use of ergogenic substances in active people?
2. What has contributed to the widespread use of ergogenic substances in our society?
3. What are the ethical implications of ergogenic substance use?
4. How can one effectively evaluate the efficacy of an ergogenic substance?

At the end of the chapter, we briefly review two popular ergogenic substances—carnitine and creatine—and discuss proposed mechanisms of their action and evidence of their effectiveness. We hope that you will gain the ability to review media claims and research studies with a critical eye—and that widespread critical evaluation of ergogenic substances will help reduce the flood of mythical information about them.

Ergogenic Substances in Sport and Exercise

Bucci (1993) defines **ergogenic substances** as those "used to improve exercise and athletic performance by improving the production of energy." Theoretically there are potentially thousands of substances that could fit this defi-

nition. Carbohydrates, protein, fat, and vitamin or mineral supplements, in addition to other "nutritional" products, can be defined as ergogenic based on their theorized or proven functions. In addition, many drugs are classified as **ergogenic drugs.** What is the difference between an ergogenic substance and an ergogenic drug? The Food and Drug Administration (FDA) has specified that substances claimed to prevent, alleviate, or cure a physical or mental illness, or affect the structure or function of the body, are classified as drugs (Cowart 1992; Lightsey and Attaway 1992); according to this definition, some products classified as ergogenic substances could also be considered drugs under certain circumstances.

Many drugs, ergogenic and otherwise, are banned by both the National Collegiate Athletic Association (NCAA) and the International Olympic Committee (IOC). Table 16.1 provides a short list of drugs that are banned by the NCAA and IOC (for complete lists of banned drugs, see Wagner 1991). The United States Olympic Committee (Soop et al. 1988) has published a definition of drug use or **doping.** To be classified as a drug by the IOC, a substance

- must be foreign to the body, *or* must be a physiological substance taken in abnormal quantity or by an abnormal route into the body; *and*
- must be taken with the sole intention of increasing, in an artificial manner, performance in competition.

While **banned substances** include drugs that may affect performance and may be harmful to the individual, substances used to avoid detection of drug use are also banned, as are practices such as blood doping. *Blood doping is the practice of infusing extra red blood cells into the body in an attempt to increase oxygen-carrying capacity.* While many other available substances are not banned, scientific experts and health practitioners have questioned the safety and ethics surrounding the use of these substances.

Prevalence of Use

How prevalent is the use of ergogenic substances? This is a very difficult question to answer. A number of surveys have assessed substance abuse and anabolic steroid use in high school and college students (Anderson and McKeag 1985, 1989; Buckley et al. 1988;

Table 16.1   Drugs Banned by the International Olympic Committee (IOC) and/or National Collegiate Athletic Association (NCAA)[1]

Drug	Examples
Stimulants	Caffeine,[2] ephedrine, cocaine
Narcotic analgesics	Codeine, morphine, heroin
Anabolic steroids	Testosterone,[3] stanozolol
Beta-blockers	Atenolol, metaprolol, propranolol
Diuretics	Furosemide, triamterene
Peptide hormones and analogues	Growth hormone, erythropoietin

[1]Complete lists of substances can be found in Wagner 1991.
[2]Urine concentrations must exceed 12 mg/L for IOC and 15 mg/L for NCAA.
[3]Ratio of total urine concentration of testosterone to epitestosterone must exceed 6.

Johnson et al. 1989). The surveys show that student athletes use and abuse a wide variety of drugs, both ergogenic and recreational. In two separate surveys among college students, 4 and 5% of the students reported using anabolic steroids, 88 and 89% reported using alcohol, and 36 and 28% reported using marijuana (Anderson and McKeag 1985, 1989). Many of the students who used ergogenic and recreational drugs in college reported beginning drug use before entering college. Buckley et al. (1988) and Johnson et al. (1989) found the incidence of steroid use among high school students to be 6-11%. Alarmingly, many of these students started using steroids by 15 years of age (Buckley et al. 1988).

Athletes have used vitamin and mineral supplements for years. Many believe the supplements are critical for optimal performance. Sobal and Marquart (1994) reviewed 51 papers that reported the use of vitamin/mineral supplements by athletes in a variety of sports. Of the 10,274 athletes surveyed, 46% reported using supplements. Elite athletes, women athletes, and those involved in sports that emphasize muscle size (e.g., weight lifting and bodybuilding) reported greater supplementation use. Multivitamin supplements were most frequently used, followed by vitamin C and iron.

A number of researchers have documented use of supplements and other ergogenic substances by bodybuilders (Bazzarre et al. 1990; Brill and Keane 1994; Faber et al. 1986; Kleiner et al. 1990; Kleiner et al. 1989; Lamar-Hildebrand et al. 1989), who report regular use of vitamin and mineral supplements, amino acid supplements, and other products claimed to enhance strength and muscle mass. While these athletes are also known to use anabolic steroids, an accurate assessment of the number who use them is difficult to obtain because many athletes refuse to answer questions regarding drug use.

An accurate estimate of the prevalence of ergogenic substance use by the general U.S. population is not available at the present time. While people may be willing to answer questions about vitamins and other nutritional supplement products, they are less open about their use of illegal or banned substances. According to Philen et al. (1992), the widespread availability of and large quantity of advertisements for ergogenic substances suggest that many people (including nonathletes) are using them.

Reasons for Use

Why do athletes and nonathletes use ergogenic substances? While many athletes use these substances in an attempt to enhance performance, there are other reasons why even the general public may find them attractive:

- To improve physical appearance
- To prevent or treat injuries
- To treat or cure illness or disease
- To be accepted by peers
- To help cope with stress

Many of these substances are readily available and highly promoted in magazines and fitness facilities. A survey of 33 supplement companies found more than 800 performance claims were made for 624 supplements (Grunewald and Bailey 1993). Benefits attributed to these products include weight or muscle gain, increases in strength, loss of body fat, increases in energy and endurance, and enhanced recuperation. People with limited knowledge of sport nutrition, or who are looking for a "magic bullet" to success, are among those susceptible to advertisers' claims. Even individuals with knowledge of proper nutrition may be tempted to try these products "just in case they may work" in an attempt to gain a competitive edge.

Ethical Issues

Williams (1994) suggested there are three primary foundations on which individuals or groups can base their ethical decisions concerning use of ergogenic substances:

- The moral principles of a particular *school of thought*—for example, the Olympic ideal that athletes should succeed in sport through their own unaided efforts.

- The rules of conduct recognized in certain *associations*—for example, rules of conduct defined by a specific sports organization, such as the IOC or the NCAA.

- The moral principles by which an *individual* is guided.

Williams observed that an athlete who wants to win at any cost will be driven to gain an unfair advantage, resulting in violation of the **ethics** of the Olympic ideal and the sports governing bodies. Even if the behavior of this athlete is consistent with his or her own personal ethics, it is contrary to the ethics put forth by the athletic governing organizations.

Is it acceptable for athletes to use any means available, including ergogenic substances, in order to gain the competitive edge? A simple answer to this question does not exist, and the ethical issues surrounding the use of ergogenic substances will be a heated topic of discussion for many years. Interestingly, Smith and Perry (1992) found that many athletes consider ergogenic drugs an essential component of successful competition—most likely because in order to continue to set world records, athletes must find ways to push the limits of human performance. And because many record-setting athletes may be using these substances, the attitude prevails among other athletes that they also must use them to compete "fairly" with others.

It is unlikely that the use of ergogenic substances will ever disappear. Athletes will continue to find ways, many unethical, to be the very best in their sport. This situation appears similar to the nuclear arms race. Once one country has nuclear weapons, others feel they need them in order to protect themselves or to be competitive. Asking all countries to get rid of their weapons is ineffective because of the fear that some countries will secretly keep a few weapons. Since it is impossible to detect all ergogenic substances, these products will continue to be a part of many athletes' lifestyles.

Another important issue is whether it is ethical to use nutritional products that are not banned or illegal (Williams 1994). According to the definition of drug use provided earlier in this chapter, any physiological substance taken in abnormal quantities with the intent of increasing performance in an artificial manner is considered a drug. Since many nutritional substances are taken in this specific manner

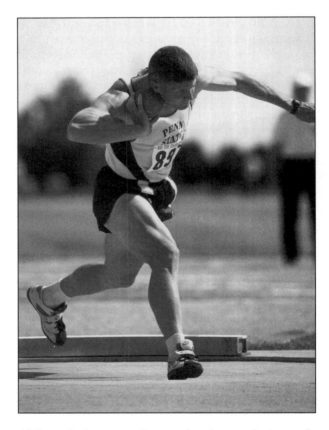

Although increased muscle size and strength can be achieved through diet and exercise alone, competitive athletes are susceptible to advertisements for ergogenic aids that are reported to improve muscle development.

and since some may actually improve performance, one has to question whether taking these substances is unethical. Should a nutritional product be banned or its intake limited if it is found to enhance performance? While it is not within the scope of this text to answer this question, this issue should provide a lively debate topic in the classroom, at scientific meetings, and throughout the world of athletics.

Evaluating Ergogenic Substances

According to the companies who manufacture and market ergogenic substances, using their products will result in numerous physiological changes. These claims include not only improvements in performance-related characteristics but also reduced risks for diseases. Do these products meet the published claims? How can sport nutrition practitioners help lay people evaluate the plethora of ergogenic products on the market? In this section, we discuss three areas in which one can evaluate ergogenic aids: marketing claims, research studies, and safety issues.

Marketing Claims

The primary goal of an advertisement is to present information about a product in a way that convinces consumers to purchase it. Unfortunately, companies often use deceptive tactics.

Lightsey and Attaway (1992) published an evaluation of ergogenic products by the National Council Against Health Fraud (NCAHF) task force on ergogenic aids and athletic performance. The focus of the NCAHF is health fraud, misinformation, and quackery with public health problems; the task force on ergogenic aids was established to evaluate claims that products enhance performance. Table 16.2 provides a partial list of the products that were reviewed.

Lightsey and Attaway (1992) reviewed the nine most common tactics manufacturers use to sell ergogenic substances (see "Nine Deceptive Advertising Practices Frequently Used to Market Ergogenic Aids" on page 443).

It is clear that objective representation of these products is not available from the companies that sell them. The burden of proof that a substance does or does not work falls upon research scientists.

Research Studies

Understanding how to properly evaluate the literature on ergogenic substances will help sport nutrition professionals advising athletes about the products. It is unrealistic to expect the general public to possess the knowledge and to access the necessary resources to adequately evaluate ergogenic substances. One important role of the sport nutrition professional is to act as a conduit of reliable, accurate information about the substances that are available.

Butterfield (1996) reviewed the issues surrounding the evaluation of ergogenic substances, providing a list of criteria one should follow to evaluate the research literature (table 16.3).

Remember that many athletes care little, if at all, about the science or plausibility of a particular product. Their primary concern is whether the product enhances performance. In order to establish rapport with athletes and gain their respect and trust regarding your evaluation of an ergogenic substance, take the following steps (Butterfield 1996):

1. Assess the athletes' level of knowledge and belief about the product.

2. Do not demand that athletes stop using all ergogenic substances—you may come off as "out of touch," and they may not feel comfortable discussing products with someone who is adamantly against the use of all substances.

3. Accept practices that are not harmful or illegal—recommend changes *gradually*.

4. Assess the role that the substance plays in athletes' overall diets; determine if you need to address their dietary practices.

5. Focus on enhancing practices that are critical to performance.

6. Commend the athletes for practicing sound nutrition principles.

7. Address questionable supplementing practices only after you have established trust and rapport with the athletes.

Safety Issues

Many safe ergogenic products are available. They generally do not enhance performance in healthy, active individuals who regularly eat a well-balanced diet, but they may play a critical role in optimizing the nutritional and

Table 16.2 Partial List of Ergogenic Aids Reviewed

Product	Promoted use
Inosine	Increase energy, strength, and recovery
Carnitine	Increase endurance
Dibencozide (cobalimides)	Steroid alternative; increase stamina
Organic germanium	Increase oxygen transport; strengthen immunity
Betaine	Lipolytic
Chromiun picolinate	Anabolic, lipolytic
Boron	Anabolic
Citrulline	Anabolic
Ferulic acid	Anabolic; antioxidant; lipotropic; decrease fatigue
Succinates	Reduce lactic acid; maintain ATP production
Tryptophan/piperidine	Lipolytic
L-phenylalanine	Stimulant to increase noradrenaline production
Nicotinic acid	Anabolic
Pyridoxine HCL	Anabolic
Coenzyme Q_{10}	Optimize ATP production to increase energy and stamina
Aspartates	Increase energy
Gamma linolenic acid, eicosapentaenoic acid	Steroid alternative; increase energy and endurance
Ornithine, arginine, glycine, lysine	Anabolic
Branched-chain amino acids (leucine, isoleucine, valine)	Anabolic; increase recovery; decrease muscle catabolism
Protein powder	Anabolic; increase recovery; decrease muscle catabolism
Arginine pyroglutamate/lysine	Anabolic
Mexican sarsaparilla root	Increase energy and recovery; anabolic; lipolytic; steroid alternative
Sterols	Anabolic
Ginseng	Increase energy and recovery; decrease fatigue
Eleutherococcus senticosus	Increase energy and recovery; decrease fatigue
Yohimbe bark	Steroid alternative; increase energy
Gamma oryzanol	Anabolic; lipotropic; decrease fatigue
Guarana	Increase energy
Adrenal cortex extract	Increase energy
Potassium with herbs	Cure-all, do-all product
Chinese herbs	Cure-all; increase energy, recovery time, and weight loss

Reprinted from Lightsey and Attaway 1992.

energy needs of many people who cannot regularly meet the demands of training and performance through diet alone. For instance, endurance runners generally benefit from the use of carbohydrate (e.g., glucose polymer) drinks and energy bars, while many female athletes with relatively low energy intakes benefit from multivitamin/mineral and calcium supplements.

Unfortunately, there are risks associated with the use of numerous ergogenic substances, particularly when people consume them in supraphysiologic doses. Note also that, since supplemental products are not subject to strict safety regulations, mass-marketed products are sometimes unsafe. The following risks are sometimes associated with use of ergogenic substances:

• *Low energy intake:* People attempt to compensate for poor energy and nutrient intakes by taking supplements. They fail to real-

Table 16.3 Criteria for Reviewing Research Literature on Ergogenic Substances

Component of study	Criteria to be evaluated
Author	√ Are the researcher and laboratory experienced and reputable? √ Is there any conflict of interest between the scientist/laboratory and the company making the product?
Abstract	√ Is the abstract succinct, and does it accurately describe the objectives and results? √ Does the abstract include information that cannot be substantiated?
Research design	√ Is the purpose of the study based on scientifically valid (i.e., biologically plausible) information? √ Was the appropriate study design employed (e.g., double-blind, placebo-controlled)? √ Were subjects properly selected (e.g., gender, training status) and randomly assigned to treatment groups? √ Were confounding variables (e.g., prior diet, diet during intervention, exercise patterns) controlled as completely as possible? √ Do the researchers rely only on correlative relationships (with no cause-and-effect data available)? √ Is the sample size large enough to find a physiologically significant effect? √ Was a randomized, matched control group studied (or were subjects used as their own controls)?
Research methods	√ Were the methods used (e.g., performance tests) appropriate for the product being tested? √ Were the methods used reliable; was the reliability of the methods reported? √ Were the methods sufficiently described or referenced so that they can be repeated? √ Were the statistics employed clearly specified and appropriate for the study design?
Results	√ Were the results clearly presented in tables and graphs? √ Were statistically significant differences indicated? √ Do the results make sense, and are they appropriately applied to the original objectives?
Discussion	√ Is the discussion presented objectively? √ Are both conflicting and similar data from other investigators presented? √ Are the limitations of the methods discussed as well as the implications these limitations may have on the interpretation of the results? √ Are references other than the author's included? √ Are the final conclusions drawn directly from the data, and is speculation kept to a minimum?
Conclusion	√ Is the conclusion specific to the purpose of the study, and is it consistent with the reported findings?

Adapted from Butterfield 1996; Rangachari and Mierson 1995; Sherman and Lamb 1995.

■ HIGHLIGHT ■

Nine Deceptive Advertising Practices Frequently Used to Market Ergogenic Aids

1. General misrepresentation
   - Misuse of genuine research: Published research is taken out of context; conclusions are extrapolated beyond the published findings or applied in an unproven manner.
   - Claims that product is university tested: If the study is legitimate and approved by a university, a specific professor may be named in the advertisement. The "research" is often conducted by a naive university staff member (not a trained researcher) with the firm controlling all aspects of the study. In some cases, the research has never been done.

(continued)

- Claims of endorsement by professional organizations: A member of a professional team may use the product, and the manufacturer uses this to suggest that the product is endorsed by the entire organization (which is many times not the case).

2. Claims that company is currently doing blind research work
   - This statement is commonly used in advertisements, but rarely is it true. Firms are very seldom able to provide specific information about studies claimed to be in progess.

3. Research not available for public review
   - There is no rationale to "hide" research information; consumers have the right to obtain documentation about performance claims.

4. Testimonials
   - These are based on the placebo effect. There is at least a 40% chance that a benign substance will enhance mental or physical performance. Testimonials can be faked, bought, or embellished. Even if truthful, the benefit suggested by the person testifying may be a result of the placebo effect or coincidence.

5. Patents
   - Patents are not granted based on the effectiveness of a product; they only indicate distinguishable differences among products. Patents do not demonstrate that a product is effective or safe, and they can be obtained upon no more than a theoretical model of a product. Sometimes no objective research has been conducted.

6. Inappropriately referenced research
   - References to unpublished research: Many of these studies have very poor research designs and lack adequate scientific control.
   - References to Eastern European research: Often there are no tangible research data; the research is not available for peer review; and it may be based upon unconfirmed reports or rumors.
   - Poorly controlled research: Ads quote only one published report that has not been verified by subsequent research. The availability of only one study indicates that the results are preliminary, and more studies are needed to substantiate the product.
   - Outdated research: Ads cite old research even though newer, appropriately controlled studies refute outdated claims.
   - Results taken out of context: Data are extrapolated from findings that have no relation to the product's effectiveness.
   - Publications not peer reviewed: References are to "studies" published in popular magazines, variety journals, or for direct distribution to the consumer. These are not adequately controlled or reviewed and should be considered invalid.

7. Media
   - Advertising companies use mass-media marketing videos, and infomercials are popular tools. False claims in advertising are regulated by the Federal Trade Commission; the Food and Drug Administration (FDA) regulates false labeling.
   - Publicity: Some communications are not recognizable as advertising (e.g., editorial comments, talk show interviews, and stories planted in the press). While publicity is not regulated as strictly as advertising, companies can be prosecuted if they use intentional deception to sell a product. Unfortunately, products are generally only investigated if they pose significant danger to the public.

8. Mail-order fitness evaluations
   - Most of these evaluations are too subjective to be of use to the consumer, and their accuracy should be questioned due to the generic nature of the information obtained. They are provided only to convince consumers to buy products.

9. Anabolic measurements
   - Some companies use in-house methods (e.g., amino acid chromatography and nitrogen balance) to study changes in protein balance. The methods may be used inappropriately. The manufacturer can claim that negative nitrogen balance occured, supporting the use of their product, but fail to mention that this change is a normal response to training. Nitrogen balance returns to baseline levels or may become positive with further training. In addition, other nutritional factors can affect the results, and these factors may not be adequately controlled.

Adapted from Lightsey and Attaway 1992.

444

ize the necessity of consuming adequate energy derived from carbohydrates, protein, and fat. Food also supplies the essential micronutrients the body needs to function properly, many of which cannot be purchased in a bottle (USOC 1988).

• *Toxicity effects:* Taking large doses of single micronutrients can lead to nutrient overload and toxicity symptoms, in addition to inhibiting the absorption of other nutrients. For example, large doses of zinc can inhibit the absorption of copper, and high intakes of folate can mask the signs of vitamin B_{12} deficiency or pernicious anemia (USOC 1988). Individual supplements are commonly formulated with large doses of a particular nutrient, which can lead to toxic effects with regular consumption of the manufacturers' recommended dose (Philen et al. 1992).

• *Poor quality control:* There are no rigorous standards or manufacturing controls for supplements and nutritional products, and no safety testing is required (Cowart 1992). There is no way to know if a product contains the ingredients listed on the label. After analyzing several mail-order supplements, Cowart (1992) found significant discrepancies between the claims on the labels and the actual products.

• *Incomplete labels and untraceable products:* Philen et al. (1992) attempted to identify the ingredients in various supplements advertised in health and bodybuilding magazines. These researchers were unable to find any information on many of the ingredients listed on the labels. Also, the labels seldom listed possible side effects and rarely mentioned groups that may be at risk from using the products (e.g., people with hypertension or women who are pregnant, etc.). Often the labels did not list the amounts of ingredients in the products, and the labels made false claims of "natural" and "organic" even though most ingredients were from manufactured or chemically derived sources.

• *Illness and death:* As there is minimal quality control of ergogenic products, these substances may contain contaminants or may react in an additive or synergistic way with other products or medications a person is taking (Kleiner 1991). In some cases, the product itself may be poisonous or harmful. The stimulant ephedra has been banned due to its potentially fatal effect related to elevations in heart rate and blood pressure. Philen et al. (1992) found a plant, hydrangea, listed as an ingredient on some supplements. The leaves and buds of this plant contain cyanogenic glycosides, which could induce cyanide poisoning.

Due to many risks associated with taking large doses of supplement products, the American Medical Association recommends that vitamins used as supplements shouldn't contain more than 150% of RDA, and vitamins used as therapeutic agents not exceed 10 times the RDA. The products used as therapeutic agents should be used only with a physician's recommendation (Council on Scientific Affairs 1987).

Review of Two Ergogenic Substances

This section briefly reviews two popular ergogenic substances, creatine and carnitine. We do not intend to discuss all of the studies involving these substances. Rather, our purpose is to familiarize you with their proposed mechanisms of action and to discuss whether they are effective. We have included references for people interested in learning more about these substances.

Carnitine

Carnitine is widely touted in fitness magazines as a "fat burner." Carnitine supplements are claimed to induce loss of body fat, spare glycogen, postpone fatigue, increase $\dot{V}O_2max$, and decrease lactate production. In this section we address the validity of these claims.

What Is Carnitine?

Carnitine is a short-chain carboxylic acid containing nitrogen that is required for the transport of long-chain fatty acids into the mitochondria. It is not an essential nutrient as it is synthesized in the body from the two essential amino acids lysine and methionine. Meat, poultry, fish, and dairy products are food sources high in carnitine. L-carnitine is the active form, the D-isomer being biologically inactive. Administration of D-carnitine depletes L-carnitine stores in the body and may be harmful in that it can result in carnitine deficiency (Keith

1986). Carnitine is found in most tissues of the body, with approximately 98% found in skeletal and cardiac muscle in humans (Engel and Rebouche 1984). Heinonen (1996) and Kanter and Williams (1995) have written excellent reviews of carnitine and its role in exercise. Carnitine supplementation appears to be safe. Doses ranging from 500 mg/d to 6 g/d (the typical dose being 2 g/d), taken up to 4 weeks, appear to cause no adverse effects.

How Does Carnitine Work?

Carnitine has two primary functions in the body:

- To transport long-chain fatty acids into mitochondria so they can be used for energy.
- To transport excess CoA intermediates out of the mitochondria to prevent inhibition of mitochondrial enzyme activities and to detoxify the inner mitochondrial milieu.

Fatty acids are critical sources of energy during resting metabolism and low- and moderate-intensity exercise. The biochemical pathways participating in the production of energy from fatty acids include β-oxidation, the TCA cycle, and the electron transport chain. These pathways are located inside the mitochondria, but because fatty acids cannot cross the mitochondrial membrane, they first must be activated as CoA esters and then esterified with carnitine to be carried into the mitochondria (see chapter 3). The latter reaction is catalyzed by the enzyme **carnitine-acyl-transferase I.** As figure 16.1 illustrates, this fatty-acid carnitine (FA-carnitine) complex, called **acyl-carnitine,** can cross the mitochondrial membrane. **Carnitine translocase** is the transport protein.

Once inside the membrane, the acylcarnitine is reconverted to carnitine and acyl-CoA through the action of **carnitine-acyl-transferase II**. The acyl-CoA can then go through β-oxidation to form acetyl-CoA, which is oxidized in the citric acid cycle to produce energy. The carnitine resulting from this conversion process is recycled and transported outside of the mitochondria to continue its transport function with other fatty acids. Because carnitine plays such a critical role in fat metabolism, and because carnitine levels correlate positively with fat oxidation in muscle cell preparations (Cederblad et al. 1976), it has been theorized that supplemental carnitine will enhance fat metabolism and result in body fat loss.

The second function of carnitine is to prevent CoA intermediates in the mitochondria from accumulating to toxic levels. These intermediates accumulate during times of abnormal metabolism such as exercise, fasting, diabetes, and ischemia (Rebouche 1992; Siliprandi 1986). Excess accumulation of the intermediates reduces the acyl-CoA:free CoA ratio, which theoretically can inhibit pyruvate dehydrogenase activity. Inhibition of pyruvate dehydrogenase could ultimately result in lactate accumulation—leading to reduced anaerobic power and heightened fatigue. Carnitine helps restore the acyl-CoA:free CoA ratio by binding with the acyl groups, thus increasing the amount of free CoA. This role of carnitine has led to speculation that supplemental carnitine could reduce lactate production, thus increasing time to fatigue and anaerobic power. While the factors limiting the use of fatty acids as a substrate during more intense exercise are not clear, one potential factor is a limitation in transporting fatty acids into the mitochondria (Kanter and Williams 1995). Thus, carnitine supplementation theoretically could spare glycogen and decrease lactate production by increasing fatty acid availability in the mitochondria. None of these theories, however, has been vindicated by experimental data (see "Does Carnitine Supplementation Enhance Performance and Reduce Body Fat?" on page 448).

Why does carnitine supplementation fail to reduce body fat and enhance exercise performance? In large part, it is because the theoretical basis for carnitine's role in body fat loss is not as sound as it superficially appears. Despite claims in popular magazines, active people do not have an increased need for carnitine: carnitine excretion with exercise is minor, and *exercise does not lead to loss of carnitine in muscle.* Carnitine supplementation does not appear to benefit healthy humans; however, supplementation can improve exercise performance in individuals with carnitine deficiency, such as certain patients with peripheral arterial disease (Cederblad et al. 1976; Hiatt et al. 1992). Despite shifts in the amounts of free carnitine and acylcarnitine during exercise, *total carnitine remains unchanged, and adequate levels of carnitine are maintained in the muscles during exercise* (Heinonen 1996). Thus, regular exercise does not cause carnitine deficiency, and carnitine levels should not be a concern for healthy active people. Overall, there is no support for the use of carnitine supplements

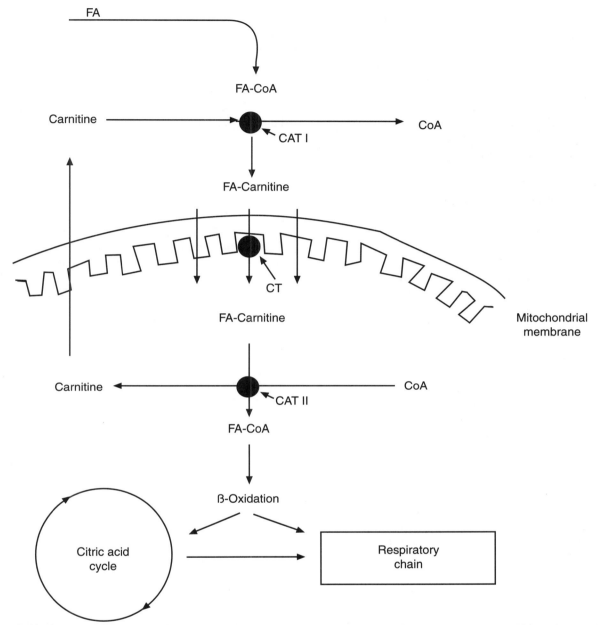

Figure 16.1 Carnitine as a carrier of long-chain fatty acids (FA) into the mitochondria. CoA = coenzyme A; FA-carnitine = fatty-acid carnitine (or simply "acylcarnitine"); CAT I = carnitine-acyl-transferase I; CAT II = carnitine-acyl-transferase II; CT = carnitine translocase.

Adapted from Heinonen 1996.

to improve body composition or athletic performance.

Creatine

Creatine supplements have become extremely popular. Numerous anecdotal reports on the effectiveness of creatine supplementation have prompted researchers to formally study this

metabolite. Nearly 200 research articles related to creatine and exercise were published between 1995 and 1998. It is beyond the scope of this chapter to provide a complete review of creatine. We encourage anyone interested in learning more about creatine to conduct a thorough literature search; a number of articles on creatine and exercise are published every month. In this section we briefly describe creatine's mechanism of action and review its effects on performance.

What Is Creatine?

Creatine phosphate (also called **phosphocreatine, or PCr**) occurs predominantly in skeletal muscle. The term **"creatine"** actually refers to free creatine in the muscle or to the supplement form of creatine. Creatine is obtained in part from the diet, with meat being the predominant dietary source; the liver and pancreas also synthesize creatine, which is then transported to the skeletal muscle. About 95% of the body's creatine pool is found in skeletal muscle, with the remainder in brain, kidney, liver, and testes (Hunter 1922; Myers and Fine 1915). Creatine can also be taken in supplement form—**creatine monohydrate** is the form studied in relation to exercise performance.

How Does Creatine Work?

Phosphocreatine is a reservoir of high-energy phosphate bonds. PCr serves to resynthesize ATP, as shown in the following reaction (Hunter 1922):

$$PCr + ADP + H^+ \leftrightarrow ATP + creatine$$

Approximately 60% of creatine is in the form of PCr at rest (Greenhaff 1997). Creatine and PCr function together to maintain ATP availability; they also buffer hydrogen ion accumulation during muscular contraction. Creatine has been linked with exercise performance due to its role in ATP regeneration. Depletion of PCr is thought to be one primary contributor to muscle fatigue during intense contractions as its depletion causes ADP concentration to increase; excess ADP inhibits cross-bridge formation in the muscle, causing fatigue. In addition, the rate of PCr resynthesis during recovery is associated with exercise performance during a single bout of maximal exercise (Casey et al. 1996a). In theory, creatine supplementation would be beneficial to performance by delaying depletion of PCr and the rate of ADP accumulation and also by increasing PCr resynthesis during recovery (Greenhaff 1997).

Does Creatine Supplementation Enhance Performance?

While many ergogenic products do not influence exercise performance, creatine does appear to enhance exercise performance in some instances. Creatine supplementation increases the PCr content of muscle, particularly in type II, or fast-twitch, muscle fibers (Casey et al. 1996b). The result of PCr enhancement is that force or work output can be sustained during maximal exercise, and this is especially true during repeated bouts of exercise.

Numerous papers have addressed the impact of creatine supplementation on performance. We discuss only a few of the most important studies here. Creatine supplementation has been shown to improve sprint performance in swimming, running, and cycling (Balsom et al. 1995; Grindstaff et al. 1997; Harris et al. 1993; Kreider et al. 1998) and to increase work performed during resistance exercise (Almada et al. 1997; Earnest et al. 1995; Kreider et al. 1998; Volek et al. 1999). Some researchers, however,

■ HIGHLIGHT ■

Does Carnitine Supplementation Enhance Performance and Reduce Body Fat?

Overall, carnitine supplementation has not been found to be effective in enhancing performance or reducing body fat in humans. One study reported an increase in $\dot{V}O_2$max with carnitine supplementation (Marconi et al. 1985); later research, however, did not replicate those results (Greig et al. 1987; Sobal and Marquart 1994). Oyono-Enguelle et al. (1988) failed to find beneficial changes in fat oxidation, exercise tolerance, or performance with carnitine supplementation. Carnitine supplementation appears to have no effect on lactate accumulation (Grieg et al. 1987; Marconi et al. 1985; Oyono-Enguelle et al. 1988). There is also no evidence that carnitine decreases body fat (Grunewald and Bailey 1993). Heinonen (1996) has thoroughly reviewed the published studies on carnitine and exercise performance.

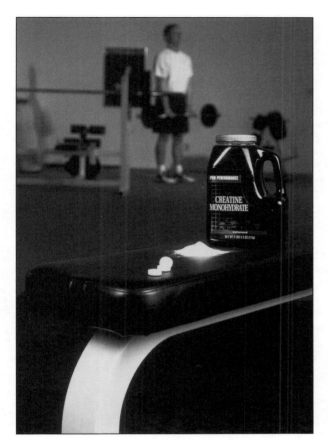

Creatine monophosphate is one of the most popular ergogenic aids on the market today.

that there is a limit to the amount of creatine muscle tissue can store. Long-term supplementation with creatine does not result in exceeding this maximal capacity. People with the lowest presupplementation creatine content (e.g., vegetarians and vegans) benefit most from supplementation in that they have a greater increase in muscle creatine content and show greater performance improvements. Thus, individuals who are already taking creatine supplements do not benefit from larger doses. Taking 20 g/d for 5 d is reported to be effective and has minimal risks for healthy individuals. Taking larger doses for longer periods may simply be a waste of money (Greenhaff 1995).

Creatine supplementation, while considered safe, may not be without risk. Anecdotal reports have included adverse effects such as kidney damage and muscle cramps. The only published account of adverse effects to date is renal dysfunction in a British soccer player (Pritchard and Kaira 1998). In contrast, Poortmans and Francaux (1999) found that long-term oral creatine supplementation (i.e., 10 mo to 5 years) had no adverse effect on the renal function of nine athletes. More research is needed to determine the safety of long-term and high-dose creatine supplementation.

Chapter in Review

Ergogenic substances include any substance used to enhance performance and increase energy production. There are significant ethical and legal implications related to the use of ergogenic substances, making this topic highly controversial. A plethora of substances are advertised to enhance performance and alter body composition. While many of them are harmless and ineffective, others may lead to health risks. You should be able to critically evaluate these substances and to assist the general public in assessing the true effectiveness and safety of these products.

have found no effect of creatine supplementation on exercise performance (Balsom et al. 1993; Burke et al. 1996; Godly and Yates 1997). Reasons for the discrepancies among these studies may include differences in prescribed creatine dose, differences among the subjects (e.g., presupplementation creatine status, skill level, etc.), and differences among specific exercise protocols and recovery periods.

Presupplementation muscle content of creatine can be a limiting factor in studies of exercise performance. Greenhaff (1995) reported

KEY CONCEPTS

 1. Describe the issues surrounding the use of ergogenic substances.

Ergogenic substances are used with the sole intention of artificially increasing performance in competition. Many ergogenic substances are banned due to safety concerns and ethical issues—yet their use appears widespread among athletes. Reasons for their use include potential improvements in performance and body composition, prevention and treatment of injuries, and stress reduction. The ethical issues surrounding the use of ergogenic substances are highly controversial, and it is unlikely that use of these products will ever be eliminated.

2. Understand how to evaluate currently available ergogenic substances.

Thoroughly investigate all marketing claims. To adequately evaluate published research, you must assess (1) the quality of the investigators and of the laboratory; (2) the research design and the methods used; (3) the accuracy and appropriateness of the results; and (4) the appropriateness of the conclusion in light of the data. In addition, you should be aware of the risks associated with ergogenic substances, including poor dietary practices, potential toxicity, poor quality control, incomplete labels, and untraceable products. Always investigate reports of illness or death in a person who has been taking an ergogenic product since in some cases even athletes' physicians or families are not aware that they are taking supplements.

3. Discuss two popular ergogenic aids.

Carnitine and creatine are widely used ergogenic products. Carnitine has not been shown to enhance athletic performance or to improve body fat levels. Creatine can improve sprint performance for some people in certain sports and, in some cases, can increase the work performed during resistance exercise. Additional studies of creatine that are currently underway should help to clarify its influence on athletic performance.

KEY TERMS

acylcarnitine
banned substance
carnitine
carnitine-acyl-transferase I
carnitine-acyl-transferase II
carnitine translocase
creatine

creatine monohydrate
creatine phosphate
doping
ergogenic drug
ergogenic substance
ethics
phosphocreatine (PCr)

References

Almada A, Kreider R, Ferreira M, et al. Effects of calcium β-HMB supplementation with or without creatine during training on strength and sprint capacity. FASEB J 1997;11:A374.

Anderson WA, McKeag DB. The substance use and abuse habits of college student-athletes: College of Human Medicine, Michigan State University, East Lansing, Michigan. Presented to the National Collegiate Athletic Association, January 1985.

Anderson WA, McKeag DB. Replication of the national study of the substance use and abuse habits of college student-athletes: College of Human Medicine, Michigan State University, East Lansing, Michigan. Presented to the National Collegiate Athletic Association, October 1989.

Balsom PD, Harridge SDR, Söderlund K, Sjödin B, Ekblom B. Creatine supplementation per se does not enhance endurance exercise performance. Acta Physiol Scand 1993;149:521-3.

Balsom PD, Söderlund K, Sjödin B, Ekblom B. Skeletal muscle metabolism during short duration high-intensity exercise: influence of creatine supplementation. Acta Physiol Scand 1995;1154:303-10.

Bazzarre TL, Kleiner SM, Litchford MD. Nutrient intake, body fat, and lipid profiles of competitive male and female bodybuilders. J Am Coll Nutr 1990;9:136-42.

Brill JB, Keane MW. Supplementation patterns of competitive male and female bodybuilders. Int J Sport Nutr 1994;4:398-412.

Bucci L. Nutrients as Ergogenic Aids for Sports and Exercise. Boca Raton, FL: CRC Press, 1993:xv.

Buckley WE, Yesalis CE, Friedl KE, Anderson WA, Streit AL, Wright JE. Estimated prevalence of anabolic steroid use among high school seniors. J Am Med Assoc 1988;260:3441-5.

Burke LM, Pyne DB, Telford RD. Effect of oral creatine supplementation on single-effort sprint performance in elite swimmers. Int J Sport Nutr 1996;6:222-33.

Butterfield G. Ergogenic aids: evaluating sport nutrition products. Int J Sport Nutr 1996;6:191-7.

Casey A, Constantin-Teodosiu D, Howell S, Hultman E, Greenhaff PL. The metabolic response of type I and II muscle fibres during repeated bouts of maximal exercise in humans. Am J Physiol 1996a;271:E38-E43.

Casey A, Constantin-Teodosiu D, Howell S, Hultman E, Greenhaff PL. Creatine supplementation favourably affects performance and muscle metabolism during maximal intensity exercise in humans. Am J Physiol 1996b;271:E31-E37.

Cederblad G, Bylund A-C, Holm J, Scherst'en T. Carnitine concentration in relation to enzyme activities and substrate utilization in human skeletal muscles. Scand J Clin Lab Invest 1976;36:547-52.

Clarkson PM. Nutrition for improved sports performance: current issues on ergogenic aids. Sports Med 1996;21(6):393-401.

Council on Scientific Affairs, American Medical Association. Vitamin preparations as dietary supplements and as therapeutic agents. J Am Med Assoc 1987;257:1929-36.

Cowart VS. Dietary supplements: alternatives to anabolic steroids? Phys Sportsmed 1992; 20(3):189-98.

Earnest CP, Snell PG, Rodriguez R, Alamada AL, Mitchell TL. The effect of creatine monohydrate ingestion on anaerobic power indices, muscular strength and body composition. Acta Physiol Scand 1995;153:207-9.

Engel AG, Rebouche CJ. Carnitine metabolism and inborn errors. J Inherit Metab Dis 1984;7(1 suppl):38-43.

Faber M, Benade AJS, Van Eck M. Dietary intake, anthropometric measurements, and blood lipid values in weight training athletes (body builders). Int J Sports Med 1986;7:342-6.

Godly A, Yates JW. Effects of creatine supplementation on endurance cycling combined with short, high-intensity bouts. Med Sci Sports Exerc 1997;29:S251.

Greenhaff PL. Creatine and its application as an ergogenic aid. Int J Sport Nutr 1995; 5:S100-S110.

Greenhaff PL. The nutritional biochemistry of creatine. J Nutr Biochem 1997;8:610-8.

Greig C, Finch KM, Jones A, Cooper M, Sargeant AJ, Forte CA. The effect of oral supplementation with L-carnitine on maximum and submaximum exercise capacity. Eur J Appl Physiol 1987;56:457-60.

Grindstaff PD, Kreider R, Bishop R, Wilson M, Wood L, Alexander C, Almada A. Effects of creatine supplementation on repetitive sprint performance and body composition in competitive swimmers. Int J Sport Nutr 1997;7:330-46.

Grunewald KK, Bailey RS. Commercially marketed supplements for bodybuilding athletes. Sports Med 1993;15(2):90-103.

Harris RC, Viru M, Greenhaff PL, Hultman E. The effect of oral creatine supplementation on running performance during maximal short term exercise in man. J Physiol 1993;467:74P.

Heinonen OJ. Carnitine and physical exercise. Sports Med 1996;22(2):109-32.

Hiatt W, Wolfel E, Regensteiner J, Brass E. Skeletal muscle carnitine metabolism in patients with unilateral peripheral arterial disease. J Appl Physiol 1992;73:346-53.

Hunter A. The physiology of creatine and creatinine. Physiol Rev 1922;2:586-99.

Johnson MD, Jay MS, Shoup B, Rickert VI. Anabolic steroid use by male adolescents. Pediatrics 1989;83:921-4.

Kanter MM, Williams MH. Antioxidants, carnitine, and choline as putative ergogenic aids. Int J Sport Nutr 1995;5:S120-S131.

Keith RE. Symptoms of carnitine like deficiency in a trained runner taking DL-carnitine supplements. J Am Med Assoc 1986;255:1137.

Kleiner SM. Performance-enhancing aids in sport: health consequences and nutritional alternatives. J Am Coll Nutr 1991;10(2):163-76.

Kleiner SM, Bazzarre TL, Litchford MD. Metabolic profiles, diet and health practices of championship male and female bodybuilders. J Am Diet Assoc 1990;90:962-7.

Kleiner SM, Calabrese LH, Fiedler KM, Naito HK, Skibinski CI. Dietary influences on cardiovascular disease risk in anabolic steroid-using and non-using bodybuilders. J Am Coll Nutr 1989;8:109-19.

Kreider RB, Ferreira M, Wilson M, et al. Effects of creatine supplementation on body composition, strength, and sprint performance. Med Sci Sports Exerc 1998;30:73-82.

Kreider RB, Miriel V, Bertun E. Amino acid supplementation and exercise performance: analysis of the proposed ergogenic value. Sports Med 1993;16(3):190-209.

Lamar-Hildebrand N, Saldanha L, Endres J. Dietary and exercise practices of college-aged female bodybuilders. J Am Diet Assoc 1989; 89:1308-10.

Lightsey DM, Attaway JR. Deceptive tactics used in marketing purported ergogenic aids. Natl Strength Cond Assoc J 1992;14(2):26-31.

Marconi C, Sassi G, Carpinelli A, Cerretelli P.

Effects of L-carnitine loading on the aerobic and anaerobic performance of endurance athletes. Eur J Appl Physiol 1985;54:131-5.

Myers VC, Fine MS. The metabolism of creatine and creatinine. VII. The fate of creatine when administered to man. J Biol Chem 1915;21:377-83.

Oyono-Enguelle S, Freund H, Ott C, et al. Prolonged submaximal exercise and L-carnitine in humans. Eur J Appl Physiol 1988;58:53-61.

Philen RM, Ortiz DI, Auerbach SB, Falk H. Survey of advertising for nutritional supplements in health and bodybuilding magazines. J Am Med Assoc 1992;268(8):1008-11.

Poortmans JR, Francaux M. Long-term oral creatine supplementation does not impair renal function in healthy athletes. Med Sci Sports Exerc 1999;31:1108-10.

Pritchard NR, Kaira PA. Renal dysfunction accompanying oral creatine supplements. Lancet 1998;351(9111):1252-3.

Rangachari PK, Mierson S. A checklist to help students analyze published articles in basic medical sciences. Am J Physiol 1995;268 (Adv Physiol Educ 13):S21-S25.

Rebouche CJ. Carnitine function and requirements during the life cycle. FASEB J 1992;6:3379-86.

Sherman WM, Lamb DR. Introduction to ergogenic aids supplement. Int J Sport Nutr 1995;5:Siii-Siv.

Siliprandi N. Carnitine in physical exercise. In: Benzi G, Packer L, Siliprandi N, eds. Biochemical Aspects of Physical Exercise. Amsterdam: Elsevier, 1986:197-206.

Smith DA, Perry PJ. The efficacy of ergogenic agents in athletic competition: Part II. Other performance-enhancing agents. Ann Pharmacother 1992;26:653-9.

Sobal J, Marquart LF. Vitamin/mineral supplement use among athletes: a review of the literature. Int J Sport Nutr 1994;4:320-34.

Soop M, Björkman O, Cederblad G, Hagenfeldt L, Wahren J. Influence of carnitine supplementation on muscle substrate and carnitine metabolism during exercise. J Appl Physiol 1988;64:2394-9.

United States Olympic Committee (USOC). Guide to banned medications. Sportsmediscope 1988;7:1-5.

Volek JS, Duncan ND, Mazzetti SA, et al. Performance and muscle fiber adaptations to creatine supplementation and heavy resistance training. Med Sci Sports Exerc 1999;31:1147-56.

Wagner JC. Enhancement of athletic performance with drugs: an overview. Sports Med 1991;12(4):250-65.

Williams MH. The use of nutritional ergogenic aids in sport: is it an ethical issue? Int J Sport Nutr 1994;4:120-31.

Williams MH, Branch JD. Creatine supplementation and exercise performance: an update. J Am Coll Nutr 1998;17:216-34.

APPENDIX A

Nutritional Recommendations

Appendix A.1 Food and Nutrition Board, National Academy of Sciences–National Research Council Recommended Dietary Allowances,[a] Revised 1989 (Abridged)

Designed for the maintenance of good nutrition of practically all healthy people in the United States

Category	Age (years) or condition	Weight[b] (kg)	Weight[b] (lb)	Height[b] (cm)	Height[b] (in.)	Protein (g)	Vitamin A (μg RE)[c]	Vitamin E (mg α-TE)[d]	Vitamin K (μg)	Vitamin C (mg)	Iron (mg)	Zinc (mg)	Iodine (μg)	Selenium (μg)
Infants	0.0-0.5	6	13	60	24	13	375	3	5	30	6	5	40	10
	0.5-1.0	9	20	71	28	14	375	4	10	35	10	5	50	15
Children	1-3	13	29	90	35	16	400	6	15	40	10	10	70	20
	4-6	20	44	112	44	24	500	7	20	45	10	10	90	20
	7-10	28	62	132	52	28	700	7	30	45	10	10	120	30
Males	11-14	45	99	157	62	45	1000	10	45	50	12	15	150	40
	15-18	66	145	176	69	59	1000	10	65	60	12	15	150	50
	19-24	72	160	177	70	58	1000	10	70	60	10	15	150	70
	25-50	79	174	176	70	63	1000	10	80	60	10	15	150	70
	51+	77	170	173	68	63	1000	10	80	60	10	15	150	70
Females	11-14	46	101	157	62	46	800	8	45	50	15	12	150	45
	15-18	55	120	163	64	44	800	8	55	60	15	12	150	50
	19-24	58	128	164	65	46	800	8	60	60	15	12	150	55
	25-50	63	138	163	64	50	800	8	65	60	15	12	150	55
	51+	65	143	160	63	50	800	8	65	60	10	12	150	55
Pregnant						60	800	10	65	70	30	15	175	65
Lactating	1st 6 mo					65	1300	12	65	95	15	19	200	75
	2nd 6 mo					62	1200	11	65	90	15	16	200	75

Note: This table does not include nutrients for which Dietary Reference Intakes have been recently established [see *Dietary Reference Intakes for Calcium, Phophorus, Magnesium, Vitamin D, and Fluoride* (1997) and *Dietary Reference Intakes for Thiamin, Riboflavin, Niacin, Vitamin B₆, Folate, Vitamin B₁₂, Pantothenic Acid, Biotin, and Choline* (1998)].

[a] The allowances, expressed as average daily intakes over time, are intended to provide for individual variations among most normal persons as they live in the United States under usual environmental stresses. Diets should be based on a variety of common foods in order to provide other nutrients for which human requirements have been less well defined.

[b] Weights and heights of reference adults are actual medians for the U.S. population of the designated age, as reported by NHANES II. The median weights and heights of those under 19 years of age were taken from Hamill PVV, Drizd TA, Johnson CL, Reed RB, Roche AF, Moore WM. Physical growth: National Center for Health Statistics Percentiles. Am J Clin Nutr 1979;32:607-29. The use of these figures does not imply that the height-to-weight ratios are ideal.

[c] Retinol equivalents. 1 retinol equivalent = 1 μg retinol or 6 μg β-carotene.

[d] α-tocopherol equivalents. 1mg/d α-tocopherol = 1 α-TE.

Reproduced from Food and Nutrition Board, Institute of Medicine. Recommended Dietary Allowances, 10th ed. National Academy Press, Washington, DC, 1989.

Appendix A.2 Food and Nutrition Board, Institute of Medicine–National Academy of Sciences Dietary Reference Intakes: Recommended Levels for Individual Intake

Life-stage group (years)	Calcium (mg/d)	Phosphorus (mg/d)	Magnesium (mg/d)	D (μg/d)[a,b]	Fluoride (mg/d)	Thiamine (mg/d)	Riboflavin (mg/d)	Niacin (mg/d)[c]	B_6 (mg/d)	Folate (μg/d)[d]	B_{12} (μg/d)	Panthothenic acid (mg/d)	Biotin (μg/d)	Choline[e] (mg/d)
Infants														
0-5 mo	210*	100*	30*	5*	0.01*	0.2*	0.3*	2*	0.1*	65*	0.4*	1.7*	5*	125*
6-11 mo	270*	275*	75*	5*	0.5*	0.3*	0.4*	4*	0.3*	80*	0.5*	1.8*	6*	150*
Children														
1-3	500*	460	80	5*	0.7*	0.5	0.5	6	0.5	150	0.9	2*	8*	200*
4-8	800*	500	130	5*	1*	0.6	0.6	8	0.6	200	1.2	3*	12*	250*
Males														
9-13	1300*	1250	240	5*	2*	0.9	0.9	12	1.0	300	1.8	4*	20*	375*
14-18	1300*	1250	410	5*	3*	1.2	1.3	16	1.3	400	2.4	5*	25*	550*
19-30	1000*	700	400	5*	4*	1.2	1.3	16	1.3	400	2.4	5*	30*	550*
31-50	1000*	700	420	5*	4*	1.2	1.3	16	1.3	400	2.4	5*	30*	550*
51-70	1200*	700	420	10*	4*	1.2	1.3	16	1.7	400	2.4f	5*	30*	550*
>70	1200*	700	420	15*	4*	1.2	1.3	16	1.7	400	2.4f	5*	30*	550*
Females														
9-13	1300*	1250	240	5*	2*	0.9	0.9	12	1.0	300	1.8	4*	20*	375*
14-18	1300*	1250	360	5*	3*	1.0	1.0	14	1.2	400g	2.4	5*	25*	400*
19-30	1000*	700	310	5*	3*	1.1	1.1	14	1.3	400g	2.4	5*	30*	425*
31-50	1000*	700	320	5*	3*	1.1	1.1	14	1.3	400g	2.4	5*	30*	425*
51-70	1200*	700	320	10*	3*	1.1	1.1	14	1.5	400g	2.4f	5*	30*	425*
>70	1200*	700	320	15*	3*	1.1	1.1	14	1.5	400	2.4f	5*	30*	425*
Pregnancy														
≤18	1300*	1250	400	5*	3*	1.4	1.4	18	1.9	600h	2.6	6*	30*	450*
19-30	1000*	700	350	5*	3*	1.4	1.4	18	1.9	600h	2.6	6*	30*	450*
31-50	1000*	700	360	5*	3*	1.4	1.4	18	1.9	600h	2.6	6*	30*	450*

(continued)

Appendix A.2 (continued)

Life-stage group (years)	Calcium (mg/d)	Phosphorus (mg/d)	Magnesium (mg/d)	D (μg/d)[a,b]	Fluoride (mg/d)	Thiamine (mg/d)	Riboflavin (mg/d)	Niacin (mg/d)[c]	B6 (mg/d)	Folate (μg/d)[d]	B12 (μg/d)	Panthothenic acid (mg/d)	Biotin (μg/d)	Choline[e] (mg/d)
Lactation														
≤18	1,300*	1250	360	5*	3*	1.5	1.6	17	2.0	500	2.8	7*	35*	550*
19-30	1,000*	700	310	5*	3*	1.5	1.6	17	2.0	500	2.8	7*	35*	550*
31-50	1,000*	700	320	5*	3*	1.5	1.6	17	2.0	500	2.8	7*	35*	550*

Note: This table presents Recommended Dietary Allowances (RDAs) in bold type and Adequate Intakes (AI) in ordinary type followed by an asterisk (*). RDAs and AIs may both be used as goals for individual intake. RDAs are set to meet the needs of almost all (97-98%) individuals in a group. For healthy breastfed infants, the AI is the mean intake. The AI for other life-stage and gender groups is believed to cover their needs, but lack of data or uncertainty in the data prevents clear specification of this coverage.

[a] As cholecalciferol. 1 μg cholecalciferol = 40 IU vitamin D.

[b] In the absence of adequate exposure to sunlight.

[c] As niacin equivalents. 1 mg of niacin = 60 mg of tryptophan; 0-5 mo = preformed niacin (not mg NE).

[d] As dietary folate equivalents (DFE). 1 DFE = 1 μg food folate = 0.6 μg of folic acid (from fortified food or supplement) consumed with food = 0.5 μg of synthetic (supplemental) folic acid taken on an empty stomach.

[e] Although AIs have been set for choline, there are few data to assess whether a dietary supply of choline is needed at all stages of the life cycle, and it may be that the choline requirement can be met by endogenous synthesis at some of these stages.

[f] Since 10-30% of older people may malabsorb food-bound B12, it is advisable for those older than 50 years to meet their RDA mainly by consuming foods fortified with B12 or a B12-containing supplement.

[g] In view of evidence linking folate intake with neural tube defects in the fetus, it is recommended that all women capable of becoming pregnant consume 400 μg of synthetic folic acid from fortified foods and/or supplements in addition to intake of food folate from a varied diet.

[h] It is assumed that women will continue consuming 400 μg of folic acid until their pregnancy is confirmed and they enter prenatal care, which ordinarily occurs after the end of the periconceptional period—the critical time for formation of the neural tube.

Reproduced from Food and Nutrition Board, Institute of Medicine. *Dietary Reference Intakes: Calcium, phosphorus, magnesium, vitamin D, and fluoride.* National Academy Press, Washington, DC, 1998.

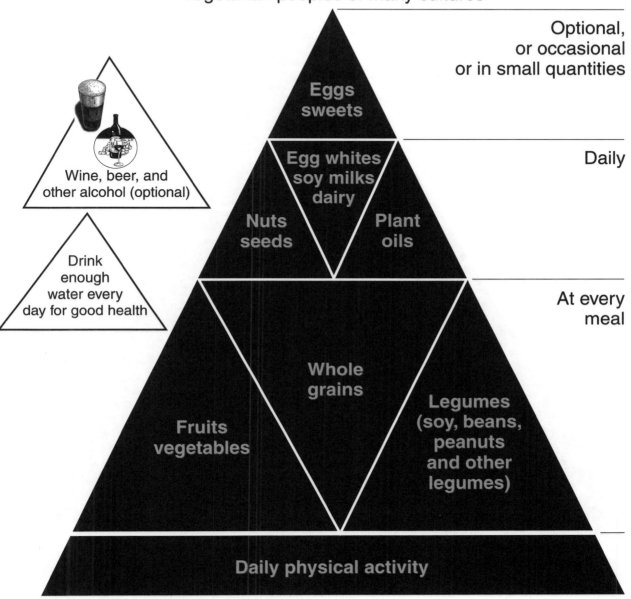

Vegetarian Diet
Based on traditional eating patterns of healthy vegetarian peoples of many cultures

Optional, or occasional or in small quantities

Daily

At every meal

Eggs sweets

Egg whites soy milks dairy

Nuts seeds

Plant oils

Whole grains

Fruits vegetables

Legumes (soy, beans, peanuts and other legumes)

Daily physical activity

Wine, beer, and other alcohol (optional)

Drink enough water every day for good health

©1997 Oldways preservation & exchange trust

This Healthy Traditional Vegatarian Diet Pyramid reflects vegetarian dietary traditions historically associated with good health. It is one of a group of food pyramids developed in a series of conferences—Public Health Implications of Traditional Diets—that consider diverse traditions around the world. These pyramids, a principal objective of the conferences, are intended to stimulate greater dialogue and interest in cultural models for healthy eating and to provide the basis for effective healthy eating guidelines. This Vegetarian Diet Pyramid is subject to revision in light of ongoing nutrition research.

Appendix A.3 Vegetarian Diet Pyramid.
Reprinted from Gifford 1998.

The Traditional Healthy Asian Diet Pyramid

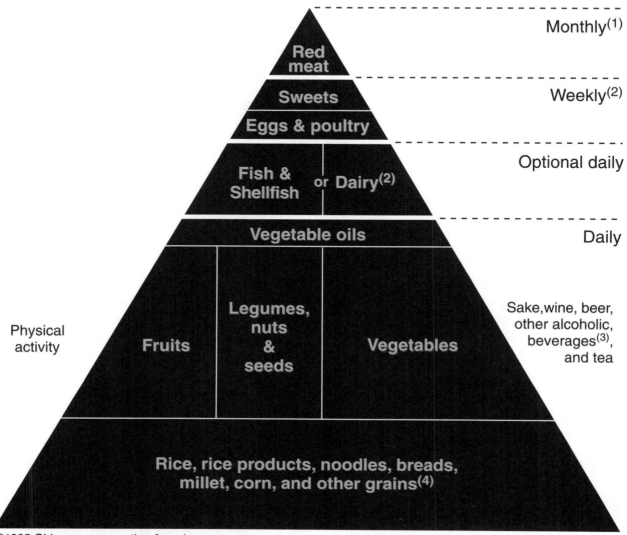

Monthly[1]

Weekly[2]

Optional daily

Daily

Red meat

Sweets

Eggs & poultry

Fish & Shellfish   or Dairy[2]

Vegetable oils

Fruits

Legumes, nuts & seeds

Vegetables

Sake, wine, beer, other alcoholic, beverages[3], and tea

Physical activity

Rice, rice products, noodles, breads, millet, corn, and other grains[4]

(1) Or more often in very small amounts.
(2) Dairy foods are generally not part of the healthy, traditional diets of Asia, with the notable exception of India. If dairy foods are consumed on a daily basis, low-fat dairy products should be used.
(3) Wine, beer, and other alcoholic beverages should be consumed in moderation and primarily with meals, and avoided whenever consumption would put an individual or others at risk.
(4) Minimally refined whenever possible.

Appendix A.4   The Traditional Healthy Asian Diet Pyramid.
Reprinted from Gifford 1998.

The Traditional Healthy Latin American Diet Pyramid

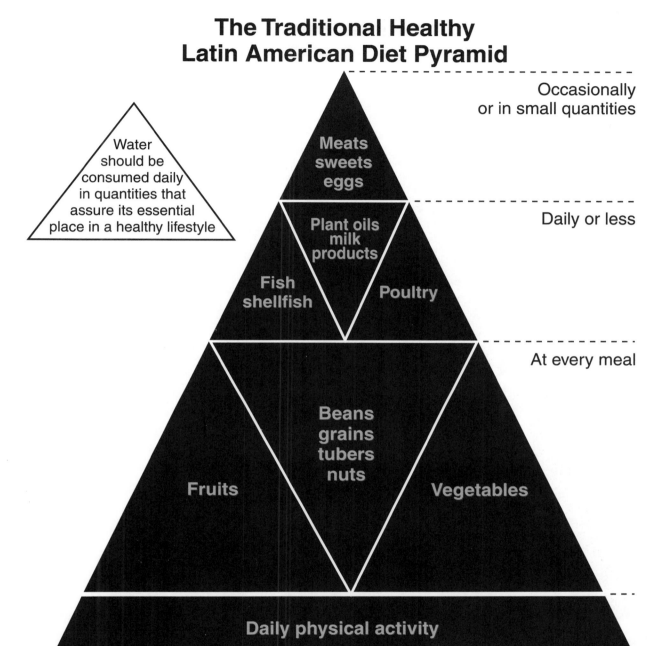

Occasionally or in small quantities

Daily or less

At every meal

Water should be consumed daily in quantities that assure its essential place in a healthy lifestyle

Meats sweets eggs

Plant oils milk products

Fish shellfish

Poultry

Beans grains tubers nuts

Fruits

Vegetables

Daily physical activity

Alcohol may be consumed by adults in moderation and with meals, but consumption should be avoided during pregnancy and whenever it would put the individual or others at risk.

Appendix A.5 The Traditional Healthy Latin American Diet Pyramid.
Reprinted from Gifford 1998.

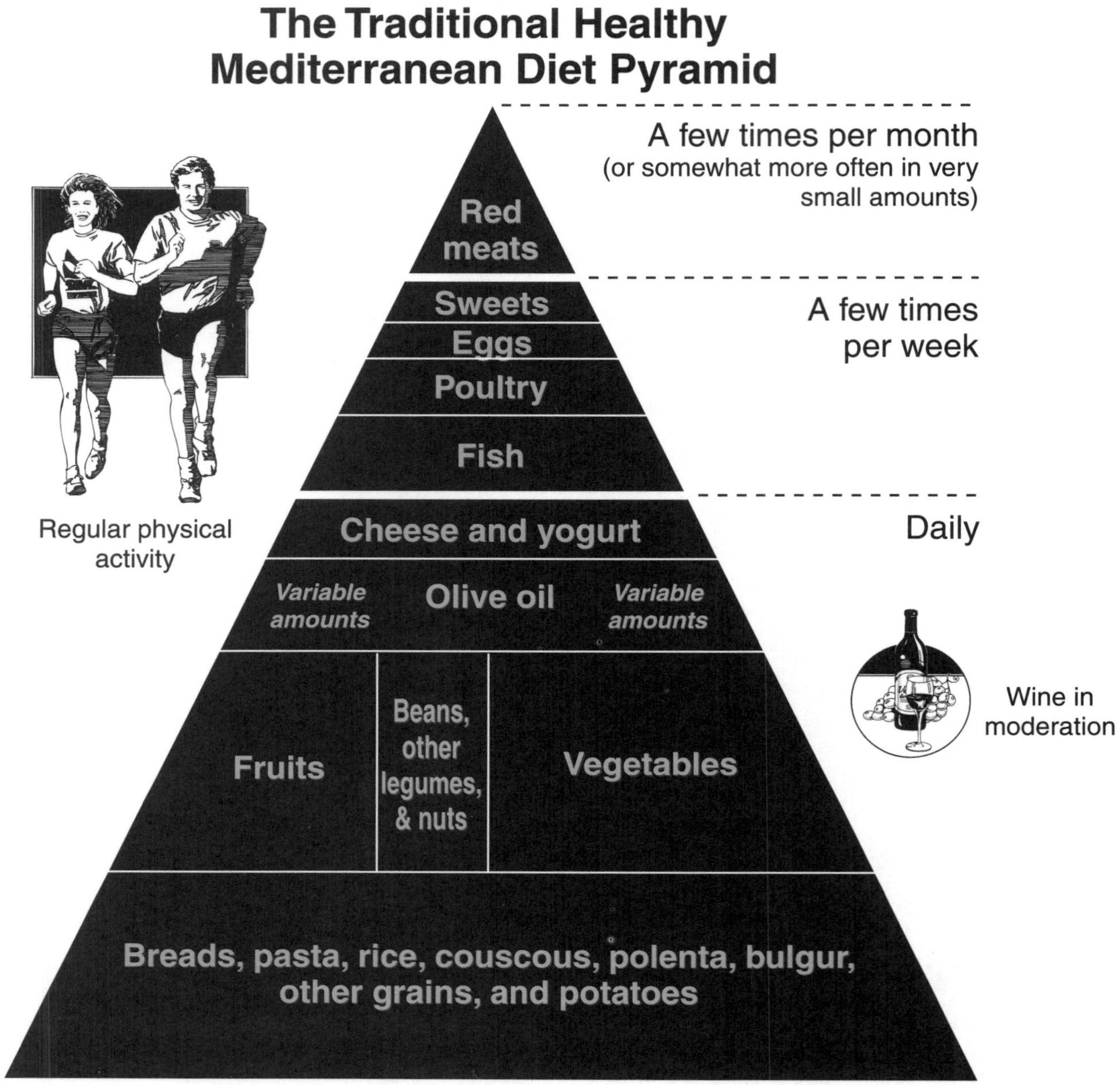

The Traditional Healthy Mediterranean Diet Pyramid

A few times per month
(or somewhat more often in very small amounts)

Red meats

A few times per week

Sweets

Eggs

Poultry

Fish

Daily

Cheese and yogurt

Olive oil

Variable amounts

Variable amounts

Fruits

Beans, other legumes, & nuts

Vegetables

Breads, pasta, rice, couscous, polenta, bulgur, other grains, and potatoes

Regular physical activity

Wine in moderation

Figure A.6 The Traditional Healthy Mediterranean Diet Pyramid.
Reprinted from Gifford 1998.

APPENDIX A.7

RESOURCES LIST FOR AGENCIES INVOLVED IN HEALTHY PEOPLE 2000 AND HEALTHY PEOPLE 2010

Physical Activity and Fitness Resource list

Federal and National Information Sources

U.S. DEPARTMENT OF EDUCATION

National Diffusion Network
555 New Jersey Avenue, NW, Room 510
Washington, DC 20208-5645
202-219-2134; 202-219-1407 Fax

Makes educational programs available to schools, colleges, and other institutions. Lists of facilitators and programs are free.

U.S. DEPARTMENT OF HEALTH AND HUMAN SERVICES

Public Health Service

Centers for Disease Control and Prevention (CDC)
Public Inquiries
1600 Clifton Road, NE
Mailstop A23
Atlanta, GA 30333
404-639-3534; 404-639-1537 Fax

Refers inquiries from the public and professionals to the appropriate area at CDC.

National Center for Chronic Disease Prevention and Health Promotion
4770 Buford Highway, NE
Mailstop K13
Atlanta, GA 30333
404-488-5080; 404-488-5962 Fax

Plans, directs, and coordinates national programs for the prevention of premature mortality, morbidity, and disability due to chronic illnesses and conditions. Call for electronic product information.

National Institutes of Health

National Arthritis and Musculoskeletal and Skin Diseases
  Information Clearinghouse
P.O. Box AMS
9000 Rockville Pike
Bethesda, MD 20892
301-495-4484

Provides patient education materials and information related to arthritis and musculoskeletal and skin diseases. Publications list available.

National Diabetes Information Clearinghouse
Box NDIC
9000 Rockville Pike
Bethesda, MD 20892
301-654-3327

Provides patient and professional educational materials on diabetes-related topics. Call for electronic product information.

National Heart, Lung, and Blood Institute (NHLBI) Education Programs
    Information Center
P.O. Box 30105
Bethesda, MD 20824-0105
301-251-1222; 301-251-1223 Fax

Provides information about NHLBI education programs on high blood pressure, cholesterol, obesity, asthma, and heart attack. Offers information on cardiovascular disease prevention and heart-health promotion to consumers and professionals. Call for electronic product information.

National Institute on Aging
Public Information Office
Building 31, Room 5C27
9000 Rockville Pike
Bethesda, MD 20892
301-496-1752; 800-222-2225 Publications
800-438-4380 Alzheimer's information; 301-496-1072 Fax

Answers questions and distributes free consumer publications about the diseases of older people, including Alzheimer's, the aging process, and safety. Publishes a series of fact sheets, Age Pages, which address health concerns applicable to the elderly. Publications list available.

Office of Minority Health Resource Center
P.O. Box 37337
Washington, DC 20013-7337
800-444-6472; 301-589-0884 Fax

Responds to inquiries about major health problems among minority populations. Assists in locating materials, programs, and technical assistance through an automated Resource Persons Network and materials database.

President's Council on Physical Fitness and Sports
701 Pennsylvania Avenue, NW
Suite 250
Washington, DC 20004
202-272-3424; 202-504-2064 Fax

Works with schools, clubs, recreation agencies, and employers on physical fitness and exercise program design and implementation. Produces informational materials on exercise, school physical education programs, corporate fitness, and physical fitness for youth, adults, and senior citizens.

National Sources

American Alliance for Health, Physical Education, Recreation, and Dance
1900 Association Drive
Reston, VA 22091
703-476-3400; 703-476-8316 Fax

Develops special programs including fitness for older persons, activity programs for people with handicaps, and exercise programs for youth and adults. Promotes school health and physical education programs. Distributes materials for professionals.

American College Health Association
P.O. Box 28937
Baltimore, MD 21240-8937
410-859-1500; 410-859-1510 Fax

Publishes and distributes a series of pamphlets and videotapes for college students on a variety of health topics, including acquaintance rape, AIDS, and sexually transmitted diseases.

American College of Sports Medicine
P.O. Box 1440
Indianapolis, IN 46206-1440
317-637-9200; 317-634-7817 Fax

Publishes materials, including position statements, on physical activity, physical fitness, and other sports medicine and exercise science topics.

American Heart Association
7272 Greenville Avenue
Dallas, TX 75231-4599
214-373-6300; 800-AHA-USA1
214-706-1341 Fax

Sponsors research, community programs, and professional education on cardiovascular diseases and stroke. Catalog of materials available.

Boys and Girls Clubs of America
1230 West Peachtree Street, NW
Atlanta, GA 30348-5771
404-815-5759; 404-815-5757 Fax

Publishes materials and promotes physical activity and health programs that include participation in the lives of America's youth and the Keystone Conference.

National Eldercare Institute on Health Promotion
601 E Street, NW, Fifth Floor, Building B
Washington, DC 20049
202-434-2200; 202-434-6474 Fax

Supports states and agencies in the development and implementation of health promotion programs for older adults. Provides resource lists, publications, and referrals.

National Handicapped Sports
451 Hungerford Drive, Suite 100
Rockville, MD 20850
301-217-0960; 301-217-0968 Fax
301-217-9836 Electronic bulletin board

Provides sports and recreation activities for persons with orthopedic, spinal cord, neuromuscular, and visual impairments through more than 90 community-based chapters. Free bulletin board.

National Recreation and Park Association
2775 South Quincy Street, Suite 300
Arlington, VA 22206
703-820-4940; 703-671-6772 Fax

Increases public awareness of the role of physical fitness in health, encourages recreation among the elderly, and establishes standards for recreation services for people with handicaps.

YMCA of the USA
Health and Physical Education
101 North Wacker Drive, 14th Floor
Chicago, IL 60606
800-USA-YMCA; 312-977-0031; 312-977-9063 Fax

Provides fitness training, conditioning, and group fitness programs for all ages. Distributes brochures.

YWCA of the USA
726 Broadway
New York, NY 10003
212-614-2700; 212-614-2703 Fax

Provides fitness training, conditioning, and group fitness programs for all ages. Distributes brochures.

Nutrition Resource List

Federal and National Information Sources

U.S. DEPARTMENT OF AGRICULTURE (USDA)

Food and Nutrition Information Center
National Agricultural Library
10301 Baltimore Boulevard, Room 304
Beltsville, MD 20705
301-504-5719; 301-504-6409 Fax

Provides print and audiovisual materials for consumers and bibliographies and resource guides for professionals on topics in human nutrition. Call for electronic product information.

Food and Consumer Service (FCS)
3101 Park Center Drive
Alexandria, VA 22302
703-305-2276; 703-305-1117 Fax

Administers the Special Supplemental Food Program for Women, Infants, and Children (WIC). Provides food, nutrition education, and health care referrals. Publications list available. Some titles available in Spanish and other languages. Orders should be placed through regional FCS/USDA offices.

Food Safety and Inspection Service
Office of USDA Meat and Poultry Hotline
14th and Independence Avenue, SW
Room 2925 South
Washington, DC 20205
202-720-3333; 202-690-2859 Fax
800-535-4555 Meat/poultry hotline

Administers the meat and poultry inspection program to ensure a safe, wholesome, and truthfully labeled product. Produces pamphlets and other educational materials on food safety, food poisoning, labeling, food additives, and the inspection program. Publications list available.

Agricultural Research Service
Survey Systems/Food Consumption Laboratory, USDA Center
4700 River Road, Mail Unit 83
Bethesda, MD 20837
301-734-8450; 301-734-5496

Conducts applied research in food consumption, nutrition knowledge and attitudes, and food composition. Conducts the Continuing Survey of Food Intakes by
Individuals and the Diet-Health Knowledge Survey.

U.S. DEPARTMENT OF HEALTH AND HUMAN SERVICES (DHHS)

Public Health Service

Food and Drug Administration (FDA)
Center for Food Safety and Applied Nutrition
200 C Street, SW
Washington, DC 20204
202-205-5004; 202-401-3532 Fax
800-FDA-4010 FDA seafood hotline

Regulates all food and cosmetic products other than meat and poultry. Responsible for food safety, nutrition, food labeling, and economic fraud. Provides educational information.

Office of Consumer Affairs
5600 Fishers Lane (HFE-88)
Rockville, MD 20857
301-443-3170

Answers inquiries on food and cosmetics. Publications available on federal regulations, drug development process, drug labeling, and pharmaceuticals.

Health Resources and Services Administration
National Maternal and Child Health Clearinghouse
8201 Greensboro Drive, Suite 600
McLean, VA 22102-3810
703-821-8955, ext. 254 or 265; 703-821-2098 Fax

Provides information on maternal and child health topics including nutrition.
Distributes federal programs directories, topical resource guides, and provides
referrals.

Indian Health Service
Communications Office
Parklawn Building, Room 6-35
5600 Fishers Lane
Rockville, MD 20857
301-443-3593; 301-443-0507 Fax

Provides a comprehensive health services delivery system for American Indians
and Alaska Natives. The system features many special programs, including nutrition. Gathers and publishes information about the health status of American
Indians and Alaska Natives.

National Institutes of Health (NIH)
Division of Nutrition Research Coordination
National Institute of Diabetes and Digestive and Kidney Diseases
Natcher Building, Room 5AN-32
45 Center Drive, MSC 6600
Bethesda, MD 20892-6600
301-594-8822

National Institutes of Health (NIH)
National Cancer Institute
Cancer Information Service
Building 31, Room 10A16
9000 Rockville Pike
Bethesda, MD 20892-3100
800-4-CANCER; 301-402-2594 Fax

Provides a nationwide telephone service for the public and health care professionals and disseminates publications. Spanish-speaking staff members are available.

NIDDK Weight Control Information Network (WIN)
7910 Woodmont Avenue, Suite 300
Bethesda, MD 20814
301-951-1120; 301-951-1107 Fax

Provides support for the National Task Force on Prevention and Treatment of Obesity, develops fact sheets, disseminates information for consumers, and performs communication research through the Boston Obesity and Nutrition Research Center. For health messages, call 800-WIN-8098.

National Heart, Lung, and Blood Institute (NHLBI) Education Programs
  Information Center
P.O. Box 30105
Bethesda, MD 20824-0105
301-251-1222; 301-251-1223 Fax

Provides information on NHLBI education programs on high blood pressure, cholesterol, obesity, asthma, and heart attack. Offers information on cardiovascular disease prevention and heart-health promotion to consumers and professionals. Call for electronic product information.

Office of Minority Health Resource Center
P.O. Box 37337
Washington, DC 20013-7337
800-444-6472; 301-589-0884 Fax

Responds to inquiries about major health problems among minority populations. Assists in locating materials, programs, and technical assistance through an automated database.

National Sources

American Association of Retired Persons
601 E Street, NW
Washington, DC 20049
202-434-2277; 202-434-2588 Fax

Offers national programs and materials for older people and sponsors community programs. Provides consumer education pamphlets on nutrition and the elderly.

American Cancer Society
1599 Clifton Road, NE
Atlanta, GA 30329
800-ACS-2345

Distributes materials for consumers and professionals on the link between diet and cancer.

American Diabetes Association
1660 Duke Street
Alexandria, VA 22314
800-232-3472; 703-549-1500

Provides information and services for consumers and professionals. Publications catalog available.

The American Dietetic Association
216 West Jackson Boulevard, Suite 800
Chicago, IL 60606-6995
312-899-0040; 312-899-1758 Fax

Provides consumers and nutrition professionals with objective, credible food and nutrition information.

American Heart Association
7272 Greenville Avenue
Dallas, TX 75231-4599
214-373-6300; 800-AHA-USA1; 214-706-1341 Fax

Sponsors research, community programs, and professional education on cardiovascular diseases and stroke. Catalog of materials available.

American School Food Service Association
1600 Duke Street, 7th Floor
Alexandria, VA 22314
703-739-3900; 703-739-3915 Fax
303-762-1144 Fax (Publications)

Promotes improvement in school food and nutrition programs. Distributes information on school food service and nutrition programs and child nutrition legislation. Call for electronic product information.

American School Health Association
7263 State Route 43
Kent, OH 44240
216-678-1603; 216-678-4526 Fax

Promotes comprehensive school health programs. Provides referral services and distributes materials. Publications list available.

Center for Science in the Public Interest
1875 Connecticut Avenue, NW, Suite 300
Washington, DC 20009
202-332-9110; 202-265-4954 Fax

Provides information about food, nutrition, the food industry, food safety, alcohol, and regulations. Publications list available.

National Academy of Sciences
Food and Nutrition Board
2101 Constitution Avenue, NW
Washington, DC 20418
202-334-1732; 202-334-2316 Fax

Advises public agencies on nutrition research, including food safety, food protection, meat and poultry inspections, and surveys of food additives. Publications list available.

As the Healthy People 2000 goals are evaluated and the Healthy People 2010 objectives determined, check the following web sites for the latest information.

For general information on Healthy People 2000 and Healthy People 2010:

Office of Disease Prevention and Health Promotion
U.S. Public Health Service
330 C Street, SW, Room 2132
Washington, DC 20201
202-205-8583

Web site: **http://web.health.gov/healthypeople/2010**
Web site: **http://odphp.osophs.dhhs.gov/pubs/hp2000**

For Healthy People 2000 and 2010 publications, please write to:

ODPHP National Health Information Center
P.O. Box 1133
Washington, DC 20013-1133

APPENDIX B

Artificial Sweeteners and Fat Replacers

Appendix B.1 Low-Kilocalorie and Reduced-Kilocalorie Sweeteners Commonly Used in the United States

Acesulfame K (brand name Sunnet)—a noncaloric sweetener (white, odorless, crystalline structure) discovered in Germany in 1967. It is 200 times sweeter than sucrose and may be blended with other low-kilocalorie sweeteners in foods. Acesulfame K is not metabolized by the body and is excreted by the kidneys unchanged. It is most frequently used in dry beverage mixes, instant coffee and tea, chewing gum, dairy product analogs, and as a tabletop sweetener.

Aspartame—a nutritive sweetener made from two amino acids (L-phenylalanine and L-aspartic acid). It is 180 times sweeter than sucrose. Although aspartame is made up of amino acids, so little is needed to sweeten products that it is virtually noncaloric. It is digested like protein. It has a sugar-like taste and actually enhances some flavors when added to products. When aspartame is combined with other low-kilocalorie sweeteners, they have a synergistic effect so that the combined effect is sweeter than the sum of the individual sweeteners. Aspartame cannot be used in products exposed to high temperatures because heat denatures the molecule. Individuals with phenylketonuria (PKU) should restrict aspartame intake since it contains phenylalanine. Aspartame is most frequently used as a tabletop sweetener and in carbonated soft drinks, frozen desserts, puddings, and yogurt-type products. Aspartame is sold under the brand name Nutrasweet. As a tabletop sweetener, it is packaged and sold under the brand name Equal.

Saccharin—a noncaloric sweetener discovered in 1879 and used commercially since the early 1900s. It is not metabolized by the body and is excreted by the kidneys unchanged. Saccharin is 300 times sweeter than sucrose and has a stable shelf life. As with aspartame, saccharin combines synergistically with other low-kilocalorie sweeteners to produce an effect sweeter than the sum of the individual sweeteners. It is used in soft drinks, tabletop sweeteners, and a wide variety of foods and beverages. It is also used in cosmetic and pharmaceutical products. Saccharin has an aftertaste that is reduced when saccharin is combined with other low-kilocalorie sweeteners. Although the Food and Drug Administration (FDA) proposed a ban on saccharin in the United States to further study its safety, the ban never went into effect. In 1991, the FDA withdrew the proposed ban. Saccharin continues to be used in 100 countries. It is sold under the brand name of Sweet'N Low.

Sorbitol—a sugar alcohol formed through the hydrolysis of sugar. It is approximately 0.5-0.7 times as sweet as sugar (sucrose) and is used in special dietary foods, candies, and gum marketed to diabetics. The FDA reports an energy value of 2.6 kcal/g; thus, this sweetener provides some energy, but its energy content is lower than the 4 kcal/g found in sucrose. Excessive consumption of sorbitol (50-80 g/d) can cause gastrointestinal distress and have a laxative effect.

Sucralose—the newest non-nutritive sweetener (approved by the FDA in the spring of 1998). Sucralose is a disaccharide made from sucrose in a five-step process that selectively substitutes three atoms of chlorine for three hydroxyl groups in the sugar molecule. The result is a high-intensity sweetener that is 98% pure and is 320-1000 times sweeter than sugar, depending on the food application. The majority of ingested sucralose is excreted unchanged in the feces; most of what is absorbed appears unchanged in the urine. Therefore, sucralose adds sweetness without adding calories. It is currently approved for a number of uses including baked goods, beverages, gum, desserts, candy, jams, puddings, and milk products. It can also be used as a tabletop sweetener.

Xylitol—sugar alcohol derived from fruits and vegetables (e.g., strawberries, carrots). It has the same sweetness and bulk as sucrose, but the energy content is 2.4 kcal/g. Xylitol is frequently used in chewing gum, gum drops, hard candies, and in pharmaceutical and oral health products.

Types of fat replacers

Names on the ingredient list	Foods that may contain fat replacers
The following ingredients may be added to replace the amount of fat required to make the product.	These foods can contain any combination of fat replacers to reduce or eliminate the amount of fat required to make the product.

Carbohydrate-based fat replacers:

Provide kilocalories similar to carbohydrate (1-4 kcal/g): corn syrup solids, dextrin, hydrolyzed corn starch, maltodextrin, modified food starch, polydextrose (Litesse), tapioca dextrin, oatrim (Beta-Trim, TrimChoice)	baked goods, candy, cheese, chewing gum, salad dressing, frozen dessert, gelatin, meat-based products, puddings, sauces, sour cream, yogurt
Provide negligible kilocalories (dietary fibers): carrageenan, cellulose gel, cellulose gum, guar gum, inulin, pectin, sugar beet fiber or powder, fiber (Z-Trim, Oat fiber, Ultracel)	

Protein-based fat replacers:

microparticulated protein (Simpless), egg white and mild protein (K-Blazer, Ultra-Baket), modified whey protein concentrate (Dairy-Lo)	butter, cheese, sour cream, mayonnaise spreads, baked goods, salad dressings

Fat-based fat replacers:

caprenin, olestra (Olean), salatrim (Benefat), mono- and diglycerides, emulsifiers (Dur-Lo)	soft candy, candy coatings, chips, crackers

Descriptions of carbohydrate-based fat replacer listed above:

• Dextrins, maltodextrins, tapioca dextrin, modified food starch: These are bland, nonsweet carbohydrates made from hydrolyzed starches, which can mimic the texture and mouth feel of fat due to their gel-like structure. Can provide 1 to 4 kcal/g and can completely replace the fat in food.

• Oatrim: A beta-glucan (type of soluble fiber) derived from oat fiber, which can replace fat and add the additional cholesterol-lowering benefit of oat bran. Provides 4 kcal/g.

• Z-Trim: A noncaloric, bland mix of insoluble fiber made from the crushed hulls of corn, oats, and rice. Can replace some of the fat and carbohydrate in foods such as chocolates, brownies, cheese, and ground beef.

• Polydextrose: This is a nonsweet starch polymer made from food-grade dextrose and small amounts of sorbitol and citric acid. Can be used to replace up to half the fat in a product. Most polydextrose passes through the body undigested, with only 5-10% digested, and provides only 1 kcal/g. Polydextrose bulking agents are used in baked goods, puddings, hard and soft candies, chocolates, salad dressings, nutrition bars, frozen dairy desserts, syrups, chewing gums, jams, jellies, and spreads.

• Microcrystalline cellulose: Made from wood pulp, noncaloric. Can be used to replace 100% of the fat in a product.

• Gum: A type of dietary fiber that mimics the functional properties of fat when water is used to replace fat in goods. Gums are not digested except by gut bacteria, which make their caloric contribution negligible.

Descriptions of protein-based fat replacers listed above:

• Simpless: A protein-based fat replacer made by the NutraSweet Company and approved for use in frozen desserts, mayonnaise, sour cream, salad dressings, refrigerated desserts, yogurt, and cheese. Made from milk and/or egg white proteins, water, sugar, pectin, and citric acid. Supplies 1 to 2 kcal/g.

Descriptions of fat-based fat replacers listed above:

• Olestra (Olean): Produced by Proctor and Gamble Co., and it is one of the most studied fat replacers on the market. Formed by the esterification of sucrose with six to eight long-chain fatty acids from edible oils. Olestra is not sweet; has the appearance, taste, texture, and mouth feel of fat; and can be used in fried, cooked, and baked products. Currently approved for snack foods like chips and crackers. Because it is not digested, Olestra is calorie free, but it may reduce the absorption of fat-soluble vitamins and cause some gastrointestinal distress if consumed in large amounts. Foods made with olestra have added vitamins A, D, E, and K.

- Salatrim (Benefat): Developed by Nabisco, sold by Cultor Food Service, Inc. Represents a family of reduced-fat triglycerides containing only 4-6 kcal/g compared with normal dietary fats at 9 kcal/g. Salatrim is a real fat made by combining short-chain fatty acids (either acetic, propionic, or butyric) and one long-chain fatty acid (stearic) to a glycerol backbone. The energy content is lower than regular fat because short-chain fatty acids contain only 4 kcal/g, and stearic acid is not completely absorbed by the body. Made in either liquid or solid form and used in ice cream, cheese, sour cream, margarine, spreads, chocolate bars and chips, cookies, and snacks.

References: Calorie Control Council (CCC) National Consumer Survey. Most popular reduced-fat products. Atlanta, GA: CCC, 1998.

Dreher M, Leveille GA, Auerback M, Callen C, Klemann L, Jones K. Salatrim: a triacylglycerol-based fat replacer. Nutr Today 1998;33:164-70.

Hudnall MJ, Conner SJ, Conner WE. Position of the American Dietetic Association: fat replacements. J Am Diet Assoc 1991;91:1285-8.

APPENDIX C

Energy Balance

Appendix C.1 Equations Used to Determine Energy Expenditure (kcal/min) From Indirect Calorimetry

Weir (1949): [a]

$$\text{kcal/min} = 3.941 \, (\dot{V}O_2 \, [\text{L/min}]) + 1.106 \, (\dot{V}CO_2 \, [\text{L/min}])$$

$$\text{kcal/min} = 3.941 \, (\dot{V}O_2 \, [\text{L/min}]) + 1.106 \, (\dot{V}CO_2 \, [\text{L/min}]) - 2.17 \, (\text{g/min urinary N})$$

where ($\dot{V}O_2$ = oxygen consumed; $\dot{V}CO_2$ = carbon dioxide produced.

Consolazio et al. (1963):

$$\text{kcal/min} = 3.78 \, (\dot{V}O_2 \, [\text{L/min}]) + 1.16 \, (\dot{V}CO_2 \, [\text{L/min}]) - 2.98 \, (\text{g/min urinary N})$$

Peters and Van Slyke (1946):

$$\text{kcal/min} = 3.82 \, (\dot{V}O_2 \, [\text{L/min}]) + 1.22 \, (\dot{V}CO_2 \, [\text{L/min}]) - 2.01 \, (\text{g/min urinary N})$$

Jequier et al. (1987):

$$\text{kcal/min} = [4.686 + 1.096 \, (\text{NPRQ} - 0.707)] \times \text{NP}\dot{V}O_2 + 4.60 \times \text{P}\dot{V}O_2$$

where: NPRQ is the nonprotein respiratory quotient = $\text{NP}\dot{V}CO_2/\text{NP}\dot{V}O_2$
NP$\dot{V}O_2$ is the nonprotein oxygen consumption (L/min)
P$\dot{V}O_2$ is the protein oxygen consumption (L/min)
NP$\dot{V}CO_2$ is the nonprotein CO_2 production (L/min)
P$\dot{V}CO_2$ is the protein CO_2 production (L/min)
P$\dot{V}O_2$ = N $\times$ 6.25 $\times$ 0.996 where N is the total urine nitrogen (g/min)
P$\dot{V}CO_2$ = N $\times$ 6.25 $\times$ 0.774
NP$\dot{V}O_2$ = $\dot{V}O_2$ − P$\dot{V}O_2$
NP$\dot{V}CO_2$ = $\dot{V}CO_2$ − NP$\dot{V}CO_2$

when: NPRQ = 0.707, NP$\dot{V}O_2$ is entirely due to lipid oxidation, and the calorie equivalent of 1 L of oxygen consumed is 4.686 kcal (or 19.61 kJ).

[a] The difference in energy expenditure calculated by these two equations is less than 3%.

References for Appendix C.1

Consolazio CJ, Johnson RE, Pecora LJ. Physiological measurements of metabolic functions in man. New York: McGraw-Hill, 1963.

Jequier E, Acheson K, Schultz Y. Assessment of energy expenditure and fuel utilization in man. Ann Rev of Nutr 1987;7:187-208.

Peters JP, Van Slycke DD. Quantitative clinical chemistry interpretations. Vol 1. Baltimore: Williams & Wilkins, 1946.

Weir JB. New methods for calculating metabolic rate with special reference to protein metabolism. J Physiol 1949;109:1-9.

Appendix C.2 Various Factorial Methods for Calculating Total Daily Energy Expenditure (TDEE)

1. Activity factor method 1

- Predict RMR using one of the prediction equations listed in table 5.4 (page 152).

- Multiply RMR by one of the following activity factors (AF):

- Use this method if you are using only one AF to estimate the whole day.

Factors for Estimating Daily Energy Allowance at Various Levels of Physical Activity for Men and Women (Ages 19-50 Years)

Level of activity	Activity factor ($\times$ RMR)	Energy expenditure (kcal/kg/d)
Sedentary/confined to bed	1.2	25
Very light activity		
Men	1.3	31
Women	1.3	30
Light activity		
Men	1.6	38
Women	1.5	35
Moderate activity		
Men	1.7	41
Women	1.6	37
Heavy activity		
Men	2.1	50
Women	1.9	44
Exceptional activity		
Men	2.4	58
Women	2.2	51

The activity factor 1.3 $\times$ RMR is a minimum value, reflecting 10 h/d at rest and 14 h of very light activity. Thus, TDEE = RMR(AF).

Example: An active woman (age 41 years, height 163 cm, weight 64.4 kg, body fat 17.2%) who exercises approximately 7.5 h/week in both aerobic activities and weight training. Using the Harris-Benedict equation to predict RMR (see table 5.4, page 152).

RMR = 655.1 + 9.56 (64.4 kg) + 1.85 (163 cm) − 4.68 (41 years) = 1380 kcal/d

TDEE = 1380 kcal/d (AF)

= 1380(1.6) (using a moderate activity factor of 1.6)

= 2208 kcal/d

473

References for Method 1

Food and Nutrition Board, National Academy of Sciences. Recommended Dietary Allowances, 10th ed. Washington, DC: National Academy Press, 1989:27.

Zeman FJ, Ney DM. Applications of Clinical Nutrition. Englewood Cliffs, NJ: Prentice Hall, 1988:27.

2. Activity factor method 2

- Record typical 24-h activities; group amount of time spent in each activity according to the activity categories listed in the table on page 472.
- Multiply the amount of time spent in each activity by the appropriate activity factor to calculate a weighted RMR factor. See example below.
- Average the weighted RMR factors to provide a mean activity factor for the day.
- Multiply the mean activity factor by RMR to provide TDEE.

Example: An active woman (age 41 years, height 163 cm, weight 64.4 kg, body fat 17.2%) who exercises approximately 7.5 h/week in both aerobic activities and weight training. Activity factors are derived from the table on page 472. This individual sleeps and rests for 9 h/d; works at a desk and cooks for 9 h/d; does housecleaning, child care, and walking for 5 h/d; and does aerobics for 1 h/d.

Activities as multiples of RMR	Activity factor	Duration (h)	Weighted activity factor
Rest	1.0	9	9.0
Very light activity	1.5	9	13.5
Light activity	2.5	5	12.5
Moderate activity	5.0	0	0.0
Heavy activity	7.0	1	7.0
Total		24 h	42
Mean activity factor			1.75 (42 ÷ 24 h)

RMR is estimated using the Harris-Benedict equation from table 5.4 (page 152).

$$RMR = 655.1 + 9.56(64.4 \text{ kg}) + 1.85(163 \text{ cm}) - 4.68(41 \text{ years})$$

$$TDEE = 1380 \text{ kcal/d (AF)}$$

$$= 1380(1.75) \text{ (using the estimated activity factor of 1.75)}$$

$$= 2415 \text{ kcal/d}$$

Reference for method 2

Food and Nutrition Board, National Research Council, National Academy of Sciences. Recommended Dietary Allowances, 10th ed. Washington, DC: National Academy Press, 1989:27.

3. Combination method: general and specific activity factors

- Record typical 24-h activities. Divide activities into two categories: general activities (amount of time spent walking, sitting, reading, resting, etc.) and specific activities (amount of time spent running 60 min at an 8-mph pace, lifting weights for 30 min, or cycling 15 mi at a 20-mph pace).
- Estimate RMR from one of the equations in table 5.4 (page 152).

- Determine a general activity factor (GAF) for the time the individual is not participating in specific activities. Multiply this activity factor by predicted RMR.
- Determine the amount of energy expended in the specific activities; this is called the specific activity factor (SAF). Use the table provided in appendix E.4 to do this. This table gives the amount of energy expended in kcal/kg/ min. Multiply this number by the kilogram body weight of the individual and the number of minutes spent in the activity.
- Add the GAF and SAF values (kcal/d). For example, RMR(GAF) + (SAF).
- Multiply the above value by 10% to determine the thermic effect of food (TEF). Add this number to the value obtained in the previous step.
- TDEE = RMR(GAF) + (SAF in kilocalories) + 10% for TEF

Example: A male long distance runner (age 23 years, weight 80 kg, height 179 cm, body fat 13%) is a graduate student who trains 2 h/d. When he is not training, he is relatively sedentary and spends his time walking to class, sitting in class, studying, and working at the computer.

1. Determine RMR.

$$RMR = 66.47 + 13.75(wt) - 5(ht) - 6.76(age) \text{ (see table 5.4)}$$

$$RMR = 66.47 + 13.75(80 \text{ kg}) + 5(179 \text{ cm}) - 6.76(23 \text{ years})$$

$$= 1906 \text{ kcal/d}$$

2. Determine energy expended for GAF by multiplying RMR by GAF. A GAF of 1.3 will be used (see table in example 2) since this individual is relatively inactive outside of the daily running.

$$1906 \text{ kcal/d } (1.3) = 2478 \text{ kcal/d}$$

3. Determine energy expended for SAF. These values are obtained from the example table provided in appendix E.4.

60 min/d running 10 mph (6-min mi) at 0.252 kcal/kg/min

$$0.252 \times 80 \text{ kg} \times 60 \text{ min} = 1209 \text{ kcal}$$

60 min/d running 8 mph (7:30-min mi) at 0.208 kcal/kg/min

$$0.208 \times 80 \text{ kg} \times 60 \text{ min} = 998 \text{ kcal}$$

Total calories spent in SAF = 2207 kcal/d

4. Add values from steps 2 and 3. Thus, 2478 + 2207 = 4685 kcal/d.
5. Add cost of TEF at 10% to total calories needed (see step 4).

$$TEF = 4685 \times 10\%$$

= 468 kcal/d expended in TEF. Add this to the value in step 4.

6. TDEE = RMR(GAF) + SAF (kcal/d) + 10% TEF

$$= 2478 + 2207 + 468$$

$$= 5153 \text{ kcal/d required to cover energy expenditure}$$

4. Specific activity factor method

- Determine all activities in a 24-h period. It is best if 24-h activities can be recorded for 7 d and then averaged.
- Using the energy expenditure table given in appendix E.4, calculate the number of calories expended in each activity the subject engaged in (kcal/ kg body weight/min).
- Add calories expended in each activity over the 24-h period. This should give you TDEE.

Example: A male long distance runner (age 23 years, weight 80 kg, height 179 cm, body fat 13%) is a graduate student who trains 2 h/d. When he is not training, he is relatively sedentary and spends his time walking to class, sitting in class, studying, and working at the computer.

Activity	Duration of activity (h)	Energy expenditure (kcal/kg/min)	Total energy expended in activity (kcal/d)
Sleeping	7	0.020	672.0
Sitting quietly	6	0.021	604.8
Walking, normal pace	1.5	0.080	576.0
Standing quietly	1	0.027	129.6
Cleaning	0.25	0.058	69.6
Cooking	0.25	0.048	57.6
Eating (sitting)	1	0.023	110.4
Lying at ease	2	0.022	211.2
Playing the piano	1	0.040	192.0
Typing at computer	2	0.031	297.6
Running 6 min/mi	1	0.252	1209.6
Running 7:30 min/mi	1	0.208	998.4
Totals	24 h		5129 kcal/d

Thus, TDEE for this individual using the specific activity method is 5129 kcal/d. Many computer programs (Food Processor Plus, ESHA Research, Salem, OR and Nutritionist 4, California) calculate TDEE using this method.

Appendix C.3 Effect of Exercise on Resting Metabolic Rate (RMR) in Trained Versus Untrained Young Men

Reference	Subjects	Mean $\dot{V}O_2$max (ml/kg/min)	Mean RMR (kcal/kg FFM)	% diff. in RMR	Significant difference
Almeras et al. (1991)	CC skiers (n = 7)	—	26.75	5.2%	NS
	Controls (n = 8)	—	25.36		
Broeder et al. (1992)	Trained (n = 10)	70.1	30.17	3.4%	NS
	Controls (n = 21)	41.1	29.47		
Bullough et al. (1995)	Trained (n = 8)	62.9	27.73 ↑flux day	16%[a]	$p < 0.01$
	Controls (n = 8)	43.0	23.27		
Horton and Geissler (1994)	Trained (n = 10)	[b]	26.75	5.3%	NS
	Controls (n = 10)	[b]	25.33		
Poehlman et al. (1988)	Trained (n = 9)	70.5	28.32	11.0%	$p < 0.05$
	Controls (n = 9)	53.0	25.20		
Poehlman et al. (1990)	Trained (n = 22)	60.2	26.50	4.2%	$p < 0.05$
	Controls (n = 20)	50.4	25.40		
Tremblay et al. (1983)	Runners (n = 8)	69.2	34.12	4.8%	NS
	Controls (n = 8)	47.7	32.48		

Reference	Subjects	Mean $\dot{V}O_2$max (ml/kg/min)	Mean RMR (kcal/kg FFM)	% diff. in RMR	Significant difference
Tremblay et al. (1986)	Runners/skiers (n = 20)	68.4	26.95	5.4%	NS
	Controls (n = 39)	50.8	25.50		

NS = not significant.

[a] Differences between groups found only when trained group was in a high-flux period (exercising at least 90 min/d at 75% $\dot{V}O_2$max and compared to untrained subjects who were not exercising). No differences were found between groups when trained subjects were in a low-flux period (no exercise for 3 d). Values estimated from paper.

[b] Subjects were classified as sedentary or highly active on the basis of their habitual exercise patterns.

References for Appendix C.3

Almeras N, Mineault N, Serresse O, Boulay MR, Tremblay A. Non-exercise daily energy expenditure and physical activity patterns in male endurance athletes. Eur J Appl Physiol 1991;63:184-7.

Broeder CE, Burrhus KA, Svanevik LA, Wilmore JH. The effects of aerobic fitness on resting metabolic rate. Am J Clin Nutr 1992;55:795-801.

Bullough RC, Gillette CA, Harris MA, Melby CL. Interaction of acute changes in exercise energy expenditure and energy intake on resting metabolic rate. Am J Clin Nutr 1995;61:473-81.

Horton TJ, Geissler CA. Effect of habitual exercise on daily energy expenditure and metabolic rate during standardized activity. Am J Clin Nutr 1994;59:13-19.

Poehlman ET, Melby CL, Badylak SF. Resting metabolic rate and postprandial thermogenesis in highly trained and untrained males. Am J Clin Nutr 1988;47:793-8.

Poehlman ET, McAuliffe TL, VanHouten DR, Danforth E. Influence of age and endurance training on metabolic rate and hormones in healthy men. Am J Physiol 1990;259:E66-E72.

Tremblay A, Cote J, LeBlanc J. Diminished dietary thermogenesis in exercise-trained human subjects. Eur J Appl Physiol 1983;52:1-4.

Tremblay A, Fontaine E, Poehlman ET, Mitchell D, Perron L, Bouchard C. The effect of exercise-training on resting metabolic rate in lean and moderately obese individuals. I J Obesity 1986;10:511-7.

Appendix C.4 Effect of Exercise Training on Posttraining Resting Metabolic Rate (RMR) in Previously Untrained Individuals

Reference	Subjects and type of training	Pretraining RMR (kcal/kg FFM)	Posttraining RMR (kcal/kg FFM)	% RMR difference ([post–pre] ÷ pre)	Significant differences
Broeder et al. (1992)	Males (n = 22) ET for 12 weeks	28.95	29.19	<1%	NS
Broeder et al. (1992)	Males (n = 22) RT for 12 weeks	29.17	29.48	<1%	NS
Goran and Poehlman (1992)[a,b]	Males (n = 6) and females (n = 5) ET for 8 weeks	32.22	34.99	8.6%	$p < 0.01$
Poehlman and Danforth (1991)[a]	Males (n = 13) and females (n = 6) ET for 8 weeks	24.48	27.36	11.8%	$p < 0.01$

(continued)

Appendix C.4   *(continued)*

Reference	Subjects and type of training	Pretraining RMR (kcal/kg FFM)	Posttraining RMR (kcal/kg FFM)	% RMR difference ([post–pre] ÷ pre)	Significant differences
Tremblay et al. (1986)[b]	Obese females (n = 8); ET for 11 weeks	26.64	28.51	7.0%	$p < 0.01$

ET = endurance training; RT = resistance training; NS = not significant.
[a] Subjects were >60 years of age.
[b] Relative RMR values estimated for graphs and tables.

References for Appendix C.4

Broeder CE, Burrhus KA, Svanevik LA, Wilmore JH. The effects of either high-intensity resistance or endurance training on resting metabolic rate. Am J Clin Nutr 1992;55:802-10.

Goran MI, Poehlman ET. Endurance training does to enhance total energy expenditure in healthy elderly persons. Am J Phyisol 1992;263:E950-E957.

Poehlman ET, Danforth E. Endurance training increases metabolic rate and norepinephrine appearance rate in older individuals. Am J Physiol 1991;261:E233-E239.

Tremblay A, Fontaine E, Poehlman ET, Mitchell D, Perron L, Bouchard C. The effect of exercise-training on resting metabolic rate in lean and moderately obese individuals. I J Obesity 1986;10:511-7.

Appendix C.5   Effect of Type of Exercise and Exercise Intensity on Magnitude and Duration of Excess Post-Exercise Oxygen Consumption (EPOC)

Reference	Subjects: type of exercise training and fitness level	Exercise: intensity and duration	% EPOC or duration of EPOC (min or h)
Bahr et al. (1987)	ET males (n = 6) $\dot{V}O_2$max = 54 ml/kg/min	70% $\dot{V}O_2$max for 20 min 70% $\dot{V}O_2$max for 40 min 70% $\dot{V}O_2$max for 80 min	5.1% at 12 h 6.8% at 12 h 14.4% at 12 h
Bahr and Sejersted (1991)	ET males (n = 6) $\dot{V}O_2$max = 50 ml/kg/min	29% $\dot{V}O_2$max for 80 min 50% $\dot{V}O_2$max for 80 min 75% $\dot{V}O_2$max for 80 min	0.3 h 3.3 h 10.5 h
Bahr et al. (1992)	Males (n = 6) $\dot{V}O_2$max = 49 ml/kg/min	2 min at 108% $\dot{V}O_2$max 1× 2 min at 108% $\dot{V}O_2$max 2× 2 min at 108% $\dot{V}O_2$max 3×	30 min 60 min 4 h
Bielinski et al. (1985)	ET males (n = 10) $\dot{V}O_2$max = 63 ml/kg/min	50% $\dot{V}O_2$max for 3 h	O_2 ↑ 4-5 h post-ex.; RMR ↑ by 4.7% after 24 h
Brehm and Gutin (1986)	ET subjects (n = 8) and controls (n = 8)	6.4 mph walking for 2 mi	42 min
Chad and Quigley (1989)	UT females (n = 5)	55% $\dot{V}O_2$max for 90 min	O_2 still ↑ after 60 min
Chad and Quigley (1991)	ET females (n = 5) and UT females (n = 5)	50% $\dot{V}O_2$max for 3 h 70% $\dot{V}O_2$max for 3 h	O_2 still ↑ after 3 h for both groups but highest after 50% $\dot{V}O_2$max

Reference	Subjects: type of exercise training and fitness level	Exercise: intensity and duration	% EPOC or duration of EPOC (min or h)
Elliot et al. (1992)	ET and RT males (n = 4) and females (n = 5); $\dot{V}O_2$max = 45-48 ml/kg/min	40 min cycling at 80% MHR; 40 min circuit training at 50% maximum repetition; 40 min heavy resistance at 80-90% maximum repetition	↑ 10% 30 min post-ex. ↑ 19% 30 min post-ex. ↑ 21% 30 min post-ex.
Freedman-Akabas et al. (1985)	ET subjects (n = 12) and controls (n = 7)	20 min at individual anaerobic threshold	Return to baseline by 40 min
Freedman-Akabas (1985)	ET males (n = 4) and females (n = 3)	40 min at 2 mph faster than anaerobic threshold	Return to baseline by 40 min
Gillette et al. (1994)	ET and RT males (n = 10) $\dot{V}O_2$max = 52 ml/kg/min	100 min weight lifting equaling 588 kcal 64 min at 50% $\dot{V}O_2$max cycling equaling 536 kcal	5-h EPOC ↑ 12.5% for weight lifting; ↑ 4.5% for cycling
Gore and Withers (1990a)	ET males (n = 9) $\dot{V}O_2$max = 63 ml/kg/min	30, 50, 70% $\dot{V}O_2$max at 20, 50, and 80 min	After 8 h EPOC only slightly ↑ (1-8.9%; mean = 4.8%)
Gore and Withers (1990b)	ET males (n = 9) $\dot{V}O_2$max = 63 ml/kg/min	30, 50, 70% $\dot{V}O_2$max at 20, 50, and 80 min	After 8 h no EPOC after 30% $\dot{V}O_2$max ex.; ↑ EPOC for 50 & 70% $\dot{V}O_2$max exercise
Melby et al. (1992)	RT males (n = 6)	40 min weight lifting	↑ 12% at 30 min and ↑ 6% at 60 min post-exercise
Melby et al. (1993)	RT males (n = 13)	90 min weight lifting	↑ O_2 after 2 h by 11-12%; RMR ↑ by 4.7-9.7% after 24 h
Pacy et al. (1985)	Lean subjects (n = 4)	35-55% $\dot{V}O_2$max for 4 h	Return to baseline by 60 min
Sedlock et al. (1989)	ET males (n = 10)	high intensity-short duration low intensity-short duration low intensity-long duration	33 min 20 min 28 min
Sedlock (1991a)	Females (n = 7) moderately ET	40% $\dot{V}O_2$max for 200 kcal 60% $\dot{V}O_2$max for 200 kcal	28 min 18 min
Sedlock (1991b)	Females (n = 8); $\dot{V}O_2$max = 40 ml/kg/min	60% $\dot{V}O_2$max for 200 kcal	19 min
Smith and McNaughton (1993)	ET males (n = 8) and females (n = 8)	40% $\dot{V}O_2$max for 30 min 50% $\dot{V}O_2$max for 30 min 70% $\dot{V}O_2$max for 30 min	27-31 min 36-42 min 39-48 min

ET = endurance training; RT = resistance training; UT = untrained; MHR = maximal heart rate.

References for Appendix C.5

Bahr R, Gronnerod O, Sejersted OM. Effect of supramaximal exercise on excess postexercise O_2 consumption. Med Sci Sport Exer 1992;24:66-71.

Bahr R, Ingnes I, Vaage O, Sejersted OM, Newsholme EA. Effect of duration of exercise on excess postexercise O_2 consumption. J Appl Physiol 1987;62(2):485-90.

Bahr R, Sejersted OM. Effect of intensity of exercise on exercise post-exercise O_2 consumption. Metabolism 1991;40:836-41.

Bielinski R, Schutz Y, Jequier E. Energy metabolism during the post-exercise recovery of man. Am J Clin Nutr 1985;42:69-82.

Brehm BA, Gutin B. Recovery energy expenditure for steady state exercise in runners and nonexercisers. Med Sci Sports Exer 1986;18:205-10.

Chad K, Quigley B. The effects of substrate utilization, manipulated by caffeine, on post-exercise oxygen consumption in untrained female subjects. Eur J Appl Physiol 1989;59:48-54.

Chad KE, Quigley BM. Exercise intensity: effect on postexercise O_2 uptake in trained and untrained women. J Appl Physiol 1991;70(4):1713-9.

Elliot DL, Goldberg L, Kuchl KS. Effect of resistance training on excess post-exercise oxygen consumption. J Appl Sport Sci Res 1992;6:77-81.

Freedman-Akabas S, Colt E, Kissileff HR, Pi-Sunyer X. Lack of sustained increase in VO_2 following exercise in fit and unfit subjects. Am J Clin Nutr 1985;41:545-9.

Gillette CA, Bullough RC, Melby CL. Postexercise energy expenditure in reponse to acute aerobic or resistive exercise. IJSN 1994;4:347-60.

Gore CJ, Withers RT. Effect of exercise intensity and duration on postexercise metabolism. A Appl Physiol 1990a;68(6):2362-8.

Gore CJ, Withers RT. The effect of exercise intensity and duration on the oxygen deficit and excess post-exercise oxygen consumption. Eur J Appl Physiol 1990b;60:169-74.

Melby C, Scholl C, Edwards G, Bullough R. Effect of acute resistance exercise on postexercise energy expenditure and resting metabolic rate. J Appl Physiol 1993;75(4):1847-53.

Melby CL, Tincknell T, Schmidt WD. Energy expenditure following a bout of non-steady state resistance exercise. J Sports Med Phy Fitness 1992;32:128-35.

Pacy PJ, Barton N, Webster JD, Garrow JS. The energy cost of aerobic exercise in fed and fasted normal subjects. Am J Clin Nutr 1985;42:764-8.

Sedlock DA, Fissinger JA, Melby CL. Effect of exercise intensity and duration on postexercise energy expenditure. Med Sci Sports Exer 1989;21:662-6.

Sedlock DA. Effect of exercise intensity on postexercise energy expenditure in women. Br J Sports Med 1991a;25(1):38-40.

Sedlock DA. The effect of acute nutritional status on postexercise energy expenditure. Nutr Research 1991b;11:735-42.

Smith J, McNaughton L. The effects of intensity of exercise on excess postexercise oxygen consumption and energy expenditure in moderately trained men and women. Eur J Appl Physiol 1993;67:420-5.

Appendix C.6 Equations for Estimating Resting Metabolic Rate (RMR) (kcal/24 h) in Obese Individuals [a,b,c]

Age (y)	Men	Women	Age (y)	Men	Women
Kilocalories per square meter of body surface according to Robertson and Reid (1952)			Kilocalories per square meter of body surface according to Fleisch		
			1	53.0	53.0
			2	52.4	52.4
3	60.1	54.5	3	51.3	51.2
4	57.9	53.9	4	50.3	49.8
5	56.3	53.0	5	49.3	48.4
6	54.2	51.8	6	48.3	47.0
7	52.1	50.2	7	47.3	45.4
8	50.1	48.4	8	46.3	43.8
9	48.2	46.4	9	45.2	42.8
10	46.6	44.3	10	44.0	42.5
11	45.1	42.4	11	43.0	42.0
12	43.8	40.6	12	42.5	41.3
13	42.7	39.1	13	42.3	40.3
14	41.8	37.3	14	42.1	39.2
15	41.0	36.8	15	41.3	37.9
16	40.3	36.0	16	41.4	36.9
17	39.7	35.3	17	40.8	36.3
18	39.2	34.9	18	40.0	35.9
19	38.8	34.4	19	39.2	35.5
20	38.4	34.3	20	38.5	35.5
21	38.1	34.1			
22	37.6	34.0			
23	37.5	34.0			
24	37.3	33.9			
25	37.1	34.0	25	37.5	35.2
26	37.0	34.0			
27	36.8	34.0			
28	36.6	34.0			
29	35.5	34.1			
30	35.4	34.1	30	36.8	35.1
31	35.3	34.0			
32	35.2	33.9			
33	35.1	33.8			
34	35.0	33.7			
35	35.9	33.5	35	36.5	35.0
36	35.3	33.3			
37	35.7	33.1			
38	35.7	32.9			
39	35.6	32.5			
40	35.5	32.5	40	36.3	34.9
41-44	34.5	32.5	45	36.2	34.5
45-49	34.1	32.2	50	36.3	33.9
50-54	33.8	31.9	55	35.4	33.3
55-59	33.4	31.6	60	34.9	32.7
60-64	33.1	31.3	65	34.4	32.2
65-69	32.7	31.0	70	33.8	31.7
70-74	32.4	30.7	75	33.2	31.1
75 or more	32.0	—	80	33.0	30.9

[a] The Robertson and Reid and the Fleisch equations are recommended for clinical use with obese patients by Heshka et al. 1993.
[b] Equations use body surface area (BSA). BSA (m2) = 0.007184 (wt in kg)$^{.425}$ × (ht in cm)$^{.725}$. RMR = BSA × 24 × tabled value.

Adapted with permission from Robertson and Reid 1952; Fleisch 1951.

APPENDIX D

Body Fat Percentages for Athletes

Sport	Level of competition	Gender	% Fat ± SD	Age (years)
Method	Reference			
Basketball	Collegiate postseason	Female	20.4 ± 0.9	20 ± 1
UWW[1]	Johnson et al. 1989			
DXA[2]	Collegiate	Female[4]	29.0 ± 5.2	19 ± 1
	Nichols et al. 1995			
Skinfolds	Not reported	Female	23.2 ± 3.4	—
	Mokha and Sidhu 1987			
BIA[3]	Collegiate	Female	24.4 ± 3.2	19 ± 1
	Nowak et al. 1988			
Skinfolds	U17 National Team	Female	18.0 ± 1.8	16 ± .4
	Bale 1991			
UWW	Collegiate	Female	20.5 ± 2.3	20 ± 1
	Siders et al. 1991			
BIA	Collegiate	Male	10.6 ± 3.4	19 ± 1
	Nowak et al. 1988			
Skinfolds	Collegiate	Male	7.7(no SD)	Not reported
	Bolonchuk et al. 1991			
UWW	Collegiate	Male	10.5 ± 3.8	21 ± 1
	Siders et al. 1991			
Volleyball	Collegiate	Female[4]	27.1 ± 3.9	19 ± 1
DXA	Nichols et al. 1995			
Skinfolds	Not reported	Female	23.1 ± 3.6	—
	Mokha and Sidhu 1987			
UWW	Collegiate	Female	20.9 ± 2.8	20 ± 1
	Johnson et al. 1989			
Swimming	Collegiate (preseason) (peak training)	Female	18.3 ± 3.6 15.7 ± 3.4	19 ± 1
UWW	Meleski and Malina 1985			
UWW	Collegiate	Female	21.4 ± 3.4	19 ± 1
	Siders et al. 1991			
UWW	National Team (synchronized)	Female	24.0 ± 4.8	20 ± 2
	Roby et al. 1983			
UWW	Collegiate	Female	22.2 ± 4.2	19 ± 1
	Johnson et al. 1989			
UWW	Collegiate	Male	14.3 ± 3.1	20 ± 1
	Siders et al. 1991			
Distance running	Not reported	Female	19.7 ± 3.0	—
Skinfolds	Mokha and Sidhu 1987			
	Recreational	Female[4]	18.8 ± 1.7	23 ± 5

Sport		Level of competition	Gender	% Fat ± SD	Age (years)
	Method	Reference			
	UWW	Phillips et al. 1993			
		Collegiate	Female	14.3 ± 4.3	21 ± 1
	UWW	Johnson et al. 1989			
		Moderate mileage	Male	11.2 ± 1.6	32 ± 6
	Skinfolds	Lucia et al. 1996			
		Recreational	Male	10.5 ± 1.2	23 ± 4
	UWW	Phillips et al. 1993			
Gymnastics		Elite (and figure skaters)	Female[8]	17.5 ± 3.1	17 ± 1
	DXA and UWW[7]	Fogelholm et al. 1995			
		Collegiate	Female[4]	22.6 ± 3.7	19 ± 1
	DXA	Nichols et al. 1995			
		High school	Female	13.1 ± 1.4	15 ± 1
	UWW	Moffatt et al. 1984			
		Collegiate (preseason)	Female	21.4 ± 6.2	20 ± 3
		(postseason)		13.3 ± 5.9	
	Skinfolds	Vercryssen and Shelton 1988			
		Collegiate	Female	14.5 ± 3.5	19 ± 1
	UWW	Johnson et al. 1989			
Soccer		National	Female[4]	25.8 ± 3.0	18 ± 2
	DXA and UWW	Fogelholm et al. 1995			
		Collegiate, national, and professional	Male	9.1 to 15.7	17 to 27
	Not reported	Kirkendall 1985			
		Professional (team A)	Male	12.2 ± 2.4	26 ± 4
		Professional (team B)	Male	13.0 ± 2.5	23 ± 4
	Not reported	Maughn 1997			
Cycling		Professional	Male	9.4 ± 0.7	26 ± 2
	Skinfolds	Lucia et al. 1996			
		Amateur	Male	15.0 ± 3.0	55 ± 5
		Amateur	Male	15.0 ± 3.0	24 ± 6
	BIA	Giada et al. 1995			
Triathlon		Elite	Male	9.4 ± 0.5	26 ± 3
	Skinfolds	Lucia et al. 1996			
		European or World Champion	Male	8.2 ± 2.3	18 ± 2
	Skinfolds	Bunc et al. 1996			
		European or World Champion	Female	10.4 ± 2.6	17 ± 1
	Skinfolds	Bunc et al. 1996			
Power sports		High school	Male	16.8 ± 7.3	17 ± 1
	Skinfolds	Nindl et al. 1995			
		High school	Female	26.1 ± 5.6	16 ± 1
	Skinfolds	Nindl et al. 1995			
		Not reported (throwers)	Female	23.8 ± 3.5	—
	Skinfolds	Mokha and Sidhu 1987			
		Not reported (jumpers)	Female	19.2 ± 2.9	—
	Skinfolds	Mokha and Sidhu 1987			
Rowing		Elite (heavyweight)	Female	20.7 ± 4.0	26 ± 4
	UWW	Pacy et al. 1995			
		International winners	Male	6.5 ± 0.5	26 ± 0.6
	Not reported	Secher et al. 1983			
		International competitors	Male	8.3 ± 0.4	25 ± 0.5
	Not reported	Secher et al. 1983			
Wrestling		Collegiate	Male	9.8 ± 0.5	18 to 21
	Skinfolds	Enns et al. 1987			
		Collegiate	Male	10.9 ± 1.9	18 to 24
	Skinfolds	Song and Cipriano 1984			
		Collegiate	Male	11.4 ± 3.2	20 ± 1
	UWW	Siders et al. 1991			

(continued)

Sport	Level of competition	Gender	% Fat ± SD	Age (years)
Method	Reference			
Football	Collegiate	Male	13.7 ± 4.2	20 ± 2
UWW	Siders et al. 1991			
	Collegiate	Male	12.4 ± 3.2	—
Football *(continued)*	Bolonchuk and Lukaski 1987			
Skinfolds	Collegiate (backs)	Male	7.3 to 13.8	—
Not reported	Pincivero and Bompa 1997			
	Collegiate (linemen)	Male	13.2 to 21.8	—
Not reported	Pincivero and Bompa 1997			
	Professional (backs)	Male	5.7 to 18.5	—
Not reported	Pincivero and Bompa 1997			
	Professional (linemen)	Male	15.5 to 18.7	—
Not reported	Pincivero and Bompa 1997			
Running/triathlon	Highly competitive	Female[4]	15.9 ± 1.3	31 ± 1
		Female[5]	16.0 ± 1.5	26 ± 2
DXA	Laughlin and Yen 1996	Female	20.8 ± 1.1	20 ± 1
Swimming/running/ triathlon	Mixed (collegiate, local, and national)	Female	16.3 ± 1.7	34 ± 1
		Female[7]	22.6 ± 2.1	45 ± 1
DXA	Ryan et al. 1996			
Endurance training	Not reported	Male—young	10.9 ± 1.4	27 ± 1
		Male—middle aged	19.5 ± 3.4	52 ± 2
UWW	Meredith et al. 1989			
Swimming/ Nordic skiing	Collegiate	Male	8.6 ± 0.2	27 ± 1
Skinfolds	Enns 1987			
Cross-country skiing	World-class	Male	12 ± 1	26 ± 2
	World-class	Female[6]	18 ± 3	25 ± 2
Deuterium dilution	Sjödin et al. 1996			
Ice hockey	Elite (professional)	Male	14.4 ± 0.6	24 ± 1
		Male	13.9 ± 0.7	25 ± 1
Skinfolds	Tegelman et al. 1996			
Field hockey	Not reported	Female	22.3 ± 4.1	—
Skinfolds	Mokha and Sidhu 1987			
Tennis	Collegiate	Female[4]	30.2 ± 3.5	22 ± 4
DXA	Nichols et al. 1995			
Ballet dancing	Classically trained	Female	16.4 ± 4.0	15 ± 1.6
UWW	Clarkson et al. 1985			
Baseball	Professional	Male	16.2 ± 3.2	26 ± 3
Skinfolds	Gurry et al. 1985			
Rugby	National	Male	9.1 ± 2.7	28.1 ± 3.1
Skinfolds	Maud and Schultz 1984			
Golf	Professional	Female	24.0 ± 4.0	33.3 ± 6.8
Skinfolds	Crews et al. 1984			

[1]Underwater weighing.
[2]Dual-energy x-ray absorptiometry.
[3]Bioelectrical impedence.
[4]Subjects reported to be regularly menstruating.
[5]Subjects reported to be amenorrheic.
[6]One subject reported to have prior history of anorexia nervosa.
[7]80% of these athletes were postmenopausal.
[8]25% of these athletes were oligomenorrheic; 17% were amenorrheic.

APPENDIX E

Nutrition and Fitness Assessment

Appendix E.1 Sample Food Intake Recording Form

Date ____/____/____   Day of the week _____

Time and Place (AM/PM)	Foods and beverages Include: fresh, frozen, low-fat, etc.	Amount	Method of preparation (baked, fried, broiled, etc.)	Food exchanges

Food Intake Diary   Name:

Appendix E.2 Sample Recording Form for 24-Hour Activity Records

Name _____

Energy Expenditure Grid

Date _____

Minutes	0	5	1 0	1 5	2 0	2 5	3 0	3 5	4 0	4 5	5 0	5 5	6 0
AM 6													
7													
8													
9													
10													
11													
Noon													
PM 1													
2													
3													
4													
5													
6													
7													
8													
9													
10													
11													
Midnight													
AM 1													
2													
3													
4													
5													

Appendix E.3 Food Frequency Questionnaire

	Weight (g)	Medium amount	Frequency[a] D	W	M	Y	Portion[b] N	S	M	L	Frequency per day	Grams per day
Fruits												
Apples	138	medium										
Bananas	119	small										
Peaches (canned or frozen)	128	1/2 cup										
Peaches (fresh)	152	medium										
Cantaloupe	136	1/6th										
Watermelon	300	slice										
Strawberries (fresh)	75	2/3 cup										
Oranges	145	medium										
Orange juice	187	3/4 cup										
Grapefruit (fresh)	134	1/2 med.										
Grapefruit juice	188	6 oz										
Tang or other fruit drink	250	9 oz										
Any other fruit including berries or fruit cocktail	128	2/3 cup										
Vegetables												
String beans or green beans	70	2/3 cup										
Peas	85	1/2 cup										
Beans (baked or pintos or kidney or lima)	185	3/4 cup										
Corn	83	1/2 cup										
Mixed vegetables	94	2/3 cup										
Winter and baked squash	108	3/4 cup										
Tomato juice	182	5 oz										
Tomatoes (raw)	62	3 slices										
Broccoli	93	2/3 cup										
Cauliflower or brussels sprouts	100	1/2 cup										
Spinach (raw)	28	2/3 cup										
Spinach (cooked)	103	2/3 cup										
Cole slaw or cabbage or sauerkraut	60	1/2 cup										
Carrots raw or cooked	62	1/2 cup										
Green salad	93	1 cup										
French fries or fried potatoes (1-2 in. strips)	57	18										
Sweet potatoes or yams	114	medium										
Other potatoes including boiled or baked or mashed	122	medium										
Rice, cooked	175	3/4 cup										
Eggs, meat, and fish												
Hamburger or meatloaf	113	3 oz										
Beef (steaks or roasts)	112	4 oz										
Beef stew	245	1 1/3 cup										
Pot pie with vegetables	227	1 (8 oz)										

	Weight (g)	Medium amount	Frequency[a]					Portion[b]			Frequency per day	Grams per day
			D	W	M	Y	N	S	M	L		
Organ meats (liver, etc.)	112	4 oz										
Pork (including chops or roasts)	56	med. chop										
Chicken, fried	112	1 leg or 2 drumsticks or 1/2 breast										
Chicken, baked or broiled	112	4 slices										
Turkey, baked or broiled	112	4 slices										
Shellfish or shrimp or lobster	43	2.5 oz										
Tuna fish	80	2.5 oz										
Other fish (haddock, etc.)	112	5 oz										
Eggs (large)	64	1										
Bacon (med. sliced)	16	2 slices										
Sausage (links)	45	2 links										
Weiners (small)	66	2										
Ham or luncheon meats	67	3 oz										
Mixed dishes and soups												
Spaghetti or lasagna or other pasta with tomato sauce	375	1 cup										
Pizza (slices)	152	2 slices										
Mixed dishes with cheese (macaroni and cheese)	200	1 cup										
Vegetable soup or vegetable-beef or minestrone or tomato soup	245	1 1/4 cup										
Creamed soup	245	1 1/4 cup										
Breads, snacks, and spreads												
White bread or rolls	44	1 1/2 slices										
Dark bread or rolls	34	2 slices										
Crackers	15	5										
Muffins	62	medium										
High fiber cereals	43	2/3 cup										
Other cold cereals	20	1 cup										
Cooked cereals	240	1 1/4 cup										
Sugar added to cereal		1 tsp										
Salty snacks (chips, etc.)	18	1 cup										
Peanuts	36	1/3 cup										
Peanut butter	16	1 tbsp										
Butter	7	2 tsp										
Margarine	9	2 tsp										
Salad dressing or mayonnaise	14	1 tbsp										
Gravies	71	1/4 cup										
Pancakes	81	3 medium										
Sweets												
Ice cream	133	3/4 cup										
Sweet rolls or doughnuts	43	1										
Cookies	25	3										

(continued)

Appendix E.3 *(continued)*

	Weight (g)	Medium amount	Frequency[a] D	W	M	Y	N	Portion[b] S	M	L	Frequency per day	Grams per day
Cake	66	1 slice										
Pies (8 pieces/pie)	118	1/8 pie										
Pudding	99	1/3 cup										
Chocolate candy	32	1/8 cup										
Licorice	23	1 pc										
Hard candy	10	2										
Jelly or jam or syrup	18	1 tbsp										
Dairy products												
Whole milk	183	5 oz										
2% milk	245	6 oz										
Skim milk	245	5 oz										
Cottage cheese	113	1/2 cup										
Other cheese and spreads	28	2 cubes										
Flavored yogurt	227	3/4 cup										
Beverages and other foods												
Coffee (decaffeinated)	240	1 cup										
Coffee (not decaffeinated)	240	1 cup										
Tea	240	1 cup										
Nondairy creamer in coffee or tea		2 tsp										
Milk in coffee or tea		1 tbsp										
Cream in coffee or tea (creamers)		1 tbsp										
Sugar in coffee or tea		1 tsp										
Artificial sweetener in coffee or tea		0.5 tsp										
Wine	174	5 oz										
Beer (12-oz bottle)	360	1 bot										
Whiskey or vodka or rum	56	1.5 oz										
Brewer's yeast	19	0.5 oz										
Wheat germ	43	2/3 cup										
Bran	25	1/3 cup										

[a]D = daily; W = weekly; M = monthly; Y = yearly; N = never. [b]S, M, L = Small, Medium, Large.

Reprinted with permission from Gibson 1993.

References

Anderson SA. Guidelines for Use of Dietary Intake Data. Bethesda, MD: Life Sciences Research Office, Federation of American Societies for Experimental Biology, 1986.

Block G, Hartman AM, Dresser CM, Carroll MD, Gannon J, Gardner L. A data-based approach to diet questionnaire design and testing. Am J of Epidemiology 1986;124:453-69.

Gibson RS. Nutrition Assessment: A Laboratory Manual. Oxford: Oxford University Press, 1993.

Howarth CC. Food frequency questionnaires: a review. Aust J of Nutr and Diet 1990;47:71-6.

Jain MG, Harrison L, Howe GR, Miller AM. Evaluation of a self-administered dietary questionnaire for use in a cohort study. Am J of Clin Nutr 1982;36:931-5.

Pao EM, Fleming KH, Guenther P, Mickle S. Foods commonly eaten by individuals. Amount per day and per eating occasion. Home Economics Research Report No. 44, 1982.

Sabray JH. Nutrition Canada Food Consumption Portion Data. Guelph, Ontario: Department of Family Studies, University of Guelph, 1981.

Appendix E.4   Energy Cost Values for Various Activities

Activity	kcal/kgBW/min	Energy expenditure (kcal/min) for a specific body weight			
		50 kg (110 lb)	60 kg (132 lb)	70 kg (154 lb)	80 kg (176 lb)
Bicycling					
10-11.9 mph, leisurely	0.1	5.0	6.0	7.0	8.0
16-19 mph, racing	0.2	10.0	12.0	14.0	16.0
Conditioning exercise					
Stationary cycling, 100 W	0.092	4.583	5.5	6.417	7.333
Stationary cycling, 200 W	0.175	8.75	10.5	12.25	14.0
Weight lifting					
Light to moderate effort	0.05	2.5	3.0	3.5	4.0
Power lifting	0.10	5.0	6.0	7.0	8.0
Hatha yoga	0.067	3.333	4.0	4.667	5.333
High-impact aerobics	0.117	5.833	7.0	8.167	9.333
Running					
12 min/mi	0.133	6.667	8.0	9.333	10.667
10 min/mi	0.167	8.333	10.0	11.667	13.333
8 min/mi	0.208	10.417	12.5	14.583	16.667
6 min/mi	0.267	13.333	16.0	18.667	21.333

Adapted with permission from Ainsworth BE, Haskell WL, Leon AS, Jacobs DS Jr., Montoye HJ, Sallis JF, Paffenbarger RS Jr. Compendium of physical activities: classification by energy costs of human physical activities. Med Sci Sports Exerc 1993;25:71-80.

Appendix E.5   Commonly Reported Clinical Laboratory Values for Adults (Reference Ranges Can Vary; Refer to the Specific Laboratory Ranges Reported)

Test	Reference range	Purpose of test
Fasting glucose	65-110 mg/dL	Test for diabetes.
Glycosylated hemoglobin (HbA$_{1c}$)	5.5-8.5% (for nondiabetic)	Test for diabetes/control of disease for diabetic client.
Serum sodium	135-145 mmol/L	Detects changes in salt and water balance.
Serum potassium	3.5-5.3 mmol/L	Detects acid-base and water imbalances.
Serum chloride	98-106 mmol/L	Detects acid-base and water imbalances.
BUN (blood urea nitrogen)	7-18 mg/dL	Gross index of renal function.
Serum creatinine	0.6-1.3 mg/dL	Detects impaired renal function.
Uric acid	3.5-7.2 mg/dL (men) 2.6-6.0 mg/dL (women)	Indicator of renal failure, gout, and leukemia.
Serum calcium (total)	8.6-10.0 mg/dL	Assesses parathyroid function, calcium metabolism.
Inorganic phosphorus	2.5-4.5 mg/dL	Evaluated in relation to calcium levels.
Alkaline phosphatase	17-142 U/L	Index of liver and bone disease.
GGT (glutamyltransferase)	5-85 U/L (men) 5-55 U/L (women)	Detects liver cell dysfunction and alcohol-induced liver disease.
Bilirubin (total)	0.2-1.0 mg/dL	Evaluates liver function and hemolytic anemias.

(continued)

Test	Reference range	Purpose of test
Serum glutamic-oxaloacetic transaminase (SGOT) or aspartate transaminase (AST)	5-40 U/L	Evaluates liver and heart disease.
Serum glutamic-pyruvic transaminase (SGPT) or alanine transaminase (ALT)	7-56 U/L	Detects liver diease.
Serum lactate dehydrogenase (LDH)	313-618 U/L	Used to confirm myocardial or pulmonary infarction in conjunction with other test results.
Serum cholesterol	<200 mg/dL	Detects blood lipid disorders and is a potential risk factor for coronary artery disease.
Serum triglycerides	<200 mg/dL	Detects potential coronary artery disease and measures body's ability to metabolize fat.
HDL (high-density lipoprotein)-cholesterol	37-70 mg/dL (men) 40-85 mg/dL (women)	Assesses coronary artery disease risk; increased values are inversely proportional to disease.
LDL (low-density lipoprotein)-cholesterol	<130 mg/dL	Assesses coronary artery disease risk.
Total serum protein	6.0-8.0 g/dL	Detects liver and immune dysfunctions.
Serum albumin	3.8-5.0 g/dL	Detects liver and immune dysfunctions.
Serum globulin	0.7-1.6 g/dL	Indicative of chronic infections, liver and immune diseases, and leukemia and other cancers.
Serum iron	75-175 μg/dL (men) 65-165 μg/dL	Assists in diagnosis of various anemias and hemochromatosis.
Total iron-binding capacity (TIBC)	240-450 μg/dL	Assists in diagnosis of various anemias, iron insufficiency, and hemochromatosis.
Transferrin (% saturation)	0-5% (men) 15-50% (women)	Assists in diagnosis of various anemias, iron insufficiency, and hemochromatosis.
Ferritin	18-270 ng/ml (men) 18-160 ng/ml (women)	A more sensitive test than iron or TIBC for diagnosing iron insufficiency or overload.
Thyroid tests: T3 (triiodothyronine) uptake	25-35%	Assesses thyroid function.
Serum T4 (thyroxine)	5.4-11.5 μg/dL	Assesses thyroid function.
T7 index (free thyroxine)	1.5-4.5 (arbitrary units)	Assesses thyroid function.
TSH (thyroid stimulating hormone)	0.2-5.4 μU/ml	Assesses thyroid function.
WBC (white blood cell count)	5-103/μL	Indicates increased susceptibility to infection.
RBC (red blood cell count)	$4.2\text{-}5.4 \times 10^6/\mu L$ (men) $3.6\text{-}5.0 \times 10^6/\mu L$ (women)	Detects anemia.
Hemoglobin	14.0-17.4 g/dL (men) 12.0-16.0 g/dL (women)	Indicates severity of anemia.
Hematocrit	42-52% (men) 36-48% (women)	Determines red cell mass and helps in diagnosing anemia.
MCV (mean corpuscular volume)	82-98 fl (femtoliters)	Indicates volume of a single red blood cell; used in diagnosing anemia.

Values from Fischbach FA. Manual of Laboratory and Diagnostic Tests. 5th ed. Philadelphia: Lippincott, 1996.

Date ___/___/___   Day of the week _____

Food Intake Diary		Name:	*Tammy*	
Time and Place (AM/PM)	**Foods and beverages Include: fresh, frozen, low-fat, etc.**	**Amount**	**Method of preparation (baked, fried, broiled, etc.)**	**Food exchanges**
9:30 a.m.	Café mocha	12 fl. oz.	cafeteria	
	cinnamon raisin bagel - cold	1 small		
12 p.m.	Mountain Dew	12 fl. oz.	can	
	Quaker Caramel Corn Rice Cakes/ no salt	30g (1.06 oz)		
6 p.m.	Whopper Jr. with cheese	1 sandwich	Burger King- flame broiled	
	small fries	1 order	fried	
	Hawaiian Punch	12 fl. oz.	can	

(continued)

Serving size: 1464.5 g (51.66 oz)
Serves: 1
Cost: —

Amount for 1 serving	Food item	Cost	Food list ESHA code
12 fl oz	Swiss mocha coffee mix + water	—	20043
1 each	Cinnamon raisin bagel	—	42100
12 fl oz	Mountain Dew soda pop	—	20271
30 g	Unsalted mini rice cakes	—	44063
1 each	Burger King Whopper Jr sandwich + cheese	—	57000
1 each	French fries, small svg	—	6142
12 fl oz	Fruit punch drink, canned	—	20024

Nutrients per serving

Calories	1447.76	Fat, total	45.27 g
Protein	36.77 g	Saturated Fat	16.26 g
Carbohydrates	229.10 g	Vitamin A RE	93.85 RE
Dietary fiber	8.89 g	Vitamin C	135.71 mg
% Calories from fat	28 %	% Calories from CHO	62 %

% Comparison to: Tammy

Basic components

Calories	1447.76	63%
Protein	36.77 g	95%
Carbohydrates	229.10 g	69%
Dietary fiber	8.89 g	39%
Soluble fiber	0.58 g	
Sugar, total	107.06 g	
Monosaccharides	27.32 g	
Disaccharides	23.44 g	
Other CHO	89.86 g	
Fat, total	45.27 g	59%
Saturated fat	16.26 g	71%
Mono fat	7.66 g	27%
Poly fat	1.25 g	5%
Trans fatty acids	0 g	
Cholesterol	76.27 mg	25%
Water	829.46 g	

Vitamins

Vitamin A RE	93.85 RE	12%
A, Carotenoid	6.81 RE	
A, Retinol	5.68 RE	
Thiamine (B_1)	0.49 mg	43%
Riboflavin (B_2)	0.34 mg	25%
Niacin (B_3)	7.53 mg	50%
Niacin equivalent	3.57 mg	24%
Vitamin B_6	0.09 mg	6%
Vitamin B_{12}	0 mcg	0%
Vitamin C	135.71 mg	226%
Vitamin D	0 mcg	0%
Vitamin E	0.03 mg	
Folate	26.14 mcg	15%
Pantothenic acid	0.11 mg	2%

Minerals

Calcium	214.08 mg	18%

Multi-column

Copper	0.45 mg	18%
Iron	8.83 mg	59%
Magnesium	80.90 mg	29%
Manganese	0.86 mg	25%
Phosphorus	223.92 mg	19%
Potassium	1026.26 mg	27%
Selenium	— mcg	
Sodium	1364.66 mg	57%
Zinc	2.22 mg	18%

Other fats

Omega-3 fatty acids	0.03 g
Omega-6 fatty acids	0.46 g

Other

Alcohol	0 g
Caffeine	136.97 mg

% Comparison to: Tammy

Bar graph

Nutrient	Value	Goal %
Basic components		
Calories	1447.76	63%
Protein	36.77 g	95%
Carbohydrates	229.10 g	69%
Dietary fiber	8.89 g	39%
Soluble fiber	0.58 g	
Sugar, total	107.06 g	
Monosaccharides	27.32 g	
Disaccharides	23.44 g	
Other CHO	89.86 g	
Fat, total	45.27 g	59%
Saturated fat	16.26 g	71%
Mono fat	7.66 g	27%
Poly fat	1.25 g	5%
Trans fatty acids	0 g	
Cholesterol	76.27 mg	25%

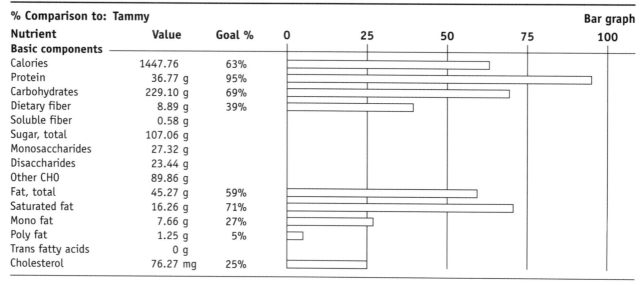

Serving size: 1464.5 g (51.66 oz)
Serves: 1
Cost: —

% Comparison to: Tammy

Bar graph

Nutrient	Value	Goal %	0	25	50	75	100
Water	829.46 g						
Vitamins							
Vitamin A RE	93.85 RE	12%					
A, Carotenoid	6.81 RE						
A, Retinol	5.68 RE						
Thiamine (B_1)	0.49 mg	43%					
Riboflavin (B_2)	0.34 mg	25%					
Niacin (B_3)	7.53 mg	50%					
Niacin equivalent	3.57 mg	24%					
Vitamin B_6	0.09 mg	6%					
Vitamin B_{12}	0 mcg	0%					
Vitamin C	135.71 mg	226%					▷
Vitamin D	0 mcg	0%					
Vitamin E	0.03 mg						
Folate	26.14 mcg	15%					
Pantothenic acid	0.11 mg	2%					
Minerals							
Calcium	214.08 mg	18%					
Copper	0.45 mg	18%					
Iron	8.83 mg	59%					
Magnesium	80.90 mg	29%					
Manganese	0.86 mg	25%					
Phosphorus	223.92 mg	19%					
Potassium	1026.26 mg	27%					
Selenium	— mcg						
Sodium	1364.66 mg	57%					
Zinc	2.22 mg	18%					
Other fats							
Omega-3 fatty acids	0.03 g						
Omega-6 fatty acids	0.46 g						
Other							
Alcohol	0 g						
Caffeine	136.97 mg						

(continued)

Energy Expenditure Grid

Name __Tammy__

Date __1-28-07__

Minutes		0	5	10	15	20	25	30	35	40	45	50	55	60
AM	6	SLEEP												
	7	SLEEP		Bath room	Shower		Dressing			Walk slow	Drive	Bath room	Walk brisk	
	8	IN CLASS (sitting writing)										IN CLASS		
	9	IN CLASS			Walk to class (brisk)			IN CLASS (sitting writing)				EAT	Walk to class (brisk)	
	10	IN CLASS												
	11	IN CLASS												
Noon		IN CLASS				Stand/Talk		IN CLASS				Walk to Practice		
PM	1	IN CLASS											Walk to Practice brisk	
	2	Bath room	Dress	Stretch			Jog 6 mph	Rest	Run 6.5 min/mile			Walk to cafeteria		
	3	Jog 6 mph	Stretch		Shower		Dress					Order food slow	Walk to class (slow)	
	4	Sit & Eat				Sit & Talk								
	5	IN CLASS (sit & write)			Bath room		Stand Talk	IN CLASS						
	6	IN CLASS					Talk					Walk to meeting		
	7	IN CLASS										Walk to meeting (brisk)		
	8	IN MEETING (sitting/talking)												
	9	IN MEETING					Walk slow				Walk slow	SHOWER		
	10	READ IN BED (lying down)						DRIVE HOME						
	11	READ IN BED			SLEEP									
Midnight		SLEEP												
AM	1													
	2													
	3													
	4													
	5													

496

24-Hour Activity Record for Tammy

Subject name: Tammy

Activity	Energy factor (kcal/kg/min)	Body wt (kg)	Energy factor (kcal/min)	Minutes spent doing activity	Total minutes for activity	Kcal for activity
Sleep	0.015	48.6	0.729	70 45 365	480	349.92
Bathroom	0.017	48.6	0.8262	5 5 5	20	16.524
Shower	0.067	48.6	3.2562	5 10 13	28	91.1736
Dress	0.042	48.6	2.0412	15 5 15	35	71.442
Walk (slow)	0.042	48.6	2.0412	3 10 10 5 3	31	63.2772
Walk (brisk)	0.067	48.6	3.2562	3 15 10 10 10	48	156.2976
In class and meetings	0.03	48.6	1.458	45 25 20 50 60 30 / 50 60 15 35 50 25	545	794.61
Eating	0.025	48.6	1.215	10 20	30	36.45
Stand and talk	0.03	48.6	1.458	10 5	15	21.87
Sit and talk	0.025	48.6	1.215	30	30	36.45
Stretch	0.067	48.6	3.2562	10 10	20	65.124
Jog (6 mph)	0.167	48.6	8.1162	7 5	12	97.3944
Stand quietly	0.03	48.6	1.458	3	3	4.374
Run (6.5 min/mi)	0.25	48.6	12.15	30	30	364.5
Stand/talk (order food)	0.03	48.6	1.458	10	10	14.58
Drive	0.033	48.6	1.6038	14 14	28	44.9064
Read in bed	0.017	48.6	0.8262	60 15	75	61.965
Total					1440	2290.858

497

Index

The italicized *f* and *t* following page numbers refer to figures and tables respectively.

About the Authors

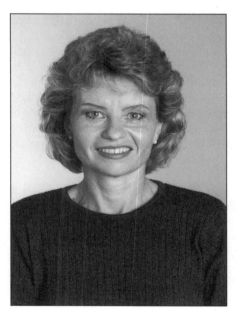

Melinda M. Manore, PhD, RD, FACSM, is currently a professor of nutrition at Arizona State University in Tempe, Arizona. She is also a graduate faculty member in the exercise science doctoral program and the exercise and wellness doctoral program. In addition to her teaching responsibilities, she conducts research and supervises graduate student research. Her areas of expertise include the interaction of nutrition and exercise as it relates to health, disordered eating, nutritional status in active individuals, women's health issues, energy balance, and obesity.

Dr. Manore has served on the editorial boards for several prestigious publications such as the *American College of Sports Medicine's Health and Fitness Journal*, *Medicine and Science in Sport and Medicine*, *Journal of the American Dietetic Association*, and the *International Journal of Sport Medicine*. She is also on the advisory boards for USA Gymnastics and Gatorade Sports Nutrition. In 1999, she was nominated for the American Dietetic Association's Foundation Award for Excellence in Research and has been a fellow of the American College of Sports Medicine since 1996. Dr. Manore is also a member of the American Society for Clinical Nutrition, American Society for Nutritional Sciences, and the North American Association for the Study of Obesity.

Dr. Manore is an avid outdoorswoman who enjoys hiking, camping, cycling, and golf. She has completed three marathons and currently participates in power walking.

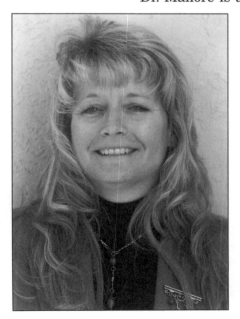

Janice L. Thompson, PhD, FACSM, is a research scientist at the University of New Mexico Health Sciences Center, Center for Health Promotion and Disease Prevention in Albuquerque, New Mexico. She is currently working in partnership with Native American communities to develop and implement physical activity and nutrition education programs to reduce the risks for chronic diseases. Dr. Thompson also provides sport nutrition education for various athletes at the University of New Mexico. Dr. Thompson has been involved in sport nutrition research for over 10 years, and she has also been very active in studying the impact of weight loss on reducing risks for chronic diseases. She has taught undergraduate and graduate courses for the past 12 years in the areas of basic nutrition, exercise physiology, sport nutrition, and health fitness. In addition, she has assessed the body composition and fitness levels of thousands of athletes and sedentary individuals and designed their training programs to promote weight loss and improve performance.

Dr. Thompson is very active in numerous health organizations. Most notably, she is a fellow of the American College of Sports Medicine, the world's leading exercise science organization, and she is a member of the American Society for Nutritional Scientists. She serves as a reviewer for scientific journals such as *Medicine and Science in Sports and Exercise, International Journal of Sport Nutrition, American Journal of Clinical Nutrition,* and *Journal of Applied Physiology*. In 1997, she won the outstanding undergraduate teaching award from the University of North Carolina at Charlotte.

In her personal time, Dr. Thompson is a distance walker and enjoys golfing and yoga.

ABOUT THE CONTRIBUTOR

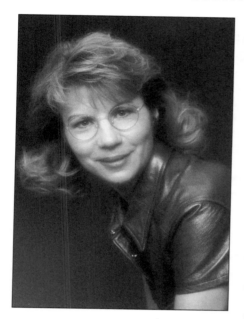

Linda B. Houtkooper, PhD, RD is a nutrition specialist and tenured faculty member at the University of Arizona. She has 15 years of research experience regarding body composition and has published several research articles on body composition assessment methods for children, adults, and elite athletes. Some of her most noted accomplishments include codirecting clinical research studies on the effects of diet and exercise on body composition in young adults and postmenopausal women, which was funded by the National Institutes of Health; directing a study on nutrition status in elite female athletes, which was funded by USA Track and Field; and presenting lectures and workshops internationally.

Dr. Houtkooper has developed a nationally distributed educational video and training manual titled *Winning Sports Nutrition*. She is a member of the American College of Sports Medicine and the American Society for Nutritional Sciences. In 1998, she received the Center for Athletes Total Success (CATS) Service Award.

Dr. Houtkooper enjoys running, hiking, alpine skiing, and swimming.